OXFORD MEDICAL PUBLICATIONS

Critical Care Nursing
Science and Practice

MEDICAL EDITOR
Mervyn Singer

Critical Care Nursing
Science and Practice

SHEILA K. ADAM

Clinical Nurse Specialist,
Department of Intensive Care, University College Hospitals, London

and

SUE OSBORNE

Department of Intensive Care, St George's Hospital, London

Oxford   Toronto   Melbourne
OXFORD UNIVERSITY PRESS
1997

Oxford University Press, Great Clarendon Street, Oxford OX2 6DP
Oxford New York

Athens Auckland Bangkok Bombay
Calcutta Cape Town Dar es Salaám Delhi
Florence Hong Kong Istanbul Karachi
Kuala Lumpur Madras Madrid Melbourne
Mexico City Nairobi Paris Singapore
Taipei Tokyo Toronto
and associated companies in
Berlin Ibadan

Oxford is a trade mark of Oxford University Press

Published in the United States
by Oxford University Press Inc., New York

A catalogue record for this book is available from the British Library

Library of Congress Cataloging in Publication Data
Adam, Sheila K.
Critical care nursing : science and practice | Sheila K. Adam,
Sue Osborne : [medical editor, Mervyn Singer].
p. cm. – (Oxford medical publications)
Includes bibliographical references and index.
1. Intensive care nursing. I. Osborne, Sue. II. Singer, Mervyn.
III. Title. IV. Series.
[DNLM: 1. Critical Care–methods. 2. Nursing Care–methods.
WY 154 A193c 1997]
RT120.I5A35 1997
610.73'61–dc20
DNLM/DLC
for Library of Congress 96-19320 CIP

ISBN 0 19 263022 9 (pb)
0 19 263023 7 (hb)

Typeset by Hewer Text Composition Services, Edinburgh
Printed in Great Britain by The Bath Press, Bath

Preface

This book has been written as a practical guide to nurses working in intensive care. Our aim is to combine relevant theory with the clinical skills required to work effectively in this area both as a novice and when greater proficiency is attained. All the contributors have many years' experience in the intensive care field and hope to pass on their knowledge and clinical acumen. This book is not intended to serve as a fully comprehensive reference work or to cover every possible cause of admission to intensive care. Rather, it should be seen as a starting point for a cross-section of nurses, from the novice and those undertaking post-registration specialist courses in intensive care to those who have worked for some time in the specialty.

Broad-based foundation chapters will introduce the problems of the intensive care environment and the critically ill patient, and there is a final chapter on the evaluation of care.

Each chapter initially discusses underlying physiology where appropriate, followed by identification of the priorities and principles of caring for a critically ill patient. There will then be an overview of the problems and needs associated with specific disorders or dysfunction. The practice described is research-based where possible or a product of the combined clinical skills of the authors.

The book is based on the style of nursing and the management of critically ill patients in the United Kingdom but will also have relevance in other countries with similar values and attitudes. Its philosophy reflects caring, competence, and clinical skills, supported by comprehensive knowledge and research-based practice.

It is hoped that the book will act as a clear and concise reference for immediate use in the clinical area.

London   S.K.A.
July 1996   S.O.

Acknowledgements

This book would not have materialized without the hard work and expertise of Dr Mervyn Singer (Medical Editor) who has donated considerable amounts of time and thought to reading, correcting, and in some cases contributing to each chapter.

We would like to acknowledge three other contributors to the book:
Amanda Sheppard (author of Chapters 1 and 8), and Patsie Barrie-Shevlin and Debbie Field (contributors to Chapter 9). Their expertise and skill have been invaluable.

It would not have been possible for Sheila Adam to complete the book without the support and enthusiasm of her husband, David Fathers, who gave encouragement when it was badly needed.

Finally, our thanks to the patient and supportive staff at OUP who have been a source of help and advice throughout.

Contents

List of abbreviations

A-a gradient	alveolar–arterial oxygen gradient
ABC	Airway, Breathing, and Circulation
ACE	angiotensin converting enzyme
ACh	acetylcholine
ACT	activated clotting time
ACTH	adrenocorticotrophic hormone
ADH	antidiuretic hormone
AF	atrial fibrillation
AFLP	acute fatty liver of pregnancy
ALL	acute lymphoblastic leukaemia
AML	acute myeloid leukaemia
ANCA	antineutrophil cytoplastic antibody
APACHE	acute physiology and chronic health evaluation
APTT	activated partial thromboplastin time
ARDS	acute respiratory distress syndrome
ATP	adenosine triphosphate
AST	aspartate transaminase
ATN	acute tubular necrosis
BP	blood pressure
BPI	bactericidal permeability-increasing protein
BPM	beats per minute
BSA	body surface area
C-ANCA	C form of antineutrophil cytoplasmic antibody
CAL	chronic airflow limitation
CBF	cerebral blood flow
CFAM	cerebral function analysis monitor
CI	cardiac index
CK	creatine kinase
CLL	chronic lymphocytic leukaemia
CML	chronic myeloid leukaemia
CNS	central nervous system
CO	cardiac output, and carbon monoxide
COAD	chronic obstructive airways disease
COP	colloid osmotic pressure
COHb	carboxyhaemoglobin
CMV	cytomegalovirus
CPAP	continuous positive airway pressure
CPB	cardiopulmonary bypass
CPK	creatine phosphokinase
CPP	cerebral perfusion pressure
CPR	cardio-pulmonary resuscitation
CSF	cerebrospinal fluid
CSU	catheter specimen of urine
CT	computed tomography
CUPID	continuous ultrafiltration with periods of intermittent dialysis
CVA	cerebrovascular accident
CVP	control venous pressure
CVS	cardiovascular system
CXR	chest X-ray
DC	direct current
DIC	disseminated intravascular coagulation
DDAVP	1-desamino-8-D-arginine-vasopressin
DKA	diabetic ketoacidosis
DNR	do not resuscitate
DoH	Department of Health
2,3-DPG	2,3,diphosphoglycerate
DVT	deep venous thrombosis
ECF	extracellular fluid
ECG	electrocardiogram
ECM	external cardiac massage
ECMO	extracorporeal membrane oxygenation
EDV	end diastolic volume
$ECCO_2R$	extracorporeal carbon dioxide removal
EDTA	ethylenediamine tetraacetic acid
EEG	electroencephalogram
EF	elongation factor
ET	endo-tracheal
$ETCO_2$	end-tidal carbon dioxide

F_iO_2	fractionated inspired oxygen	IV	intravenous
FDP	fibrin degradation products	IVC	inferior vena cava
FES	fat embolism syndrome	IVOX	intravascular oxygenator
FFP	fresh frozen plasma	IVS	intravascular space
FG	French gauge		
FRC	functional residual capacity	KUF	ultrafiltration coefficient
GI	gastrointestinal	LA	left atrial
GTN	glyceryltrinitrate	LAP	left atrial pressure
G6PD	glucose-6-phosphate	LDH	lactate dehydrogenase
	dehydrogenase	LFT	liver function tests
		LV	left ventricular
H^+	hydrogen ion	LVEDP	left ventricular end diastolic
HD	haemodialysis		pressure
HELLP	haemolysis, elevated liver function,	LVEDV	left ventricular end diastolic volume
	low platelets		
HFJV	high frequency jet ventilation	MAOI	monoamine oxidase inhibitor
HFO	high frequency oscillation	MAP	mean arterial pressure
HFPPV	high frequency positive pressure	MAST	medical antishock trousers
	ventilation	MI	myocardial infarction
HHNKC	hyperosmolar, hyperglycaemic,	MMV	mandatory minute volume
	non-ketotic coma	MODS	multiple organ dysfunction
HITS	heparin-induced thrombocytopenia		syndrome
	syndrome	MOF	multiple organ failure
HLA	human leucocyte antigen (system)	MPAP	mean pulmonary artery pressure
HME	heat-moisture exchanges	MRB	manual resuscitation bag
HOCM	hypertrophic obstructive	MRI	magnetic resonance imaging
	cardiomyopathy	MS	mass spectrometry
HR	heart rate	MV	minute volume
HRS	hepatorenal syndrome		
5-HT	5-hydroxytryptamine	NG	naso-gastric
		NIDDM	non-insulin-dependent diabetes
IABP	intra-aortic balloon pump		mellitus
ICP	intracranial pressure		
ICS	intracellular space	P_aCO_2	partial pressure of carbon dioxide in
ICU	intensive care unit		arterial blood
IDDM	insulin-dependent diabetes mellitus	P_aO_2	partial pressure of oxygen in arterial
IHD	ischaemic heart disease		blood
IL	interleukins	P_AO_2	partial pressure of alveolar oxygen
IMV	intermittent mandatory ventilation	PA	pulmonary artery
INR	international normalized ratio	P-ANCA	P form of antineutrophil
IPPV	intermittent positive pressure		cystoplastic antibody
	ventilation	PADP	pulmonary artery diastolic
ISS	interstitial space, and injury severity		pressure
	score	PAF	platelet-activating factor
ITP	ideopathic thrombocytopenic	PAP	pulmonary artery pressure
	purpura	PASP	pulmonary artery systolic pressure

PAWP (PAOP, PCWP)	pulmonary artery wedge pressure (occlusion, capillary)	SAH	subarachnoid haemorrhage
		SAPS	simplified acute physiology score
		SBE	subacute bacterial endocarditis
PC-IRV	pressure-controlled inverse ratio ventilation	SDD	selective digestive decontamination
		SIMV	synchronized intermittent mandatory ventilation
PD	peritoneal dialysis		
PE	pulmonary embolism	SIRS	systemic inflammatory response syndrome
PGE_1	prostaglandin		
PGI_2	prostacyclin	SLE	systemic lupus erythematosus
PMN	polymorphonuclear (leucocytes)	SV	stroke volume
PEEP	positive end expiratory pressure	SVC	superior vena cava
pH_i	intramucosal pH	S_vO_2	mixed venous oxygen saturation
PNS	peripheral nervous system	SVR	systemic vascular resistance
PSV	pressure support ventilation	SVT	supraventricular tachycardia
PSVT	paroxysmal supraventricular tachycardia		
		T_3	triiodothyronine
P_vO_2	partial pressure of oxygen in venous blood	T_4	thyroxine
		TENS	transcutaneous electrical nerve stimulation
PT	prothrombin time		
PTH	parathyroid hormone	TISS	therapeutic intervention scoring system
PTT	partial thromboplastin time		
PVR	pulmonary vascular resistance	TMP	transmembrane pressure
P_vCO_2	partial pressure of carbon dioxide in venous blood	TNF	tumour necrosis factor
		tPA	tissue plasminogen activator
		TPN	total parenteral nutrition
RAA	renin-angiotensin-aldosterone	TRH	thyroid-releasing hormone
RA	right atrial	TRISS	trauma injury severity score
RAP	right atrial pressure	TSH	thyroid stimulating hormone
RBC	red blood cell	TTP	thrombotic thrombocytopenic purpura
REM	rapid eye movement		
RICP	raised intracranial pressure	T_XA_2	thromboxane
RNA	ribonucleic acid		
ROM	range of movement	UTI	urinary tract infection
RS	respiratory system		
rTPA	recombinant tissue plasminogen activator	VC	vital capacity
		VF	ventricular fibrillation
RV	right ventricular	V/Q	ventilation/perfusion
		VSD	ventricular septal defect
S_aO_2	peripheral tissue oxygen saturation	VT	ventricular tachycardia

1. The intensive care environment

Introduction

The recognition and subsequent development of intensive care began in the 1950s and was influenced by a number of factors, significantly; (i) the advent of mechanical ventilation in response to the polio epidemic; (ii) the development of cardiac surgery with the requirement for post-operative care; and (iii) the general advances in technology that occurred following in the Second World War. As the speciality has progressed since those early beginnings, so too have the associated requirements and specifications for the intensive care environment.

What is intensive care?

There are numerous definitions of intensive care in existence which by their very nature are brief, precise statements which may not necessarily provide a comprehensive understanding, or picture of the speciality. However, the following definitions do share some common themes.

- To provide care for severely ill patients with potentially reversible conditions.

- To provide care for patients who require close observation and/or specialized treatments that cannot be provided in the general ward.

- To provide care for patients with potential or established organ failure, commonly the lungs.

- To reduce avoidable morbidity and mortality in critically ill patients.

To achieve these objectives, intensive care must be a clearly defined area within a hospital where the skills of specialist personnel and technology can be successfully combined in the management and care of critically ill patients.

Which patients benefit from intensive care?

There are a number of reasons why intensive care should be offered only to those patients who are likely to receive any benefit.

- Intensive care is potentially traumatic for patients in emotional, social, and psychological terms and the cost must always be weighed against the potential benefit.

- The combination of technology and specialist staff is expensive, which is significant when health care is increasingly subject to financial constraint.

- In the United States, intensive care beds number approximately 15% of acute hospital beds compared to 1% in the United Kingdom. This, in effect, limits the availability of the service in the United Kingdom (Jennett 1984).

- Intensive care can be physically uncomfortable and potentially hazardous for patients.

It can be extremely difficult to identify or predict those patients who will not benefit from intensive care. Frequently, patients are admitted to the intensive care unit (ICU) as a consequence of medical/surgical intervention, or in an emergency, where diagnosis or reason for clinical deterioration is uncertain and refusal to admit to the ICU would be inappropriate. Once the patient has been admitted to the ICU and treatment has been implemented, moral, professional, and ethical dilemmas can cloud any decision-making process if it is subsequently felt that the patient is unlikely to benefit from continuation of treatment.

The discontinuation of treatment is always a difficult decision in health care and in intensive care there are specific problems (see Chapter 15 for further details). Most patients do not expect to be admitted to the ICU and therefore are unlikely to have discussed their wishes prior to any deterioration in their condition with their relatives. As the majority of severely ill patients in the ICU are unconscious and not able to participate in discussion, decision-making and advocacy rests with the relatives and staff. This unenviable position in part underlines the necessity of identifying those patients who are unlikely to benefit from intensive care preferably before admission to the ICU. This can be facilitated by the development of admission policies (Spangenberg *et al.* 1990). It is important to recognize that such policies can never address every conceivable situation and consequently should represent a set of guidelines rather than rules. It is not uncommon for patients to be referred to the ICU by medical staff who are relatively junior and/or have little experience in the speciality. It is more appropriate for these patients to be assessed by the intensive care team, who are in the best position to determine whether admission to the ICU is justified. This method of assessment can be a component of an admission policy. Once the patient has been admitted, any decisions regarding the discontinuation of treatment should be made as quickly as is appropriate or possible.

Jennett (1984) describes the effects of procrastination over these patients who do not survive intensive care as: first, a prolonged death, and secondly, an increase in intensive care costs.

Spangenberg *et al.* (1990) outline three common admission errors to the ICU:

1. *The patient is too healthy*, resulting in overtreatment and therefore a decreased efficiency (e.g. a patient who would receive equal benefit from a high dependency unit).

2. *The patient is too ill on admission*, resulting in undertreatment and reduced effectiveness (e.g. a delayed referral to the ICU).

3. *The patient is dying on admission*, resulting in zero effectiveness (e.g. an extremely delayed referral to the ICU or an inappropriate referral in terms of the particular disease proces).

There are no easy solutions to the perennial problem of which patient should or should not be offered intensive care. The King's Fund report (1989) highlighted the distinct lack of data in the United Kingdom relating to the potential advantages and disadvantages of intensive care and recommended that units should collect information about clinical outcome and cost. Clinical outcome must include not only survival from the ICU but also hospital and long-term survival to enable a valid analysis to be made. This type of data would assist clinicians in these difficult decisions by providing objective, clinical information. In addition, scoring systems such as the Acute Physiology and Chronic Health Evaluation (APACHE) have in part been developed (see Chapter 15 for further details) to identify patients who are likely or unlikely to receive benefit.

Levels of intensive care

Oh (1990) suggests a stratification of ICUs which allows for a more efficient organisation and utilization of resources.

Level 1 ICU

• situated in small district hospitals

• provide close observation, non-invasive monitoring, and resuscitation

• short-term ventilation (24–48 hours) may be provided

• may also be termed high dependency units (HDUs)

Level 2 ICU

• situated in larger hospitals to support surgery, the main hospital and accident and emergency departments

• mechanical ventilation and invasive monitoring routinely performed

• more formal organization of medical staff and support services

---

Level 3 ICU

• Situated in major tertiary referral centres,

• All aspects of intensive care provided, as dictated by the tertiary role,

• more complex investigations and technology provided,

• participates in formal intensive care medical and nurse training

• undertakes research

The Intensive Care Society (1990) suggested an additional level, that being the 24-hour post-operative recovery unit. This avoids the transfer of patients having undergone emergency surgery back to general wards during 'out of hours' periods when staffing levels are proportionately lower and therefore limits any capacity for close patient observation. In addition, the use of a recovery unit avoids inappropriate admission to the HDU or ICU.

This stratification also allows for a 'progression of care' (AAGBI 1988), whereby patients are cared for in clearly defined areas according to their degree of illness and not their clinical speciality. Unfortunately, in many hospitals, level 1, in particular, is performed on general wards which can be inefficient, uneconomical, and furthermore, can have a dilutional effect on expertise

(AAGBI 1988). The HDU should also provide a 'step-down' facility for patients who are discharged from the ICU but not yet able to return to the general ward environment.

The development of intensive care has been unco-ordinated and haphazard over the past three decades. Partly as a result of this, many units are a combination of all three levels of intensive care in varying proportions.

The intensive care unit as part of a hospital

Ideally, the ICU should be situated where it is in close proximity to the source of the patients and to the support services that are most frequently required (Hopkinson 1994).

Patient source ⟵ ICU ⟶ Support services	
Accident and emergency	Radiology
Operating theatres	Laboratories
Acute wards	Operating theatres

Any distance between the source of patients or support services and the ICU should be facilitated by the provision of dedicated lifts which are spacious enough to accommodate critically ill patients and any accompanying equipment.

Communications should be enhanced with direct telephone lines and/or intercom systems.

There should be recognized equipment used only for the transport of patients in and out of the ICU (see Chapter 2 for details).

The intensive care unit

Unfortunately, many ICUs have either not been purpose-built or have not had the involvement of clinicians during the planning stages. It must be remembered that a great deal of foresight, in terms of future service and equipment requirements, is required when planning an ICU as there is usually a time delay of several years between the planning, building and commissioning stages. The publication of a revised building note (HBN 27 1992) by the Department of Health (DoH) updated the guidelines for planning an ICU according to the recommendations of the DoH. This is an important basic document for the construction of any ICU.

General requirements for an intensive care unit

The AAGBI (1988) suggest that a unit with less than 200 admissions per year, less than 4 beds, and/or bed occupancy of less than 60% is not economical. In addition, Oh (1990) suggests that a unit with more than 12 to 16 intensive care beds is difficult to manage.

Most ICUs have a combination of beds situated in open plan areas and beds in cubicles. The ICS (1990) recommend that there should be no more than 3 beds in cubicles per every 10 beds. There are certain advantages and disadvantages associated with open plan units:

Advantages:
Easier observation of patients.
Quicker mobilization of staff and equipment.
More economic to maintain/more effective use of resources.
Improved staff support and motivation.
Can be beneficial in the reorientation of patients.

Disadvantages:
Less privacy for patients and relatives.
Increased cross-infection risks (Abizanda 1990).
Can be noisier and contribute to sensory overload.

In an open plan environment it is recommended that each patient bed area be at least 18.5 square metres (Oh 1990). Bed areas within cubicles should be slightly larger, at 20 square metres.

Safety

While it is imperative that safety measures are adhered to in all parts of a hospital, there are significant factors that further heighten safety awareness in the ICU.

1. The abundance of electrical equipment.

2. The dependence of the patients.

3. The presence of oxygen (a combustible gas).

This requires:

● All equipment to be checked prior to use.

● All equipment to be regularly maintained.

● Accepted precautions to be taken in relation to oxygen (e.g. no naked flames, antistatic flooring and footwear, increased humidity).

- All staff to be aware and regularly updated in health and safety procedures, including the action required in the event of fire.

- Equipment to be available at each bedside for potential evacuation in the event of fire (e.g. fire mattresses, rebreathing bags, etc.).

- The facility to turn off gas supplies within the unit.

- Equipment to be available in the event of power or gas failure (e.g. torches, battery-operated equipment, back-up gas supply).

Cleaning and infection control

The most important source of cross-infection is un-washed hands. Compared to the risks from poor hand-washing technique, the design of the ICU will do little to affect the incidence of cross-infection (Rey-brouck 1983; Gould 1991).

Hand-basins should be available in all single cubicles. If patients are in either source or protective isolation, a second hand-basin should be situated outside the cubicle. In open areas there should be no less than one hand-basin per two beds. Each basin should have a supply of liquid soap and agreed antiseptic scrub solutions. Ideally, all taps and dispensers should be elbow- or foot-operated.

A storage space should be designated for cleaning materials and equipment. Floors should be swept and mopped at least daily. Patient areas and equipment should be damp dusted on a daily basis and there should be agreed protocols for the cleaning of bed areas following patient discharge.

Staff facilities

Within the ICU there should be a rest room for staff which has facilities for making refreshments and snacks — this should be separate from any patient food preparation area.

There should be changing rooms within the unit that have showering facilities. There should be sufficient space for an office, teaching equipment, and a bedroom for medical staff.

Visitors facilities

Visitors to the ICU need a general waiting room, preferably slightly apart from the main unit to avoid observation of any potentially disturbing situations. The room should have toilets, telephones, and refresh-ment facilities. In some cases, relatives require a room in which to stay overnight and this should be available as near as possible to the unit.

General decor

The decoration of an ICU should promote a relaxed and restful atmosphere for patients, staff, and visitors. It should be of a colour that does not camouflage spillages and of a material that is easy to clean. All materials should be fire-resistant. Any paint work, especially on ceilings should be of a matt (not gloss) finish to avoid reflection. There should be wall-mounted clocks that are in easy view of not only the staff but also the patients to assist during re-orientation phases.

Noise

Noise levels can be high in ICUs, mainly due to the amount of equipment and constant activity. This can significantly contribute to sensory overload for the patient (see Chapter 2). Telephones must be in a position where they can be heard and answered by staff but also so as to cause minimum disturbance for patients. Portable telephones are useful if staff are not in the immediate vicinity and for patients to speak with callers. However, mobile phones should not be used in the vicinity of medical electrical equipment as their signal can cause artefacts and alarm conditions (Clifford et al. 1994). Equipment alarm parameters should be set appropriately and on the lowest possible audible setting. Alarms should always be attended to promptly as the potential for increased background noise is enormous. Continuous or frequent alarms tend to become part of background noise and may not be attended to in real emergencies. Materials for walls and floors can be selected for noise absorption capabilities.

Temperature and air-conditioning

In patient areas, the temperature should be adjustable between 22 and 26 °C. There should be a minimum of six air changes per hour with two changes an hour of outside air. The relative humidity should be kept between 30% and 60% to prevent risks from static electricity.

Access

Access into the ICU must be controlled, either by the presence of a continuously staffed reception area or an intercom/video entry system. The unit should not be used as a route to other areas of the hospital.

Lighting

It is desirable for ICUs to have windows allowing natural daylight. If the unit is situated on a lower floor and there are windows, there must be the facility to ensure privacy and provide shade. This can best be achieved with blinds between two layers of glass. Blinds and curtains external to the glass can be a source of cross-infection. Good-quality general lighting must be provided in all areas with additional examination lights, mobile theatre lights for procedures, night lights (or dimmer control of main lights), and emergency lighting in the event of a main power failure.

Storage areas

Many ICUs suffer from inadequate storage space. Oh (1990) suggests an area of 25% of all patient and central station areas to be allocated to storage and HBN 27 (1992) includes storage areas for many items previously unaccounted for such as mobile X-ray equipment. Separate areas should be designated for the following:

- monitoring/respiratory/cardiovascular equipment,
- sterile/disposable goods,
- linen,
- stationery,
- fluids/drugs.

Utility areas

There should be provision of clean utility and completely separate dirty utility/sluice areas. If possible, access to dirty utility areas should not be via the main unit or patient areas.

Technical areas

Designated space should be made available for technical development, repair, and maintenance. A restricted access laboratory should be within the unit for, as a minimum, the analysis of arterial blood gases and electrolytes.

Emergency equipment

Each unit should have at least one defibrillator, designated cardiac arrest drugs, and resuscitation equipment in a central, recognized location. This may or may not include intubation equipment which can also be kept at each bed area.

ICUs with cardiothoracic patients should have equipment for emergency thoracotomy (see cardiac surgery chapter), to include:

- a thoracotomy pack (including internal defibrillation paddles),
- sutures,
- diathermy machine,
- suction equipment.

Requirements for specific bed areas in the ICU

- A bed with adjustable position, removable bed head, tilting facility, and cot sides.

- Patient monitoring to allow continuous measurement of: ECG, up to 3 transduced pressures, core and skin temperatures, arterial oxygen saturation.

- Ventilator, rebreathing bag, anaesthetic facemask, oropharyngeal airway (intubation equipment either at each bed or on a central trolley), humidification equipment.

- Wall-mounted sphygmomanometer.

- At least 24 electric sockets with emergency generator back-up within close proximity of the bed, at least 90 cm from the floor.

- At least 3 oxygen, 2 compressed air, and 3 vacuum outlets situated on either side of the bed (or form a ceiling-or floor-mounted column), but at least 1.5 m above the floor.

- One oxygen outlet should have an oxygen flow-meter and rebreathing bag permanently attached for emergencies.

- One vacuum outlet should have a suction unit permanently attached and set up for endotracheal suction.

- Provision for charts, documentation, and drug preparation on appropriately situated, surfaces allowing easy view of the patient.

- Storage space for linen and disposable goods (e.g. needles and syringes).

- Space for patient's possessions and hygiene requirements.

Many units find that central trolleys equipped for the insertion of intercostal drains and central venous cannulae are effective.

Each patient bed area must have a form of emergency call button or alarm which can be heard throughout the unit, except in the visitors' areas.

The equipment kept in the ICU, in addition to that already listed, will depend on the level and services offered by the particular unit.

The following list reflects the requirement of a major, level 3 intensive care unit (Oh 1990):

Monitoring

- Cardiac output computers.
- Mixed venous oxygen analysers.
- 12-lead ECG machine.
- Cerebral function/EEG machine.
- Blood glucose analyser.
- Blood gas analyser.
- Sodium/Potassium analyser.
- Patient/bed weighing machine.
- Patient lifting hoist.
- Expired CO_2 analyser.

Respiratory

- CPAP flow generators/circuits.
- Fibreoptic bronchoscope.

Renal equipment

- Continuous arteriovenous haemofiltration sets, or.
- Haemofiltration/Diafiltration machines.

Radiology

- Portable X-ray machine.
- X-ray viewers.
- Image intensifier.

Cardiovascular

- Intra-aortic balloon pump.
- Infusion/syringe pumps.
- Pacing boxes.

Miscellaneous

- Autoclave.
- Drip stands.
- Dressing trolleys.
- Heating/cooling mattresses.
- Blood/fluid warming devices, pressure bags, and scales.
- Nasogastric feeding pumps.
- Commodes/Bedpans.
- Blood fridge.

Some ICUs may also have direct computer links with other parts of the hospital which facilitate such tasks as pharmacy ordering, retrieval of laboratory results, and medical record-keeping.

The staffing of an intensive care unit

The variety, number, and inherent skills of the staff required for an ICU should reflect the level and activity of the unit. In general, the four main groups of staff are:

1. Medical.
2. Nursing.
3. Technical.
4. Administration and clerical.

These groups are then supported by physiotherapists, pharmacists, dietitians, radiographers, speech therapists, occupational therapists, and social workers.

1. Medical staff

An ICU should, ideally, have resident medical staff 24 hours a day who have no other commitments in the hospital.

Patients are admitted to the ICU from a variety of sources and during their stay may require the attention of a number of medical specialities. It is vital that the clinical care is co-ordinated by a director who is trained as an intensivist (Brown and Sullivan 1989). It has been suggested that a full-time intensivist can reduce mortality rates and improve efficiency (Pollack *et al.* 1988).

The ICS (1990) recommend that medical training for intensive care should be at the higher professional training level. In the United Kingdom, there are relatively few training programmes for medical staff wishing to specialize in intensive care medicine. This may reflect the slow acceptance in the United Kingdom of intensive care as a speciality in its own right — it is frequently still perceived as a branch of anaesthesia.

Junior doctors who are training in intensive care should have gained at least six months anaesthetic experience to provide a foundation for resuscitation skills. (ICS 1990). The European Society of Intensive Care Medicine has now developed a European Diploma of Intensive Care Medicine. Doctors who have trained for at least two years in intensive care and four to five years in their basic speciality are eligible to apply. Both written and oral examinations are taken for the diploma (Burchardi and Atkinson 1990).

2. Nursing staff

A balance has to be struck within the nursing establishment between the number of intensive care nurses and those who are training in intensive care. The ICS (1990) suggest that 75% of the nurses are trained in the speciality. Those who are in a training role (whether undertaking a nationally accepted course, such as the English National Board 100 general intensive care nursing course, or an 'in-house' training course) require supervision and facilitation which is demanding of staff time.

The nursing group should be managed by a nurse manager. In larger units with a high number of staff, clinical and professional leadership and development may need to be provided by a clinical nurse specialist. A combination of the two roles is more appropriate in smaller ICUs (ICS 1990). The nursing establishment comprises a significant proportion of the overall budget and therefore must be managed efficiently and cost-effectively. Maintenance of standards of nursing care must be balanced with staffing requirements and the dependency of the patients admitted to the ICU.

Education of nursing staff within the ICU

The validation and training of post-registration nurses in ICU comes under the auspices of the four national boards of England, Scotland, Wales, and Northern Ireland. The common current structure of a course in general intensive care is a 24-week period of clinical experience and study, culminating in the presentation of a certificate in clinical studies. However, the publication of the UKCC post-registration education and practice project (PREPP) opened up the possibility of providing training in different ways and culminating in accumulation of different numbers of points towards academic qualification at degree or diploma standard. These points are allocated by the Council for National Academic Awards and are known as the credit accumulation transfer system (CATS).

In the future, the development of advanced clinical practitioners will be supported by Master's level education either full- or part-time. This will improve the level of research-based nursing practice and strengthen academic nursing departments' clinical links.

3. Technical staff

Technicians play a major role in the maintenance, problem-solving, and selection of technical equipment for the ICU.

4. Administration and clerical staff

The use of ancillary and administrative staff can be highly effective in expanding the capability of nurses to concentrate purely on nursing responsibilities and reduce the dilution of the nursing role by non-nursing clerical and domestic tasks.

Smaller units may employ a ward receptionist who can also act in a secretarial capacity, but it is often necessary in larger units to have a receptionist and a secretary. The role of the health care assistant in the ICU has yet to be fully explored. It seems likely that with skills that cover a range of tasks, from answering the telephone to assisting the ICU nurse to turn patients, they will have much to offer.

The multidisciplinary team that is involved with the care of a critically ill patient is large and needs co-ordination for continuity and direction of care. The clinical management of a patient should be on a 'shared care' basis, involving all relevant clinicians, but it is essential that the director of intensive care co-ordinates all the various inputs. There need to be sufficient forums for communication both regarding patient management and between professions. The daily ward round is the ideal setting for all groups who are involved to discuss patient care and for the organization of that care to be agreed.

The individual professional groups, namely, the medical staff, nurses, and technicians, need their own communication networks to discuss their particular professional developments and problems. Further to this, regular meetings should be held for all groups of staff to provide information, invite feedback, and to highlight common problems.

Indeed, despite the plethora of equipment to be found in an ICU, it is the nurturing, organization, and co-ordination of the multidisciplinary team that will exert greatest effect upon patient care.

Environmental considerations must progress in parallel with further developments within a speciality. There will doubtless be new items of equipment developed (e.g. a new ventilator). Prior to the purchase of the machine, there are a surprising number of issues to be considered. These include:

  (i) the space required around the bed,

  (ii) the amount of electricity and gas required,

  (iii) the level of staff required to operate it,

  (iv) the staff needed to repair or maintain it,

  (v) education and training required to use the equipment,

  (vi) any supplementary equipment needed, such as disposable circuits or humidifiers, and their cost.

This underlines the importance of viewing the intensive care unit globally: as a structure, the equipment within it, and the staff, when making decisions which involve any or all of them.

References

AAGBI Association of Anaesthetists of Great Britain and Ireland (1988). *Intensive care services — Provision for the future.* AAGBI, London.

Brown, J. and Sullivan, G. (1989). Effect on ICU mortality of a full time critical care specialist. *Chest*, **96**, 127–9.

Burchardi, H. and Atkinson, B. (1990). Education and training. In *Management of intensive care. Guidelines for better use of resources*, (ed. D. Williams, A. Reis Miranda, and P. Loirat), pp. 125–64. Kluwer, Dordrecht.

Clifford, K.J., Joyner, K.H., Stroud, D.B., Wood, M., Ward, B., and Fernandez, C.H. (1994). Mobile telephones interfere with medical electrical equipment. *Australasian, Physics, Engineering Science and Medicine*, **17**, 23–7.

Gould, D. (1991). Nurses' hands as vectors of hospital-acquired infection: a review. *Journal of Advanced Nursing*, **16**, 1216–25.

Hopkinson, R. B. (1994). How to plan an ICU. *Care of the Critically Ill*, **10**, 57–62.

HBN (*Hospital Building Note*) 27, (1992). Intensive Therapy Unit, NHS estates. HMSO, London.

ICS (Intensive Care Society) (1990). *The intensive care service in the UK.* London.

Jennett, B. (1984). Inappropriate use of intensive care. *British Medical Journal*, **289**, 1709–11.

King's Fund Panel (1989). *Intensive care in the United Kingdom.* King's Fund, London.

Oh, T.E. (ed.) (1990). *Intensive care manual*, (3rd edn), pp. 1–6. Butterworths, Sydney.

Pollock, M.M., Katz, R.W., Ruttimann, U.E., and Gerson, P.R. (1988). Improving the outcome and efficiency of intensive care: the impact of an intensivist. *Critical Care Medicine*, **16**, 11–17.

Reybrouck, G. (1983). Role of the hands in the spread of nosocomial infections. 1. *Journal of Hospital Infection*, **4**, 103–10.

Spangenberg J., *et al.* (1990) Management control in the ICU. In *Management of intensive care. Guidelines for better use of resources*, (ed. D. Williams, A. Reis Miranda, and P. Loirat), pp. 103–23. Kluwer, Dordrecht.

2. The patient in intensive care

Introduction

The value of a holistic approach to the critically ill patient cannot be overemphasized. Many of the patient's needs and problems will be forgotten or negated if he is simply viewed as a collection of organs with varying levels of dysfunction. The equipment and its numerical representations of the state of organ dysfunction can assume inappropriate importance if the patient as an individual is disregarded. A considerable part of the skill attached to nursing these patients concerns the ability to relate all of the information available to the patient as a whole and to view any change in their condition in context rather than in isolation.

This chapter will address the priorities of caring for critically ill patients, including their common needs and problems, as well as those of their families. Two particular concepts are important to the understanding of the critically ill patient: homeostasis and stress.

Homeostasis

Homeostasis is a process of self-regulation and maintenance of uniformity (Greek: *homoios*, similar and *sta*, stand). Homeostatic mechanisms are triggered by any change in the genetically determined normal value of a given physiological variable. The aim of the homeostatic mechanism is always to return the variable to a steady state. This is achieved by negative feedback. Most of the physiological variables of the body are governed by homeostasis and invoke numerous complex mechanisms in order to maintain them within usually very narrow limits. An example is the maintenance of blood pH (the negative logarithm to the base 10 of hydrogen ion concentration, see Chapters 3 and 8) between the limits of 7.35 and 7.45. Any deviation from this will trigger a series of mechanisms including respiratory changes, metabolic changes, and renal changes in order to compensate for the change and return the level to normal.

Many critically ill patients have reached the limits of their body's compensatory mechanisms; interventions are then necessary in order to return the variable to the physiological normal. Unfortunately, these interventions have no governing negative feedback mechanisms

and can only be controlled by external monitoring of the variable involved, followed by manipulation of the variable by the nursing or medical staff. An example is the infusion of sodium bicarbonate for an unresponsive acidosis. Arterial blood gases must be taken following infusion in order to monitor blood pH. Further bicarbonate may be given according to the result. Limited as the possible manipulations are, the maintenance of homeostasis is one of the most important aspects of caring for the critically ill patient. This provision of support for failing systems allows time for the patient's organs to respond to treatment or recover from the initial insult.

Stress

All critically ill patients are stressed to a greater or lesser degree during their time in intensive care. There is a limit to the level of stress that each person can tolerate; while many stressors cannot be reduced or eliminated there are some inherent in the ICU environment that can be relieved by appropriate nursing intervention. An example of this is the delivery of sufficient, understandable information to the patient so that he can make sense of his surroundings. The patient's physiological response to stress can cause considerable added strain on failing organs. Some nursing interventions may be able to reduce the patient's level of stress and attenuate some of its effects.

Selye's general adaptation syndrome

There are three phases to the response to stressors:

1. Alarm reaction — a transient phase which cannot be sustained.

2. Resistance or adaptation — this produces either a successful adaptation to the stressor or entry to phase 3.

3. Exhaustion and death.

Controlled stress or a degree of stimulation is essential to life and growth but excessive or maladapted levels of stress are harmful.

The limbic system (a rim of cortical tissue surrounding the hilum of the cerebral cortex and other associated deep structures) is involved in the relay of emotional states to the endocrine system. It has connections with the cerebral cortex for transmissions of social and emotional influences, and connections with the hypothalamus for control of endocrine activity. Thus, hypothalamic activation of sympathetic nervous activity and adrenaline secretion is stimulated via the limbic system (Figure 2.1).

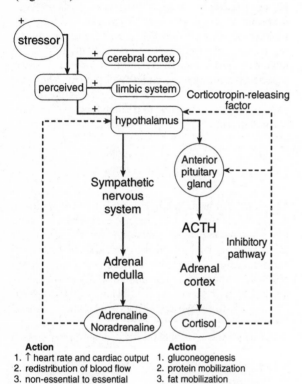

Action
1. ↑ heart rate and cardiac output
2. redistribution of blood flow
3. non-essential to essential
   ↑ oxygen consumption
4. ↑ metabolic rate
5. ↑ glycogen breakdown
6. ↑ glucose uptake by tissues
7. dilation of pupils
8. ↑ gut motility and digestion
9. constriction of GI and bladder
   sphincters

Action
1. gluconeogenesis
2. protein mobilization
3. fat mobilization
4. stabilization of lysosomes
5. ↑ tissue utilization of glucose
6. suppression of the
   inflammatory response
7. inhibition of granulation tissue
8. general CNS effect—increased
9. rate of learning
10. ↑ extracellular fluid volume
    through ↑ sodium and water
    absorption

Fig. 2.1 Stress, the hormonal response (↑ = increase).

Although the effects of the stress response are appropriate and useful in the short-term response to injury; in the long term, the same effects are likely to be detrimental to recovery. The continued breakdown of protein stores will lead to muscle wasting and fatigue, the suppression of the inflammatory response will lead to superinfection, the inhibition of tissue granulation will prevent healing and the increased extracellular fluid volume will produce oedema and altered fluid balance. A major nursing goal must be to reduce or eliminate extraneous stressors to allow the body to respond appropriately to injury but to prevent further complications associated with the stressed state.

Anxiety and fear

Anxiety is a state of disequilibrium or tension caused by apprehension of possible misfortune that prompts attempts at coping. It is an almost universal feature of patients admitted to an ICU. Most patients will respond using personal coping mechanisms if they are able to help themselves, or using the help and support of all members of the caring team and family if they are not. Fear is a state of distress and apprehension causing sympathetic arousal. Anxiety or fear can occur as a result of any stress threatening personal security and balance/control.

The response to fear and anxiety

The physiological response is that of sympathetic arousal, that is, increased circulating catecholamines, increased heart rate, increased blood pressure, increased respiratory rate, dilated pupils, dry mouth (decreased saliva production), peripheral, and splanchnic vasoconstriction. The behavioural response depends on individual background, culture, and social conditioning. All behaviours are aimed at coping with the stressor. Many of the stressors associated with being critically ill (fear of pain and death, isolation, loss of family support, physical discomfort) cannot be completely eliminated and patients frequently require help with coping. The following strategies can be used:

● Support and augment the patient's coping mechanisms.

● Communicate caring and understanding to the patient through attentiveness, tone of voice, touch, etc.

● Provide information repeatedly and in sufficient detail for the patient to understand and make sense of what is going on.

● Encourage and support relatives in reassuring patients and reiterating information. Allow the relatives as much time with the patient as is possible.

Table 2.1 Patient's coping mechanisms for anxiety

- Denial
- Substitution of positive thoughts for negative
- Retention of control (often via the nurse) of aspects of care and the environment (e.g. position, lighting, personal hygiene)

Sensory imbalance and disorientation

Sensory imbalance or disorientation occurs when the level of sensory stimuli received by the individual is either too great or too minimal to be meaningful or recognizable. A number of predisposing factors, including many of the drugs used, are associated with the critically ill patient in the ICU (Easton and Mackenzie 1988). There are five main types of sensory alteration according to Clifford (1985). All can apply to patients in the ICU:

(i) reduction of the amount and variety of stimuli.

(ii) monotony of indistinct, meaningless stimuli.

(iii) isolation, either physical or social.

(iv) confinement, immobilization or restriction of movement.

(v) increased sensory input.

Types (i)–(iv) will cause sensory deprivation and type (v) will cause sensory overload.
The causes of types (i)–(iv) are:

- loss of caring touch (although there may be an overload of procedural touch),
- increased confinement due to drains, IV lines, catheters, and sedation,
- isolation (either physical or social),
- limited visual stimuli.

The causes of type (v) are:

- continuous high noise levels due to equipment alarms, telephones, buzzers, staff conversation, etc. Levels of noise in the ICU have been recorded peaking as high as 80 decibels and to run continuously at a minimum of 50 decibels throughout the night (Topf and Davis 1993),
- unfamiliar and frequently incomprehensible sounds,
- stressful environment with loss of meaningful sounds/ environment from which the patient can orientate,
- frequent uninvited touch and invasion of personal space,
- constant lighting.

Predisposing factors to sensory imbalance

- Alcohol/drug addiction
- Previous cerebral damage
- Psychological illness
- Chronic cardiovascular, respiratory, metabolic, or renal illness
- Increasing age
- Previous episodes of delirium
- Previous psychological stressors

Implicated pharmacological agents

- Atropine and anticholinergics
- Aminocaproic acid
- Anticonvulsants
- Barbiturates
- Penicillin and cephalosporins
- Steroids
- Morphine
- Lignocaine
- Diazepam
- Digoxin

At its worst, sensory imbalance will produce delirium. This is a state of fluctuating consciousness characterized by: fatigue, distraction, confusion, disorientation, restlessness, clouding of consciousness, incoherence, fear, anxiety, excitement, illusions, hallucinations, and delusions.

The nurse has an important part to play in the prevention or alleviation of sensory imbalance. Many of the interventions controlled and initiated by nurses will have marked effects on the patient's sensory load.

Illusion: a false interpretation of external (usually auditory or visual) stimuli.

Hallucination: a false sensory perception occurring without external stimulus.

Delusion: a fixed irrational belief not consistent with cultural mores. It may include persecutory, grandiose, nihilistic, or somatic ideas.

Strategies that will assist in optimizing the patient's response to sensory stimuli are to:

- assess the patient for predisposing factors (see box),
- provide pre-operative visits and information to elective admission patients to reduce anxiety associated with the unknown,
- give repeated, frequent orientation to time, place, person, and events,
- establish an appropriate day/night differentiation and accentuate markers of daily routine such as morning toilet, meals, etc.,
- make the patient comfortable for the night with attention to analgesia, sedation, positioning, warmth, and reduced light,
- limit and cluster interventions during the night to allow periods of at least 90 minutes of uninterrupted sleep (Closs 1988a,b),
- reduce unnecessary 'meaningless' noise,
- use large clocks and calendars within the patient's sight,
- introduce the patient to staff entering the patient's bed space,
- have formal greeting and leavetaking from the nurse caring for them on each shift,
- use family photos and familiar objects from home to create a less hostile environment,
- encourage involvement of family members in conversation,
- obtain information about topics of patient's interest and include the patient in conversation,
- play music appropriate to the patient's taste (Chlan 1995),
- use television, radio, newspapers, magazines, and conversation to provide meaningful stimulation,

- include caring touch in communicating with the patient,
- ensure patient can see out of windows and use natural light as much as possible,
- provide explanations and information on the ICU environment to assist the patient in interpretation and understanding,
- encourage autonomy in self-care where possible and provide explanations and information so that the patient may participate in decisions about daily care.

Disturbance of diurnal (circadian) rhythm

Humans possess a 24-hour cycle that is resistant to change. Long-term disruption of this can be fatal. It is an unfortunate feature of the ICU that care and interventions must continue round the clock. This makes the patient vulnerable to sleep and diurnal rhythm disturbance. In the ICU, disturbance is due to:

(i) the constant need for interventions to the patient throughout the 24-hour cycle and the high level of continuous noise (Topf and Davis 1993),

(ii) loss of REM sleep,

(iii) loss of the regenerative phase of non-REM sleep,

(iv) inappropriate ICU routine where morning baths may be carried out at a time when patients are at their lowest ebb (between 2 a.m. and 5 a.m.),

(v) inadequate pain relief; this is a major sleep-disturbing factor (Jones et al. 1979)

Functions of sleep

- Mental restoration.
- Anabolic processes:
  - protein synthesis is inhibited by cortisol, glucagon, and catecholamines which reach their highest level during the day
  - during sleep, energy expenditure falls and energy is stored within cells. Levels of ATP rise high enough for protein synthesis to occur
  - growth hormone (which stimulates protein and RNA synthesis and amino acid uptake) reaches peak secretion rates during slow wave sleep

The effects on the patient are (Closs 1988a,b)

- irritability and anxiety,
- physical exhaustion and fatigue,
- disruption of metabolic functions.

Once again, there are many interventions under the nurse's control which will limit the detrimental effects of 24-hour care:

- Assess the patient's sleep pattern by observing sleep/wake states overnight. Nurse observers' assessments were found to be accurate in 82% of cases allowing early recognition of potential problems (Edwards and Schuring 1993)
- Dim the lights and reduce environmental noise for the night period.
- Provide protected periods of uninterrupted sleep of at least 90 minutes.
- Carry out only vital observations and interventions at night.
- Avoid procedures likely to add to patient stress between the hours of 2 a.m. and 5 a.m. (lowest levels of cortisol and other stress-related hormones are secreted during this time).
- Ensure pain relief and sedation are sufficient to allow rest.

Communication

Communication is a universal need and a universal problem in the ICU. The normal processes are disrupted by sedation, opiates, endotracheal and tracheostomy tubes, fluctuating conscious levels, and fear. One of the greatest skills required by an ICU nurse is the ability to communicate. It requires patience, motivation, a perception of the patient as an individual, perseverance, and experience to provide the patient with an appropriate level of understanding and response. Barriers to communication experienced by ICU patients have been identified by Borsig and Steinacker (1982):

(1) *Psychical and psychological conditioned causes*
Previous psychiatric illness, psychiatric disturbance related to the ICU environment.

(2) *Social conditioned causes*
Hospitalization and unfamiliarity of the environment, use of jargon, ethnic differences, social isolation.

(3) *Chemically conditioned causes*
Drugs such as sedatives, narcotics, and muscle relaxants.

(4) *Environmental causes*
Sensory deprivation, sensory overload, isolation, loss of familiar environment, and contact with the outside world.

(5) *Organic and therapeutic causes*
Fatigue, breathlessness, presence of endotracheal or tracheostomy tube, neuropathy, head injury, and other aspects of illness or treatment. Effective and therapeutic communication is a vital aspect of nursing intervention. Insufficient communication can invoke feelings of isolation, frustration, anxiety, and fear (Bergbom-Engberg and Haljamäe 1993).

There are a wide variety of alternative methods and aids which should be utilized to assist the patient in communicating.

Strategies

Speech, writing, symbols, mime, touch.

- Assess the patient's ability to see, hear, touch, respond, understand, use sign language, speak.
- Identify the most appropriate communication device(s) according to patient ability (see Table 2.2)
- In pre-operative visits prepare the patient for communication difficulties, agree gestures for minimal communication, and document them.
- Use positive feedback such as smiling, nodding attentively, giving the patient full attention, touch.
- Orientate the patient to time, place, and identify who is speaking to them.
- Use appropriate questions: open questions for the patient who is able to speak/communicate more fully; closed questions for patients who can only gesture and nod.
- Include patient's visitors and family in planning methods of communication.

Table 2.2 Communication devices

• Electronic communicator	• Possum portascan
• Pen/pencil and paper	(uses the ability to suck
• Lip-reading	or press to alter
• Alphabet board	indicators on a screen)
• Symbol board/book	• Touch
• Computer	• Mime/gesture/facial
	expression
	• Eye contact

An important adjunct to finding and using an appropriate method of communication is the need to record and pass on this information to other members of the caring team. Effective patient-orientated documentation is essential. The patient's feelings of isolation, alienation, and fear can and should be reduced by the promotion of effective communication from all members of staff (Ashworth 1980).

Patients' perceptions of their stay in the ICU

Much can be gained in understanding the problems facing the critically ill by listening to survivors' accounts of their intensive care experience. There are a number of problems which affect the patient's ability to perceive and make sense of what is going on around them. Their ability to communicate this problem is often seriously limited (see above) and staff may only become aware of it when the patient finally becomes well enough to describe it. Personal accounts of intensive care experiences by ex-patients are a valuable source of information about the sort of problems that occur.

Follow-up studies have shown that 63% of patients have little or no recollection of their stay in the ICU (Friedman *et al.* 1992). However, those who do remember their stay have several important points to make (Heath 1989). The main themes from research are outlined below followed by suggestions for limiting the specific problems identified:

Presence of endotracheal tube and discomfort

Patients describe the presence of the endotracheal tube as very uncomfortable, particularly during turning or movement. Oral tubes are felt to cause a continuous gagging sensation but keep the mouth moist by stimulating saliva. Nasal tubes are felt to be less uncomfortable although the degree of discomfort is related to the level of trauma on intubation.

(i) Mouth care is important.

(ii) Support of the tube during movement or turning is essential to prevent further discomfort.

Disconnection from the ventilator

Patients who have long-term ventilation develop considerable psychological dependence on the ventilator. They describe the situation of disconnection from the ventilator as terrifying and feel that it seems an intolerable length of time before they are reconnected. These feelings are bound up with the level of confidence they have in the staff caring for them.

The ventilator alarms are also a source of distress as

patients are often unable to identify if they emanate from their ventilator or that of another patient. If the alarm is allowed to continue for any length of time it can cause considerable stress to the patient listening to it.

(i) A level of trust and confidence must be developed between the patient and his/her nurse.

(ii) Disconnection from the ventilator should only be carried out after full explanation to the patient and reassurance that it will not continue any longer than necessary.

(iii) Ventilator alarms should be cancelled as quickly as possible and their cause and its remedy explained to the patient.

Communication

Patients express great frustration at their inability to speak and are warmly appreciative of patient and persistent efforts by nursing staff to understand them. In particular, lip-reading is mentioned as an important factor in relieving the patient's distress at being unable to speak.

(i) Communication by the patient should be given a high priority by the nurse.

(ii) Patient, persistent attempts at understanding are valued by the patients.

(iii) Perfecting the ability to lip-read (in orally intubated patients) is an essential achievement (Drane 1986).

The importance of touch

Patients describe the comfort of human touch and hand holding in particular. It is an important indicator to the patient that they are cared for (Estabrooks 1989).

(i) Use hand-holding and touch to communicate caring and comfort.

Staff noise and talking at the bedside

The high noise levels associated with ICUs have already been discussed. While some patients find a level of background noise comforting, many found difficulty in sleeping and felt generally disturbed by high levels of noise. In particular, 'radios played at high volumes', 'staff chatter', and 'nurses who raise their voices unnecessarily when talking to patients' were mentioned.

(i) Aim to keep background noise levels low.

(ii) Use normal level of speech when talking to patients.

(iii) Do not play radios loudly unless it is music played specifically for the patient.

(iv) Reduce levels of noise during night hours (see above).

Sensory deprivation and temporal disorientation
Many patients report an inability to distinguish the passage of time. They find high levels of fluorescent light unpleasant and appreciate natural daylight where possible.

(i) Where possible, long-term patients should be nursed where natural light is available.

(ii) Methods of marking the time and the day should be used (see above).

Dreams and hallucinations
Patients frequently refer to dreams and/or hallucinations that they have experienced during their critical illness. Many of them have a prison, depersonalization or torture theme (Daffurn *et al.* 1994). This sounds a reasonable rationalization of some of the events which they have experienced. However, they provide a frightening and distressing perception of the situation.

(i) It is difficult to help the patient in these situations — use of anxiolytics and sedatives with amnesic properties may be of benefit.

(ii) Touch, verbal reassurance, comfort, and communication may help.

Transition to the ward
Many patients who have spent a lengthy period in intensive care express great fear of transfer to the ward (Jones and O'Donnell 1994). They feel that the loss of an individual nurse caring for them means a period of neglect while they are still unable to perform most of their care needs themselves.

(i) Use of a step-down care facility, such as a high dependency unit, may be of help.

(ii) High levels of liaison and communication between ward and unit staff may smooth the transition. A visit from key ward staff to the patient on the unit prior to transfer may also benefit.

(iii) Appropriately timed discharge (i.e. not in an emergency to make way for a new admission) is also important.

Pain experience
Intensive care patients identify pain as one of the biggest stressors associated with intensive care. Many indicate that analgesia did not bring total relief (Puntillo 1990) and that communicating their pain was difficult.

(i) Regular assessment of pain using visual analogues (see below).

(ii) Evaluation of efficacy of analgesia following administration

(iii) Use of alternative methods of pain relief such as warmth, massage, imagery, etc. (See Chapter 9 for further details.)

Supporting and maintaining patient/family relationships

The term 'family' includes all those who provide the patient's intimate social support structure. Problems are due to:

• Loss of normal communication and interaction.

• Increased levels of stress related to the patients illness.

• Family anxiety about outcome.

• In emergency admissions, the shock of the sudden critical illness and removal of the patient from his/her family role.

• The threat to family stability and loss of normal family rituals and day-to-day routine.

Family needs have been identified by a body of research (Rukholm *et al.* 1991; Price *et al.* 1991; Forrester *et al.* 1990; Leske 1991; Wilkinson 1995). Leske's meta-analysis of the research (1991) identified five common factors:

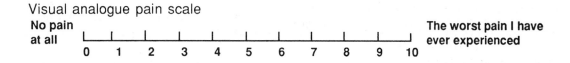

(1) The need for support.

(2) The need for comfort.

(3) The need for information.

(4) The need for proximity.

(5) The need for assurance.

It may not be possible to fulfil all these needs, particularly with regard to patient prognosis, but an awareness of them will direct efforts to support the family and to meet them as far as is possible.

Family support network

● Nursing staff

● Medical staff

● Social work department

● Spiritual support

● Extended family, friends, neighbours

● Specialist support groups (e.g. Headway)

● Community workers (e.g. GP, distinct nurse)

Unfortunately, little research into interventions to meet family needs has been carried out but some suggested strategies based on experience and on suggestions made by researchers are listed below:

● The care of the family should be a multidisciplinary responsibility preferably co-ordinated by the nursing staff as they are the point of continuity.

● The family should be given repeated, detailed updates of the patient's condition, progress, and, where possible, prognosis.

● A common approach must be sought from all support staff and particularly between medical and nursing staff with constant intercommunication about contacts with the family.

● A common record should be kept of all support staff's approaches to the family (Wilkinson 1995).

● Questions should be answered honestly.

● Where possible, the family should be included in planning and carrying out the patient's non-therapeutic care.

● The family should have encouragement and education in communicating, touching, and caring for the patient.

● The strengths and weaknesses within the family coping mechanisms should be identified. Support should be aimed at accentuating strengths and moderating or diminishing weaknesses.

● The family should have open access to the patient but be encouraged to take time away from the patient in order to rest when necessary and have time to themselves (Dracup 1993).

● In the longer-term intensive care patient the family may need encouragement and assistance to resume a modified form of daily life.

● The support team should monitor family members closely for signs of failure to cope, overwhelming stress, and exhaustion.

Overall, the aim should be to establish a positive, supportive relationship with the family.

Family support can be time consuming and emotionally draining but is an essential part of maintaining the patient's coping mechanisms and morale. It should be considered to be one of the most important aspects of nursing the critically ill patient.

Models for delivery of nursing care

Conceptual nursing models or frameworks are designed to guide the application of nursing practice. Riehl and Roy (1980) define a nursing model as: 'a systematically constructed, scientifically based, and logically related set of concepts which identify the essential components of nursing practice, together with the theoretical basis of the concepts and values required for their use by the practitioner'.

The proliferation of different models in recent years has illustrated one fundamental point: no single model of nursing will reflect all areas of nursing practice. It is appropriate to use different models for different types of patients and even for different periods during the patient's course of illness. The use of a nursing model should be viewed as an enhancement of nursing practice rather than a theoretical outline to be applied without thought or alteration to all types of patients. Similarly, the use of the medical model in some circumstances should not be dismissed out of hand. It can be particularly useful for refining priorities in acute situations where the patient's physiological problems require urgent action.

It is not appropriate to include an exhaustive description of nursing models currently used in intensive care in this chapter. However, the process of identifying a model or framework of care will be described.

Nursing philosophy

The primary step in development of nursing theory is to establish a philosophy for the unit. The philosophy should contain:

(i) the values, ideals and goals of the nursing staff,

(ii) a synopsis of how the staff view the patient and his/her needs,

(iii) the environment in which care is delivered, and

(iv) any other significant external issues which will affect the delivery of care.

The key issues that need consideration in forming a philosophy are:

(1) The nature of care — caring is seen as the foundation of nursing practice.

(2) Social viability — does the philosophy meet the expectations of society, is it seen as important by society and does it have value for the profession of nursing?

(3) The extrinsic environment of care — the philosophy should reflect the nature of the environment in which it is carried out (i.e. an intensive care philosophy will bear different hallmarks to a community care philosophy).

(4) The intrinsic environment of care — this refers to the way nursing or the delivery of care is organized within the environment.

Multidisciplinary philosophy

Many intensive care units work primarily as multidisciplinary teams and it is important that the philosophy reflects the whole team's approach and not simply that of the nursing staff. If it does not, then it is likely that the values and views expressed within the philosophy will remain an abstract rather than a real exercise.

Nursing models

The key points of the philosophy should then be reviewed and used as a basis either for matching a published nursing model or for building a new model.

Certain concepts are central to nursing as a discipline and are the foundation stones for building any model. They are known as metaparadigm concepts and include: person, environment, health, and nursing (as an activity).

Nursing metaparadigm concepts (Fawcett 1989)

Person — the recipient of nursing actions

Environment — the recipient's significant others and surroundings

Health — the wellness or illness state of the recipient

Nursing — the actions taken by nurses either on behalf of or which the recipient

---

Application of these concepts to intensive care carries problems which require special consideration:

1. The barriers to communication involved in intensive care mean that the patient as a person may be difficult to know and assess. Information regarding aspects other than physical state may be obtainable only second-hand through relatives or friends. Similar problems relate to the patient's environment. These aspects must be taken into account and the nursing model chosen should neither discount them completely nor place too heavy an emphasis on them.

2. Intensive care nursing accentuates the importance of the physical state of the patient as this forms the basis for admission. The nurse is frequently working in critical situations where other aspects must take second place. However, these priorities will change in different circumstances and it is important that physical aspects give way to psychological or social needs where it is appropriate and beneficial to the patient to do so.

    One of the real values of a well-thought out framework of care is the ability to switch emphasis appropriately without diminishing the patient's physical and psychological well-being.

3. The complexity of the physical and physiological problems of the critically ill patient requires a framework which will allow a clear and succinct approach to assessment, intervention and evaluation. One of the reasons the medical model has been so useful to intensive care nurses is its clarity of structure and suitability to physical and physiological problems.

The key components of nursing models (Aggleton and Chalmers 1986) are the:

- nature of people (people and their needs),
- causes of problems likely to require nursing intervention,
- nature of the assessment process,
- nature of the planning and goal-setting process,
- focus of intervention during the implementation of the care plan,
- nature of the process of evaluating the quality and effects of nursing care given,
- role of the nurse.

The influence of the model on delivery of care

The emphasis of the model chosen will have an influence on the care given. If the model is chosen to reflect the unit nursing philosophy then that emphasis will be in accordance with the values and ideals encompassed in the philosophy. However, it is not the only factor influencing care and although important, must take its place amongst numerous others such as medical interventions and values, education, research, new therapies, nursing staffing, and skill mix.

Priorities of care

Good intensive care practice seeks to prevent critical situations where possible, by employing close observation and monitoring of the patient and skilled interpretation of the information obtained. Early warning of impending problems and appropriate treatment based on this can prevent some emergencies. There will always be a proportion of sudden overwhelming disasters but many potentially life-threatening events can be circumvented by the skill and knowledge of the nurse who identifies these early signs. By the nature of their critical illness, patients in the ICU are more likely to develop life-threatening problems and emergency situations.

Emergency equipment

A major priority for the nurse must be ensuring emergency equipment at the bedside is functioning and to hand. Unit emergency equipment, such as defibrillators and pacing systems, should be checked by a designated nurse on each shift.

The following equipment/skills provide a minimum basic standard of safety for emergency events and will at least allow the nurse to maintain patient's vital functions until help arrives.

1. Equipment for airway protection

- Check the suction is functioning by occluding the end of the suction tubing and ensuring a vacuum pressure builds up.
- Ensure the correct size suction catheters are available for the size of the patient's endotracheal or tracheostomy tube (see Chapter 3).
- An oropharyngeal (Guedel) airway of a size appropriate to the patient (usually 2 for women and 3 for men) and a Yankauer sucker should also be available.

2. Equipment for support of patient's breathing

- Check the manual resuscitation or rebreathe bag is functioning and leak-free by occluding the end of the valve outlet with the valve screwed tight. The bag should inflate to a taut pressure without air escaping.
- Any nurse responsible for a ventilated patient should be competent to ventilate them with a manual resuscitation bag. It is the only method of ensuring adequate ventilation and oxygenation if the ventilator or gas supply fails. It may also be necessary to manually ventilate the patient in the event of emergency evacuation.
- Check the bag has the correct attachment to allow ventilation. There should be a catheter mount if the patient is intubated and an anaesthetic facemask if he is not.
- An anaesthetic facemask should also be available at the bedside at all times in case of accidental extubation.
- Check any portable oxygen cylinders to ensure they are at least half full.

3. Equipment for support of the patient's circulation

- Check that the arterial line is functional and accurate or that any non-invasive blood pressure monitoring is functional and accurate.
- Every nurse caring for a patient should be competent in external cardiac massage (see Chapter 6). The cardiac arrest call button should be functioning or help should be within easy calling distance.
- In almost all intensive care patients some form of IV access should be available and patent.
- As a basic precaution, every nurse should run through these checks at the beginning of each shift and whenever they take over the care of a patient.

Common core problems for patients in the ICU

Many of the patient's problems exist as a result of the body's response to critical illness and the nature of the ICU environment. There are, therefore, a number of problems which are experienced by most ICU patients. These are listed in Table 2.3. These common core problems are discussed in this chapter if they constitute a global problem or in the chapters listed if they refer specifically to a system.

Table 2.3 Common core problems for intensive care patients

Problem	Chapter
Airway maintenance	Respiratory problems (Chapter 3)
Support of ventilation	Respiratory problems (Chapter 3)
Support of circulation	Cardiovascular problems (Chapter 5)
Fluid balance	Renal problems (Chapter 8)
Nutrition	Gastrointestinal and nutrition chapter
Elimination	Gastrointestinal problems, and nutrition (Chapter 10)
Pain relief	Neurological problems (Chapter 9)
Communication Anxiety/fear Maintenance of sensory balance Support of the family Alterations in diurnal rhythm Prevention of the effects of limited mobility Personal hygiene	These topics are discussed in this chapter

Personal hygiene

Mouth care

This is a high priority in the critically ill patient because of the loss of normal cleaning mechanisms and the increased vulnerability of the patient to infection. The presence of an oral endotracheal tube will cause pressure problems and impede full assessment of and access to the oral cavity. This is due to:

- a decreased or absent oral fluid intake,
- dehydration of the buccal mucosa related to inhaling dry gases, systemic dehydration, stress, and tachypnoea,
- decreased salivary stimulation due to loss of food as a stimulating factor and increased sympathetic arousal,
- an increased number of contributory factors to mouth care problems such as antibiotics, renal failure, vitamin deficiency, xerostomic drugs (e.g. atropine and catecholamines),
- decreased host defence mechanisms giving rise to an increased risk of mouth infection, particularly *Candida*, herpes simplex virus, and *Streptococcus viridans*,
- inability to perform own oral hygiene,
- continued formation of plaque and debris on teeth whether the patient is eating or drinking or not.

Little research has been performed on mouth care problems in the critically ill and even less on the efficacy of different mouth care procedures (Roth and Creason 1986). However, work in the dental and periodontal fields can be extrapolated in some cases to identify the correct tools and cleansing agents, and the few studies that do exist can provide some guidelines for oral hygiene in the critically ill (Howarth 1977). See Table 2.4 for assessing the condition of the mouth.

Management
- Frequency and type of hygiene should be based on assessment of the oral cavity (see Table 2.4) rather than routine care.
- A small, soft toothbrush moistened in water to provide a neutral pH (Gooch 1985) and used in a circular motion, or with short horizontal strokes has been shown to be more effective than foam sticks or swabs in removing debris (DeWalt 1975).
- Dilute hydrogen peroxide (20% vol.) solution diluted 1:4 with water) or sodium bicarbonate (0.5 teaspoon to 1 pint (500 cc) water) can be used for removing debris and dissolving tenacious mucus.
- If there is evidence of infection, such as stomatitis or gingivitis, use of an antimicrobial mouthwash or toothpaste such as chlorhexidine gluconate 1% may

help but the major intervention is preventive removal of plaque (Kite and Pearson 1995).

- Lips should be protected from drying out with either vaseline or KY jelly.

- A neutral mouthwash solution (non-hygroscopic) may be used for patient comfort but has not be shown to have any effect on maintenance of mucosal integrity.

- Limited use (2–3 times/day) of lemon and glycerin hygroscopic mouthwash may help stimulate salivary production (Warner 1986).

- If the mouth is very dry and fluids are limited or difficult to swallow artificial saliva spray may be of help.

- Dentures should be removed overnight — cleaning and soaking should be performed during this period.

- Adequate fluid hydration of the patient will help with xerostomia.

Table 2.4 Assessment of the oral cavity (adapted from Richardson 1987; Crosby 1989)

Oral cavity	Normal	Abnormal
Mucosa	Pink, moist, intact, smooth	Reddening, ulceration, other lesions
Tongue	Pink, moist, intact, papillae present	Coated, absence of papillae with smooth shiny appearance, debris, lesions, crusted, cracks, blackened
Lips	Clean, intact, pink	Dry skin, cracks, reddened, encrusted, ulcerated, bleeding
Saliva	Watery, white or clear	Thick, viscous, absent, blood-stained
Gingiva (gums)	Pink, moist, firm	Receding, overgrowing, oedematous, reddened, bleeding
Teeth	White, firm in sockets, no debris, no decay	Discoloured, decayed, debris present, wobbly

Severe oral problems can cause considerable distress to patients as well as providing a reservoir of organisms such as *Candida albicans* which can lead to systemic infection.

Eye care

The healthy eye is protected from dehydration and infection by the production of tears. The tear film is made up of three layers, the outer lipid layer, the middle water-based layer, and the inner mucilaginous layer. Each layer has a specific purpose. The outer layer retards fluid evaporation and prevents tear film overflow. The middle layer contains oxygen, electrolytes, and proteins including antibacterial agents. The inner layer aids wetting of the cornea. The normal rate of production of tears by the lacrimal gland is about 1–2 µl/min and these are spread over the surface of the cornea by the blink reflex.

Ventilated and sedated patients are particularly susceptible to eye care problems due to:

(i) Their reduced or absent ability to blink.

(ii) Incomplete lid closure.

(iii) Decreased tear production as a side-effect of certain drugs including atropine, phenothiazines, disopyramide, and tricyclic antidepressants.

(iv) Decreased resistance to infection and increased likelihood of cross-infection from respiratory pathogens (Hilton *et al.* 1983). This is related to poor suction technique where the catheter is removed from the ET tube over the top of the eye, disseminating droplets containing organisms into the cornea (Ommeslag *et al.* 1987).

(v) An increased likelihood of orbital oedema due to the high intrathoracic pressures produced by positive pressure ventilation reducing venous return. This is exacerbated if the patient is nursed flat during periods of instability or if the tapes securing tracheostomy or endotracheal tubes are tied too tightly. The dependent areas are affected and fluid is forced into the periocular tissues and the conjunctival membrane.

(vi) Dehydration reduces tear production.

There are two common eye care problems associated with the ventilated or unconscious patient: dry eyes and exposure keratopathy.

1. *Dry eyes*, this problem is due to:

- any, or all, of the above factors (i)–(vi),

- incorrect positioning of CPAP mask. This can quickly dry corneal surfaces even when the blink reflex is intact.

2. *Exposure keratopathy*:

- exposure of the corneal surface due to incomplete lid closure leads to drying, epithelial erosions, and, ultimately, corneal ulceration. The risk of infection is also increased.

Management

- Assess the following aspects to determine frequency of intervention:

  (i) the patient's ability to close the eyelid voluntarily or involuntarily,

  (ii) patient position,

  (iii) the patient's hydration status,

  (iv) the condition of the cornea — look for evidence of infection (purulent or crusting exudate), clouding, haemorrhage, etc.,

  (v) evidence of discharge,

  (vi) drugs.

- Use sterile water for cleansing (saline has been found to disrupt the normal tear film structure and increase the rate of evaporation).

- If corneal wetting is inadequate use artificial tears up to ½-hourly.

- If the corneal surface is constantly exposed, close lids using hydrogel pads, paraffin gauze, or eye shields. Taping eyes is traumatic to the eyelid and can be unsightly for the patient's family although some ophthalmologists feel that this is the only secure method of keeping the patient's eyes shut.

- Care should be taken when withdrawing suction catheters to avoid droplet transference of respiratory organisms to the corneal surface (Ommeslag *et al.* 1987).

- If the eye is discharging or obviously infected take a swab for culture and sensitivity and apply appropriate topical antibiotic drops or ointment as prescribed.

Prevention of problems associated with urinary catheterization

Most critically ill patients are catheterized to allow close monitoring of urinary output. However, the presence of a urinary catheter has a number of problems associated with it.

1. *Increased risk of urinary* tract infection
Infection rates in catheterized patients can be as high as 62%. This is due to:

- Trauma associated with the catheter insertion. This creates breaks in mucosal integrity allowing bacterial colonization.

- Contamination during insertion and afterwards due to poor hand-washing/hygiene procedures.

- Bypassing the normal defence mechanisms of the urethra

- Use of larger than necessary catheters which cause pressure on the urethral wall and ischaemia.

- Use of larger than necessary balloons which cause pressure on the bladder wall and an increase in residual urine.

- Obliteration of the natural urethral mucosal cleansing which occurs during voiding. The flow of urine in the normal condition discourages pathogen migration.

- Patient susceptibility to infection is increased due to any serious underlying pathology.

- The intensive care environment has an increased level of bacteria (see risks in ICU, p. 24).

(*Note*: 55% of patients catheterized develop bacteriuria within 48 hours.)

2. *Trauma and discomfort associated with the presence of the catheter*
This is due to (Lowthian 1989):

- Use of larger than necessary catheters.

- Movement/dragging of the catheter.

- Use of larger than necessary balloons.

3. *Blockage of the catheter from debris or blood*
This is due to:

- Poor urinary flow allowing debris to collect in the bladder.

- Urinary tract infection producing large amounts of debris.

Management

- Strict asepsis for catheter insertion.

- Hand-washing prior to any manipulation of the catheter.

- Maintenance of closed urinary drainage system with minimal manipulation of any part (Platt *et al.* 1983).

- Maintenance of unimpeded urinary flow with no reflux (positioning of the drainage bag is all important to ensure gravity aided flow) (Mulhall *et al.* 1988).

- Strict asepsis for collection of CSU through specimen port. (*Note*: the drainage system should never be disconnected for this.)

- Avoidance of bladder irrigation unless absolutely necessary. If possible, irrigate through the specimen port using a needle rather than disconnection of the drainage system (Burgener 1987).

- Use the smallest size catheter that will drain adequately. This is usually 12–14 Ch (=4–4.5 mm external diameter) (Rees-Williams *et al.* 1988).

- Only use the 5 ml balloon catheter, unless immediately following bladder or prostatic surgery when a larger balloon may be necessary (Belfield 1988).

- Attach the catheter to the inner aspect of the thigh using a device specifically designed for this to prevent drag.

- Daily or more frequent if necessary, meatal cleansing with soap and water or saline. There is no evidence to support the use of antiseptic solutions for cleansing (Mulhall *et al.* 1988)

- Ensure the catheter used is appropriate to the likely length of catheterization (i.e. pure silicone for long-term use, Hyrogel or PVC for short-term use) (Rees-Williams *et al.* 1988).

- Ensure the foreskin does not remain retracted, which can cause a painful phimosis.

Prevention of the effects of restricted mobility

Most critically ill patients are either unable to move themselves or have only limited movement of their limbs. They remain in one position unless moved by their nurses and when unstable are frequently nursed flat or with the head of the bed at a 30–45 degree angle. The effects of immobility are a major problem to the critically ill patient and prevention can make the difference between recovery and death. The quality of life of any surviving patient may also be reduced if these problems are ignored.

The effects of restricted mobility

1. *An increased risk of chest infection.*
This is due to:

   (i) basal collapse;

   (ii) increased secretions;

   (iii) decreased sputum clearance, and

   (iv) ventilatum to perfusion (V/Q) mismatch secondary to atelectasis, dependent lung oedema, and alterations due to positioning.

Lung volumes (FRC and residual volumes) are reduced when lying supine due to the rise in the diaphragm associated with the change in position of abdominal contents. Impaired ability to cough, decreased ciliary movement and weak thoracic muscles cause stasis and pooling of secretions. Production of alveolar surfactant may be impaired during periods when the patient is flat and the ratio of ventilation to perfusion is also altered by the supine, lateral, and prone position.

2. *An increased risk of deep vein thrombosis and peripheral oedema.*
This is due to:

   (i) decreased venous return,

   (ii) venous stasis, and

   (iii) increased coagulability associated with loss of muscle pumps.

Loss of muscle movement means that the normal pumping mechanism returning venous blood to the heart is reduced. Pooling occurs which increases intracapillary hydrostatic pressure. This rise increases movement of fluid through the capillary membrane into the interstitial tissues. The extracapillary shift of fluid increases the viscosity of the blood causing further stasis and increased risk of platelet aggregation and coagulation.

3. *Muscle atrophy due to disuse*
The rate of muscle atrophy is rapid in the early immobilization phase and is often accelerated by the catabolic nature of the patient's illness. The muscles of the thigh and calf usually exhibit the greatest reduction and lead to weakness and fatigue requiring long periods of convalescence to rebuild.

4. *Joint stiffness and contractures*
The particular risk lies with flexion as the flexor muscles are stronger than the extensors. If normal range of movement exercises do not occur the muscle becomes

permanently shortened resulting in limb contractures. Common sites include plantar flexor, hip, and knee joints.

5. Demineralization and loss of density in the long bones
Loss of weight-bearing pressure within the long bones results in decreased osteoblastic (bone forming and repair) activity. Osteoclastic (bone destruction) activity continues resulting in loss of bone density and ultimately osteoporosis. Hypercalcaemia and hypercalciuria are seen within one to two days of immobility and have been associated with prolonged immobility in all age groups in spite of adequate calcium intake.

6. Peripheral nerve injury
The particular risk is ulnar nerve injury due to incorrect positioning. Pronation of the forearm in the supine position traps the ulnar nerve in the cubital tunnel and flexion of the elbow in this position will add further pressure on the ulnar nerve. Risk factors include diabetes mellitus, bedrest for more than 22 a day, age of patient, more than 50 years, and alcoholism (Chuman 1985).

7. Increased risk of pressure sores
This is due to pressure on dependent areas and inability to change position as required.

Development is dependent on the product of the level of pressure exerted and the time it is exerted for. The higher the pressure, the less time is required for a sore to develop. The most vulnerable areas are the tissues over bony prominences (See box and diagram).

Pressure points (see diagram)

(1) occiput	(7) sacrum
(2) acromion processes	(8) ischial tuberosities
(3) scapulae	(9) coccyx
(4) spinous processes	(10) medial epicondyles
(5) olecranon processes	(11) medial and lateral
(6) iliac crests	malleoli
	(12) calcaneus

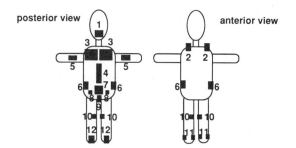

posterior view   anterior view

Critically ill patients are particularly vulnerable to pressure sores due to a number of factors (see box).

Pressure sore risk factors present in the critically ill
- Immobility
- Emaciation and muscle wasting
- Altered sensory function (often due to sedation)
- Decreased cardiac output
- Increased vasoconstriction
- Reduced venous return, tissue hypoperfusion

Batson *et al.* (1993) found five factors in a critically ill population which were specifically related to the development of pressure sores:

- diabetes,
- infusion of noradrenaline,
- infusion of adrenaline,
- restricted movement (e.g. traction, continuous venovenous haemofiltration, intra-aortic balloon pump),
- patient too unstable to turn.

Relief of pressure simply by a two-hourly change of position can be inadequate in the acutely ill and other methods of support may be required.

8. Increased risk of urinary tract infection
This is due to:

(i) urinary stasis,

(ii) bladder distension,

(iii) increase in urinary pH,

(iv) decreased immune function, and

(v) presence of a urinary catheter.

The supine position results in the renal pelvis filling with urine before drainage via the ureter occurs. This urinary stasis acts as a focus for bacterial growth and the formation of renal calculi. There will also be an accumulation of urine in the bladder in the supine position due to filling of the dependent portion of the bladder prior to drainage via the urethra. This may be relieved by the presence of a urinary catheter. There may be an increase in urinary pH due to increased calcium and phosphate excretion which will increase the infection risk.

9. *Increased incidence of nephrolithiasis*
This is due to: increased urinary calcium excretion related to bone degeneration.

Hypercalcaemia occurs as a result of degeneration of bone from disuse (see above) and this produces an increase in renal excretion of calcium and phosphorus in the first week of bedrest. This can continue for up to 5 weeks.

10. *Decreased gut motility and constipation*
Muscle wasting and loss may include the muscles controlling excretion (diaphragm, abdominal muscles, and levator ani). Reduced gut motility may occur as a result of loss of stimuli such as the presence of food passing through the oesophagus.

The degree of immobility relates to the severity of illness, the need for sedation and paralysis, haemodynamic instability, spinal injuries, direct result of the illness, such as acute polyneuropathy (Guillain–Barré), syndrome and loss of muscle function due to muscle wasting.

Management

Central to the prevention of problems associated with immobility is the need to alter patient position frequently. This cannot always happen due to reasons such as haemodynamic instability, changes in ventilation/perfusion ratios due to shunting in certain positions, and spinal or pelvic trauma. In these situations other goals take priority but an awareness of the problems caused by periods of immobility will allow interventions to support and limit the effects during the rehabilitation phase.

- Regular turning and repositioning of the patient. Knowledge of the correct alignment and positioning of limbs to prevent joint injury.

- Use of specialist beds and mattresses which relieve pressure over susceptible points and spread the pressure load.

- Regular full inspection of skin integrity, with particular attention to the high-risk dependent areas.

- Passive limb movements and full range of movement (ROM) exercises for joints to maintain joint mobility.

- Where possible, active, isotonic limb and ROM exercises will maintain muscle strength and mass as well as joint mobility.

- Active chest physiotherapy, use of adequate humidification, etc. (see Chapter 3).

- Close observation of bowel function.

- Early commencement of feeding (especially enteral).

- Scrupulous attention to infection control measures.

- Early and frequent mobilization.

Prevention of the complications associated with immobility is unlikely to alter the patient outcome but may contribute significantly to the rate of rehabilitation and the degree of morbidity following discharge.

Infection risks in intensive care

Intensive care patients have a high incidence (between 10% and 15%) of nosocomial infection. Maki (1989) has shown nosocomial infection to be two to five times higher in ICU patients than non-ICU hospitalized patients. ICU patients are particularly vulnerable to primary bacteraemias (mostly from intravenous cannulae), pneumonias (usually as a result of intubation and IPPV), intra-abdominal infections, and urinary tract infections. Most invasive devices facilitate colonization by nosocomial organisms and greatly increase vulnerability to infection. As well as the high level of susceptibility the increased incidence of antibiotic usage in the ICU creates resistant strains which can be transmitted from patient to patient.

Opportunistic and fungal infections can also occur as a result of compromised host defence mechanisms and the use of antibiotics, which reduce indigenous bacterial flora, allowing overgrowth of other organisms.

Significant risk factors for infections in ICU patients (Craven *et al.* 1988)	
Risk factor	*Increase in risk*
Presence of urinary catheter > 10 days	3.2-fold
Stay in ICU > 3 days	2.5-fold
Intracranial pressure monitor *in situ*	2.5-fold
Arterial line	1.5-fold
Shock	2.5-fold

The high risk of infection in the ICU patient is due to:

1. Patient-related problems:

- invasive procedures and monitoring,

- abnormal humoral immunity,

- abnormal phagocytic function,

- abnormal antibody function.

2. Environment-related problems:

- high numbers of high-risk patients in one area,

- high usage of antibiotics encourages growth of resistant bacteria,

- if staffing levels fall to less than 1:1, cross-infection may be increased.

Intravascular devices

These comprise central venous catheters, arterial and peripheral venous cannulae, and pulmonary artery flotation catheters.

Any intravascular cannula left *in situ* will provide a direct portal of entry for microorganisms into the circulation. Local and systemic infections can occur even with peripheral cannulae, particularly if they are plastic, inserted as an emergency, or by cut-down technique, and left *in situ* for more than 72 hours (Maki 1989).

Patients with central venous catheters are likely to have a 9.2-fold increase in risk if there is cutaneous colonisation of the site. The most common site of origin of organisms causing catheter tip infections and bacteraemia is the catheter hub (Linares *et al.* 1985). There is conflicting evidence as to the infection rates associated with multi-lumen as opposed to single lumen central venous catheters with some studies reporting no difference in rates (Gil *et al* 1989; Powell *et al.* 1988) and some reporting a significant difference. The variation may be related to the severity of illness involved in the study populations, with some studies using non-randomized samples. Multi-lumen cannulae are commonly used due to the decreased need for manipulation and use of multiple connection devices, and the reduction in number of invasive procedures required with their use.

Use of systems, such as the 'klick-lock' piggy-back system allowing access to IV cannulae without breaking the circuit, may well reduce infection rates but current research in this area is limited.

Routes of infection in intravascular devices

- Hub contamination leading to transfer of organisms down the cannula

- Connections between giving set and cannula such as three-way taps

- Site contamination

- Thrombosis of cannula providing a medium for organism growth

---

Nosocomial pneumonia

Pneumonia is the leading nosocomial cause of death with a mortality rate of up to 60% (Bihari 1992). Relevant risk factors involved in development of nosocomial pneumonia are frequently present in critically ill patients and include:

(i) presence of an endotracheal tube,

(ii) chronic ill health particularly chronic pulmonary disease,

(iii) malnutrition,

(iv) use of H_2 (histamine receptor) antagonists to prevent stress ulceration (see Chapter 10),

(v) use of antibiotics,

(vi) smoking,

(vii) prolonged upper abdominal or thoracic surgery,

(viii) impaired upper airway reflexes such as the cough reflex,

(ix) advanced age and obesity.

Mechanisms of infection

(i) contamination of inspired air (e.g. respiratory therapy equipment),

(ii) spread from contiguous (neighbouring) infected tissue,

(iii) blood-borne spread from distant infections or tricuspid valve vegetations,

(iv) oropharyngeal and gastric colonization with transmission to the trachea probably by aspiration (Pingleton 1991).

Aspiration is the most frequent cause of infection in ventilated patients due to the presence of endotracheal (ET) tubes. ET tubes provide protection from large volume aspiration but may actually facilitate transfer of tiny amounts of aspirate by preventing closure of the vocal cords and bypassing the cough reflex. Bacterial translocation (the passage of organisms from the lumen of the gut into the blood) has been proposed as an alternative route to aspiration for infection (Fiddian-Green and Baker 1991). It is discussed in more detail in Chapter 10. The presence of enteral feed in the stomach and the resultant rise in gastric pH may also be related to overgrowth of bacteria and an increase in aspiration pneumonia (Jacobs *et al.* 1990).

Most nosocomial pneumonias are due to Gram-negative organisms (Santamaria 1990). Prevention is the aim, as identification and treatment of the causative organism can be difficult and ineffective.

Preventative measures

1. Ventilator and circuits:

    (i) use of heat–moisture exchange (HME) humidifiers rather than water bath humidifiers,

    (ii) regular change of ventilator circuits and manual ventilation systems at least every 48 hours if HME humidifiers are not used,

    (iii) scrupulous hand-washing prior to endotracheal suctioning,

    (iv) use of disposable nebulizers or scrupulous washing and drying of reusable nebulizers between use,

    (v) use of closed suction catheter systems.

2. The patient:

    (i) regular change of position allowing maximum basal lung expansion from supine to left and right lateral,

    (ii) regular chest physiotherapy (see Chapter 3).

Urinary tract infections

Nosocomial urinary tract infections (UTIs) are the most frequent infections seen in ICUs (Bihari 1992). Nearly all infections are related to the presence of an indwelling urinary catheter. The incidence of infection increases with the length of time the catheter remains *in situ* and the severity of illness. Women and the elderly are more at risk of developing a UTI.

The most important preventative measure is to avoid urinary catheterization unless absolutely essential, although this will have little effect in the ICU where most patients require catheterization. If catheterization is necessary, early removal should be a major goal although this is frequently impractical in the critically ill patient.

Catheter insertion should always be performed aseptically and thorough hand-washing carried out prior to any manipulation of the drainage system. Closed circuit drainage systems should always be used. Use of topical

antibiotics for irrigation and meatal cleansing have not been shown to have any effect.

Hand-washing

One of the major preventable routes of transmission of nosocomial infection is via the hands of unit personnel (20–40% of infections) and the single most important factor in preventing transmission is a scrupulous hand-washing technique (Turner 1993). Environmental factors, such as positioning of wash-basins with easy access from each bed area, and sufficient numbers of wash-basins to allow unrestricted access are important in supporting hand-washing.

Individual unit policy may vary on infection control procedures but the following guidelines give a synopsis of the policies identified as reducing the level of nosocomial infection in intensive care.

Management to reduce infection risks
- Strict adherence to local infection control policies.

- Hand-washing between patient contacts.

- Strict aseptic technique for dressings, line insertions, invasive procedures, etc.

- Limitation of manipulation of IV lines, urinary catheters, dressings.

- Policy of immediate removal of IV lines if infection is suspected.

- Infection control standards/protocols for staff.

- Feedback from microbiology regarding infection rates.

- Avoidance of antacid ulcer prophylaxis and H_2 blockers in combination.

- Avoidance of endotracheal intubation wherever possible by use of CPAP (see Chapter 3) and other forms of non-invasive ventilation.

- Adherence to a locally defined antimicrobial policy.

Transfer of critically ill patients

Secondary transfer refers to transfer from or within a hospital setting. The transfer of critically ill patients requires thought, preparation, appropriate equipment, and a high level of expertise. Unfortunately, this is rarely seen when patients are rushed from one hospital to another and may be a contributory factor in the increased morbidity associated with such moves. Bion *et al.* (1988) showed that most journeys are inadequately prepared for, hurriedly undertaken, noisy, traumatic and frequently lead to a discontinuation of vital monitoring or therapy. Waddell (1975) found a high incidence of deterioration in the patient's condition directly accountable to being moved.

However, with the limited number of intensive care beds and suggested moves towards increasing centralization of costly and limited resources, the number of inter-hospital transfers is likely to increase.

It is therefore imperative that the safest possible environment for transfer is created and the nurse should be responsible for ensuring that this is done before the journey starts. These journeys may constitute either accompanying a patient from one ICU to another, or going out from a specialist ICU to pick up a patient from another ICU.

Suggested procedure

- Transfer should be handled by experienced, suitably qualified personnel.

- The equipment used should be designed for transport with reliable performance and battery back-up.

- Monitoring should consist of a minimum of ECG, pulse oximetry, invasive or non-invasive blood pressure and end tidal CO_2 (Hope and Runcie 1993).

- Staff should be familiar with the equipment used.

- The patient should be stabilized prior to transfer.

- If it is likely that intubation or other therapeutic manoeuvres may be needed, these should be carried out prior to transfer.

- Ideally, mobile flying squads should be established to stabilize and then transfer patients.

- The patient's infective status should be checked in order that adequate precautions may be taken in the event of such problems as MRSA.

Care prior to and during transport

1. Ensure patient safety prior to and during transfer

- Check all equipment for:
  - performance,
  - battery life, and
  - functioning alarm systems.

- Set up and use appropriate alarm settings.

- Ensure all staff transferring patient are familiar with all equipment including emergency equipment.

2. Stabilize patient prior to transfer and monitor patient during transfer (Table 2.5)

Any patient with respiratory problems should be assessed prior to the journey by an experienced intensivist or anaesthetist for possible intubation and elective ventilation prior to transfer. If the patient is not intubated he/she should be accompanied by someone experienced in intubation.

Use of rebreathe bags over a long journey are likely to result in hypercapnia but are acceptable for short journeys.

3. Notification of relatives

Ensure relatives are aware of the reason for transfer, the approximate journey time, the details of the receiving hospital and the name of the receiving consultant. If possible, provide a copy of the unit information booklet for patient's relatives and, if necessary, supply directions.

4. Collection of copies of documentation

The following are important: notes, X-rays, diagnostic reports, charts, nursing documentation, prescription chart.

If copies cannot be obtained, a synopsis should be produced by the transferring hospital.

5. Arrangements for transfer

- These should be carried out only when the patient is virtually ready for transfer.

- Notify ambulance control, and the police, if necessary.

- Inform the receiving hospital immediately prior to departure of an estimated time of arrival.

(*Note*: Inter-hospital transfer by helicopter or aircraft is a specialized procedure which should only be carried out by trained teams.)

Elective vs. emergency admissions to the ICU

Most ICUs will admit a mixture of elective and emergency admissions. Preparation for these two types of patients is different and their needs and prognosis will also differ.

Elective patients

Admissions are usually post-operative but may occasionally be pre-operative if haemodynamic optimisation is required.

Table 2.5 Preparing the critically ill patient for transfer

Problem	Prior to transfer	During transfer
Airway and O_2 requirements	<ul><li>ABGs</li><li>CXR</li><li>Insert chest drains if necessary</li><li>Intubate if necessary</li><li>Chest physiotherapy and suction</li></ul>	<ul><li>Portable ventilator (ideally)</li><li>Pulse oximetry</li><li>Portable suction and catheters</li><li>Oxygen supply with at least 1 hour over calculated requirements</li><li>Rebreathe bag or Ambu bag</li></ul>
Cardiovascular support	<ul><li>Insert any central venous access/arterial lines</li><li>Correct any electrolyte or pH abnormality (as far as possible)</li><li>Set up support drug infusions</li><li>Check temperature</li><li>Insert pacing wire if necessary</li></ul>	<ul><li>ECG and systemic BP monitoring</li><li>If possible, CVP monitoring facility</li><li>Continuous drug infusion via battery-operated pump</li><li>Portable defibrillator and emergency drugs to hand</li><li>Adequate bed linen for patient</li></ul>
Maintenance of fluid balance	<ul><li>Insert urinary catheter</li><li>Set up required infusions</li><li>Place nasogastric tube if necessary</li></ul>	<ul><li>Carry appropriate fluid for infusion plus extra colloid and crystalloid</li><li>Continue urinary and nasogastric drainage during transfer</li></ul>
Patient anxiety and fear of journey	<ul><li>Introduce transfer team to patient</li><li>Inform patient of reasons for transfer, location of receiving hospital, approx. journey time</li><li>Reassure patient about relatives, visiting, and any other queries</li></ul>	<ul><li>Continue to reassure the patient and inform them of progress</li><li>Ensure the patient is secure and comfortable on the trolley</li></ul>
Pain control and sedation	<ul><li>Assess patient's pain</li><li>Ensure adequate supplies of analgesia for journey</li><li>Set up analgesic/sedative infusions if required</li></ul>	<ul><li>Reassess pain: sedation as necessary</li></ul>
Miscellaneous	<ul><li>Insert wound drains</li><li>Stabilize fractures</li><li>Assess pressure areas</li></ul>	<ul><li>Carry adequate drainage containers</li><li>Transfer on pressure-relieving mattress</li></ul>

1. The patient is usually prepared for admission, he/she may have visited the ICU and will have been given information from nursing and medical staff as well as physiotherapy and possibly other specialist staff. It is likely that relatives will also be well informed and may have met ICU staff prior to admission. The elective patient has some defence or coping mechanisms to aid him in making sense of the environment.

2. The admission is usually only for a short period of time (frequently overnight) and the effects of ventilation, the ICU environment, close observation and monitoring, and sensory disturbance are likely to be minimal.

3. Recovery is usually swift unless complications develop and the patient may have only limited recollection of the time spent in the ICU due to a combination of anaesthesia and analgesia.

These factors make elective admission patients far less vulnerable to the problems associated with being in intensive care providing that care is taken to prepare them adequately and to prevent complications occurring.

Emergency admissions

1. By the nature of the crisis which precipitated admission, these patients are often sicker and have a poorer

prognosis. Patient scoring systems, such as APACHE II (see Chapter 15), carry weighting which reflects this.

2. The lack of preparation increases fear and decreases the ability of the patient to cope with the stresses of the ICU environment. They are therefore highly vulnerable to the problems associated with an admission to ICU.

3. Recovery is frequently prolonged and less likely to occur although this varies with the cause of admission.

4. The emergency produces shock and distress in both patient and relatives who must cope with this unexpected life-threatening event.

Strategies ·

1. Intensive and repeated information-giving is essential. People do not process information or retain it when distressed or shocked. It is therefore important to limit the amount of information given but repeat it frequently.

2. Support is often limited to the relatives when the patient is first admitted as the serious nature of the illness make it impossible to establish two-way communication. However, information-giving for the patient should continue and reassurance that care and treatment are being carried accompanied by caring touch may help the patient.

3. Alternative support agencies for both relatives and patients should be considered and used where appropriate (see section on family needs, p. 15)

The dying ICU patient

Intensive care is associated with a high mortality rate which will vary from week to week but which is likely overall to be between 15% and 25% of patients (Rowan *et al.* 1993). In some cases, death will occur as a fairly immediate event following emergency admission to the unit and there will be little time to prepare either the patient or the family. In the majority of cases, death will occur after a period of several days on the unit and will be an expected outcome. In a small number of patients it will become evident that further intervention and the continuation of treatment is both distressing for the patient and futile. The ethics of decisions regarding withdrawal of treatment are discussed fully in Chapter 15, on the evaluation of patient care. However, care of the dying patient and his family will be discussed here.

Withdrawal of treatment

It is generally accepted that once it has been decided that additional medical intervention will not assist the patient the priorities change to those of care and comfort.

Analgesia and sedation may have been carefully controlled to limit cardiovascular side-effects and important but uncomfortable treatment, such as physiotherapy and suction, may have been carried out on a frequent basis to assist the patient in achieving a cure. Once the decision is taken to withdraw or to limit further interventions then care as opposed to cure becomes the priority and the patient's physical and psychological needs should supersede any other considerations. Analgesia should be given at levels that ensure pain relief, and unnecessary interventions, such as suction, should be limited to the minimum required to maintain patient comfort.

Comfort, psychological care, and support are paramount, not only for the patient but also for the patient's family. Where the patient is able to respond, any decisions on pain relief, movement, personal hygiene, and comfort should be discussed with them.

Use of alternative methods of pain relief and dealing with anxiety should be considered (see Chapter 9 for details). The patient may feel that they would prefer to be alert and able to communicate with their family as long as possible. In this case, they may negotiate a tolerable level of pain in order to avoid the drowsiness and disorientation associated with increased quantities of analgesia.

Supporting the family/friends of the dying patient

The phrase 'family/friends' will be used to cover all those with relationships of importance to the patient.

Breaking the news of impending death

The family/friends should be told by a senior member of the medical staff who is familiar with the patient and family/friends. A member of the nursing staff should be present and, if appropriate, other professional support such as the chaplain or a counsellor.

The setting should be private, available for as long as necessary, and away from the hubbub of the unit (Dyer 1993).

Details may have to be repeated a number of times. The family/friends are usually distressed and may be able to take in only minimal information.

Supporting the family in coping with death

The news that the patient is dying will usually destroy any hope that the family may have cherished for recovery. Having their deepest fears expressed as a certainty provides a trigger for a crisis point and it is often only then that they will break down.

Responses range from grief to denial and anger.

Some people use denial as a coping mechanism and will be unable to accept what is said to them. Their response may seem inappropriate to the gravity of the situation and staff may need to assess the individual to determine whether forcing them to face reality or retain their defence is appropriate.

Anger may also be expressed as a response to the situation and should be dealt with using understanding and tact.

Communication

Frequent communication and an open and honest relationship between staff and the family/friends are important aspects of support. Any conversation with the family/friends may include cues for help, information, and support, so listening is as vital as saying the right things at the right time. Use of non-verbal communication — touch, facial expression, sitting with the family is comforting and expresses concern. Sometimes, it may be as helpful to sit in silence and it is useful for the nurse to become comfortable with this.

Participation in care of the patient

This should be discussed with the family/friends as well as the patient where possible and areas of care which are appropriate should be defined. Support and encouragement as well as education and direction in the delivery of care should be given. Examples include:

- Mouth care

- Massage

- Hair washing and brushing

- Reading to the patient

- Positioning limbs

- Caressing and holding

- Helping to take oral fluids

Continuity of care

The family/friends should not have to establish relationships with members of staff they do not know at this stage. It is important to provide continuity of care from a few nurses who are known to the family and who may express a sense of affinity to them. This will help the family to feel supported and relieve some of the stress they may feel. However, it is likely to increase the stress that these nurses experience and they may well require extra support from those in charge, or their peers.

Establishing delivery of care to suit the patient, family, and friends

The nurse should discuss with the family whether they prefer privacy with the patient or the company of the nurse and they should arrange their care accordingly. If the family prefer privacy the nurse should withdraw from the immediate area but reassure the family that he/she is readily available should they or the patient need him/her.

The family/friends should also be approached as to whether they wish to be present at the patient's death and if there is anyone else they would wish to be there (e.g. the chaplain or their own minister). This information should be recorded and communicated clearly between all those looking after the patient so that whenever death occurs their wishes can be met.

If the family/friends have expressed the desire to be present at the patient's death every effort should be made to ensure that they are informed in time for them to reach the hospital. Many people experience guilt associated with bereavement and failing to arrive in time to be with their loved one at their death can only add to this.

The family/friends should be supported in deciding how they wish to organize the interim time. All may wish to stay or they may take it in turns to remain with the patient until death is near.

After death has occurred

Interventions that will help the bereaved to eventually come to terms with the loss include:

(a) Viewing the body after death. This facilitates grief and ultimate acceptance of the loss.

(b) Avoidance of euphemisms for death.

If there is a follow-up counselling service available offer this further help.

Give clear details of what is required for registering the death and arranging removal of the body by the undertakers. Ideally, there should be an information sheet with these details to give to the family, but if not, make sure they are written down.

The effect of caring for the dying patient on the nurse

There is no doubt that coping with the experience of

death is stressful for any one. The work of Glaser and Strauss (1965) showed that the majority of nurses at that time coped by avoidance of the dying patient. This is not a possible alternative for the intensive care nurse and most will have to develop other coping mechanisms.

Support groups and networks available either within the unit itself or the hospital are a useful external release and have the added advantage of being confidential.

Peer group support can be important but can also work negatively for some individuals. Unit atmosphere is an important factor. An open, accepting environment where all staff feel able to express their feelings will help the majority to cope. Team feeling and concern for co-workers is also supportive.

There will always be those who require more than this. Senior staff should be constantly aware and able to intervene if necessary to provide a safety net for those vulnerable to the stress of caring for the dying patient.

The quality of care the patient and family receive in the ICU will have a major impact on their lives, not only at the time but also for many years afterwards. It is a part of the caring aim of nursing to ensure that their experience is as benign as possible in the circumstances.

References and bibliography

Aggleton, P. and Chalmers, H. (1986). *Nursing models and the nursing process*. Macmillan, London.

Albarran, J. (1991). A review of communication with intubated patients and those with tracheostomies within an intensive care environment. *Intensive Care Nursing*, 7, 179–86.

Ashworth, P. (1980). *Care to communicate*. Royal College of Nursing, Research Series, London.

Barrie-Shevlin, P. (1987) Maintaining sensory balance for the critically ill patient. *Nursing*, 3, 597–601.

Batson, S., Adam, S., Hall, G., and Quirke, S. (1993). The development of a pressure area scoring system for critically ill patients: a pilot study. *Intensive and Critical care Nursing*, 9, 146–51.

Baun, M.M. and Flones, M.J. (1984). Cumulative effects of three sequential endotracheal suctioning episodes in the dog model. *Heart and Lung*, 13, 148–54.

Belfield, P.W. (1988). Urinary catheters. *British Medical Journal*, 296, 836–7.

Bergbom-Engberg, I. and Haljamäe, H. (1989). Assessment of patients' experience of discomforts during respirator therapy. *Critical Care Medicine*, 17, 1068–71.

Bihari, D.J. (1992). Nosocomial infections in the intensive care unit. *Hospital Update*, 266–76.

Bion, J.F., Wilson, I.H., and Taylor P.A. (1988). Transporting critically ill patient by ambulance: audit by sickness scoring. *British Medical Journal*, 296, 170.

Borsig, A. and Steinacker, I. (1982). Communication with the patient in the intensive care unit. *Nursing Times Supplement*, 78, 2–11.

Burgener, S. (1987). Justification for closed intermittent urinary catheter irrigation/instillation: a review of current research and practice. *Journal of Advanced Nursing*, 12, 229–34.

Chlan, L.L. (1995). Psychophysiologic responses of mechanically ventilated patients to music: a pilot study. *American Journal of Critical Care*, 4, 233–8.

Chuman, M.A. (1985). Risk factors associated with ulnar nerve compression in bed-ridden patients. *Journal of Neurosurgical Nursing*, 17, 338–342.

Clifford C. (1985). Helplessness: A concept applied to nursing practice. *Intensive Care Nursing*, 1, 19–24.

Closs, J. (1988a). Patient's sleep-wake rhythms in hospital, part 1. *Nursing Times Occasional Papers* 84, 48–50.

Closs, J. (1988b). Patient's sleep-wake rhythms in hospital, part 2. *Nursing Times Occasional Papers*, 84, 54–5.

Crosby, C. (1989). Method in mouth care. *Nursing Times*, 85, 38–41.

Daffurn, K., Bishop, G.F., Hillman, K.M., and Bauman, A. (1994). Problems following discharge after intensive care. *Intensive and Critical Care Nursing*, 10, 244–251.

DeWalt, E. (1975). Effect of timed hygienic measures on oral mucosa in a group of elderly subjects. *Nursing Research*, 24, 104–8.

Dracup, K. (1993). Challenges in critical care nursing. Helping patients and families cope. *Critical Care Nurse*, (suppl.), August.

Drane, L. (1986). Watch my lips. *Nursing Times*, 82, 52.

Dyer, L.L. (1989). Training and development of the ICU nurse for critical care transport. *Critical Care Nurse*, 9, 74–80.

Dyer, I.D. (1993). Breaking the news: informing visitors that a patient has died. *Intensive and Critical Care Nursing*, 9, 2–10.

Easton, C.E. and Mackenzie, F. (1988). Sensory-perceptual alterations: Delirium in the intensive care unit. *Heart and Lung*, 17, 229–37.

Edwards, G.B and Schuring, L.M. (1993). Pilot study: Validating staff nurses' observations of sleep and wake states among critically ill patients using polysomnography. *American Journal of Critical Care*, 2, 125–31.

Estabrooks, C.A. (1989). Touch: A nursing strategy in the intensive care unit. *Heart and Lung*, 18, 392–401.

Fawcett, J. (1989). *Analysis and evaluation of conceptual models of nursing*, (2nd edn.). F.A. Davis, Philadelphia.

Fiddian-Green, R.G. and Baker, S. (1991). Nosocomial pneumonia in the critically ill: Product of aspiration or translocation? *Critical Care Medicine*, 19, 763–9.

Forrester, D.A., Murphy, P.A., Price, D.M., and Monaghan, J.F. (1990). Critical care family needs: Nurse–family member confederate pairs. *Heart and Lung*, 19, 655–61.

Friedman, B.C., Boyce, W., and Bekes, C.E. (1992). Long-term follow up of ICU patients. *American Journal of Critical Care*, 1, 115–17.

Gil, R.T., Kruse, J.A., Thill-Baharozian, M.C. and Carlson, R.W. (1989). Triple- vs. single-lumen central venous catheters. *Archives of Internal Medicine*, **149**, 1139–43.

Glaser, B.G. and Strauss, A.L. (1965). *Awareness of dying*. Aldine Press, Chicago.

Gooch, J. (1985). Mouthcare. *Professional Nurse*. **1**, 77–78.

Heath, J. (1989). What the patients say. *Intensive Care Nursing*, **5**, 101–8.

Hilton, E., Uliss, A., Samuels, S., *et al.* (1983). Nosocomial bacterial eye infections in intensive-care units. *Lancet*, **i**, 1318–20.

Hope, A., and Runcie, C.J. (1993). Inter-hospital transport in the critically ill adult. *British Journal of Intensive Care*, **3**, 187–92.

Howarth, H. (1977). Mouth care procedures for the very ill. *Nursing Times*, **73**, 354–5.

Jacobs, S. Chang, R.W.S., Lee, B., and Bartlett, F.W. (1990). Continuous enteral feeding: A major cause of pneumonia among ventilated intensive care unit patients. *Journal of Parenteral and Enteral Nutrition*, **14**, 353–6.

Jones C. and O'Donnell, C., (1994). After intensive care — what then? *Intensive and Critical Care Nursing*, **10**, 89–92.

Jones, J., Hoggart, B., Withoy, J., Donaghue, K., and Ellis, B.W. (1979). What the patient's say: A study of reactions to an intensive care unit. *Intensive Care Medicine*, **5**, 89–92.

Kite, K. and Pearson, L. (1995). A rationale for mouth care: the integration of theory and practice. *Intensive and Critical Care Nursing*, **11**, 71–6.

Kuch, K. (1990). Anxiety disorder and the ICU. *Clinical Intensive Care*, **1**, 7–11.

Larson, E. (1985). Infection control issues in critical care: An update. *Heart and Lung*, **14**, 149–55.

Leske, J. (1991). Internal psychometric properties of the critical care family needs inventory. *Heart and Lung*, **20**, 236–44.

Linares, J., Sitges-Serra, A., Garau, J., Pérez, J.L. and Martin, R. (1985). Pathogenesis of catheter sepsis: a prospective study with quantitative and semiquantitative cultures of catheter hub and segments. *Journal of Clinical Microbiology*, **21**, 357–360.

Lloyd, F. (1990). Eye care for ventilated or unconscious patients. *Nursing Times*, **86**, 36–7.

Lowthian, P. (1989). Preventing trauma. *Nursing Times*, **85**, 73–5.

Mackereth, P.A. (1987). Communication in critical care areas: competing for attention. *Nursing*, **15**, 575–8.

Maki, D.G. (1989). Risk factors for nosocomial infection in intensive care. *Archives of Internal Medicine*, **149**, 30–3.

Molter, N.C. (1979). Needs of relatives of critically ill patients: a descriptive study. *Heart and Lung*, **8**, 332–9.

Moore, T. (1989). Sensory deprivation in the ICU. *Nursing*, **3**, 44–7.

Mulhall, A., Chapman, R., and Crow, R. (1988). The aquisition of bacteriuria and meatal cleansing. *Nursing Times*, **84**, 66–9.

Ommeslag, D., Colardyn, F., and De Laey, J. (1987). Eye infections caused by respiratory pathogens in mechanically ventilated patients. *Critical Care Medicine*, **15**, 80–1.

Pingleton, S.K. (1991). Enteral nutrition and infection: Benefits and risks. In *Update in intensive care and emergency medicine*, (ed. J.L. Vincent), Vol. 14, pp. 581–9. Springer, Berlin.

Platt, R., Murdock, B., Polk, F., and Rosner, B. (1983). Reduction of mortality associated with nosocomial UTI. *Lancet*, **i**, 893–6.

Powell, C., Fabri, P.J., and Kudsk, K.A. (1988). Risk of infection accompanying the use of single-lumen vs. double-lumen subclavian catheters: a prospective randomized study. *Journal of Parenteral and Enteral Nutrition*, **12**, 127–9.

Price, D.M., Forrester, D.A., Murphy, P.A., and Hanaghan, J.F. (1991). Critical care family needs in an urban teaching medical center. *Heart and Lung*, **20**, 183–8.

Puntillo, K. (1990). Pain experiences of intensive care unit patients. *Heart and Lung*, **19**, 526–33.

Rees-Williams, C., Meyrick, M., and Jones, M. (1988). Making sense of urinary catheters. *Nursing Times*, **84**, 46–7.

Richardson, A. (1987). A process standard for oral care. *Nursing Times*. **83**, 38–40.

Riehl, J.P., and Roy, C. (1980). *Conceptual models for nursing practice*, (2nd edn). Appleton-Century-Crofts, New York.

Roth, P.T. and Creason, N. (1986). Nurse administered oral hygiene: is there a scientific basis? *Journal of Advanced Nursing*. **11**, 323–31.

Rowan, K.M., Kerr, J.H., Major, E., McPherson, K., Short, A. and Vessey, M.P. (1993). Intensive Care Society's APACHE II study in Britain and Ireland — II: Outcome comparisons of intensive care units after adjustment for casemix by the American APACHE II method. *British Medical Journal*, **307**, 977–81.

Rukholm, E., Bailey, P., Boutu-Wakulczyk, G., and Bailey, W.B. (1991). Needs and anxiety levels in relatives of intensive care patients. *Journal of Advanced Nursing*, **16**, 920–8.

Russell, M.T. and McElwee, M.R. (1987). Compensating for xerostomia in the critically ill patient. *Critical Care Nurse*, **7**, 98–103.

Santamaria, J. (1990). Nosocomial infections. In *Intensive care manual*, (ed. T.E. Oh), (3rd edn) pp. 409–21. Butterworths, Sydney.

Simpson, T.F., Armstrong, S., and Mitchell, P. (1989). AACN demonstration project: Patient's recollections of critical care. *Heart and Lung*. **18**, 325–32.

Stanton, D.J. (1991). The psychological impact of intensive therapy: the role of nurses. *Intensive Care Nursing*, **7**, 230–5.

Szaflarski, N.L. (1993). Immobility phenomena in critically ill adults. In *Critical care nursing*, (ed., J.M., Glochesy, C., Breo, S., Cardin, E.B., Rudy and A. Whittaker), pp. 31–54. W.B. Saunders, Philadelphia.

Topf, M. and Davis, J.E. (1993). Critical care unit noise and rapid eye movement (REM) sleep. *Heart and Lung*, **22**, 252–8.

Turner, J. (1993). Hand-washing behavior versus hand-washing guidelines. *Heart and Lung*, **22**, 275–7.

Waddell, G. (1975). Movement of critically ill patients within hospital. *British Medical Journal*, **2**, 417–19

Warner, L.A. (1986) Lemon-glycerine swabs should be used for routine oral care. *Critical Care Nurse*, **6**, 82–3.

Wilkinson, P. (1995). A qualitative study to establish the self-perceived needs to family members fo patients in a general intensive care unit. *Intensive and Critical Care Nursing*, **11**, 77–86.

3. Respiratory problems

Physiology and anatomy

The primary function of the respiratory system is to supply oxygen to the metabolically active tissues and remove the waste product, carbon dioxide. This function takes place in complete interdependence with the circulatory system's prime role of blood transport.

$$O_2 + Fuel = Energy + CO_2 + H_2O$$

Respiration can be divided into four components:

(1) Mechanical movement of gases into and out of the lungs.
(2) Exchange of these gases across a membrane.
(3) Carriage of gases to and from the tissues.
(4) Metabolic process of the cell to produce energy.

1. Movement of gases

This is usually referred to as ventilation and is the product of the movement of the chest wall and diaphragm. Movement of the gases is brought about by the creation of a pressure gradient between mouth and alveoli.

The trans-airway pressure (P_{ta}) is the difference between pressure at the mouth and that at the alveoli. It can be negative (as in normal breathing) or positive (as in positive pressure ventilation) and this gradient will initiate gas flow.

Transpulmonary pressure (P_{tp}) is the difference between alveolar pressure and pleural pressure. It is always negative and maintains lung expansion. The lungs are thus maintained in a neutral position by the slightly negative pressure (-5 mmHg) between the parietal pleura lining the chest wall and the visceral pleura covering the lung (Fig. 3.1).

Inspiration occurs when the diaphragm and the intercostal muscles contract, pulling the lungs downwards and outwards. This increases the volume within the lungs creating a negative pressure (-3 mmHg) which sucks air in. During deep inspiration it is possible for the negative pressure to reach -35 to -40 mmHg (Des Jardins 1988).

Expiration occurs when the inspiratory muscles relax and the elastic nature of the lung tissue forces a recoil to the neutral position. A slightly positive pressure is then exerted on the lung and air is forced out.

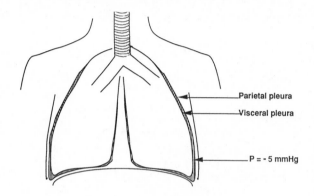

Fig. 3.1 Maintenance of positive pleural pressure.

The elasticity of the lung is an important feature and depends on two factors. The first is the high surface tension of the alveoli which acts as a potent force pulling the alveoli closed and resisting expansion. The surface tension is decreased by the secretion of surfactant, a lipoprotein substance produced by the epithelial lining. A number of elements can affect the production of this substance with serious consequences to the ability to expand alveoli (see Table 3.1). The problems associated with neonatal respiratory distress syndrome are in part due to the inability of immature lungs to produce surfactant leading to poor elasticity and a vastly increased work of breathing. The second factor affecting elasticity is the elastic fibres of the lung itself which tend to contract.

Table 3.1 Causes of pulmonary surfactant deficiency (after Des Jardins 1988)

General	Specific
Acidosis	Acute respiratory distress syndrome (ARDS)
Hypoxia	Infant respiratory distress syndrome (IRDS)
Hyperoxygenation	Pulmonary oedema
Atelectasis	Pulmonary embolus
Pulmonary vascular congestion	Excess pulmonary lavage/ hydration
Starvation	Drowning
	Extracorporeal oxygenation

When breathing becomes difficult, or increased during exercise, other respiratory muscles may be used to increase ventilation. These are known as the accessory muscles of respiration. They consist of the neck, trapezius, pectoral, and external intercostal muscles in inspiration and the abdominal and internal intercostal muscles in expiration.

Work of breathing

The degree of effort involved in moving a specific volume of air into and out of the lungs is known as the work of breathing and can be affected by:

(1) The resistance of the airways to flow of air.

(2) The elasticity of the lung tissue.

(3) Any obstruction to flow.

(4) Chest wall compliance.

These factors comprise the compliance of the respiratory system which is expressed as the change in volume of the lung over the change in pressure required to produce that change in volume ($\Delta V/\Delta P$ ml/cm H_2O). It is the inverse of the degree of stiffness of the lung (i.e. when a lung is compliant it will expand easily but when non-compliant it will be more resistant to expansion). The greatest compliance is where small changes in pressure reflect the greatest change in volume.

Lung compliance can be classified into static and dynamic compliance:

(i) *Static compliance*, as the name suggests, refers to compliance of the lung measured under static conditions produced by occlusion of the airway for a brief period at the end of inspiration. This allows an assesment of compliance without the pressure associated with flow resistance. It is measured by occluding the airway at end inspiration for a minimum of 2 seconds to allow the plateau pressure to be reached.

$$Cst_{rs} = \frac{\Delta V}{\text{End inspiration occluded (plateau) pressure}}$$

where Cst_{rs} = static compliance of the respiratory system and ΔV = tidal volume.

The normal range is 60–100 ml/cm H_2O (Tobin 1991).

(ii) *Dynamic compliance* refers to the change in pressure from end inspiration to end expiration:

$$Cdyn_{rs} = \frac{\Delta V}{\text{end inspiratory pressure (immediate)} - \text{end expiratory pressure}}$$

where $Cdyn_{rs}$ = dynamic compliance of the respiratory system and ΔV = tidal volume.

In healthy lungs there is little difference between static and dynamic compliance at all respiratory rates. In patients with airway obstruction, the dynamic compliance decreases rapidly as the respiratory rate rises while there is little change in the static compliance. (Table 3.2).

Table 3.2 Causes of alteration in lung compliance (Oh 1990)

Lung compliance is decreased by:
Pulmonary congestion
Increased pulmonary smooth muscle tone
Increased surface tension
Pulmonary fibrosis, infiltration or atelectasis
Pleural fibrosis
Lung compliance is increased by:
Pulmonary oligaemia (deficient blood volume)
Decreased pulmonary smooth muscle tone
Augmented surfactant release
Destruction of lung tissue (e.g. emphysema)

2. Gas exchange

Not all airways are available for gas exchange which only takes place in the respiratory lobule. Areas of the lung not available for gas exchange are known as dead space. There are three types of dead space.

(i) *Anatomical dead space*. The volume of the airway in which gas exchange cannot take place is known as the anatomical dead space. It consists of the nose, pharynx, trachea, and bronchi and is usually about 150 ml in a normal-sized adult. This means that of any tidal volume inspired ($\sim$ 5–8 ml/kg for a normal spontaneous breath), 150 ml is not able to either oxygenate or remove carbon dioxide.

(ii) *Alveolar dead space*. This refers to alveoli which are ventilated but not perfused with pulmonary blood. They are therefore unable to contribute to gas exchange.

(iii) *Physiological dead space*. This is the sum of the anatomical and alveolar dead space. It can be increased by old age, anaesthesia, controlled ventilation, and chronic lung disease. It can be increased acutely by pulmonary embolism. Hypoventilation will increase the ratio of dead space to tidal volume though not the actual dead space volume.

Table 3.3. Lung volumes

Term	Volume	Definition
Tidal volume (V_T)	5–9 ml/kg ($\sim$ 500 ml)	Volume of gas/air that will move in or out of lungs in a normal quiet breath
Minute volume (MV)	5–9 ml/kg $\times$ 12 ($\sim$ 5–6 l) calculated by multiplying V_T by respiratory rate	Volume of gas/air that will move in and out of lungs over the period of one minute
Vital capacity (VC)	3000–4800 ml	Maximum volume of gas that can be exhaled after a maximum inspiration
Anatomical dead space	2 ml/kg ($\sim$ 150 ml)	Volume of gas filling conducting airways (nose down to lower airways but not bronchioles)
Functional residual capacity (FRC)	1800–2400 ml	Volume of air remaining in the lungs after normal exhalation

Effective alveolar ventilation per unit time (V_A) = Expired minute volume (V_E) — physiological dead space (V_D).

Physiological dead space = anatomical + alveolar dead space.

It is variable depending on the ventilation and perfusion of alveoli thus a ratio of dead space to tidal volume is used (V_D/V_T).

The ratio of V_D to V_T is normally <0.3.

Gas exchange only takes place in those areas where the barrier between gas contained within alveoli and blood passing through the alveolar capillaries is thin enough to allow movement across the pulmonary capillary membrane. An enormous surface area of approximately 70 m^2 is provided for the movement of gas. This area results from the convoluted surfaces of the alveoli and the distribution of a small volume of blood throughout the pulmonary membrane. The resulting close contact between individual red blood cells and the respiratory membrane enables diffusion of gases across the two membranes at a fast and efficient rate. (Figure 3.2.)

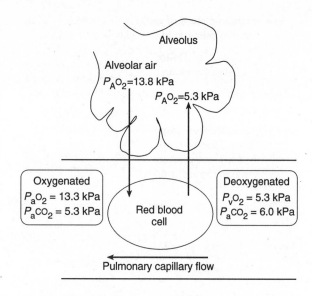

Fig. 3.2 Gas exchange in the lungs.

Gas diffusion

Diffusion is defined as the movement of molecules from an area of high concentration towards an area of low concentration. The diffusion of gases across the respiratory membrane is affected by two laws governing the physical properties of gases.

(i) Dalton's law of partial pressures
The first part of the law refers to pressure exerted by gases:

The pressure exerted by a mixture of gases is equal to the sum of the pressures which each would exert if it alone occupied the space.

The partial pressure of a gas is the force exerted by it when contained within a space and is a measure of the amount of gas.

Air is made up of three main gases, nitrogen (N_2), 79%, carbon dioxide (CO_2), 0.03%; and oxygen (O_2), 20.9%. These gases form the Earth's atmosphere and contribute to atmospheric pressure.

Atmospheric pressure is 101 kPa (760 mmHg) at sea level. The partial pressure of a gas is written as P, thus:

The partial pressure of oxygen = PO_2.
The partial pressure of carbon dioxide = PCO_2.

If the partial pressure is referred to in a specific part of the body, it is written as P with a suffix letter referring to the part of the body, e.g.

P_AO_2 = partial pressure of *alveolar* oxygen.

P_aCO_2 = partial pressure of *arterial* carbon dioxide.

The second part of Dalton's law refers to pressure exerted by saturated vapours:

The pressure exerted by a saturated vapour depends only on the temperature and the particular liquid considered.

Air is humidified on inspiration and thus contains water vapour. This will exert a pressure which will depend on body temperature. At 37 °C the pressure exerted by water vapour is 6.3 kPa

(ii) Boyle's law

The partial pressure of any gas is proportional to its percentage by volume in the mixture.

Example:

Air = Nitrogen (N_2) + Oxygen (O_2) + Carbon dioxide (CO_2)
     79%   20.9%   0.03%

Air at sea level has an atmospheric pressure of 101 kPa. Thus, according to Boyle's law, each gas will exert a partial pressure proportional to its percentage in air:

Nitrogen will exert 79% of 101 kPa   = 79.8 kPa

Oxygen will exert 20.9% of 101 kPa   = 20.9 kPa

Carbon dioxide will exert 0.03% of 101 kPa   = 0.03 kPa

If that air is humidified, as it is on inspiration, then the pressure exerted by the water vapour in the air will depend on the temperature of the body. Thus, at a body temperature of 37 °C, the pressure of the gases on entering the alveoli will equal 101 kPa − 6.3 kPa = 94.7 kPa.

When the gas enters the lung it mixes with carbon dioxide which has been excreted and the contents of alveolar gas are significantly different to the original inspired gas. The oxygen content of alveolar gas can be calculated using the alveolar gas equation (see box).

The alveolar gas equation

Alveolar PO_2 = [Inspired PO_2 × (atmospheric pressure − water vapour pressure)] − arterial PCO_2/respiratory quotient.

The respiratory quotient is the ratio of carbon dioxide produced to oxygen consumed, usually approximately 0.8.

With perfect lung function the arterial PO_2 should theoretically equal the alveolar PO_2. However, in normal lungs the difference is usually approximately 2 kPa in youth and 3.3 kPa in old age (Oh 1990). This is known as the A–a (alveolar–arterial) oxygen gradient.

The difference is due to a small amount of blood which has passed through the lungs but has not been oxygenated. An increase in the A–a oxygen gradient is evidence of an abnormality in the ventilation/perfusion ratio. The alveolar–arterial oxygen difference is calculated using the alveolar gas equation and comparing it with the measured arterial PO_2.

Factors affecting diffusion through the pulmonary capillary membrane:

(1) The difference between partial pressures of the gases in the alveoli and in the pulmonary capillary.

(2) The area of the respiratory membrane. Any factors that severely limit the area available for gas exchange such as emphysema or acute respiratory distress syndrome (ARDS) can have a severe effect on respiratory function.

(3) The thickness of the respiratory membrane. Factors affecting this, such as cardiogenic and non-cardiogenic pulmonary oedema, will impair pulmonary function.

(4) The diffusion or solubility coefficient of the gas involved.

Carbon dioxide is far more soluble than oxygen and thus diffuses at a faster and more efficient rate.

The presence of nitrogen in the inspired gas has the function of acting as a gas reservoir remaining in the alveoli as it is not soluble and does not pass into the capillaries. This maintains the expansion of the alveoli, preventing collapse (atelectasis). This function is lost with very high percentages of inspired oxygen.

Ventilation/Perfusion match

Another important determinant of gas exchange is the relationship between pulmonary capillary perfusion (Q) and alveolar ventilation (V). A well-ventilated alveolus should have a correspondingly well perfused capillary and the ratio of V/Q is ideally 1. A three-compartment model of the lungs is used to illustrate ventilation/perfusion relationships:

1. Physiological dead space — an area of wasted ventilation (i.e. V/Q > 1)

2. Perfectly matched areas of ventilation and perfusion (i.e. V/Q = 1)

3. Areas contributing to venous admixture (the mixing

of non-oxygenated with oxygenated blood after passage through the lungs) where perfusion has been wasted, for example, diffusion defects, right to left shunts (i.e. V/Q < 1).

There is normally a variation between the degree of perfusion and ventilation in different areas of the lungs. This is due to the effects of gravity which increases the amount of work required to force blood through the vessels further above the heart. Therefore, the lower lung lobes receive a better blood supply than the upper lobes in the erect position. The body adapts to this by preferentially ventilating the better perfused lower lobes. This response is lost when the patient is mechanically ventilated.

A pathological cause of hypoxaemia is the presence of a right to left shunt (venous admixture). This is where poorly ventilated areas of lung continue to be perfused (e.g. atelectasis). Thus the ratio of ventilation (V) to perfusion (Q) is decreased allowing blood to pass through the lung without being oxygenated.

Situations causing right-to-left shunts

- Obstructive lung disease (emphysema, bronchitis, asthma)

- Restrictive lung disease (ARDS, pneumonia, fibrotic lung disease)

- Hypoventilation for any reason (e.g. excess sedation, respiratory muscle weakness)

A right to left shunt is always increased when alveoli are:

(i) completely collapsed;

(ii) totally consolidated; or

(iii) filled with oedema fluid.

A ventilation/perfusion mismatch occurs when a poorly perfused area of lung continues to be ventilated (e.g. pulmonary embolus). Thus, the ratio of ventilation (V) to perfusion (Q) is increased as is the physiological dead space.

Two intrinsic responses to variations in ventilation and perfusion allow a certain amount of adjustment in order to maintain V/Q matching. The first involves the pulmonary capillary response to areas of low PO_2. If the alveolus is poorly ventilated the P_AO_2 will be low. This results in a correspondingly low P_aO_2 in the pulmonary capillaries supplying that area. This initiates a vasoconstrictor response – 'hypoxic pulmonary vasoconstriction' which reduces pulmonary blood flow to the affected region.

Causes of ventilation/perfusion mismatch include:

- Pulmonary embolus

- Partial/complete obstruction of the pulmonary artery

- Extrinsic pressure on pulmonary vessels (pneumothorax, tumour)

- Destruction of pulmonary vessels

- Decreased cardiac output

- Obstruction of the pulmonary microcirculation (ARDS)

The second involves a localized bronchoconstrictor response to low pulmonary capillary levels of carbon dioxide due to reduction in perfusion of the area (e.g. following a pulmonary embolus). The P_ACO_2 will remain low in the non-perfused area and the bronchioles will constrict thereby limiting ventilation of that region.

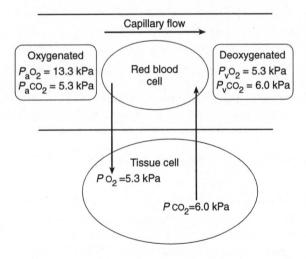

Fig. 3.3 Gas exchange in the tissues.

3. Carriage of gases

The degree of solubility of oxygen is considerably less than that of carbon dioxide. It would be impossible to deliver the quantity of oxygen required by the body if it was simply carried as a solution. The majority is therefore carried in combination with haemoglobin. At a normal level of haemoglobin (15 g/dl), 20 ml of oxygen is carried per 100 ml of blood, whereas only 0.3 ml of oxygen is carried dissolved in the plasma. The amount of oxygen dissolved in plasma is only increased by an increase in atmospheric pressure such as that produced by a hyperbaric oxygen chamber.

The chemical structure of haemoglobin allows for a varying affinity to oxygen molecules according to the environmental PO_2 of the capillary. Thus, at a PO_2 of 13.3 kPa almost all of the oxygen-binding capacity of haemoglobin is utilized and the haemoglobin is said to be approximately 98% saturated. This is the situation found in the normal lung. Oxygen-saturated haemoglobin is termed *oxyhaemoglobin* and unsaturated haemoglobin is termed *reduced haemoglobin* or *deoxyhaemoglobin*.

In the tissues, where oxygen is extracted, the saturation of haemoglobin is reduced to about 75% and oxygen will be released to the tissues. Three-quarters of the haemoglobin remains oxygenated providing a reservoir for conditions where oxygen demand exceeds supply (e.g. exercise and cardiogenic shock). More oxygen can be released from the haemoglobin, down to 20–30% saturation in extreme circumstances, in order to maintain aerobic metabolism. Where supply fails to meet demand the tissues undergo anaerobic metabolism resulting in lactate production and a metabolic acidosis. (Figure 3.4).

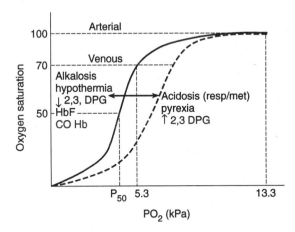

Fig. 3.4 Oxyhaemoglobin dissociation curve (Bohr). HbF = fetal haemoglobin; COHb = carbon monoxide bound to haemoglobin (carboxyhaemoglobin); P_{50} = pressure at which haemoglobin is 50% saturated; 2,3 DPG = 2, 3 diphosphoglycerate.

There are several important factors which affect oxyhaemoglobin dissociation (the detachment of oxygen from haemoglobin). In the presence of some factors the curve can shift to the right (i.e. for the same level of arterial PO_2 the haemoglobin saturation is lower therefore more oxygen is available to the tissues). However, in the presence of other factors, the curve can shift to the left (i.e. for the same level of PO_2 the haemoglobin saturation is higher therefore less oxygen is available to the tissues). In the normal range of PO_2, these shifts will have minimal effect on oxygen availability but can be highly significant in patients with a low arterial PO_2.

Shift to the right
Under conditions which shift the dissociation curve to the right, a higher level of PO_2 is required in order to maintain the same oxygen saturation of haemoglobin. Less oxygen will therefore combine with haemoglobin in the alveoli at the normal level of P_AO_2 but more oxygen will be available to the tissues where the PO_2 is low. This is the situation found in acidosis and is a compensatory mechanism to augment tissue oxygenation.

Factors causing a shift to the right:

- decreased pH,

- increased body temperature,

- increased PCO_2,

- increased 2,3-diphosphoglycerate (2,3-DPG is a substance contained within the red blood cell formed during anaerobic glycolysis. Levels are increased in response to hypoxia, anaemia, and increased pH forming a compensatory mechanism).

Shift to the left
Under conditions which shift the haemoglobin saturation curve to the left a lower level of PO_2 is required to maintain the same haemoglobin saturation. More oxygen will therefore combine with haemoglobin in the alveoli at the normal P_AO_2 but less oxygen will be available to the tissues at the normal P_aO_2.

Factors causing a shift to the left:

- increased pH,

- decreased PCO_2,

- decreased temperature,

- decreased 2,3-diphosphoglycerate,

- fetal haemoglobin (HbF). This has a greater affinity for oxygen in order to enhance transfer of oxygen across the placenta,

- carboxyhaemoglobin (COHb). Carbon monoxide combined with haemoglobin has about 250 times the affinity of oxygen for haemoglobin. Thus, a small amount of carbon monoxide can bind large amounts of haemoglobin making it unavailable for oxygen transport.

Two further points are important in the carriage of oxygen:

(i) Once haemoglobin is fully saturated, no further increase in PO_2 will increase the amount of oxygen carried by haemoglobin. The amount of oxygen carried in solution in the plasma can only be increased significantly by use of a hyperbaric oxygen chamber where atmospheric pressure can be increased.

(ii) The PO_2 can decrease quite considerably before any significant fall occurs in haemoglobin saturation. Thus the haemoglobin is still 90% saturated at around 8 kPa.

Oxygen delivery to the tissues is not only dependent on haemoglobin concentration and oxygen saturation but also on cardiac output (see Chapter 5).

Oxygen delivery (DO_2) = Cardiac output (CO) × $(Hb \times S_aO_2 \times 1.34) + (P_aO_2 \times 0.003)$ ml/min (1.34 ml O_2 is carried by each gram of haemoglobin)

Carbon dioxide transport

There are six different mechanisms for the movement of carbon dioxide from the tissues to the alveoli. (See Table 3.4)

Table 3.4 Mechanisms of carbon dioxide transport

Plasma	Red blood cells	Per cent carried
1. As dissolved CO_2	4. As dissolved CO_2	~ 10%
2. Protein bound (the carbamino compound)	5. Carbaminohaemoglobin (combined with Hb)	1% protein bound, 20% carbaminoHb
3. As bicarbonate (HCO_3^-)	6. As bicarbonate (HCO_3^-)	~ 70%

Unlike oxygen, the relationship between the amount of carbon dioxide in the blood and the PCO_2 is linear over the physiological range. Thus, changes in PCO_2 will have a more direct effect on the carbon dioxide content of the blood. Carbon dioxide binding to haemoglobin is affected by the level of saturation of haemoglobin with oxygen. Deoxygenated blood enhances the loading of carbon dioxide; this is known as the Haldane effect. It is also effective in reverse, as oxygenated blood enhances the unloading of carbon dioxide.

4. The metabolic process of the cell to produce energy

Oxygen diffuses through the capillary membrane and tissue spaces into the tissue cells. It is combined with glucose, fatty acids, and amino acids in the mitochondria of the cell to produce energy. This process produces carbon dioxide and water as end-products as well as energy. The energy released is stored as a high energy phosphate bond linking a third phosphate molecule to adenosine diphosphate (ADP) to form adenosine triphosphate (ATP). ATP can then be used to provide energy as required for cell functions.

Acid–base balance

A major effect of the process of CO_2 removal is the maintenance of the acid–base balance in the body. The level of acidity (pH) of the body must be maintained within certain well-defined limits in order for normal metabolic processes to continue. The mechanisms for maintaining these limits can be divided into three distinct responses to any abnormality in pH.

1. Buffering (immediate).

2. Respiratory response (important in first 2–3 hours).

3. Renal response (over 2–3 days).

The mechanisms of the buffering and respiratory responses will be discussed here. (For full details of the renal response see Chapter 8.)

Carbon dioxide gas in solution may be considered to contribute to increased levels of hydrogen ions as the carbonic acid (H_2CO_3) produced is able to easily dissociate into hydrogen ions and bicarbonate ions. Thus, the removal of carbon dioxide has an important function in maintaining body pH in the normal range (see Table 3.5 for definitions.)

Arterial blood gas analysis

The measurement of blood gases gives not only an indication of the respiratory status but also an important view of the metabolic environment of the body. It gauges the ability of the body to maintain homeostasis (metabolic equilibrium).

Table 3.5 Definitions of terms

Acid	A substance containing weakly held hydrogen ions which is easily split into hydrogen ions and the remaining substance	e.g. carbonic acid $H_2CO_3 \rightarrow H^+ + HCO_3^-$
Base	A substance which can combine with hydrogen ions	e.g. bicarbonate $HCO_3^- + H^+ \rightarrow H_2CO_3$
H^+ (hydrogen ions)	Extremely active metabolically and can have a major effect on cell function	
pH	The scale on which hydrogen ions are measured. It is a negative logarithm to the base 10 of the concentration of hydrogen ions	$pH = -\log10[H^+]$ (Normal pH range $= 7.35 - 7.45$)
Acidosis	An abnormal process causing a relative increase in hydrogen ions and thus decrease in pH. It can be due to an increase in acid or a decrease in base	$pH = {<}7.35$
Alkalosis	An abnormal process causing a relative decrease in hydrogen ions and thus increase in pH. It can be due to a decrease in acid or an increase in base	$pH = {>}7.45$
Buffer	A substance with the ability to bind and release hydrogen ions thus maintaining a relatively constant pH	e.g. phosphoric acid and its salts, disodium hydrogen phosphate, and monosodium dihydrogen phosphate

The variables measured in arterial blood gas sampling are PCO_2, PO_2, and pH. Derived parameters such as bicarbonate (HCO_3) and base excess can also be used for additional interpretation of results. (Table 3.6)

Table 3.6 Normal values of arterial blood gases

- pH 7.35–7.45
- PCO_2 4.6–6.0 kPa
- PCO_2 10.0–13.3 kPa
- HCO_3 22–26 mmol/l
- Base excess -2 to $+2$
- O_2 saturation $>95\%$

Standard measures of bicarbonate and base excess

Standard bicarbonate is defined as the concentration of bicarbonate in equilibrated plasma at 37 °C and a P_aCO_2 of 5.3 kPa.

Standard base excess is defined as the milliequivalent (mEq or mmol) of strong acid necessary to titrate a blood sample at 37 °C and 5.3 kPa P_aCO_2 to a pH of 7.40

Respiratory dysfunction can directly affect the acid–base balance in two ways: (i) increasing the levels of CO_2 in the body and thus increasing the level of acidity (respiratory acidosis); or (ii) by decreasing the levels of CO_2 in the body and thus decreasing the level of acidity (respiratory alkalosis).

Causes of respiratory acidosis (usually associated with hypoventilation)

- Obstructive lung disease
- Oversedation/other causes of depression of respiratory centre
- Neuromuscular disorders
- Hypoventilation during mechanical ventilation
- Pain, chest wall deformities, respiratory muscle fatigue, etc.

An alteration in pH may not simply be the result of an alteration in PCO_2. Metabolic factors may also contribute to produce abnormalities of pH. In order to differentiate metabolic from respiratory factors, measurement of standard bicarbonate (HCO_3) and base excess must be used. When a metabolic process leads to acidosis, levels of HCO_3 and other buffer substances in the body will fall, increasing the level of hydrogen ions and thus decreasing the pH.

Causes of respiratory alkalosis (usually associated with hyperventilation)

- Hypoxia
- Anxiety states
- Pulmonary embolus, fibrosis, etc.
- Pregnancy
- Hyperventilation during mechanical ventilation
- Brain injury
- High salicylate levels
- Fever
- Asthma
- Severe anaemia

The equation describing the relationship between bicarbonate (HCO_3) as a buffer and the partial pressure of carbon dioxide (PCO_2) is known as the Henderson–Hasselbalch equation.

$$pH = 6.1 + \log_{10}[HCO_3^-/0.03\ PCO_2]$$

It can be seen that if HCO_3^- falls or PCO_2 rises then the pH will fall. When measured bicarbonate has been standardized to allow for variations in PCO_2 and temperature, any abnormality must be due to metabolic causes. Thus, standard bicarbonate is an indicator of metabolic abnormality contributing to acidosis or alkalosis.

The base excess is a reflection of the levels of bicarbonate and other bases. When bicarbonate values fall below the normal range the base excess will become negative (and can be termed 'base deficit'). Conversely, when bicarbonate levels rise there will be a positive base excess.

In interpreting the cause of any abnormality in pH the PCO_2 and the HCO_3 must be referred to, as well as the pH itself. (Table 3.7)

Compensated acidosis/alkalosis

When the body responds successfully by compensating for acid–base imbalance the pH will return towards normal. This may be either by respiratory or renal compensation depending on which system is primarily affected by the cause of the abnormality. For example, respiratory acidosis caused by hypoventilation in chronic pulmonary disease will be compensated for (over a period of time) by the kidneys producing and retaining bicarbonate.

Table 3.7 Alterations in different types of acidosis and alkalosis

Acute respiratory acidosis	pH low	PCO_2 high	HCO_3 normal
Acute respiratory alkalosis	pH high	PCO_2 low	HCO_3 normal
Acute metabolic acidosis	pH low	PCO_2 normal or low	HCO_3 low
Acute metabolic alkalosis	pH high	PCO_2 normal	HCO_3 high

Note There may also be mixed or combined acidosis or alkalosis due to a combination of causes

Compensation is only complete in chronic respiratory alkalosis. In other acid–base abnormalities the pH does not usually return completely to normal. (Table 3.8.)

These compensatory mechanisms have only a limited range and if the primary abnormality continues the patient may be unable to maintain a normal pH. The treatment of acid–base imbalance usually depends on determining and treating the underlying cause (see Chapter 13).

Neuronal control of respiration

The involuntary regulation of the respiratory drive is controlled from a group of respiratory neurones in the medulla of the brain. These form what is usually termed the *respiratory centre*. (Figure 3.5.)

The respiratory centre is moderated by the further influence of two centres situated in the pons. These are the apneustic and the pneumotaxic centres. The apneustic centre is inhibited by the pneumotaxic centre and by stimuli from receptors in the lung known as the Hering–Breuer or stretch receptors (see later).

The everyday control of respiration is further modified by a number of factors, the most important of which are stimuli from the chemoreceptors:

Table 3.8 Alterations in compensated acidosis and alkalosis

Compensated respiratory acidosis	PCO_2 high	pH near normal	HCO_3 high
Compensated respiratory alkalosis	PCO_2 low	pH normal	HCO_3 low
Compensated metabolic acidosis	PCO_2 low	pH near normal	HCO_3 low
Compensated metabolic	PCO_2 high	pH near normal	HCO_3 high

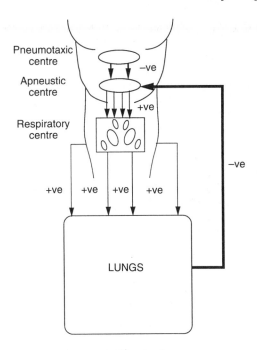

Fig. 3.5 Neuronal control of respiration.

Central chemoreceptors

These are located bilaterally and ventrally in the medulla. Some portion of the cells making up the chemoreceptors are in direct contact with the cerebrospinal fluid (CSF). The most powerful stimulus to these receptors is an increase in hydrogen ion concentration in the CSF. This can be directly related to an increase in PCO_2 in the blood supply to the brain. The chemoreceptors act directly on the respiratory centre to increase respiratory effort.

Peripheral chemoreceptors

These are groups of oxygen-sensitive cells located at the bifurcation of the internal and external carotid arteries and on the aortic arch. They stimulate the respiratory centre to increase respiratory effort when oxygen tension falls below approximately 8 kPa/90% saturation.

Peripheral chemoreceptors are sensitive to P_aO_2 rather than O_2 content so conditions where the P_aO_2 is normal yet O_2 content is low (e.g. chronic anaemia, carbon monoxide poisoning, methaemoglobinaemia) will not stimulate an increase in respiration (Figure 3.6).

There are a number of other factors which affect the response of the peripheral chemoreceptors:

  (i) increase in H^+ (not due to PCO_2), for example, lactic acidosis,

 (ii) increase in temperature,

(iii) increase in PCO_2 (minor although faster response than central chemoreceptors),

(iv) nicotine.

Peripheral chemoreceptors can also cause:

  (i) peripheral vasoconstriction,

 (ii) increased pulmonary vascular resistance,

(iii) systolic arterial hypertension,

(iv) tachycardia,

 (v) increased left ventricular perfusion.

There are several other mechanisms which can influence respiration and respiratory pattern.

Hering–Breuer inflation reflex

This is generated by stretch receptors situated in the walls of the bronchi and bronchioles. When lungs overinflate the receptors are stimulated to send impulses back to the respiratory centre terminating inspiration. This appears to be a protective mechanism preventing pulmonary damage.

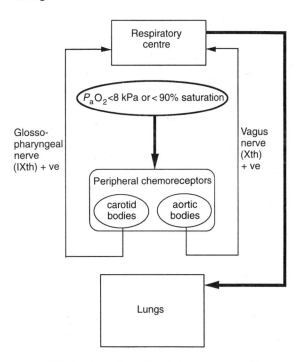

Fig. 3.6 Mechanism of peripheral chemoreceptor effect on respiration.

Deflation reflex
The rate of breathing is increased when lungs are compressed or deflated. The precise mechanism is unknown.

Irritant reflex
Receptors located subepithelially in trachea, bronchi, and bronchioles cause an increase in ventilatory rate when lungs are compressed or exposed to noxious gases. It may also cause reflex cough and bronchoconstriction.

Juxtapulmonary — capillary receptors (J-receptors)
These receptors are located in the interstitial tissues between the pulmonary capillaries and the alveoli. When they are activated they stimulate rapid, shallow breathing. They are activated by:

(i) pulmonary capillary congestion,

(ii) capillary hypertension,

(iii) oedema of the alveolar walls,

(iv) humoral agents (e.g 5-HT),

(v) lung deflation.

Baroreceptors
These have a primarily cardiovascular function but when stimulated by a low blood pressure they cause an increase in ventilatory rate as well as an increase in heart rate. When stimulated by a high blood pressure they cause a decrease in ventilatory rate.

Exercise
Neural signals from the cerebral cortex to exercising muscles appear to have a collateral transmission to the respiratory centre in the medulla producing an increased rate and depth of breathing. Movement of the limbs also transmit sensory signals up the spinal cord to the medulla.

The precise mechanism of the respiratory response to the exercise stimulus has not been fully explained.

Assessment of respiratory status

In detailing the assessment of one particular system in the patient it is very easy to forget the effect that any primary dysfunction will be having on other related systems. It is thus necessary at the outset to emphasize that any respiratory problems will have an impact on cardiovascular and nutritional status, the patient's conscious level,

and his/her emotional state. The patient's ability to perform personal needs and to maintain vital defence mechanisms will also be reduced. The nurse caring for the patient must attempt to maintain an overall view of the patient that will not neglect these other features while concentrating on the prime cause of distress. The importance of a preventative as well as a therapeutic role cannot be stressed sufficiently.

History

Patients admitted in acute respiratory distress are frequently unable to provide any detailed information and all efforts should be made to obtain as much as possible from alternative sources. These include:

- relatives and friends,

- GP letters,

- previous notes and nursing records,

- casualty notes and records,

- results of any previous investigations.

Patients in this state should not have to answer two sets of questions and so, wherever possible, the immediate nursing and medical history should be done as a collaborative process so that areas of overlap are not repeated unnecessarily. Much of the information can be obtained whilst performing other more urgent needs and priorities. (Table 3.9.)

Table 3.9 Useful information from history taking

---

1. Timespan of current problem plus any relevant past medical history, particularly the degree (if any) of chronic respiratory disability.
2. Previously tried manoeuvres found to be of benefit in reducing respiratory problems and breathlessness.
3. Current medications.
4. Type and time of occurrence of dyspnoea (e.g. on exertion only, position-related, etc.).
5. Sputum — colour, consistency, amount.
6. Pain (if any) — site, timing, modes of relief employed by patient.
7. Mood state and immediate anxieties

Physical assessment

A considerable amount of information about the patient's condition can be gained from simply observing, and listening.

Colour

This can range from pink and therefore relatively well oxygenated to frankly cyanosed. The patient suffering from carbon monoxide poisoning may have a characteristic 'cherry-red' colour due to the presence of carboxyhaemoglobin. The patient's buccal (mouth) mucosa as well as the peripheries should be viewed. Peripheral cyanosis is seen in conditions of poor circulation (vasoconstricted due to cold, poor cardiac output, arteriopaths, etc.) and does not indicate a low P_aO_2. However, central cyanosis, seen as blue lips and buccal mucosa, is indicative of a low P_aO_2. However, a grossly anaemic patient may not exhibit this clinical sign as 5 g of reduced oxyhaemoglobin per 100 ml blood must be present before cyanosis is clinically detectable.

Patient condition

This is a general assessment of the patient's level of fatigue and potential for maintaining respiration. Useful indicators of failing respiratory function are:

(i) Signs of sweating (indicates use of considerable effort to maintain function and increased sympathetic arousal),

(ii) Inability to speak or move limbs (indicates lack of breath and energy limitation due to poor respiratory function),

(iii) Restlessness and confusion as well as altered conscious level (may indicate cerebral hypoxia although this can be related to other causes and should be treated with caution). The patient's ability to protect the airway should be assessed by checking cough and gag reflex.

(iv) Distress.

(v) Posture.

Respiratory pattern

Assessment of movement of the chest wall:

(i) Both sides moving equally (pneumothorax, mechanical dysfunction, such as rib fractures and flail chest, pleural effusion, and major lobar collapse, may all cause unilateral diminished expansion).

(ii) Use of the normal muscles of inspiration (diaphragmatic splinting or paralysis, neuropathy, myopathy, Guillain–Barré syndrome and myasthenia gravis can all affect the normal ability to use the diaphragm and intercostal muscles).

(iii) Use of accessory muscles of inspiration (scalene, sternocleidomastoid, pectoralis, trapezius, and external intercostals) to assist inspiration suggest considerable extra effort required to create the increased negative pressure necessary for adequate inspiration. This can either be because inspiration is more difficult due to obstructive or restrictive disease or because the demands of the body on the lungs are greatly increased. There are other accessory muscles of expiration which include the abdominal and internal intercostal muscles. They act to increase positive pressure within the lungs to assist in expelling air when there is increased airway resistance.

(iv) Respiratory rate and depth should be observed and counted together to give a clear picture of respiration. A high respiratory rate with shallow breaths may indicate pain preventing normal inspiration whereas a high rate with normal size breaths may indicate hyperventilation.

Hypoventilation may be due to central causes including cerebrovascular accidents and head trauma. It may also be related to iatrogenic or self-administered sedatives (e.g. benzodiazepines or opiates).

It is not always possible to interpret these signs correctly without looking at other data and caution should be used before attaching too great a significance to them. (Table 3.10.)

For other respiratory patterns associated with specific neurological dysfunction see Chapter 9.

Palpation

The position of the trachea should be assessed for mediastinal shift by placing a finger either side of the trachea just above the sternal notch. Tracheal deviation is indicative of mediastinal shift caused either by large volumes of pleural air or fluid filling the pleural space and pushing the lung away from the chest wall or by lobar/lung collapse drawing the trachea towards the lung space. Tactile vocal fremitus refers to the vibrations felt when the patient speaks. Sound is usually transmitted well through solid structures and poorly through air. Thus, conditions replacing air with more solid matter in the lungs (e.g. pneumonia), may well increase the transmission of sound. If the chest is palpated with the fingertips or palm on each side and the patient is asked to speak (usually to say 'gg' several times) then a similar degree of vibration should be felt except over the heart. If there is inequality in transmission this may be due to consolidation (increased transmission) or pnuemothorax/fluid (decreased transmission).

Table 3.10   Abnormal respiratory patterns

Apnoea	Complete absence of spontaneous ventilation
Hypoventilation	Decreased alveolar ventilation with either decreased rate or depth of breaths. Results in an increased P_ACO_2 and, consequently, an increased P_aCO_2
Hyperventilation	Increased alveolar ventilation with either increased rate or increased depth of breaths. This results in a decreased P_ACO_2 and, consequently, a decreased P_aCO_2
Hyperpnoea	Increased depth of breathing, with or without increased frequency
Tachypnoea	Increased rate of ventilation
Cheyne–Stokes respiration	Periods of apnoea of between 10 and 30 seconds followed by a progressively increasing rate and volume of breaths which reach a peak and then decline to another period of apnoea. This pattern of respiration is associated with cerebral dysfunction
Kussmaul breathing	Increased rate and depth of breathing commonly associated with diabetic ketoacidosis. It produces a decrease in P_ACO_2 and, consequently, a low P_aCO_2
Biot's breathing	Short episodes of deep inspirations of the same volume and frequency followed by 10–30 seconds of apnoea. This pattern is associated with meningitis

(*Eupnoea* is the term given to normal spontaneous ventilation.)

Percussion

This is not a technique frequently used by nurses and requires some practice to become skilled. The middle phalanx of the middle finger is pressed against the chest wall and struck with the tip of the other middle finger. Different sounds may be produced:

- The normal sound over the lungs is low pitched and long and described as resonant.

- Increased density (e.g. from a pleural effusion) produces stony dull (soft, short, high-pitched) sounds.

- Decreased density (such as in pneumothorax or em-physema) causes hyper-resonant (loud, lower-pitched and longer) or tympanitic (loud, long, high-pitched, drum-like) sounds.

Auscultation

Air entry to the lung fields
This is a basic measure to ensure that there is flow of air to all areas of the lung. Causes of reduced or non-existent air entry in the self-ventilating patient vary from lobar collapse and pleural effusion to pneumothorax and hypoventilation.

Breath sounds
There are three *normal* types of breath sound heard over different parts of the chest:

  (i) *Vesicular* — low pitch, no break between inspiration and expiration, expiration is longer than inspiration, heard in the periphery of the lung.

 (ii) *Bronchial* — high pitch, loud, pause between inspiration and expiration, expiration equals inspiration, heard over the trachea.

(iii) *Bronchovesicular* — combination of the above sounds, heard over major airways in most other parts of the lung.

If bronchial sounds are heard over areas of the lung other than the trachea this may be indicative of consolidation of that area or the presence of a pleural effusion just below. This is due to the transmission of the breath sounds from the main airway through the better conducting medium of consolidated or compressed lung rather than hearing a direct flow of air. This is known as 'bronchial breathing'.

Absent or reduced/distant breath sounds may be heard over a pleural effusion or pneumothorax.

Abnormal breath sounds

  (i) *Crackles* — formerly called crepitations, these are high-pitched rustles related to the re-opening of small airways or the presence of intra-alveolar fluid. They can be heard in pulmonary oedema and pulmonary fibrosis at the end of inspiration, and in pneumonia and bronchiectasis throughout both inspiration and expiration.

 (ii) *Wheezes* — formerly known as rhonchi, these are heard on expiration as a result of expired air being forced through narrowed airways. These can be heard in asthma and other causes of bronchoconstriction (e.g toxic gas inhalation or anaphylaxis).

Rarely, wheeze may be heard in heart failure (cardiac asthma).

Inspiratory wheeze is associated with major airway obstruction such as tumour or presence of a foreign body. This is stridor and is also heard in epiglottitis and laryngeal oedema (e.g. post-extubation).

If wheezes are heard on inspiration and expiration they are often caused by excessive airway secretions.

(iii) *Pleural friction rubs* — rough, grating, and crackling sound heard on inspiration and expiration. It is found in areas of pleural inflammation (pleurisy) when the normally smooth surfaces of parietal and visceral pleura are roughened and rub on each other.

Pulse oximetry

It is now possible to obtain reasonably accurate measures of arterial oxygen saturation using the non-invasive technique of pulse oximetry. A sensor placed on the patient's skin can give an almost continuous measure of peripheral arterial oxygen saturation. The major drawback of the technique is the need for a well-perfused peripheral circulation, otherwise, the sensor is unable to detect sufficiently strong signals to give an accurate read-out. The oximeter should be used with caution in cases of smoke inhalation, heavy smokers, and patients with unexplained cyanosis as types of haemoglobin, such as carboxyhaemoglobin and methaemoglobin, decrease the accuracy of the oximeter. Readings should be checked against those obtained in a co-oximeter (see Chapter 4 for further details). This is to exclude the presence of carboxyhaemoglobin (from carbon monoxide poisoning) or methaemoglobin (e.g. following pancreatitis) (Kidd 1988).

A saturation of >95% does not imply adequate organ perfusion. The haemoglobin may be fully saturated with oxygen but an inadequate cardiac output, or a low haemoglobin, may result in an inadequate supply of oxygen to the tissues.

The probe position should always be checked if a sharp fall in saturation occurs. Transient falls in saturation may be seen following suction and repositioning of the patient; if these falls persist arterial blood gases should be checked.

Arterial blood gases

The measurement of oxygen (PO_2) and carbon dioxide (PCO_2) tension in arterial blood can give the clearest indication of the patient's respiratory function. It should not be forgotten that the results must always be interpreted in the light of the patient's clinical condition and the inspired oxygen concentration and not purely in abstract. It is possible for a severely tired and compromised patient to maintain a near normal PCO_2 until almost the point of collapse but clinical assessment of the patient will determine that this is at considerable cost and that intervention may be required. The functions are:

(i) Measurement of the oxygenation of the patient.

(ii) Determination of the acid-base status of the patient.

For further details refer back to the anatomy and physiology section.

Normal values in arterial blood for a patient breathing air	
pH	7.35–7.45
PO_2	10.0–13.3 kPa
PCO_2	4.6–6.0 kPa
Bicarbonate (HCO_3^-)	22–26 mmol/l
Base excess	−2 to +2

Tissue hypoxia

An inadequate availability of oxygen for cell metabolism. This can be due to hypoxaemia (hypoxic hypoxia), anaemia (anaemic hypoxia), circulatory impairment (circulatory hypoxia), and impairment of tissue utilization (histotoxic hypoxia). Hypoxaemia will be addressed in detail in this chapter.

Anaemic hypoxia — the oxygen tension of the arterial blood is normal but the oxygen carrying capacity of the blood is inadequate. This can be due to either a low amount of haemoglobin in the blood or a deficiency in the ability of haemoglobin to carry oxygen such as in carbon monoxide poisoning.

Circulatory hypoxia — the arterial blood that reaches the tissues may have a normal oxygen tension and content but the volume of blood (and therefore the amount of oxygen) delivered is insufficient to meet tissue needs. This is commonly due either to:

(1) *stagnant hypoxia* — slow peripheral capillary flow from either a poor cardiac output, vascular insufficiency or neurochemical abnormalities, or

(2) *arterial-venous shunt* — some tissue cells are completely bypassed by arterial blood.

Histotoxic hypoxia — impairment of the tissue cells ability to utilize oxygen. This occurs in cyanide poisoning.

Hypoxaemia

A low oxygen concentration (< 8.0 kPa) in the blood. Tissue hypoxia does not necessarily coexist, as considerable compensation may be occurring to overcome the low level of P_aO_2, for example by an increased cardiac output, increased oxygen extraction by the tissues, or (in chronic states such as chronic obstructive airways disease or living at altitude), an increased haemoglobin.

Hypocapnia

Low carbon dioxide concentration in the blood (< 4.0 kPa). Usually due to hyperventilation.

Hypercapnia

High carbon dioxide concentration in the blood (> 6.0 kPa). Causes are usually either hypoventilation or increased carbon dioxide production due to overfeeding with carbohydrate.

Methods of respiratory support

These provide a variety of levels of support from simple supplemental oxygen therapy to complete ventilatory support using mechanical ventilators (see Table 3.11). The aims of respiratory support are:

(1) To correct hypoxaemia and hypercapnia.

(2) To assist mechanical failure (including an unprotected airway).

(3) To decrease associated workload:
   (a) work of breathing,
   (b) myocardial workload.

Priorities in caring for patients requiring respiratory support

Safety
A method of back-up ventilation for the patient must be immediately to hand. This is invariably a manual ventilation bag (e.g. rebreathe bag or Ambu bag). It is essential that it is checked as a priority safety routine by any nurse responsible for the patient.

The appropriate sizes of oropharyngeal (Guedel) airways and facemask should also be available at the patient's bedside.

The concentration of inspired oxygen (F_iO_2) that the patient is actually receiving should be checked against that prescribed. This is done using an oxygen analyser either as part of the ventilator or as a separate piece of equipment. The method of delivery should also be considered; it should be capable of delivering the percentage required. Standard oxygen masks (e.g. Hudson masks are incapable of delivering an accurate level of oxygen.) Particularly when the patient has a high minute ventilation it is difficult to achieve an F_iO_2 above 0.4 using standard masks (see Table 3.11).

Equipment alarms are a very reliable way of identifying sudden or life-threatening changes in the patient's condition. They are, however, only as useful as the settings used as alarm limits, therefore the nurse must ensure that the alarms are set appropriately.

Ventilator alarms
Alarm settings on the ventilators should be checked to ensure they are on and appropriate to the patient. For most patients:

(i) Expired minute volume alarms should be set:
Upper — at 2l above current expired minute volume.
Lower — at 2l below current expired minute volume.

(ii) Airway pressure alarms should be set:
Upper — at 40 cm H_2O or as instructed by medical staff.
Lower — at 5 cm H_2O below current airway pressure reading.

(iii) Pulse oximeter alarms
These alarms should usually be set at 90% oxygen saturation. However, this may alter according to patient condition.

(iv) Cardiac monitor alarms

These settings will reflect cardiac status but will also provide a useful warning for respiratory problems and should always be set appropriately (see Chapter 5).

Suction equipment
Suction equipment is essential both as an emergency measure and in routine use for intubated or tracheostomized patients. It should always be checked to ensure it is capable of producing the appropriate level of suction and that suction catheters are the correct size for the patient's endotracheal tube and condition of secretions (see section on suction technique, p. 65).

Table 3.11 Methods of respiratory support

Mode of delivery	Oxygen percentage available	Associated problems	Safety priorities	Use
Nasal cannulae	2 l/min 23–28% 3 l/min 28–30% 4 l/min 32–36% 5 l/min 40% 6 l/min plus (max. 44%)	Limited % O_2 available. Inaccurate delivery of oxygen, particularly with high minute volumes. Requires patent nasal passages; if patient mouth-breathes then amount of oxygen delivered will be altered. Drying and uncomfortable for nasal passages.	Regular monitoring of respiratory rate and pattern. If patient unstable use pulse oximeter to monitor O_2 saturation. Positioning of cannulae inside nares. Check O_2 flow rate.	Low levels of O_2 supplementation only. Disposable.
Semi-rigid masks (e.g. Hudson, MC, etc.)	4 l/min ~35% 6 l/min ~50% 8 l/min ~55% 10 l/min ~60% 12 l/min ~65%	Inaccurate delivery of O_2, particularly with high minute volumes. Limits patient activities such as eating and drinking. Drying for patient's mucosa and for secretions. Rebreathing may occur with high minute volumes.	Regular monitoring of respiratory rate and pattern. If patient unstable use pulse oximeter to monitor O_2 saturation. Check positioning of mask and O_2 flow rate.	Low to medium levels of O_2 supplementation only. Disposable.
Venturi-type mask (high-flow system) (e.g. Ventimasks, Inspiron, etc.)	With use of appropriate venturi nozzle for each % 2 l/min 24% 4 l/min 28% 8 l/min 35% 10 l/min 40% 15 l/min 60%	Can still be drying for patient. If humidification used an extra attachment is required. Patients requiring large inspiratory flow rates may still not achieve required O_2% Limits patient activities, such as eating and drinking.	Regular monitoring of respiratory rate and pattern. If patient unstable use pulse oximeter to monitor O_2 saturation. Check positioning of mask and O_2 flow rate.	Medium to high levels of O_2 supplementation. Disposable.
Humified oxygen using nebulizer system (e.g. Aquapaks)	Varying rates of flow to deliver 28–60% O_2	Inaccurate delivery of O_2, particularly with high volumes. Limits patient activities.	Regular monitoring of respiratory rate and pattern. If patient unstable use pulse oximeter. Check positioning of mask, O_2 flow, rate and setting of O_2 percentage on nebulizer.	Low to medium levels of oxygen supplementation. Disposable.

Table 3.11   *contd*

Mode of delivery	Oxygen percentage available	Associated problems	Safety priorities	Use
Continuous positive airway pressure (CPAP) using high-flow generator or large volume balloon reservoir	40–100% with tightly fitting CPAP mask. 2.5–15 cm H_2O using adjustable or exchangeable expiratory valves.	Tightly-fitting mask causing discomfort, pressure sores, etc. Leakage of high gas flows into eyes may cause corneal drying and abrasion. Air swallowing may cause gastric discomfort and increased risk of regurgitation. Eating and drinking are very difficult. Patient may experience feelings of claustrophobia due to tightly fitting mask. Increased noise associated with high flows may disturb patient. In systems without a high-flow generator flow may be inadequate causing increased inspiratory resistance.	Pulse oximetry to monitor patient O_2 saturation. Regular monitoring of respiratory rate and pattern. Use of nasogastric tube to decompress stomach if necessary. Provision of psychological support and comfort to assist patient tolerance.	Medium to high levels of O_2 supplementation. Mask, tubing, and valve set-up disposable. Flow generator non-disposable.

Problems associated with patients undergoing respiratory support

These will be divided into problems associated with supporting the patient's own compromised respiratory function and those associated with taking over the

---

Definition of respiratory failure

Arterial blood gases

- $PO_2 < 8.0$ kPa with patient breathing air and at rest
- $+/- \ PCO_2 > 6.5$ kPa in the absence of primary metabolic acidosis
- $+/- \ $pH < 7.25 in the absence of primary metabolic acidosis

Patient

- Respiratory rate > 40 or < 6–8 breaths/min
- Deteriorating vital capacity (< 15 ml/kg)

---

patient's respiratory function using some form of mechanical ventilation. All patients requiring a form of respiratory support have some degree of respiratory failure.

Non-invasive respiratory support involves use of oxygen therapy, continuous positive airway pressure (CPAP), and intermittent positive pressure breathing through nasal mask or mouthpiece (e.g. via Bird ventilator or BromptonPac).

Hypoxaemia
Management. Oxygen therapy as per patient requirements (see Table 3.11).

Chronic carbon dioxide retainers depending on a hypoxic respiratory drive should have controlled levels of F_iO_2 with continuous observation of respiratory rate and regular monitoring of P_aCO_2 levels.

Chest physiotherapy will assist in removal of secretions. Deep breathing and coughing may also help re-open areas of collapsed lung.

Positioning of patient to optimize ventilation/perfusion matching (see section on shunting p. 38). Usually, this is upright although if the problem is unilateral, the patient should be placed on the side with the problem lung *uppermost* so that the good lung is being perfused.

Maintenance of airway and sputum clearance
Management. Humidification will assist clearance of thick, tenacious secretions and prevent the drying of mucosa and cilia associated with inhalation of dry oxygen (see section on humidification, p. 63).

Regular assistance with deep breathing and coughing will reduce the incidence of atelectasis and help the patient to clear secretions. If necessary, suctioning via the oro or nasal pharynx may assist in removal of sputum (see section on suction, p. 65). Chest physiotherapy and postural drainage are also useful.

Fatigue related to work of breathing
Management. Limit any other activity likely to fatigue. Provide periods specifically for complete rest without interference. Ensure day/night environment is preserved.

Fear and anxiety
Management. Provide comfort and reassurance by a calm and confident approach to the patient. Include the family as much as possible in care and interactions. Allow time for expression of worries and ensure the patient is given full information expressed appropriately to ensure understanding.

Poor nutritional intake due to shortage of breath and loss of appetite
Management. Provide frequent, small nutritious meals. Offer high calorie hot or cold drinks in between. Encourage the family to become involved in meals and obtain details of patient's likes and dislikes. Maintain a full record of nutritional intake and ensure medical staff are made aware of any continued deficit.

Impaired verbal communication due to shortage of breath and presence of mask
Management. Provide alternative methods of communication such as alphabet board or pen and paper. Use closed questions for specific information so that the patient can nod or shake their head to answer. Instruct the family in these methods. Anticipate the patient's information needs so that unnecessary questions can be avoided (see Chapter 2).

Drying of mouth and upper airways due to high flow of dry gases
Management. Humidify the inspired gases (see section on humidification, p. 63). Check skin turgor and condition of buccal mucosa. Provide mouthwashes and oral hygiene measures as necessary (see Chapter 2). Monitor fluid balance and avoid systemic dehydration unless the medical condition dictates otherwise.

Endotracheal intubation and tracheostomy

Positive pressure ventilation requires a closed system of delivery in the adult patient to allow effective ventilation. Thus, some form of seal in the patient's airway is essential. This is provided by the cuff of either an endotracheal (ET) tube or a tracheostomy tube. The cuff also provides some protection against the aspiration of gastric secretions, food, blood, etc., although this is not complete.

Problems associated with endotracheal tube placement

- Tracheal stenosis, ulceration, necrosis

- Tracheomalacia (degeneration of the cartilaginous rings)

- Clearance of secretions

- Loss of normal humidifying and warming mechanisms

- Loss of physiological PEEP (i.e. the resistance to expiration exerted by the pharynx and upper airways which limits alveolar collapse)

- Damage to vocal cords and trauma on insertion

- Increased risk of nosocomial (hospital-acquired) pneumonia

- Maxillary sinusitis (with nasal tubes)

Problems associated with tracheostomy tube placement

- Tracheal stenosis, fibrosis, tracheomalacia

- Loss of normal humidifying and warming mechanisms

- Loss of physiological PEEP

- Increased risk of nosocomial pneumonia

A major part of the problem of ulceration and stenosis is the need for a cuff or balloon to seal the airway. The cuffs are now designed to be high in volume and low in pressure to reduce some of the complications, and are filled with air to provide the necessary seal. Capillary occlusion pressure within the tracheal wall is approximately 30 mmHg and it is important to limit the cuff pressure to less than this. The use of manometers to measure cuff pressure is essential. They should be checked 3–4 times daily and whenever an air leak is heard in order to ensure that pressures are within this limit. Estimation by fingertip pressure on the external cuff balloon or filling until no further leak is heard is inaccurate. However, when inflation pressures are high, cuff pressures may have to be increased over the recommended levels to prevent leaks.

Care of endotracheal and tracheostomy tubes

Indications for endotracheal and tracheostomy tubes:

- to obtain or maintain a clear airway,

- to prevent aspiration of gastrointestinal contents,

- to facilitate delivery of positive pressure ventilation,

- to enable delivery of high concentrations of oxygen,

- to facilitate removal of pulmonary secretions.

Sites of insertion:

- Oral endotracheal tube — mouth to trachea.

- Nasal endotracheal tube — nose to trachea.

- Tracheostomy — percutaneous or surgical insertion below the cricoid and thyroid cartilages (usually between the 2nd and 3rd tracheal rings).

- Minitracheostomy and cricothyroidotomy — percutaneous or surgical insertion through the cricothyroid membrane.

Endotracheal tubes

Oral tubes are most commonly used in adults, being easier to insert and secure.

Nasal tubes are felt to be more comfortable for the patient and avoid the hazard of being constricted by the patient's teeth. However, a smaller size is generally necessary and the angle at the nasopharynx can cause difficulty with insertion of suction catheters. Furthermore, there is a significant associated incidence of maxillary sinusitis and this should always be considered if the patient develops an unexplained pyrexia.

Types of tube used for adults:

- Single use cuffed endotracheal and tracheostomy tubes made from silastic or PVC.

- Reuseable uncuffed silver tubes (Negus) used for long-term tracheostomized self-ventilating patients.

- Red rubber tubes should only be used for short-term situations, such as anaesthesia, as they are inflexible and irritant.

Special tubes:

- Double lumen ET tubes for asynchronous ventilation. One lumen opens into the trachea and the other into a bronchus (usually the left — this should be ascertained prior to insertion).

- Fenestrated tracheostomy tube to allow speech by diverting exhaled breath through the vocal cords. This can only be done while the patient is self-ventilating.

- Tracheostomy tube with removeable inner cannula which can be removed for cleaning to reduce encrustation

- *Note.* Endotracheal tubes for children are always uncuffed as they are highly susceptible to stenotic problems related to cuff pressure, particularly in the cricoid region which is narrowed until puberty.

Usual adult sizes of endotracheal tube		
	Oral (internal diameter)	Nasal (internal diameter)
Men:	8/9 mm	7/8 mm
Women:	7/8 mm	6/7 mm

Tube sizes routinely available range from 6.0 mm to 11.0 mm internal diameter. The tube diameter (external) should be considerably less than the cricoid diameter to decrease the risk of damage.

Note. Tube sizes for children vary with age or body weight from 2.5 mm newborn to 8.0 mm for 12- to 15-year-olds. Various formulae are available to estimate the correct diameter for age.

Length of endotracheal tubes

Oral ET tubes should be positioned at approximately 23 cm at the incisors for men and 21 cm for women. However, this position will depend on body size and neck length and requires confirmation initially by ensuring good air entry to both lungs and, subsequently, by chest X-ray. A cause of patient agitation after recovery from intubation, paralysis, and sedation can be the tube sitting on the carina or, alternatively, the cuff herniating through the vocal cords. The end of the tube should be roughly 3–5 cm above the carina.

In the United Kingdom the tubes are generally pre-cut prior to insertion to a length 2–3 cm longer than estimated to allow secure tying of the tube. This method has been used with reasonable success in preventing endobronchial intubation.

Tracheostomy tubes

The sizes routinely used for tracheostomy tubes range from 26 FG to 36 FG. They are usually of a standard length although it is possible to obtain custom-made tubes for patients with problem necks which are very short or long, or to avoid damaged areas of the trachea (e.g. tracheomalacia).

Intubation

If at all possible this should be a calm, elective procedure made in good time according to the criteria for ventilation. Ideally, the patient should not have eaten for at least 4 hours. However, it is often necessary to intubate in emergency situations so it is vital to have all equipment (see Table 3.12) readily available and kept together in one place. Safety priorities apply whether the procedure is elective or an emergency, namely:

Table 3.12 Equipment for intubation over and above available safety equipment

---

- Laryngoscopes — one curved, one straight blade (check that the light is working)
- Selection of endotracheal tubes of varying internal diameter
- Lubrication (e.g. KY jelly)
- Magill's forceps
- Introducer (Bougie)
- 10 ml syringe
- Artery forceps
- Tape to secure tube
- Catheter mount
- Cuff pressure manometer
- Sedating and paralysing agents
- A back-up manual ventilation bag and mask

- Check the manual ventilation bag and suction equipment to ensure they are functioning.

- Attach the ventilator to the gas source and check it is functioning.

- Ensure emergency drugs (see Chapter 6) are to hand and that the patient has reliable intravenous access.

Prior to intubation the procedure should be explained to the patient if there is time. In particular, the temporary loss of speech due to the presence of the tube should be emphasized to prevent anxiety.

- Prepare equipment, drugs, and ventilator.

- Pre-oxygenation via facemask for at least 5 minutes if patient's condition permits.

- Cricoid pressure (pressure on the cricoid cartilage using the finger pads of the thumb, forefinger, and middle finger to compress the pharyngeal airway) preventing reflux of gastric contents in emergency intubation may be necessary.

Before administering any drugs check:

(a) all equipment is ready and functioning (including manual ventilation bag, suction, etc.),

(b) a tube has been cut ready for insertion and an intact cuff ensured,

(c) the doctor has checked the settings on the ventilator. The inspired oxygen concentration should initially be set at a higher level than the anticipated requirements of the patient.

- Continuous observation of patient, ECG, pulse oximetry, and blood pressure is essential.

- Following insertion and cuff inflation, check air entry by auscultation then attach to ventilator.

- Secure the tube — one method is shown in Fig. 3.7.

- Check cuff pressure with manometer.

- Consider insertion of nasogastric tube.

- Carry out full set of respiratory observations.

- Ensure a chest X-ray has been arranged to confirm satisfactory tube position (tip sited 2–5 cm above the carina), and absence of pneumothorax.

- Arterial blood gases should be performed to confirm satisfactory P_aO_2 and P_aCO_2 levels after 10–15 minutes' equilibration (or sooner if indicated). Ventilator settings should then be adjusted as necessary.

Potential complications of intubation

- Inability to intubate
- Aspiration of gastric contents
- Bleeding from trauma to the airway
- Endobronchial intubation (usually right main bronchus)
- Oesophageal intubation
- Vocal cord damage
- Perforation (rare)
- Hypotension (usually due to vasodilator effects of anaesthetic agents unmasking covert hypovolaemia; occasionally due to cardiodepressant effects of same drugs)
- Arrhythmias (usually bradycardia due to hypoxia or vagal stimulation. Atropine may be required if the patient does not respond to correction of hypoxaemia)
- Dislodged teeth

Formation of tracheostomy

This may be either a surgical procedure requiring a horizontal incision between the 2nd and 3rd tracheal rings or a percutaneous approach using dilators to insert the tracheostomy tube.

Tracheostomy is a procedure which carries some risk and should not be undertaken lightly. There is some evidence to suggest that the percutaneous method has a reduced incidence of complications (Griggs *et al.* 1991). Following insertion, it is recommended that the tube be left in place for 5–7 days to allow formation of a tract from skin to trachea. It can then be changed as required. Use of tracheostomy tubes with removable inner cannulae allow cleaning of the inner tube to avoid encrustation and blockage due to secretions. The tube should be a size that is the largest that will fit comfortably into the trachea.

Peri-operative complications of tracheostomy

- Haemorrhage
- Surgical emphysema
- Pneumothorax
- Air embolism
- Cricoid cartilage damage

Specific nursing care of the intubated patient

Securing the tube
Movement of the tube can result in traumatic extubation, displacement of the tube, loss of cuff seal, and even oesophageal intubation, as well as causing considerable discomfort to the patient. Displacement of the tracheostomy tube into the pretracheal tissue is also possible. It is therefore vital to secure the tube and to check for any loosening of the tapes on a regular basis. Unplanned extubation occurs in 3–9% of patients and is associated with patient restlessness and the availability of the nurse caring for the patient (Grap *et al.* 1995).

The usual method of securing adult tubes uses cotton tapes which are looped around the ET tube or through the slits in the flange of the tracheostomy tube. These are passed round the patient's head either above or below the ears and tied at one side. They should be tight enough to allow only one finger between the tape and the patient's neck. Alternative commercially available ties use velcro flaps on soft cotton collars but these are expensive. (Figure 3.7.)

Pressure from the constricting tapes or knot is a problem. Regular changing of tapes (checking the skin and lip underneath) and foam or felt covers for the tapes are of benefit.

Note. Intracranial pressure can be increased by tight tapes occluding venous return.

Prevention of upper airway damage
Pressure within the tube cuff should be checked routinely. Ideally, cuff pressure should not exceed 30 mmHg (capillary occlusion pressure) and should be kept as low as is compatible with a good seal. High volume, low pressure cuffs should always be used for anything other than short-term intubation as the incidence of tracheal trauma is greatly reduced.

There is no evidence that periodic deflation of the cuff is of any benefit and it may actually cause problems if large amounts of saliva/secretions have collected above the cuff.

Secure fixation of the tube to prevent displacement (see above) is important in preventing tracheal damage.

The skin and lip or nostril under the tube should be checked and cleaned whenever the tapes are changed as pressure can cause severe ulceration and necrosis.

Oral hygiene
Routine oral care may have to be increased in frequency and extra care taken particularly with an oral tube. The lips may become excoriated and dry and should be protected with vaseline.

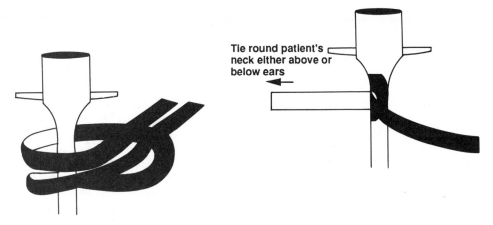

Tie round patient's neck either above or below ears

Fig. 3.7 Securing endotracheal tube (ET) tapes. (*Note*: tapes should always be tied around the plastic of the ET tube itself, not around the connector because it is possible for the connector to dislodge.)

Specific care of the patient with tracheostomy

Safety priorities
Tracheal dilators and replacement tubes of the same and a smaller size should be kept with the patient in case of accidental extubation.

Routine emergency equipment including suction, manual ventilation bag, airways, catheter mount, and black rubber mask should be immediately available and checked routinely.

Care of the stoma
Following formation, a dry dressing, such as gauze or lyofoam, is used. The stoma should be cleaned routinely ($\sim$ 8-hourly) and the site inspected for signs of infection or bleeding. This is an aseptic procedure. Normal saline is usually sufficient although other solutions, such as chlorhexidine, have been suggested. However, there is no evidence that they are more effective and therefore there is little point in their use.

If secretions from the tracheostomy are very copious, the skin should be protected with a stomahesive wafer shaped to fit and the secretions should be suctioned away as they form.

If tracheostomy tubes with removeable inner cannulae are used, these should be removed and cleaned 8-hourly. The cannula can be cleaned using mouth care sponges, small bottle brushes, or ribbon gauze soaked in antiseptic solution. If very encrusted, sodium bicarbonate may help to remove dried secretions.

Changing the tracheostomy tube

It is usual to wait 7 days or so after insertion to allow the stoma to form before changing the tube. The frequency of tube changes thereafter is usually dictated by unit policy but should be at least every 7 days in order to prevent encrustation and narrowing of the inner diameter which will increase the work of breathing. (Table 3.13.)

Table 3.13 Equipment for tracheostomy tube change

- Emergency equipment
- Tubes, one the same size, one smaller
- Tracheal dilators
- Lubricant jelly
- Sterile gloves
- Cleaning solution
- 10 ml syringe
- Tracheostomy dressing and new tapes

Tubes can be changed by an experienced nurse but medical back-up should always be readily available in case of problems.

Prior to assembling the equipment for the procedure, the patient should be prepared with an explanation of the need for a tube change and the steps involved.

Two nurses are necessary for safe procedure. It is an aseptic technique. After preparation of the equipment, the new tracheostomy tube should be checked to ensure even inflation of the cuff and easy withdrawal of the introducer. The patient should be well pre-oxygenated and have had mouth and trachea suctioned. The stoma should be cleaned as normal and the tapes cut. When all is prepared the cuff is deflated and the old tube removed. The new tube is inserted, the introducer withdrawn and the cuff inflated. The ventilator is then re-attached and air entry checked. The tube is then secured.

Removal of tracheal tubes

Extubation
Preparation of the patient should include an explanation of the procedure and securing their co-operation during removal.

Emergency equipment, as for intubation, should be checked.

If the patient has been intubated for any length of time a pulse oximeter is useful to monitor oxygen saturations during and after extubation.

Equipment for extubation

- Scissors

- Syringe

- Suction — tracheal and Yankauer

- Oxygen mask and tubing (or CPAP circuit)

- Disposable towel

- Mouthwash

The principles of extubation are:

(i) Two nurses are necessary for safe extubation.

(ii) The patient is usually most comfortable sitting up.

(iii) The patient's airway and oropharynx should be as clear of secretions as possible prior to extubation.

(iv) One nurse will cut the tapes and deflate the cuff, the other will suction and withdraw the tube.

(v) If secretions are thick or copious, suction to just below the tip of the tube should continue while the tube is withdrawn.

(vi) The patient will need assistance to cough up any further secretions and then should have a mouthwash or oral toilet to clear the mouth.

(vii) The patient will require oxygen via either an oxygen mask or CPAP depending on his/her condition.

Removal of tracheostomy tube
Preparation is as for changing the tube and preparation of the patient is as for extubation.

The equipment needed is similar to that for extubation but the mouthwash is unnecessary and an airtight dressing such as a stomahesive wafer or petroleum gauze and waterproof plaster should be added. No surgery is necessary as the stoma will close spontaneously over a number of days.

The principles of tracheostomy tube removal are:
Principles (i)–(iv) for extubation apply.

(v) The site should be cleaned prior to extubation.

(vi) The stoma should be sealed with an airtight dressing.

(vii) Attach an oxygen mask (or CPAP circuit).

(viii) A minitracheostomy may be inserted through the existing stoma after extubation if there is concern that the patient may not adequately clear secretions.

Minitracheostomy

This involves insertion of a small (4.0 mm) diameter cuffless tube through the cricothyroid membrane. It is a reasonably safe procedure employing a guidewire and dilator (Seldinger) technique for placement. Potential complications are haemorrhage, surgical emphysema, and displacement. Its uses include:

- Suction access for sputum retention in patients who do not require intubation for any other reason (a 10 FG suction catheter can be inserted through the tube).

- Emergency insertion for life-threatening airway obstruction.

Minitracheostomy is not suitable for protection of the airway in patients without a cough or gag reflex, or in patients who require ventilatory support. However, it is possible to perform jet ventilation via a minitracheostomy in some patients.

Mechanical ventilation

Mechanical ventilation includes methods of positive and negative pressure ventilation as well as high-frequency ventilation and extracorporeal support. The vast majority of ventilators used in ICUs are positive pressure ventilators. These will therefore be discussed in detail, although other types of ventilators will be described briefly and referenced for further information.

Positive pressure ventilation means that ventilatory gas is driven into the airways under a positive pressure which allows inflation of the alveoli and movement of the gas from mouth to alveoli. The force required is higher than that produced in normal ventilation and the effects of this non-physiological approach are widespread.

Furthermore, the gas mixture has to be propelled through tubing (i.e. the endotracheal tube) of a smaller diameter than the patient's own trachea (see endotracheal tube sizes, p. 52). This increases resistance to airflow and the pressures required to deliver the tidal volume are correspondingly higher.

There are three types of positive pressure ventilation:

1. *Pressure-cycled.* The ventilator allows inspiration to continue until a pre-set pressure is reached when it will cycle to expiration. It carries certain risks in that a sudden change in lung compliance or the existence of a large air leak may result in inadequate ventilation. Thus, the expired tidal volume and the inspiratory pressure must be closely monitored along with the patient's clinical status. This is the preferred mode of ventilation for small children where endotracheal tubes with a cuff to seal the airway are not used due to the potential damage to the trachea.

2. *Volume-cycled.* This is the most frequent type of ventilator setting used for the majority of adult patients. It allows a pre-set volume of air to be delivered to the patient and once this volume has been reached, expiration then occurs. The pressure generated by the delivery of this volume will be determined by the compliance of the lung, the flow rate, and the time for inspiration. It is possible to manipulate the pressure generated by manipulating the flow rate and inspiratory time. As high airway pressures are associated with an increased incidence of lung trauma, manipulation is usually aimed at minimizing airway pressure.

3. *Time-cycled.* This can be an option on ventilators that are normally volume-cycled. The time for each breath is proportioned into inspiration, expiration, and occasionally plateau sections. This gives a ratio of time for inspiration to time for expiration (I:E ratio). This is normally set at 1:2 but can be adjusted to allow a longer period for expiration in patients, such as asthmatics with outflow obstruction, or a longer period for inspiration in patients with non-compliant lungs, such as those with ARDS. In other words, the set tidal volume is delivered over shorter or longer proportions of the total time for each breath.

The mechanics of positive pressure ventilation

Most modern ventilators are driven by the pressure of compressed air, using electronic or computerized formats for control of delivery.

There are similar controls on most ventilators although there are two distinct types of ventilators available depending on their complexity and ability to incorporate weaning modes. (Table 3.14.)

Basic ventilators

1) The simpler type of ventilator tends to be used for short-stay patients without respiratory problems who will be able to recommence spontaneous ventilation without difficulty (e.g. Oxford, Brompton Manley, Blease, etc.).

Ventilators incorporating weaning modes.

2) The more sophisticated ventilator would have facilities allowing different weaning modes as well as the ability to manipulate the form of the breath taken. These are essential for patients who have altered lung mechanics in conditions such as ARDS, asthma, emphysema, etc. (Table 3.15.)

Indications for ventilatory support

- Respiratory failure which is not corrected by other forms of respiratory support (e.g. status asthmaticus, ARDS, pneumonia, pulmonary oedema).

- Support of other failing organs, especially the heart, in order to reduce its workload.

- Support of mechanical dysfunction (e.g. Guillain–Barré, flail chest, cervical fractures).

- Support of ventilatory function during use of high levels of sedation and anaesthesia necessary for other problems (e.g. status epilepticus, intra-operative anaesthesia).

- Therapeutic ventilation to reduce intracranial pressure (e.g. post head injury or extensive neurosurgery).

Physiological effects of positive pressure ventilation

The effects of positive pressure are apparent not only in the patient's respiratory status but also in a number of other systems including cardiac, renal, and vascular. Awareness of these changes is vital to any nurse caring for ventilated patients as they may have a profound effect on the patient.

Decreased cardiac output and venous return
Manifested by: hypotension, tachycardia, hypovolaemia, decreased urine output, increasing metabolic acidosis.

Table 3.14 Ventilator settings

Ventilator setting	Typical range of adult patient	Typical range of ventilation capability	Function	Alarm limits	Safety checks
Inspired oxygen (F_iO_2/%O_2)	Variable according to patient need and PO_2 from 21% to 100%.	$F_iO_2 = 0.21$–1.0. %O_2 = 21–100%.	Manipulation of inspired O_2 to produce optimal patient oxygenation.	Automatic alarm setting If F_1O_2 falls/ rises from set amount then alarm is triggered.	Use separate oxygen analyser in patient circuit to confirm setting. Check digital display of ventilator.
Respiratory rate or (frequency/min)	Usually 10–15 breaths/ minute but rate altered to manipulate MV and PCO_2/PO_2.	From 0–50 breaths/ minute (rate above 50 usually for paediatric use).	Delivery of adequate ventilation, and can be used to manipulate PO_2 and PCO_2.	Associated with expired MV alarm as resp. rate/min × V_T = V_E. MV alarms usually set manually at 2 l above (upper alarm) and 2 l below (lower alarm) set ventilator MV.	The patient's respiratory rate/min should be counted hourly. If patient on IMV/spontaneous modes then ventilator display should be checked.
Tidal volume * (V_T/ml)	10–15 ml/kg but may be altered outside this range to optimize PO_2 and PCO_2.	0–1500 ml.	Size of each breath can be altered to suit patient size and to ensure optimal alveolar ventilation without hyperinflation.	Associated with expired MV alarm as above.	Check ventilator display of expired MV or tidal volume if available. If in doubt, use separate spirometer to confirm.
Minute volume * (V_E or MV)	10–15 ml/kg × 10–15 breaths/minute = ~5–15 l/min.	0–75 l.	As above	MV alarms usually set manually at 2 l above (upper alarm) and 2 l below (lower alarm) the set ventilator MV.	Check ventilator display of expired MV. If in doubt, use separate spirometer on inspiratory and expiratory limbs.
Positive end expiratory pressure (PEEP) cmH_2O. Either feature of ventilator or added as expiratory valve.	+2 to +10 cmH_2O. Increasing levels of PEEP carry increasing risk of barotrauma and a depressant affect on cardiac output through decreased venous return.	+2 to +20 cmH_2O.	Maintenance of alveolar expansion during expiration giving increased time for gas exchange and thus increased PO_2. Also aids recruitment of collapsed areas of lung.	None. However, increased PEEP gives increasing airway pressure so upper/ lower airway press alarm limits should be adjusted to allow for PEEP.	Observe airway pressure display on ventilator. Pressure at end of expiration should not be less than set PEEP level.
Pressure support assist (for further details see ventilation modes, p. 59).	+5 to +40 cmH_2O. Levels set according to patient need as an aid to weaning and resulting airway pressure.	+5 to +40 cmH_2O.	Used to wean patients by assisting each spontaneous breath with the positive pressure set. High levels can provide complete ventilatory support.	Contributes to airway pressure and MV.	Observe airway pressure and MV. Spontaneous breaths should show a positive pressure rise of the amount set as assist.
Flow rate (V l/min)	Variable within limits: must be adjusted to ensure required V_T is reached if inspiratory time is reduced.	2–100 l/min.	1. Adjusts to achieve V_T in inspiratory time with optimal airway pressure. 2. Can be used to limit peak airway pressure by manipulation in conjunction with I:E. ratio. 3. Can manipulate I:E ratio in pressure control ventilation (see ventilation modes, p. 59).	None, but contributes to achieving set V_T and thus MV, so MV alarms as before.	Regular checks of ABGs if flow rate is altered as inadequate V_T will affect PO_2 and PCO_2 • Observe expired MV. • Particular care for COAD patients when weaning as flow must be adequate for increased inspiratory effort.

Table 3.14 *contd*

Ventilator setting	Typical range of adult patient	Typical range of ventilation capability	Function	Alarm limits	Safety checks
Inspiratory: Expiratory ratio (I:E ratio). Ratio of time for inspiration to time for expiration in each breath.	Variable from 1:1 to 1:4. Inverse ratio ventilation (see below ventilation modes) refers to inspiratory times greater than expiratory times (i.e. 2:1 up to 4:1). Normal ratio is 1:2. Asthmatics usually 1:3/1:4.	In some ventilators range is continuous from 4:1 to 1:4. In others, ratios are limited (i.e. 1:1, 1:2, 1:3, etc.).	1. Allows manipulation of peak airway pressure by altering inspiratory time. 2. Allows time for complete expiration in severe asthmatics so avoiding risk of air trapping (incomplete expiration produces build up of air in lungs).	Contributes to airway pressure so alarm limits set at 40 cm, or as instructed (upper) and 5–10 cmH$_2$O below current AP reading for lower alarm.	Observe peak airway pressure for increases. • If air trapping (incomplete expiration) is suspected, inform medical staff.
Trigger/sensitivity alters the degree of effort required by patient to trigger a positive pressure breath from the ventilator.	Negative pressure inspiratory effort of -0 to 10 cmH$_2$O.	Not always quantified on ventilator, may simply range from minimum to maximum sensitivity.	1. Assists patient weaning by altering sensitivity to patient effort, thus reducing ventilator support as patient strength increases. 2. Alters the work of breathing for the patient.	None	Careful observation of patient during weaning to ensure coping with respiratory effort. ABGs to check PO_2 and PCO_2.

Table 3.15 Table of ventilatory modes

Mode	Description	Clinical use
Controlled mechanical ventilation (CMV) (a) volume-controlled, (b) pressure-controlled	(a) Pre-set tidal volume and frequency of breaths are delivered. (b) Breaths are delivered to a pre-set pressure with tidal volume varying with lung compliance.	Patient requires complete mechanical ventilatory support.
Assist/control (triggered)	Pre-set tidal volume breaths are delivered in response to a patient attempting a spontaneous breath. A back-up delivers a pre-set rate of breaths if the patient does not achieve the required rate.	Patient is able to initiate breaths but requires ventilatory assistance to maintain oxygenation and CO$_2$ removal.
Synchronized intermittent mandatory ventilation (SIMV)	Pre-set tidal volume breaths are delivered at a pre-set rate but spontaneous breaths can be taken in between and ventilator breaths are synchronized with the spontaneous breaths.	Patient is being weaned from ventilation or for greater patient comfort/reduction of sedation requirements.
Pressure support (PSV)/Assist	Following triggering by the patient a breath is delivered to a pre-set pressure level, tidal volume delivered will thus depend on lung compliance.	Patient is being weaned from ventilation or for greater patient comfort/reduction of sedation requirements.
Mandatory minute ventilation (MMV)	A pre-set minute volume is ensured by either spontaneous or ventilator breaths. One major drawback is that this may be composed of low volume, high-frequency breaths.	Patient is being weaned from ventilation.

Caused by: increased intrathoracic pressure during inspiration reduces venous return and increases right ventricular afterload. As a result, right ventricular and, consequently, left ventricular output is reduced. If PEEP is used then pressure is positive even in expiration, and may reduce venous return further according to the level of PEEP. If the patient has been greatly distressed prior to commencing mechanical ventilation there may be a sudden reduction in peripheral vascular tone related to loss of circulating catecholamines and the effects of sedation.

Treated by: Fluid filling, using 200 ml challenges over 10–15 min until stroke volume (if measured) shows no further increase. Otherwise, fill until (CVP) increases by ⩾3 mmHg after a fluid challenge and remains increased (see Chapter 5). Inotropic support may be necessary if fluid loading is not considered clinically appropriate (see Chapter 5).

Alteration of ventilatory characteristics, such as inspiratory and expiratory time, tidal volume, level of PEEP, may also be considered.

Decreased urine output

Manifested by: oliguria.

Caused by: reduction in cardiac output invoking release of antidiuretic hormone together with the renin — angiotensin — aldosterone response leading to salt and water retention.

Treated by: fluid filling as above. Close monitoring of urine output.

Increased incidence of barotrauma (trauma caused by pressure) related to higher positive airway pressures

Manifested by: high airway pressures on inspiration.

Caused by: higher pressures are required during positive pressure ventilation to force air into airways which are resistant to airflow. Damage to the lung occurs which may be manifested clinically as pneumothorax, pneumomediastinum, etc. Resistance to flow is related to the radius of the airway to the fourth power. This is particularly relevant in the asthmatic patient, where bronchoconstriction produces greatly increased resistance to flow and greatly increased airway pressures.

Treated by: manipulation of inspiratory and expiratory times for each breath and by flow rates of inspiratory gas. The aim is to keep peak airway pressures below 35–40 cmH$_2$O.

Problems associated with mechanical ventilation (Table 3.16)

Sputum clearance and airway management
The presence of an endotracheal or tracheostomy tube means that normal humidification and warming of inspired air by the upper airway tract, in particular the nasal passages, is bypassed. The delivery of dry, cold gas, often at a high flow rate, has several deleterious effects on the trachea and bronchi:

(i) Increased viscosity of mucus which may dry and crust the airways causing inflammation and ulceration.

(ii) Depressed ciliary function.

(iii) Microatelectasis from obstruction of small airways by thickened mucus.

The overall effect of this is to grossly impair movement or clearance of secretions. This may result in obstruction of major segments of lung or blockage of the tube itself.

Two other factors contribute to the problem:

(i) The decreased ability of the intubated patient to cough. This is due either to the presence of the tube itself or to suppression of the cough reflex by sedation or analgesia.

(ii) The loss of the natural periodic sigh. This is a periodic breath of increased tidal volume which occurs at regular intervals in the spontaneously ventilating patient. It expands the base of the lungs and alveoli that may not be fully expanded during normal breathing.

If the patient is dehydrated, the moisture content of the mucus will be reduced and extra humidification will be required.

The accumulation of secretions will cause airway blockage leading to atelectasis and collapse of areas of lung with an associated shunt due to limited availability for gas exchange.

The degree to which this will cause problems is related to the underlying disease process. Thus, patients with pneumonia who are producing large amounts of purulent secretions or those with cystic fibrosis or bronchiectasis will require greatly increased intervention.

Sputum clearance requires:
1. Adequate humidification.
2. Suctioning and bronchial hygiene.
3. Chest physiotherapy.
4. Systemic hydration.
Note. The underlying disease process will affect the intensity of each intervention

---

Table 3.16 Problems associated with mechanical ventilation

High airway pressure

Manifested by: Airway pressure alarm sounds, persistent rise in peak airway pressure, evidence of patient distress, haemodynamic instability.

Causes:

(a) *Life-threatening*: (i.e. investigate and rule out/treat at once)   ET (or ventilator tubing) obstruction, pneumothorax, severe bronchospasm.

(b) *Other*:   Build-up of secretions in airway.

Patient breathing out of synchronization with ventilator ('fighting').

Patient coughing.

Increased peak airway pressure resulting from a tidal volume set too high for patient, or inspiratory time set too short, or addition of PEEP.

Displacement of the ET tube either:

(a) *downwards* – causing coughing from irritation of the carina or usually slipping down the right main bronchus and meeting smaller airways with increased resistance,

(b) *upwards* – causing cuff herniation through the larynx, resulting in patient discomfort and agitation.

Intervention:

1. If patient is severely compromised remove from ventilator and manually ventilate using rebreathe bag and 100% oxygen. Assess lung compliance (the degree of resistance to inspiration) and symmetry of inflation while bagging. Call for senior and medical help.

2. Perform suction to clear any secretions and to determine whether tube is patent. If secretions are very thick review humidification and instil 2–3 ml normal saline down ET tube prior to suctioning. Repeat as necessary.

3. If the cause is complete obstruction of the ET tube emergency re-intubation will be necessary. If there is no one immediately available to re-intubate it is possible to ventilate the patient following extubation using a Guedel airway and tight-fitting facemask with manual ventilation. It is important to have the patient's neck resting on one pillow and to lift the jaw forwards to maintain a patent airway. If trained and proficient in its use, a laryngeal mask is an alternative to either re-intubation or facemask bagging.

4. Auscultate lungs for signs of wheezing, reduction in air entry, and altered breath sounds.

5. If the cause is a pneumothorax and there is cardiovascular compromise immediate insertion of a chest drain or large needle will be necessary (by medical staff) to allow relief of tension (for details see chest drains, p. 73).

6. If the patient is stable, attempt to ascertain the cause of increased airway pressure.

7. Reassure and attempt to alleviate any cause of distress if the patient is restless and distressed by ventilation ('fighting'). This is suggested by tachypnoea, breathing out of synchronization with the ventilator, and continually coughing or gagging.

8. Check blood gases if restlessness and distress continues and/or peripheral oxygen saturation remains low. Increase F_iO_2 and consult with medical staff.

9. If the patient is restless and unable to settle on the ventilator but otherwise cardiovascularly stable with appropriate blood gases, review sedation and inform senior or medical staff if an increase $\pm$ paralysis is indicated.

10. Review ventilator settings and discuss with senior or medical staff if settings seem inappropriate or addition of PEEP appears to have caused a problem.

Low airway pressure

Manifested by: Sounds of air leak, decreased expired minute volume (MV), low airway pressure reading.

Causes:

(a) *Life-threatening*: Disconnection or major leak from the ventilator, burst cuff on endotracheal/tracheostomy tube.

(b) *Other*: Leak in the ventilator circuits, loss of seal on cuff, bronchopleural fistula (with massive air leak through chest drain), ventilator dysfunction.

Table 3.16 *contd*

Intervention:	1. Check the patient is attached to the ventilator.
	2. Check connections on ventilator tubing for leaks, tears, or cracks.
	3. Check cuff pressure to ensure a seal is present. Use cuff pressure manometer to check the cuff pressure is less than 30 mmHg. If the leak continues inflate cuff further if necessary.
	4. Check inspired tidal volume to ensure the ventilator is delivering its set amount.
	5. Check ventilator function.
	6. Check levels set for pressure alarm limits are appropriate.
	7. If low airway pressure continues and the tidal volume is not being delivered the ET tube or the ventilator may need changing. Manually ventilate the patient and inform senior nursing or medical staff.

Low minute volume

Manifested by: Low MV alarm sounding, MV read-out shows less than set MV, audible cuff leak, patient may appear distressed and haemodynamically compromised, oxygen saturation may drop and the patient may appear cyanosed.

Causes:

(a) *Life-threatening*: Disconnection from the ventilator, inappropriate ventilator settings (i.e. flow rate may be too low to allow set volume in time allocated by set respiratory rate, hole in ventilator tubing).

(b) *Other*: Leak caused by tubing connections working loose, loss of seal on cuff, presence of bronchopleural fistula with chest drain *in situ*.

Intervention:
1. Unless the cause of low MV is immediately apparent, manually ventilate patient.
2. Check ventilator tubing from machine to patient, testing connections, and looking for holes
3. Review ventilator settings to ensure MV is capable of being delivered and that ventilator is not malfunctioning.
4. Auscultate the trachea to detect any leak around the cuff. Refill cuff as before.
5. Monitor air leak through chest drain if present. If increased inform medical staff. Ventilation may have to be increased or altered to allow for leak.

High minute volume

Manifested by: Sounding of high MV alarms, patient making respiratory effort.

Causes:

(a) *Life-threatening*: Possible ventilator malfunction.

(b) *Other*: Patient making respiratory effort which is excessive, inappropriate ventilator settings.

Intervention:
1. Check causes of patient's tachypnoea such as pain, hypoxia, hypercapnia.
2. Review ventilator settings with senior and/or medical staff.

Hypoxaemia

Manifested by: Peripheral O_2 saturation $< 90\%$, arterial blood gases show fall in PO_2 to below 8–10 kPa, patient is restless (unless heavily sedated $\pm$ paralysed), tachycardic, possibly hypotensive, and cyanosed.

Causes:

(a) *Life-threatening*: Pneumothorax, pulmonary embolus, sputum plug, or other body obstructing major airway, severe haemodynamic compromise, severe bronchospasm, severe pulmonary oedema, ventilator malfunction.

(b) *Other*: Build-up of thick secretions, increase in severity of disease, atelectasis, bronchospasm, repositioning of patient causing increase in shunt, leak in ventilator tubing, patient 'fighting' ventilator, pulmonary oedema.

Intervention:
1. If hypoxaemia is severe and/or causing haemodynamic compromise ventilate patient on 100% oxygen. Call for help.
2. Check ventilator is delivering set ventilation and that alarm limits are appropriate.
3. Check arterial blood gases and ensure that pulse oximeter is picking up a good signal.

Table 3.16 *contd*

High minute volume
contd

4. Auscultate chest for air entry and abnormal breath sounds, depending on findings, suction and/or chest physiotherapy may be necessary. Observe symmetry of lung movement and consider pneumothorax.
5. Ascertain cause of hypoxaemia — reposition patient if recently placed on side, in consultation with medical staff consider need for chest X-ray, review haemodynamic causes such as decreased cardiac output. Review need for further sedation.
6. In consultation with medical staff, ventilator settings such as F_iO_2, tidal volume, I:E ratio, etc., may be altered.

Hypercapnia
Manifested by:

$PCO_2 > 6.0$ kPa, patient appears restless and agitated with tachypnoea if on weaning modes or possibly showing signs of respiratory effort if on controlled ventilation.

Note. Habitual CO_2 retainers (chronic COAD, etc.) may tolerate or even require much higher levels of CO_2 to maintain normal pH values as renal compensation will have adjusted for levels of bicarbonate. In patients with severe pulmonary disease, such as ARDS where there is risk of further lung damage with the high airway pressures necessary to reduce PCO_2, it may be preferable to tolerate high levels of CO_2 providing acidosis is adequately compensated ('permissive hypercapnia').

Causes:
Life-threatening:

No urgently life-threatening causes but long-term uncorrected hypercapnia may cause severe metabolic problems.

Other:

Inadequate MV either from patient if in weaning modes or ventilator settings. Compensation for metabolic alkalosis, carbohydrate overload, or increased CO_2 related to increased metabolic rate (see Chapter 10), air trapping (intrinsic or autoPEEP).

Intervention:

1. Ensure the patient is receiving the set mv or if weaning, that the patient is achieving the MV required.
2. Check air entry and perform suction to discount any sputum plugging or obstruction.
3. Review ventilator settings with medical staff and alter MV if necessary. A decrease in ventilation may be necessary if the patient is air-trapping.

Autopeep (intrinsic PEEP, air-trapping)
Manifested by:

Failure of alveolar pressure to return to zero at the end of exhalation (Pepe and Marini 1982). Increased resistance to airflow and increased work of breathing.

Causes:

Incomplete/impeded exhalation either as a result of high MV (> 10 l/min) or in respiratory or cardiac disease, particularly chronic airway limitation (Ruggles 1995).

Interventions:

1. Ensure low-compressible volume ventilator tubing is used.
2. Review ventilator settings with medical staff and decrease MV by decreasing respiratory rate or alter inspiratory flow rate to decrease inspiratory time and increase expiratory time.
3. Reduce metabolic workload to reduce respiratory demand.

---

1. Humidification

Ideally, the chosen method of humidification should:

(i) allow inspired gas to be delivered to the trachea at 32–36 °C with a water content of 33–43 g/m^3,

(ii) be a simple and easy to use device,

(iii) be adaptable for a variety of methods of oxygen therapy and ventilation,

(iv) avoid any increase in airway resistance or compliance,

(v) avoid any added risk of infection.

Types of humidification available:

Heat/moisture exchangers (HMEs)

These are filters which are hygroscopic on the patient side and hydrophobic on the gas source side. (Fig. 3.8.)

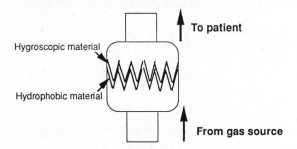

Fig. 3.8 Heat/moisture exchanger.

The hygroscopic material picks up moisture and heat from the patient's exhaled breath which is then transferred to the inhaled gas as the patient inspires.

Advantages:

- Decreased infection risk (many HMEs are bacteriostatic).
- Light and disposable.

Disadvantages:

- The level of humidification available is fixed and may be insufficient for high gas flow rates or very thick secretions.
- The presence of the HME may increase resistance to air flow in the circuit.

Nebulizers

These devices deliver aerosolized water particles. They are produced by:

- A jet of gas passed through a film of fluid or creating a suction and fine spray from a reservoir.
- A spinning disk which creates droplets using centrifugal force.
- Ultrasonic frequency-vibrating transducers.

The droplets produced are deposited in the upper airway, bronchi, and alveoli depending on their size. Particles smaller than 1 μm reach the alveoli, those of 5 μm are deposited in the bronchi, and those of 7–10 μm are deposited in the upper airway (Oh 1990, p.172).

Advantages:

- The amount of humidification can be increased and decreased according to patient need.

- The quantity of water delivered is not limited by temperature and with ultrasonic nebulizers supersaturation is possible.
- Delivery of topical medication is possible.

Disadvantages:

- Risk of infection is higher from bacterial contamination of the water (sterile water should always be used).
- Gross overhydration is possible, particularly in ultrasonic nebulizers where supersaturation may occur.
- There may be increased airway resistance due to the presence of the nebulizer in the circuit.

Hot water bath humidifiers

Gas is driven over or through a heated water bath. Humidity can only be achieved at temperatures between 45–60 °C. As the humidified gas passes through the tubing to the patient it cools and condenses producing a gas at about 37 °C which is fully saturated.

Advantages:

- Effective and efficient humidification.

Disadvantages:

- Infection is a hazard. Water temperatures of 45 °C provide an effective growth medium for contaminating bacteria such as *Pseudomonas pyocyneus*. Temperatures must be maintained near the 60 °C level to limit growth of contaminants. Water bath and tubing must be changed every 24 hours.
- Efficiency is not constant and may be altered by gas flow, water temperature, and surface area of vaporizing surface.
- There is a risk of scalding the airway. Thermostatic control and temperature sensors situated at the patient end of the circuit are vital.

Cold water humidifiers

Gas from an oxygen flowmeter passes via a Venturi system allowing alteration of oxygen concentration through a water reservoir. Most types are disposable and provide oxygen concentrations from 28% to 60%, although these are not reliable at high minute volumes. The oxygen is only partially humidified, depending on gas flow rates, but is not completely saturated.

Instillation of normal saline

Boluses of normal saline (3–5 ml) instilled into the

trachea may be used as an adjunct to other forms of humidification. They are thought to be helpful in conjunction with suction and chest physiotherapy for clearing secretions by thinning them (Bostick and Wendelgass 1987). However, the evidence for this is equivocal and an association with decreased P_aO_2 has been suggested (Ackerman 1993). There may also be lower airway contamination with upper airway organisms (Hegler and Traver 1994). Further research is required, but this method remains a useful adjunct to suction and physiotherapy.

2. Suctioning and bronchial hygiene

Removal of secretions using a suction catheter placed in the trachea is essential for maintaining airway patency. It may be performed intermittently when evidence of secretions in the large airways are heard as crackles or wheezes, or routinely in conjunction with chest physiotherapy.

An important precaution in suctioning borderline hypoxaemic patients is the use of pre-oxygenation using 100% oxygen and hyperinflation (Mancinelli-Van Atta and Beck 1992; Stone *et al.* 1989).

The deleterious effects of suctioning include:

- decreased S_vO_2 (mixed venous oxygen saturation) due to falls in cardiac output and arterial oxygen saturation (Clark *et al.* 1990),

- decreased P_aO_2,

- cardiac arrhythmias associated with vagal stimulation and hypoxia,

- microatelectasis,

- haemodynamic instability,

- increased intracranial pressure,

- laryngospasm (in the non-intubated patient),

- bronchoconstriction,

- tissue damage, haemorrhage.

Some of these problems can be reduced by the use of hyperoxygenation (usually 100%) for 1–2 minutes prior to suctioning and the use of controlled hyperinflation (1.5 times tidal volume; Stone *et al.* 1989) either via a manual resuscitation bag, rebreathe bag, or via the ventilator.

Safety principles

- Suction levels should be set below 26.6 kPa (200

mmHg) and preferably around 13.3–16 kPa (100–120 mmHg) to minimize trauma associated with suction.

- Hyperinflation should commence 3–5 breaths prior to suctioning and for 1–2 breaths after the last suction catheter is passed. This is to re-open any alveoli which may have been collapsed by the negative suction pressure.

- The technique should be aseptic:

  - Hand-washing prior to the procedure.

  - Catheters should be sterile and inserted only once prior to discarding (see later for exceptions).

  - Clean or sterile disposable gloves should be used with each catheter.

- The correct size of suction catheter is important. It should not exceed one-half of the internal diameter of the endotracheal tube.

- The catheter should be inserted to just above the carina if trauma to the trachea is to be minimized. In some patients, it may be necessary to insert the catheter further; it will usually pass into the right main bronchus due to the anatomy of the bronchi.

- Suction should be applied only as the catheter is withdrawn using a rotating movement to limit drag on the tracheal wall.

- The whole procedure of insertion and withdrawal should not take longer than 30 seconds (suction itself should be less than 15 seconds), otherwise the patient may experience hypoxaemia and distress.

- Observation of ECG and S_pO_2 (if pulse oximetry is in use) should be continuous during the procedure

- Catheters used should have an end hole and more than one side hole. A single side hole is more likely to cause tracheal trauma.

The experience is most unpleasant for the patient and has been described as feeling like choking or loss of breath (Bergbom-Engberg and Haljamäe 1989). It should therefore be performed as briefly and effectively as possible to maximize efficacy and minimize trauma.

3. Chest physiotherapy

The use of a number of techniques, such as vibration, postural drainage, percussion, and hyperinflation can all improve clearance of secretions. These techniques should

be taught by an experienced physiotherapist and practised under guidance.

Vibration

The chest wall is shaken using two hands at a frequency
of about 200 per minute throughout patient exhalation.
It is designed to loosen and move secretions into the
major airways where they can be coughed up or suctioned out.

Postural drainage

Movement of secretions using gravity by altering the
patient's position so that different areas of the lung are
drained.

Note. Remember there is increased perfusion to the
dependent lung so that the shunt/venous admixture may
increase if the dependent lung has very poor air entry.

Percussion

This technique is infrequently used in critically ill
patients because of the incidence of arrhythmias and
other problems of haemodynamic instability. It is
performed in association with postural drainage. Loosening and movement of secretions may be helped by
beating cupped hands (gently at first) over the patient's
chest from the least dependent to the most dependent
area.

Hyperinflation

Delivery of a breath to the patient which is approximately 1.5 times the tidal volume of the patient. A
rebreathing or manual ventilation bag is commonly
used to hyperinflate the lungs although some ventilators (e.g. Puritan Bennett 7200) have a hyperinflation
facility. The purpose of hyperinflation is to re-expand
collapsed areas of lung by introducing larger volume
breaths. Care must be taken to limit the airway
pressures generated by these larger breaths. The safest
method using the manual ventilation bag is to position
a manometer (pressure gauge) within the manual
ventilation bag circuit and to limit pressure generated
to less than 40 cmH_2O. The standard manual ventilation bag has a volume of about 2 litres (l) as it is
necessary to provide a reservoir of gas plus a flow rate
of 15 l/min or more. The potential volume possible in
each breath is therefore considerably larger than necessary to provide 1.5 times the normal tidal volume.
Thus, the full volume of the bag should not be used as
a guide for the size of the breath to be delivered.
During the procedure the patient's chest should be
observed to ensure inflation with the bag produces a
rise followed by a fall during deflation.

4. Patient needs

All of the above techniques involve discomfort and
distress for the patient. It should be a nursing
priority that the patient is given full explanation
prior to any intervention and as much information
as possible to explain the necessity of carrying out
these procedures.

The patient's co-operation should always be sought as
this will lessen the negative nature of these unpleasant
procedures.

Communication difficulties

These problems affect the patient themselves, the family,
and the staff who care for them.

The first priority is to explain the cause to the patient
and reassure them that it is a temporary situation which
will revert when the tube is removed. Alternative methods of communication must be sought and established so
that both patient, family, and carers become familiar
with the methods that work best.

The presence of an endotracheal or tracheostomy tube
tends to reduce communication to closed questions
requiring only a positive or negative answer. This is
obviously extremely limiting and should only be a
temporary measure until the patient can adopt an alternative method.

It is vital that the amount of information/communica-
tion offered by staff and family to the patient is not
limited and encompasses more rather than less than
would normally be communicated.

Methods of non-verbal communication

- The patient's family will need encouragement and help
  to continue talking to their relative as though they are
  able to reply fully, particularly with regard to expressing their thoughts and feelings to them.

- The speech therapy department are invaluable in
  providing assistance and technical aid and should be
  contacted early for the long-term patient. They are also
  able to assist with any swallowing or upper airway
  problems associated with the complications of tracheostomy and endotracheal tube.

- The family need involvement in determining topics of
  interest to the patient; provision of newspapers, radio,
  tapes, television, etc., will all assist the patient to
  remain in touch.

Psychological problems associated with intubation and ventilation

Most patients on ventilatory support or requiring intensive care have greatly increased levels of anxiety and stress. This is discussed in detail in Chapter 2.

Factors contributing to psychological problems

- discomfort
- fear
- loss of control
- disorientation
- disease pathology

Nutrition

This will be discussed in detail in Chapter 10, on gastrointestinal problems. Obviously, a standard oral diet is impossible for the intubated patient, although patients with tracheostomies may manage very well, particularly if the cuff can be deflated during meals. Alternative forms of nutritional support, including enteral and parenteral feeding must be utilized. The effects of malnutrition on the critically ill patient are severe and efforts should be made to establish appropriate levels of intake as soon as possible.

In the patient who is weaning from ventilation, particular problems can be encountered:

(i) Overfeeding of carbohydrate will cause the body to lay down fat stores. This process produces considerably more CO_2 than that produced by the breakdown of food for energy. The patient must therefore increase his/her minute volume in order to remove the excess CO_2. This will increase the workload the patient must perform and may prove too much for weakened respiratory muscles. In these circumstances provision of half of the non-protein calories as fat should be substituted.

(ii) Depletion of important minerals and trace elements, such as zinc, magnesium and phosphate, will also have a deleterious effect on respiratory muscle function. Repletion of muscle mass is not possible without these minerals thus respiratory muscle degeneration will not improve if supply is inadequate.

(iii) Patients exhibiting the septic response (i.e. fever, high levels of urinary nitrogen excretion, high metabolic rate; see Chapter 14), seem unable to utilize nutrition to regenerate depleted muscle mass and weaning should only be attempted slowly.

(iv) Malnourished patients have an increased risk of developing pneumonia and other complications due to the associated dysfunction of the immune system and the possible limitation of surfactant production seen with fatty acid deficiency.

(v) Malnutrition is associated with a reduced diaphragmatic mass, reduced maximal voluntary ventilation, and reduced respiratory muscle strength. All of these will seriously detract from the patient's ability to wean from the ventilator. Patients who do not require ventilatory support may also have problems maintaining adequate nutritional intake when they have oxygen masks *in situ* and experience dyspnoea when attempting to eat.

Strategies to assist the breathless patient to eat include:

- nasal cannulae to continue oxygen delivery during meals
- nutritional supplements such as high calorie (fat and carbohydrate) drinks
- small, frequent, nutritious and tempting(!) meals
- upright and comfortable positioning to eat
- thoughtful timing of meals (i.e. not just after physiotherapy!).

Increased infection risk

The presence of a 'foreign body' in the airway increases the likelihood of infection in a number of ways.

(i) The tube bypasses normal physical and physiological mechanisms of resistance such as cilia and mucous membrane of the upper airways.

(ii) Trauma associated with the presence of the tube and suctioning provides a portal for bacterial colonization. In addition the cuff of the tube is not a perfect seal and secretions from upper airways and gastric regurgitation may trickle into the lungs.

(iii) The need for interventions such as suctioning require scrupulous attention to aseptic principles in order to avoid direct delivery of any bacterial contamination to the bronchi and respiratory lobules.

(iv) Critically ill patients are usually already greatly at risk from infection due to the high level of instrumentation (cannulae etc penetrating the body for access and monitoring). They also frequently have a compromised immune response due to the underlying pathology.

Alternative modes of ventilation and respiratory support

Inverse ratio ventilation

This technique consists of reversing the normal inspiratory–expiratory ratio and controlling the inspiratory gas flow by: (i) limiting the airway pressure; (ii) slowing or decelerating the rate of inspiratory flow; or (iii) adding an additional end-inspiratory pause.

Two methods are generally used to administer inverse ratio ventilation:

(1) The ventilator is time-cycled with a pre-set inspiratory pressure limit and a long inspiratory phase. This is pressure-controlled inverse ratio ventilation (PC-IRV).

(2) The ventilator is volume-cycled with an end inspiratory pause and a slow or decelerating inspiratory flow rate. This is volume-controlled inverse ratio ventilation (VC-IRV).

Both methods ensure that inspiration occurs when there is still expiratory flow and therefore some degree of autoPEEP is maintained at the end of the expiratory phase.

Advantages of VC-IRV include:

(i) availability of this mode on all adult ventilators,

(ii) the delivery of a guaranteed tidal volume

(iii) precise manipulation of the inspiratory flow pattern,

(iv) decreased peak inspiratory flow rates with similar or lower shear force (Marcy and Marini 1991).

Disadvantages include:

changes in peak alveolar pressures may occur and may exceed the optimal level if peak inflation pressures are not carefully monitored.

Advantages of PC-IRV include:

possibly better gas distribution than constant flow VC-IRV due to the decelerating flow pattern.

Disadvantages of PC-IRV include:

(i) variation in tidal volume delivered with alterations to respiratory system compliance and resistance,

(ii) opposing pressure exerted by any level of auto-PEEP may reduce volume delivered,

(iii) compared with VC-IRV greater shear forces may be generated by the fast flow associated with the beginning of inspiration; this may contribute to tissue injury (Marcy and Marini 1991).

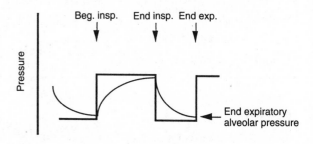

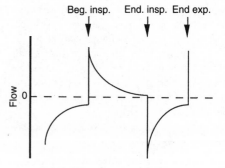

Fig. 3.9 Pressure and flow in pressure-controlled inverse ratio ventilation (= airway pressure; = alveolar pressure). (After Marcy and Matin 1991.)

Limitations of inverse ratio ventilation

(1) The breathing pattern imposed (I:E ratio of greater than 1:1) is difficult for a patient to tolerate unless well sedated and/or paralysed.

(2) Air trapping can occur in alveoli with high expiratory resistance leading to hyperinflation and possibly an increased incidence of barotrauma.

(3) In PC-IRV, the longer inspiratory time allows equilibration between alveolar and airway pressure causing an increase in peak alveolar pressure compared to volume controlled ventilation where peak airway pressure always exceeds alveolar pressure.

(4) Rises in mean airway pressure and autoPEEP may affect cardiac output and venous return as well as increasing right ventricular afterload.

Other measures for supporting respiration

In the situation where conventional ventilation is unable to support adequate PO_2 levels and ensure CO_2 excretion (even allowing for some permissive hypercapnia) there are two possible further options:

(1) High-frequency ventilation.

(2) Extracorporeal respiratory support, for example, extracorporeal membrane oxygenation (ECMO), extracorporeal carbon dioxide removal ($ECCO_2R$), and intravenous oxygenation (IVOX).

High-frequency ventilation

This refers to a group of ventilatory techniques incorporating ventilation frequencies of greater than 60–2000 breaths/minute and tidal volumes of between 1 and 5 ml/kg. Delivery requires a specialized ventilator, as conventional ventilators provide an insufficient tidal volume at high frequencies due to compression of gas within the ventilator itself. There are three types of high-frequency ventilation:

(1) high-frequency positive pressure ventilation (HFPPV),

(2) high-frequency jet ventilation (HFJV),

(3) high-frequency oscillation (HFO).

Currently, only HFJV is used in more than a few specialist centres so this is the only technique that will be described. Further details on HFPPV and HFO can be found in Villar and Slutsky (1991).

High-frequency jet ventilation (HFJV)

High-pressure air and oxygen are blended and supplied via a pneumatic valve or an electronic solenoid valve to a non-compliant injection system. The normal pressure of this gas after loss within the ventilator and blender is around 2.5 atmospheres (atm) and this is known as the driving pressure. This can be adjusted to alter the rate of flow from the maximum (2.5 atm) down to zero. In most injection systems gas entrainment is caused by the accelerating jet. This is provided for by an additional

circuit across a T-piece attached to the endotracheal tube. The entrainment circuit should provide at least 30 l/min of warmed and humidified gas at the same oxygen concentration as that delivered by the jet system. The circuit is open allowing entrainment and expiration

The usual frequency set is between 100 and 200 breaths/minute delivering tidal volumes of 2–5 ml/kg.

In an entrainment system, the tidal volume delivered by the ventilator increases with driving pressure and decreases with respiratory frequency. It remains the same with alterations in I:E ratio.

Indications for the use of high-frequency jet ventilation
(1) Bronchopleural fistula where air leak flow causes failure of conventional ventilation.
(2) Severe acute respiratory failure with high airway pressures and reduced respiratory compliance.
(3) Acute respiratory failure with circulatory shock.
(4) Emergency situations during which tracheal intubation is impossible.
(5) Synchronized with systole during acute ventricular failure to decrease LV afterload.
(6) During anaesthesia in order to minimize movement of lung fields, to allow clear access to respiratory tract surgery and to limit stone movement during lithotripsy.

Humidification
The pressure drop between driving pressure and mean airway pressure results in marked cooling of the gas within the trachea. Thus the temperature of the gases within the connecting tube has to be above 60 °C in order to reach a temperature of 37 °C within the trachea. The most effective method of humidification is the hot-plate vaporizer. A continuous infusion rate of distilled water is vaporized at 100 °C and delivered to the connecting tube during each expiratory phase. The quantity of water in ml/hour required to achieve 100% humidity can be determined by multiplying the minute volume by 2.64:

$$(H_2O \ ml/h) = \frac{MV \ (l/min) \times 60 \times 44}{1000}$$

Injection systems for high-frequency jet ventilation
There are two commonly used injection systems. One uses cannulae of approximately 4–5 cm length inserted through the adapter fixed to the standard endotracheal or tracheal tube. The other uses a special jet endotracheal

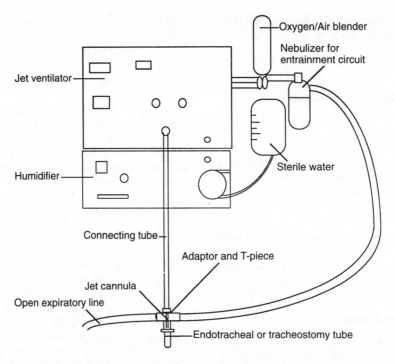

Fig. 3.10 Circuit for high frequency jet ventilation.

tube with two additional channels to the lumen of the tube. One ends 6 cm before the distal tip and is used to insufflate the jet gas and the other enables monitoring of airway pressure. There are two advantages to the distal point of jet delivery in the special jet tube:

(i) Anatomical dead space is reduced.

(ii) gas entrainment reduces, representing only 25% of the tidal volume.

This mode of ventilation has advantages for specific groups of patients but as yet there is no evidence that there is any improvement in survival or length of stay in patients who are ventilated with HFJV. It requires considerable skill to maintain a patient successfully on HFJV and as such this mode of ventilation is used only in a minority of ICUs for problem patients with specific disorders.

Extracorporeal respiratory support

Extracorporeal membrane oxygenation (ECMO) was first reported by Hill *et al.* (1972). The technique consists of an extracorporeal circuit incorporating a membrane with high surface area, a gas flow of variable percentage oxygen/air, and a blood pump. ECMO is defined as an extracorporeal system requiring 50% of cardiac output to pass via a venoarterial circuit. Exposure of venous blood to the membrane allows some oxygenation and removal of carbon dioxide across the membrane using concentration gradients. It is theoretically possible to provide adequate oxygenation and removal of CO_2 but in practice, it is usual to supplement oxygenation with mechanical ventilation of 8–12 breaths/min and F_iO_2 of <0.5.

Extracorporeal carbon dioxide removal ($ECCO_2R$) aims only to remove CO_2 by the extracorporeal circuit at flow rates of only 20–30% of cardiac output. Oxygenation is provided by apnoeic oxygenation (a continuous flow of oxygen with a respiratory rate of zero) or tracheal insufflation of oxygen (100% oxygen is delivered into the trachea via a cannula inserted to just above the carina). Some oxygen can be delivered across the extracorporeal membrane as above depending on the patient's need. Carbon dioxide can be removed through a low blood flow–high gas flow circuit as it has a much higher solubility coefficient than oxygen. The main goal of this support is to avoid elevated peak airway pressures and F_iO_2 and to abolish specific hyperventilation. Atelectasis is avoided by the use of low-frequency positive pressure ventilation (LFPPV) at a rate of 3–4 breaths/min with a limited peak airway pressure (35–45 cmH_2O) and a constant level of PEEP (20–30 cmH_2O). The theory behind the use of $ECCO_2R$ is that it will lessen further lung injury and allow time for the diseased lungs to heal.

Cannulation is usually venovenous using large (34 FG) catheters in femoral-femoral or femoral-jugular positions.

Complications

Bleeding is the most frequent complication due to the need for systemic anticoagulation to preserve the extracorporeal circuits. Heparin is infused to maintain activated clotting times (ACT) of 180–200 seconds. However, the development of heparin-bonded circuits have reduced the risk of bleeding considerably.

Infection risk is high due to the highly invasive nature of the system and scrupulous aseptic precautions are necessary, particularly if extracorporeal support continues for several days.

IVOX (intravascular oxygenator)

IVOX refers to an intravascular blood gas exchanger which consists of approximately 1000 hollow fibres which are positioned in the venae cavae. The tip lies in the superior vena cava and the bottom just above the junction of the inferior vena cava and iliac veins. When unfurled, the network of hollow fibres lie free in the venae cavae bloodstream and 100% oxygen is drawn through the fibres allowing gas exchange to occur across the membrane along the concentration gradients. P_vCO_2 is thus lowered and P_vO_2 increased.

Limitations

The small surface area of gas transfer membrane available within the venae cavae means that only one-quarter to one-third of the oxygen and carbon dioxide gas transfer requirements of most adult patients can be met (Vaca *et al.* 1993). No major improvements in blood gases have been consistently noted (Kallis *et al.* 1993).

The device can only safely be left *in situ* for 7–19 days.

Systemic anticoagulation is still required and can limit its application in some patient groups. Bleeding and thrombosis are potential problems.

The patient must have adequately sized and obstruction-free venae cavae to allow access to the current size of the device.

Further improvements in the device may enhance the use of this technique which is in the early stages of clinical evaluation. However, current results do not support its general use at present.

Weaning from mechanical ventilation

The majority of patients who are mechanically ventilated have little difficulty weaning once the disease process has been resolved. However, a small but significant group of patients prove difficult to reduce support and may never wean completely. This group includes patients with chronic airflow limitation, neuropathies, or respiratory paralysis such as myasthenia gravis, poor left ventricular function, complications following post-abdominal, and cardiac surgery (see Chapter 7), and prolonged ventilation.

Short-term weaning

- The decision to wean is made following assessment of the patient's physiological and physical status.

- The precipitating illness/factor should be resolved and the patient's haemodynamic and respiratory status should be stable. The patient should be able to make respiratory efforts and have an intact cough reflex.

- Weaning criteria may be of use (see Table 3.16) but the clinical state of the patient is as important.

- Weaning should start during the day.

- The patient should have a full explanation with the opportunity to ask any questions.

- The patient should be suctioned and made comfortable in a sitting position to allow expansion of lung bases.

- A T-piece with accurate oxygen delivery from a humidified source is attached.

- Close observation and monitoring of ECG and pulse oximetry should continue throughout the weaning period.

- Quarter-hourly respiratory rate, and tidal volume should be recorded with arterial blood gases after 20 minutes.

- If all is well after 20–30 minutes the patient is extubated.

- If the patient has not weaned after 30 minutes, CPAP with 5 cmH_2O PEEP should be attached (to compensate for the loss of laryngeal PEEP).

- If sputum clearance is a problem the patient may manage with a minitracheostomy.

Table 3.17 Factors likely to prevent weaning

- Sepsis
- Increased CO_2 production
- Electrolyte/fluid imbalance
- Decreased magnesium and phosphate levels
- Pain
- Haemodynamic instability
- Metabolic alkalosis
- Extreme malnutrition
- Untreated/unresolved respiratory problems
- Sedation
- Heart failure
- High intra-abdominal pressures
- Neurological factors such as reduced conscious level

Methods of weaning

Currently there are four methods of weaning used for long-term ventilated patients. These are IMV, MMV, PSV, and CPAP (see Tables 3.11 and 3.15). Occasionally, intermittent spontaneous breathing through a T-piece may be used.

1. If possible, the factors listed in Table 3.17 should be resolved or optimized prior to attempting weaning.

2. The first six steps of short-term weaning also apply to long-term weaning.

3. In the ventilation modes of weaning, safety is maintained by the usual ventilator alarms for apnoea, etc. However, continuous monitoring of ECG and S_aO_2 with regular arterial blood gases is important to monitor the patient.

4. If CPAP is instigated, close observation and monitoring of the patient is essential for signs of distress. ECG and pulse oximetry must be continuous. Respiratory rate, tidal, and minute volumes must be recorded quarter-hourly until the patient is evidently stable and coping with the weaning mode.

5. A full record of weaning attempts and achievement should be kept and referred to so that a logical, consistent, and structured approach can be continued.

6. The level of support provided by the chosen weaning method is gradually reduced until the patient is able to breathe without support (other than that required to overcome ventilator resistance) for more than 24 hours.

7. The patient is extubated and may be placed on mask CPAP or oxygen via mask. Observation at this point should be as per point (4).

Long-term weaning is frequently a trial and error situation with limited progress frequently followed by a set-back. No one weaning method has been shown to produce consistently superior results and each individual patient is different. The patient's psychological state has a marked effect on his/her ability to wean and a positive attitude should be fostered and maintained.

Specific respiratory problems

Pneumothorax and bronchopleural fistula

A pneumothorax is the presence of air between the visceral and parietal pleura. It occurs when trauma or a spontaneous rupture results in a hole between the alveolar or bronchial wall and the pleura, allowing air to escape into the pleural space. The loss of an area of lung for gas exchange can severely compromise patients whose lung function is already limited.

Tension pneumothorax

A tension pneumothorax can develop when the rupture in the alveolar wall acts as a one-way valve. Thus, air escapes into the pleural space on inspiration but cannot return into the lung on expiration. A build-up of air within the pleural space occurs which rapidly increases in pressure until the lung on the affected side is collapsed. Displacement of the mediastinal structures towards the unaffected lung then occurs. The clinical effects of this are life-threatening and immediate.

Clinical effects of tension pneumothorax:

- Tachycardia and rise in blood pressure followed by a fall in blood pressure as the cardiac output decreases. This is due to the rise in intrathoracic pressure which impedes venous return and compresses the heart.

- Cyanosis, respiratory distress, and agitation. If the patient is being monitored by pulse oximetry the O_2 saturation will be seen to fall rapidly.

- If ventilated, airway pressures will increase dramatically, and expired minute volume may fall.

- If not treated, cardiovascular collapse and cardiac arrest will occur.

On examination, the patient will have unilateral chest movement. Air entry and breath sounds will be greatly decreased on the affected side. There will be a displaced apex beat and hyper-resonance on percussion.

Bronchopleural fistula

A fistula connecting lung and pleural space will produce the same effect as a pneumothorax. It is, however, less likely to close spontaneously and may require surgical intervention.

Intervention:

Tension pneumothorax

This is an emergency situation and help must be sought immediately. Relief of the tension by percutaneous insertion of a large gauge needle or a 12/14 g IV cannula is performed as an emergency measure. Patients on positive pressure ventilation cannot suck in air through the needle or cannula unless they are making spontaneous breathing efforts. A chest drain is then inserted and attached to underwater seal drainage (see below).

Pneumothorax

If the pneumothorax is not life-threatening the diagnosis and position will be confirmed by CXR and a drain can then be inserted (by medical staff) in an appropriate position under aseptic conditions.

It is possible for other fluids, including effusions, to occupy the pleural space. Treatment is by needle aspiration or insertion of a chest drain or pigtail catheter.

Insertion and care of underwater seal chest drains

Chest drains are inserted into the pleural space to allow one-way drainage of:

- air,
- blood,
- pleural effusions,
- parenteral feed and other infusions,
- chyle (digested fat drained by the lymphatic system),
- empyema (pus in the pleural cavity).

Chest drains are large (18–32 FG) tubes inserted percutaneously through an intercostal space in the chest wall into the pleural space. The size of the chest drain will depend on what is to be drained, the largest sizes being required for the drainage of blood. The technique requires an aseptic procedure to cut down into the chest wall and insertion of the drain. The recommended site of insertion is in the mid or posterior axillary line. The second intercostal space of the anterior chest wall in the mid-clavicular line can be used for an anterior pneumothorax.

Insertion:

1. The patient should be informed of the procedure and explanation given.

2. If awake, the patient is usually placed in a comfortable upright or semi-upright reclining position for insertion of the drain either leaning over pillows placed on a bed-table in front of him or lying on the opposite side.

3. The underwater seal system bottle is primed with an amount of sterile water sufficient to cover the drainage tube. The initial water level should be clearly marked to allow measurement of any subsequent drainage. This prevents back-flow of fluid into the pleural space.

4. As with any insertion procedure the site is cleaned and covered with sterile towels. The area is infiltrated with local anaesthetic and a skin incision is made.

5. The chest drain is then inserted without the trocar in place to reduce the risk of significant trauma. A blunt dissection technique is used to form a track through the intercostal muscles and the parietal pleura is opened. The drain is then placed through the track into the pleural space and connected to the drainage system.

6. The drain is positioned in the uppermost chest for pneumothorax and in the dependent area for drainage of fluid. When the chest drain is correctly positioned air or fluid will drain out and there will be movement of the fluid level in the drainage tube with respiration.

7. The chest drain is sutured in and to prevent any leak of air following removal of the drain a suture (purse string) may be sewn round the site of entry at this point although this is not always necessary. A dressing of either petroleum gauze, gauze soaked in collodion, or plain gauze may be applied followed by an outer air tight strapping. This will prevent air leaks and anchor the drain firmly.

8. A CXR should be taken to check the position of the drain and lung reflation.

Problems associated with insertion and drainage

(i) Puncture of the lung is possible if the drain is inserted in the wrong position and the trochar is used; for this reason, insertion is by blunt dissection.

(ii) Any blockage of the drainage system may result in a tension pneumothorax or a build-up in pressure within the pleural space. For this reason chest drains should never be clamped and drainage of a haemopneumothorax may require milking or stripping (applying pressure to the drainage tubing with a roller) to prevent obstruction from a clot.

(iii) Milking or stripping should not be carried out routinely as the negative pressures generated can be dangerously high (-100 to -400 cmH$_2$O); (Duncan and Erickson, 1982), resulting in further trauma to the lung tissue. It should be considered if there is reason to suspect obstruction of drainage by a clot (as in haemothorax and haemopneumothorax). Irrigation of the drain with saline may be prescribed in these cases.

(iv) Leaks may occur either at insertion site, connection between drain and tubing or connection between tubing and bottle. They must be secured to prevent redevelopment of the pneumothorax.

(v) Continuous bubbling of air which continues in spite of checking for leaks may indicate a bronchopleural fistula.

(vi) Suction (usually at 5 kPa) can be added should the lung fail to re-inflate despite a well-placed drain.

(vii) If drainage is greater than 1000 ml or continues at more than 200 ml for 4 hours there may be trauma to a major blood vessel. A doctor should be informed and the patient may need referral to a thoracic surgeon.

Principles of care

Securing the drain

1. Suture at time of insertion.

2. Adhesive tape to secure at insertion site and further down the chest wall.

3. Adhesive tape can also be placed round connections between drain and tubing although this may cause problems if it becomes lax and allows connections to part but remains stuck to the tubing.

Avoiding/managing leaks and obstructions

1. Check drain, tubing, drain bottle for signs of leak. Continuous bubbling not related to respiration and leakage of fluid round connections are signs of leakage. Make all connections secure and if there is still a leak examine the site itself to ensure the drain has not slipped out. Inform medical staff.

2. Check drainage for signs of obstruction. Loss of fluid swing with respiration in the drain tubing especially if accompanied by signs of distress, and lack of drainage may be signs of obstruction. These signs may also occur as the pneumothorax or haemothorax resolves, so patient condition/situation should be evaluated. Inform medical staff.

3. Do not clamp drain or tubing if the patient is ventilated. The risk of tension pneumothorax is high. Clamping for more than a few seconds is not recommended for any patient apart from post-pneumonectomy.

4. Obstruction of the drain by blood clot may need stripping or milking and possible irrigation. This should be considered with caution as the high pressures produced can cause further trauma and discomfort.

5. The drainage bottle should always be positioned below the level of the patient's chest to avoid backflow of water into the lung.

Prevention of infection

1. The dressing should be checked daily and changed if obviously wet or soiled using routine aseptic technique.

2. Hands should be washed prior to handling the drain and gloves should be worn if disconnecting or dressing is to take place.

Removal of chest drains

1. Re-expansion of the lung should be checked on X-ray following previous discontinuation of any suction. There should be no air leak or drainage.

2. There is no need to clamp drains prior to removal but suction should be discontinued just prior to removal.

3. Full explanation is given and if possible patient co-operation is obtained. Analgesia should be given in good time prior to removal to allow it to have full effect.

4. An aseptic technique is essential.

5. If a purse string suture is used, two people are needed to remove the drain. The securing suture is removed and the ends of the purse string are freed and tied loosely.

6. The drain is removed on end-inspiration to prevent indrawing of air on removal of the drain. The purse strings are pulled tight and secured.

7. An airtight dressing, such as gauze soaked in flexible collodion or petroleum gauze, under waterproof strapping is applied.

Acute respiratory distress syndrome (ARDS)

ARDS is a form of respiratory failure resulting from a variety of direct and indirect pulmonary injuries producing similar pathophysiological changes. It is the pulmonary manifestation of multi-organ dysfunction (see Chapter 14), and reflects similar changes in other organs. The lung may be affected to a greater or lesser degree. ARDS is defined by the following clinical findings:

- Diffuse acute pulmonary infitrates seen on CXR associated with decreased pulmonary compliance

- Increased alveolar–arterial oxygen difference (despite supplemental oxygen).

- Pulmonary artery wedge pressure < 18 mmHg. (i.e. non-cardiogenic factors)

- A precipitating factor (see Table 3.18).

Table 3.18 Disorders associated with ARDS

- Infection: septicaemia, pneumonia (due to various agents)
- Trauma
- Aspiration: gastric acid, hydrocarbons, near-drowning
- Inhalation: smoke, corrosive gases
- Haematological: massive blood transfusion, post-cardio-pulmonary bypass
- Metabolic: pancreatitis, acute liver failure
- Drug overdose: heroin, barbiturates
- Miscellaneous: eclampsia, amniotic fluid embolism, etc.

Pathogenesis

Regardless of the mechanism of injury, there is an increase in permeability at the alveolar-capillary membrane. This allows leak of fluid from the capillary into the interstitial space and alveolus. The result is increased stiffness of the alveolar wall, a decrease in pulmonary compliance and interference with gas exchange due to the presence of fluid between alveolus and capillary. Furthermore, activated neutrophils and platelets are deposited in the lung capillaries causing obstruction and releasing factors which cause additional disruption and damage. These processes produce hypoxaemia in spite of supplemental oxygen and a mortality rate in excess of 40%.

Management

The main thrust of therapy is directed towards removal or treatment of the precipitating factor; this will vary for each individual patient. At present, there is no treatment *per se* for ARDS, but support of respiratory function and prevention of further complications are a major part of intensive care management.

Support

Mechanical ventilation (very occasionally CPAP)

Aims:

1. Maintenance of oxygen saturations $\geqslant 90\%$ (approximate $P_aO_2 > 8.0$ kPa) with as low an F_iO_2 as possible (ideally $\leqslant 0.6$ to avoid oxygen toxicity). PEEP may be used to support this, although its effects on reducing cardiac output and oxygen delivery, and of increasing airway pressures, may prove a limiting factor.

2. Limitation of peak airway pressure by manipulation of I:E ratio (inverse ratio ventilation) and use of pressure control. This is thought to reduce associated barotrauma.

3. In extreme situations, high-frequency jet ventilation, and extracorporeal carbon dioxide removal with low-frequency ventilation may be considered. Yet strong evidence that these techniques contribute significantly to a reduction in mortality is still lacking.

Fluid management

Aims:

1. Maintenance of intravascular fluid volume.

2. Pulmonary artery wedge pressures < 18–20 mmHg should be aimed for. In the United Kingdom, colloid is usually used to achieve optimal values of stroke volume (see haemodynamics in Chapter 5).

Although inability to oxygenate is the direct cause of death in under 5% of patients, it may become necessary in some patients to maintain low intravascular fluid volumes in order to improve oxygenation by reducing extravascular lung water. Inotropes and pressors are then used to support an adequate circulation. However, preservation of normal or even supranormal oxygen delivery is generally thought more crucial and some deterioration in P_aO_2 is usually acceptable.

Maintenance of tissue oxygen delivery

Oxygen delivery depends on the patient's oxygen saturation, haemoglobin, and cardiac output. Manipulation to maintain normal or superanormal goals in order to overcome problems with tissue oxygen extraction are discussed in Chapter 14.

Avoidance of iatrogenic complications

Barotrauma: the risk is greatly increased by the decreased compliance of the lungs.

Oxygen toxicity: gas exchange may be so poor that toxic levels of oxygen are required to sustain life. However, it is important to state that no good evidence exists in human ARDS that the use of high inspired oxygen concentrations leads directly to a higher mortality. Therefore 90–100% O_2 may be required for a number of days. Even survivors requiring a prolonged high F_iO_2 usually make a complete clinical recovery, although some abnormality may remain on lung function testing.

Nosocomial infection: increased instrumentation, suppression of immune response, and other factors increase the incidence of nosocomial infection.

Removal of secretions and prevention of atelectasis

Use of chest physiotherapy, humidification, and positioning of the patient will decrease the incidence. In severe situations, bronchoscopy may be used with caution and by an operator experienced in intensive care patients.

Acute asthma

Asthma is an acute, reversible airway restriction caused by bronchospasm in response to a range of stimuli. These include allergens, infections, and exercise.

Bronchospasm invokes smooth muscle constriction, mucosal oedema, and excessive mucus production.

Management

Reduction of bronchospasm and inflammation

1. Use of bronchodilators (β_2-agonists, e.g. salbutamol). Usually inhaled but may be given IV.

2. Steroids, such as hydrocortisone or prednisolone, are used to reduce hypersensitivity, although this takes a number of hours to begin working. Beclomethasone may also be inhaled.

3. Aminophylline given IV to relax bronchial smooth muscle.

4. Anticholinergics, such as ipratropium bromide, may be inhaled to relax smooth muscle.

5. In severe cases, adrenaline can be used either subcutaneously, by nebulizer, or inserted down the endotracheal tube.

Support of respiratory function

1. Oxygen therapy: high concentrations given as necessary.

2. Humidification and fluid hydration to avoid mucus plugging.

3. Physiotherapy and bronchoscopy, if necessary.

4. CPAP.

5. Ventilation if:

    (i) P_aCO_2 is rising,

    (ii) patient is obtunded,

    (iii) patient is fatigued,

    (iv) P_aO_2 is falling,

    (v) patient does not respond to treatment.

6. Sedatives should not be given unless the patient is about to be ventilated as they can reduce the respiratory drive causing hypoventilation and precipitating respiratory failure.

7. Antibiotics are only given if there are obvious signs of infection (fever, increased white cell count).

8. Avoidance of iatrogenic complications:

    (i) Air-trapping (intrinsic PEEP, autoPEEP).
This is evidenced by rising end expiratory pressure (see Table 3.15) and can be suggested by auscultation of expiratory wheeze continuing right up to commencement of the next breath and by increased chest girth. A long expiratory time should be used either a prolonged I:E ratio (1:3) or a slow respiratory rate, with close observation of respiratory status. Occasionally, disconnection from the ventilator and manual chest decompression is required.

    (ii) Barotrauma.
Positive pressures applied to bronchoconstricted lungs with low compliance carry a high risk of barotrauma and peak airway pressures should be kept below 40 cmH$_2$O

This can be achieved with: small tidal volumes (e.g. 6–10 ml/kg), low respiratory rate (e.g. 6–10/min), long expiratory times (1:1 or longer), acceptance of hypercapnoea, providing pH is > 7.2, low inspiratory flow rates, and adequate sedation/relaxants to prevent 'fighting' (Armstrong *et al.* 1991)

    (iii) Avoidance of drugs potentially likely to stimulate histamine release (e.g. 'natural' opiates or derivatives thereof).

(iv) Sputum plugging and lobar collapse.

Rigorous chest physiotherapy and frequent bronchial hygiene with high levels of humidification will be effective in most cases. The patient's own level of hydration is also important.

In severe cases, use of halothane or other inhalational anaesthetics has been successful and intravenous ketamine as a bronchodilator has also been tried. High-dose magnesium sulphate has also been used to relax smooth muscle.

Chronic airflow limitation (CAL)

CAL is a product of chronic bronchitis, bronchiectasis, emphysema, and asthma. Most patients have a mixture of chronic bronchitis and emphysema. Acute exacerbations usually occur as a result of infection but may also be related to atmospheric pollution or surgery (use of inhalational anaesthetics). Inappropriate use of sedatives or high concentration oxygen therapy can precipitate acute decompensation.

Management

This is similar to asthma although it may be unresponsive to steroids.

Support of respiratory function

1. Oxygen therapy.
Caution with oxygen therapy is vital as many patients with CAL have become dependent on hypoxic stimulation of respiratory drive due to chronic retention of high levels of carbon dioxide resulting in loss of their hypercapnic drive. Where this is the case, higher concentrations (those greater then 28%) should be delivered via an accurate delivery system (see Table 3.11), such as a Ventimask, and arterial blood gases should be monitored on a regular basis for evidence of increasing CO_2 retention. The level of P_aO_2 aimed for should be relative to their usual range; this may be considerably lower than that of the normal person. However, the patient should not be allowed to become excessively hypoxaemic and the question of whether or not to ventilate mechanically must be discussed, ideally at an early stage (see later). Judicious use of non-invasive ventilation, such as BIPAP, or the early use of CPAP may be of great benefit in these patients.

2. Physiotherapy.

3. Respiratory stimulants, such as doxapram or nikethimide, can be used if the P_aCO_2 continues to rise with deteriorating consciousness and it is desirable to keep the patient from being ventilated.

4. Mechanical ventilation.

The decision to ventilate patients with CAL should be carefully considered, preferably at some time well in advance of an immediate need for ventilation. Weaning from ventilation is difficult and the quality of life and survival can be very poor afterwards.

If there is a reversible precipitating factor, such as recent surgery or a treatable infection, then ventilation may provide support until recovery has taken place. However, if respiratory failure is the result of a continuing deterioration in the disease itself then ventilation simply prolongs life without prospect of improvement. Weaning may be impossible and quality of life deteriorates further. There is a need for advance discussion by all members of the team with the patient and his/her relatives to decide whether ventilation is appropriate. The responsibility for initiating this should rest with the physician rather than the intensive care team.

Ventilation should aim to maintain the patient's normal P_aCO_2 and to reduce an elevated P_aCO_2 slowly to prevent an acute alkalosis. Weaning is a prolonged process due to the patient's poor respiratory reserve and nutritional state. It benefits from the use of pressure support and gradual increase in patient effort (see ventilation modes, Table 3.15).

5. Nutrition.

Patients with CAL are usually chronically malnourished due to impairment of appetite, dyspnoea during meals, and chronic ill health. It is important to start early nutritional support.

During weaning, these patients are least likely to be able to cope with any excess CO_2 production related to carbohydrate overload (see Chapter 10). Care should be taken to ensure that equal amounts of fat and carbohydrate contribute to calorie intake.

Pulmonary embolus (PE)

PE is the occlusion of a pulmonary artery by a thrombus. The embolus is most commonly thrown off from a deep vein thrombosis of the pelvic or leg veins. The severity of effect is directly related to the size of the embolus and thus the size of the vessel which has been blocked.

Symptoms

These are tachypnoea, tachycardia, dyspnoea, and chest pain.

Diagnosis is made on clinical presentation (including a raised CVP), CXR (reduced blood flow 'oligaemia' to an area of lung, evidence of pulmonary infarction — classically a wedge-shaped shadow), ECG (right axis deviation, S1, Q3, T3 configuration, right ventricular strain pattern, partial right bundle branch block — see Chapter 5), hypoxaemia, and exclusion of other likely causes. If the patient is stable spital CTscan with contrast pulmonary angiography and V/Q scans may be performed otherwise, emergency surgery should be considered.

Management

   (i) Anticoagulation using heparin.

   (ii) Thrombolytic therapy.

   (iii) Respiratory support (oxygen, CPAP, mechanical ventilation).

   (iv) Pulmonary embolectomy.

   (v) Prevention of any further deep vein thrombosis using elastic stockings, exercises, and mobilization.

   (vi) If cardiovascular embarrassment is evident, the patient must be fluid loaded to ensure optimal right ventricular filling.

For further management see Chapter 5.

Pneumonia

Pneumonia is an inflammatory process caused by bacterial, viral, fungal, protozoan, rickettsial, and, rarely, chemical (e.g. gastric aspiration) causes. Treatment depends on aetiology and infecting agent but all patients require similar support and management.

Management

(1) Antibiotic therapy

(2) Oxygen therapy, CPAP, and mechanical ventilation may all be necessary to maintain PO_2.

(3) Chest physiotherapy and bronchial hygiene to clear secretions.

(4) Postural drainage and position changes.

(5) Adequate nutrition to prevent complications associated with malnutrition (see Chapter 10).

(6) Prevention of further infection.

References and bibliography

Ackerman, M.H. (1993). The effect of saline lavage prior to suctioning. *American Journal of Critical Care*, **2**, 326–30.

Armstrong, R.F., Bullen, C., Cohen, S.L., Singer, M., and Webb, A. (1991). *Critical care algorithms*, p. 26. Oxford University Press, Oxford.

Baun, M.M., Flones, M.J. (1984). Cumulative effects of three sequential endotracheal suctioning episodes in the dog model. *Heart and Lung*, **13**, 148–54.

Benito, S. (1991). Pulmonary compliance. In *Mechanical ventilation*, (ed. F. Lemaire), pp. 86–98. Springer-Verlag, Berlin/Heidelberg.

Bergbom-Engberg, I. and Haljamäe, H. (1989). Assessment of patients' experience of discomforts during respirator therapy. *Critical Care Medicine*, **17**, 1068.

Bethune, D. (1989) Humidification in ventilated patients. *Intensive and Critical Care Digest*, **8**(2), 37–8.

Bostick, J. and Wendelgass, S.T. (1987). Normal saline instillation as part of the suctioning procedure: effects on PaO_2 and the amount of secretions. *Heart and Lung*, **16**, 532–40.

Brathwaite, C. and Borg, U., (1990). Ventilatory support. Use of pressure modes in critically ill patients. *Critical Care Report*, **1**, 300–7.

Clark, A.P., Winslow, E.H., Tyler, D.O., and White, K.M. (1990). Effects of endotracheal suctioning on mixed venous oxygen saturation and heart rate in critically ill adults. *Heart and Lung*, **19**, 552–70.

Des Jardins, T.R. (1988). *Cardiopulmonary anatomy and physiology: essentials for respiratory care*. Delmar Publishers, New York.

Duncan, C. and Erickson, R. (1982). Pressures associated with chest tube stripping. *Heart and Lung*, **11**, 166–71.

Gift, A.G., Bolgiano, C.S., and Cunningham, J. (1991). Sensations during chest tube removal. *Heart and Lung*, **20**, 131–7.

Griggs, W.M., Myburgh, J.A., and Worthley, L.I.G. (1991). A prospective comparison of a percutaneous tracheostomy technique with standard surgical tracheostomy. *Intensive Care Medicine*, **17**, 261–3.

Grap, M.J., Glass, C., and Lindamood, M.O. (1995). Factors related to unplanned extubation of endotracheal tubes. *Critical Care Nurse*, **15**(2), 57–65.

Grossbach, I. (1986). Troubleshooting ventilator and patient-related problems, part 1. *Critical Care Nurse*, **6**(4). 58–68.

Grossbach, I. (1986). Troubleshooting ventilator and patient-related problems, part 2. *Critical Care Nurse*, **6**(5), 64–78.

Guyton, A. (1985). *Anatomy and physiology*. Holt Saunders, Japan.

Hegler, D.A. and Traver, G.A. (1994). Endotracheal saline and suction catheters: sources of lower airway contamination. *American Journal of Critical Care*, **3**, 444–7.

Hill, J.D., O'Brien, T.G., and Muray, J.T. (1972). Prolonged extracorporeal oxygenation for acute post-traumatic respiratory failure (shock-lung syndrome) *New England Journal of Medicine*, **286**, 629–34.

Hubmayr, R., Abel, M., and Rehder, K. (1990). Physiologic approach to mechanical ventilation. *Critical Care Medicine*, **18**, 103–13.

Kallis, P., al-Saady-N.M., Bennett, E.D., and Treasure, T. (1993). Early results of intravascular oxygenation. *European Journal of Cardiothoracic Surgery*, **7**, 206–10.

Kidd, J.F. (1988). Pulse oximeters: basic theory and operation. *Care of the Critically Ill*, **4**, 10–13.

Lemaire, F. (ed.) (1991). *Mechanical ventilation*. Springer-Verlag, Berlin.

Mancinelli-Van Atta, J. and Beck, S.L. (1992). Preventing hypoxemia and hemodynamic compromise related to endotracheal suctioning. *American Journal of Critical Care*, **3**, 62–79.

Marcy, T.W. and Marini, J.J. (1991). Inverse ratio ventilation in ARDS: rationale and implementation. *Chest*, **100**, 494–504.

Matthay, M.A. (1989). New modes of mechanical ventilation for ARDS: How should they be evaluated. *Chest*, **95**, 1175–6.

Oh, T.E. (ed.) (1990). *Intensive care manual*, (3rd edn). Butterworths, Sydney.

Owen, R. (1987) Endobronchial intubation: A preventable complication. *Anesthesiology*, **67**, 255–7.

Pepe, P. and Marini, J. (1982). Occult positive end expiratory pressure in mechanically ventilated patients with airflow obstruction. *American Review of Respiratory Disease*, **126**, 166–71.

Pierce, J.D., Piazza, D., and Naftel, D.C. (1991). Effects of two chest clearance protocols on drainage in patients after myo-cardial revascularization surgery. *Heart and Lung*, **20**, 125–30.

Richless, C. (1990). Current trends in mechanical ventilation. *Critical Care Nurse*, **11**(3), 41–50.

Rinaldo, J. and Heyman, S. (1990). ARDS, A multisystem disease with pulmonary manifestations. *Critical Care Report*, **1**, 174–83.

Ruggles, L. (1995). Auto-PEEP: Measurement issues and nursing interventions. *Critical Care Nurse*, **15**(2), 30–38.

Spector, N. (1989). Nutritional support of the ventilator-dependent patient. *Nursing Clinics of North America*, **24**, 407–14.

Stone, K.S., Vorst, E.C., Lanham, B., and Zahn, S. (1989). Effects of lung hyperinflation on mean arterial pressure and postsuctioning hypoxemia. *Heart and Lung*, **18**, 377–85.

Sykes, K. (1986). Advances in ventilatory support in acute lung disease. *Care of the Critically Ill*, **2**, 50–6.

Teraillon, A. (1990). Tracheobronchial suctions during mechanical ventilation. In *Update in intensive care and emergency medicine* 10, (ed. J.L. Vincent), pp. 196–8. Springer-Verlag, Berlin.

Tobin, M.J. (1991). Weaning assessment. in *Ventilatory failure* (*Update in intensive care and emergency medicine* 15), (ed. J.J. Marini and C. Roussos). Springer-Verlag, Berlin.

Vaca, K.J., Reedy, J.E., Lohmann, D.P., Moroney, D.A., and Swartz, M.T. (1993). Nursing care of the patient with an intravascular oxygenator. *American Journal of Critical Care*, **2**, 478–88.

Villar, J. and Slutsky, A.S. (1991). Alternative modalities for ventilatory support. In *Update in intensive care and emergency medicine 14*, (ed. J.L. Vincent), pp. 345–56. Springer-Verlag, Berlin.

4. Monitoring the critically ill patient

Introduction

Monitoring of physiological variables is essential in the care of the critically ill patient. The aims of monitoring are:

- To detect changes in the patient's clinical condition.
- To assess the response to treatment strategies.
- To act as a diagnostic tool.

Monitoring may be continuous or intermittent. Although individual readings can be significant for both types of monitoring, it is important to analyse trends from serial data, and to assimilate and interpret information from all forms of patient monitoring including clinical observation.

In order to act correctly on information provided by the various monitoring devices, the nurse must have a thorough understanding of the relevant physiology, practical expertise in the procedures, and an awareness of the reliability of the equipment or technique involved.

Reliability and safety of monitoring devices

- All monitoring devices are manufactured to specific standards and recommendations are given for the conditions of their use. It is important that these are adhered to in order to ensure the accuracy of information obtained.
- Most monitoring devices are powered by mains electricity and/or rechargeable battery units. The immediate area surrounding the patient therefore often contains a large number of electrical items. Cables must be treated with care to avoid undue stretching or tension and vital plugs, such as to the ventilator, should be easily identifiable. Extreme care must be taken not to allow spillage of fluid on to plugs and sockets (particularly if using extension leads). Position equipment so that leads do not drape across the patient and ensure there is easy access around the bed area.

- Some items of monitoring equipment are very heavy and care must be taken when attaching them to items, such as drip stands, in order to avoid breakage or injury to the patient or staff.
- When large amounts of monitoring equipment surround the bed area they must be positioned such that their visual displays can be seen by the nurse at all times.
- If alarm systems are incorporated within the monitoring devices these must used and the alarm limits set according to the patient's condition. Alarm settings should be checked at the beginning of every shift and reviewed if the patient's condition changes.

Types of monitoring

Methods of monitoring may be non-invasive or invasive. Details of specific neurological, metabolic, and respiratory monitoring devices are discussed in the relevant chapters.

Non-invasive monitoring

Simple monitoring of the patient can be achieved without the use of equipment. The nurse can obtain a great deal of clinical information by merely watching, touching, and listening to the patient. The patient's posture, facial expressions, behaviour, and conscious level can all reveal important information (see Table 4.1).

For respiratory observations see Chapter 3.

Monitoring fluid balance

All critically ill patients should have their fluid intake and output measured, at minimum, on an hourly basis. This includes wound and nasogastric drainage, urine output, all drug, and fluid infusions (preferably administered via volumetric pumps or syringe drivers to aid accuracy). Fluid balance must be reviewed and assessed regularly in combination with haemodynamic and respiratory data.

Table 4.1 Non-invasive monitoring: Observation

Observation	Appearance	Possible cause
Skin		
Touch	• Dry • Cool, clammy	• Hypovolaemia • Hypoperfusion states
	• Hot, flushed	• Pyrexia, vasodilatation
	• Tense and pitting	• Oedema
Colour	• Pale • Cherry pink • Cyanosed (peripheral or central)	• Anaemia • Carbon monoxide poisoning • Hypoxaemia (for central cyanosis) • Poor perfusion (for peripheral cyanosis) or vasoconstriction
	• Jaundiced	• Biliary obstruction, haemolysis, liver dysfunction
Other	• Petechiae, bruising, bleeding from puncture/ cannulae sites • Decreased limb perfusion (white, cold, mottled, loss of pulse) • Limb warm, painful, swollen • Blisters, rashes	• Clotting disorders • Arterial occlusion, rhabdomyolysis, compartment syndrome • Venous occlusion • Allergic reactions (drugs, dressings)
Neurological		
Conscious level	• Reduced	• Neurological deterioration • Drug therapy • Uraemia • Metabolic causes • Hypoperfusion states
Behaviour	• Restlessness, agitation, aggressiveness, confusion	• Hypoxaemia • Sepsis • Neurological deterioration • Metabolic causes • Pain, discomfort • Need to open bowels • Full bladder or stomach • Haemorrhage • Reaction to the environment and illness • Drug therapy
Expression	• Grimacing, worried	• Pain, discomfort fear, anxiety

Investigations

Regular haematological, microbiological, and biochemical investigations enable the early identification of physiological deterioration or improvement and must be evaluated in conjunction with data from other monitoring devices.

Routine blood tests will include arterial blood gas analysis, full blood count, clotting studies, glucose, urea, creatinine, and electrolytes, liver function tests, and urinary electrolytes, and creatinine. Many other investigations, such as amylase and endocrine function tests, may also be performed depending on the patient's presumptive diagnosis.

Most units will routinely send specimens of sputum, urine, blood, wound discharge, etc., for microbiological culture if infection is suspected. Many other specific investigations, such as computerized tomography, ultrasound, echocardiography, and X-rays, also play an important part in the monitoring and identification of disease processes and are used according to the patient's clinical condition.

The electrocardiogram (ECG)

All critically ill patients will require continuous ECG monitoring. The aims of cardiac monitoring are:

1. The early detection of changes in heart rate and rhythm.

2. To assess the effectiveness of treatment strategies.

There are many types of cardiac monitors but the essential components of ECG monitoring are the same.

Basic principles of ECG monitoring

- Electrodes are placed on the chest wall which detect the electrical activity initiated by the heart. Electrical activity that is moving towards an electrode will produce an upward (positive) deflection on the recording and activity that is moving away from the electrode will produce a downward (negative) deflection. The baseline (isoelectric line) is where the positive and negative deflections begin and end.

- The electrodes are connected by a patient cable to an oscilloscope which displays a continuous waveform reflecting each phase of the heart's electrical activity.

- The impulses produced by the cardiac activity would be too small to be seen on an oscilloscope naturally and

are therefore amplified by the monitor so that their height is increased about a thousand times.

- The waveform on the monitor can be adjusted so that the optimal size, brightness and position of the ECG is seen. A choice of leads are possible but lead II is usually selected. This is because the direction of electrical current as it passes through the ventricles is directed towards lead II, resulting in a large, positive waveform which can be easily interpreted.

Placement of ECG electrodes

The electrodes are small, disposable, adhesive pads. These are pre-gelled (to facilitate conduction) and are attached to the chest wall by simply peeling off the backing paper and pressing firmly to the skin. The skin must be clean and dry and it may be necessary to shave chest hair to facilitate contact. It is imperative to have good contact between the skin and electrode or the ECG waveform will be distorted and artefacts will appear.

Usually, three electrodes are used (see Fig. 4.1), but some equipment may require four or five electrodes to allow multiple views of the heart.

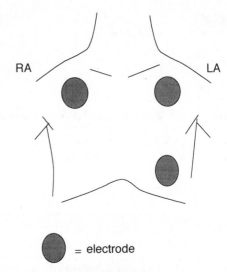

RA   LA

= electrode

Fig. 4.1 Placement of ECG electrodes.

The electrodes can remain *in situ* for several days as the gel does not usually dry out. However, skin irritation can occur due to the adhesive used on the electrode or the conducting jelly. The electrode positions should be rotated regularly to avoid soreness, and the skin checked for sensitivity.

Thin wires snap or clamp on to the electrodes and are connected to designated leads on the patient cable. These are usually designated RA (right arm), LA (left arm), and RL (right leg or earth) and should be connected to the corresponding electrode. The patient cable is then connected to the cable socket of the monitor.

Adjusting the monitor

The displayed waveform must be clear and distinct. Fine adjustments to the brightness and size of the waveform can be made on the monitor. The amplitude of the R wave is of particular importance as the monitor calculates the heart rate by recognizing and counting this wave. If the height of the wave cannot be increased sufficiently to record an accurate heart rate the position of the electrodes, or the lead displayed, may need to be changed to obtain a greater electrical potential.

High and low rate alarm limits should be set according to the patient's clinical condition. Frequent false alarms undermine the rationale for alarm setting and may cause the patient undue anxiety.

Most rate meters count the number of ventricular beats (R waves) per minute and display this as the heart rate. In fact, most meters will count all large, upward deflections as they are unable to distinguish ventricular beats from muscle potentials caused by contraction of skeletal muscle. This means that often movement by the patient or muscle tremors will cause falsely elevated heart rate readings.

False high rates can also be seen if the R and T wave of the ECG waveform (p. 84) are the same size and the monitor is recognizing both as the R wave. To rectify this the amplitude of the waveform should be increased until the R wave is higher than the T wave, or the electrode positions or ECG lead displayed should be changed.

False low heart rates will occur if the R wave is of insufficient size to be detected by the monitor (the amplitude should be increased until this is recognized), or if there is a disturbance in the transmission of the signal from the skin to the monitor. This may be due to a defective electrode, separation of the electrode from the skin, or disconnection of one of the patient leads.

Electrical interference can occur from other electrical devices at the bedside. This will appear as a series of fine, rapid spikes (artefact) which distort the baseline of the ECG. This may be due to incorrect earthing and the device responsible should be identified and checked. Artefact may also be caused by shivering of the patient (particularly if the electrodes are positioned over skeletal muscle) or loose connections at the patient's cable.

A wandering baseline can occur when the isoelectric line regularly moves up and down rather than in a straight line. This is invariably due to movement of the chest wall during respiration. The only solution is to alter the patient's position and place the electrodes to the lowest ribs and apex of the chest. (Table 4.2.)

Table 4.2 Summary of problems associated with EGG monitoring

Problem	Cause	Action
False high rate	• Patient movement, fitting, tremors	• Ensure electrodes are not placed over skeletal muscle
	• T wave same height as R wave	• Increase amplitude, change position of electrodes
False low rate	• Lead disconnection	• Check leads
	• Separation of electrode from skin	• Check/replace electrodes
	• Insufficient height of R wave	• Increase amplitude, change position of electrodes
Artefact	• Shivering, tremors	• Ensure patient is warm
	• Electrical equipment	• Check other electrical equipment in use at bedside (e.g. electric razors, fans)
	• Poor connection of leads or electrodes	• Check all connections are firm, change electrodes
Wandering baseline	• Respiration causing chest wall movement	• Adjust patient position
		• Reposition electrodes to lowest ribs to minimize effect

Arrhythmias and conduction disturbances

Disorders of cardiac rhythm are one of the commonest problems experienced by critically ill patients. Monitoring of the ECG allows prompt recognition of these disorders and immediate intervention where necessary. It is worth remembering, however, that all ECG rhythms should be examined in the context of the patient's clinical condition and intervention decided on according to this, rather than the rhythm itself.

ECG definitions

There are a number of definitions which provide a background for understanding the ECG:

Sinus rhythm: a rhythm originating in the sinoatrial node of > 60 and < 100 beats per minute (bpm).
Sinus tachycardia: a rhythm originating in the sinoatrial node of > 100 (bpm).
Sinus bradycardia: a rhythm originating in the sinoatrial node of < 60 bpm. (The above rhythms usually reflect either a normal heart or a normal physiological response to an external factor.)
   Tachycardia: heart rate > 100 bpm.
   Bradycardia: heart rate < 60 bpm.
Isoelectric line: the baseline of the ECG tracing (i.e. no electrical activity is occurring).
   Positive deflection: upward movement of the ECG tracing from the baseline.
   Negative deflection: downward movement of the ECG tracing from the baseline.
The P wave corresponds to atrial depolarization and is seen in normal sinus rhythm (see later). P waves are best seen in leads II, III, VI, and V2. (No P waves are seen in atrial fibrillation while a peaked wave is classically seen with chronic pulmonary hypertension and an M-shaped wave with mitral valve disease.)

The PR interval should be in the range 0.12–0.2 seconds. A longer interval (> 0.2 s) is seen with first degree heart block while a shorter interval (< 0.12 s) is seen with rapid atrioventricular conduction (e.g. Wolff–Parkinson–White syndrome).

The QRS complex corresponds to ventricular depolarization and the width should be less than 0.12 s. A greater width is seen with delayed conduction through the ventricular conducting system (e.g. bundle branch block). The QRS height is useful in assessing left or right ventricular hypertrophy (see later). A pathological Q wave is seen in myocardial infarction and should be at least 25% of the height of the following R wave and exceed 0.04 s in width (see myocardial infarction, p. 140).

The Q–T interval varies with heart rate and is approximately 0.35–0.43 s long when the heart rate is 60 bpm. It is prolonged in hypocalcaemia and shortened by hypercalcaemia.

The ST segment is elevated (in convex shape) from the baseline ('isoelectric line') in myocardial infarction and depressed during myocardial ischaemia (see later). Concave ST segment elevation is seen in pericarditis.

The T wave corresponds to ventricular repolarization and should normally be 'positive' (i.e. pointing upwards) in leads I, II, V4, V5, and V6. An inverted T wave may be seen in myocardial ischaemia and infarction, and in types of bundle branch block (see later). It is peaked during hyperkalaemia and flattened by hypokalaemia.

Timing of the ECG

The paper used to record the ECG trace is made up of small and large squares. Each small square measures 1 mm and each large square measures 5 mm. The paper is then run at a standard speed of 25 mm per second. Thus, each small square takes 0.04 seconds to pass the recording pen and each large square takes 0.2 seconds. This allows the timing and rate of the ECG trace to be calculated.

Systematic analysis of the ECG rhythm strip

When first attempting to identify arrhythmias it is helpful to use a step-by-step sequence to ensure all aspects of the rhythm are analysed and to avoid missing important information. Ideally, a recorded strip (traditionally, of lead II but any monitoring lead can be used) should be taken and used to analyse the rhythm systematically.

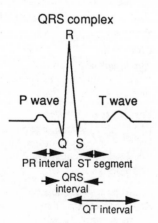

Fig. 4.2

One suggested sequence is:

(1) determine the rate,

(2) determine the regularity of the rhythm,

(3) identify the P wave and its shape,

(4) identify the QRS complex,

(5) determine the relationship between P waves and QRS complexes (i.e. is there 1 P wave to every QRS?),

(6) calculate the P–R interval,

(7) examine the shape and width of the QRS complex.

Classification of arrhythmias

Two broad classifications of arrhythmias are:

1. Disorders of impulse formation

This may be due to dysfunction of the pacemaker rate of the sinoatrial node allowing escape rhythms from other pacemakers. In conjunction, excessively rapid impulse generation may produce atrial, junctional, and ventricular tachycardias via re-entry pathways (see Table 4.3). These are discussed below.

Table 4.3 Disorders of impulse formation

Ventricular	Junctional	Supraventricular
Ventricular ectopic beats	A–V nodal (junctional) premature beats	Sinus arrhythmia
Ventricular tachycardia	A–V nodal (junctional) tachycardia	Sinus bradycardia
Torsades de pointes		Sinus tachycardia
Ventricular fibrillation		Atrial ectopic beats
		Atrial flutter
		Atrial fibrillation (AF)
		Sick sinus syndrome

2. Disorders of impulse conduction

This refers to situations where conduction is either slowed, blocked, or uses an alternative pathway (see Table 4.4).

Table 4.4 Disorders of impulse conduction

Slowed or blocked conduction	Alternative pathways
First degree atrioventricular block	Wolff–Parkinson–White (WPW) syndrome
Second degree atrioventricular block	Lown–Ganong–Levine syndrome
Third degree atrioventricular block	
Bundle branch block	

Precipitating causes of arrhythmias

As well as the focal arrhythmias associated with cardiac disease itself, alterations of underlying physiology may also precipitate arrhythmias. The patient's condition should always be reviewed for precipitating treatable causes. These include:

(1) Myocardial ischaemia due to poor coronary perfusion related to (i) low cardiac output states, (ii) hypoxaemia, (iii) sepsis.

(2) Autonomic control may be affected by central neurological damage.

(3) Alterations in electrolyte and acid–base balance (e.g. hypo and hyper-kalaemia, -calcaemia, -magnesaemia, -phosphataemia; metabolic and respiratory acidosis.

(4) Endocrine influence, particularly thyroid and adrenal.

(5) Effects of drugs.

Table 4.5 Arrhythmias caused by metabolic changes

Hyperkalaemia	Tall ('tented') T waves, $\pm$ wide QRS complexes $\pm$ absent P waves
Hypokalaemia	Flattened T waves, U waves (wave seen after T wave)
Hypercalcaemia	Short Q–T interval
Hypocalcaemia	Prolonged Q–T interval
Hypothermia	J wave (small wave appearing immediately after QRS complex), bradycardia
Digoxin effect	ST depression and inverted T wave ('reverse tick'); *not* a sign of toxicity Any arrhythmia may occur with toxicity

Disorders of impulse formation

(1) Sinus arrhythmia

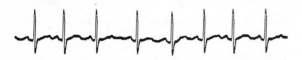

Fig. 4.3

Spacing between normal P and QRS complexes varies regularly, usually with respiration in young patients due to increased venous return on inspiration.

Aetiology. It is physiological in most young patients but is occasionally associated with inferior myocardial infarction (Lloyd in Oh 1990, p. 46).

Treatment. None.

(2) Sinus tachycardia

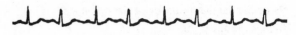

Fig. 4.4

The P and QRS complexes are normal but the rate is increased to greater than 100 bpm.

Aetiology. It is physiological in exercise and emotional states.

It is pathologically associated with underlying fever, fluid volume deficit, heart failure, anaemia, thyrotoxicosis, stimulants, such as amphetamines, and drugs, such as atropine, adrenaline, and isoprenaline.

Treatment. This is directed at finding and treating the underlying cause.

(3) Sinus bradycardia

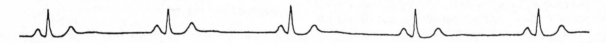

Fig. 4.5

Normal P and QRS complexes but the rate is less than 60 bpm.

Aetiology. It is physiological in athletes and fit people. It is pathologically associated with myocardial infarction, sick sinus syndrome, myxoedema, obstructive jaundice, raised intracranial pressure, glaucoma, and drugs, such as beta blockers, digoxin, verapamil, and cholinergic drugs.

Treatment. Usually only necessary if the blood pressure is compromised or where cardiac failure means the patient will be unable to compensate for the slow rate with increased myocardial contraction. Atropine 0.3 mg, followed by supplemental doses as necessary may be used to block vagal tone or isoprenaline given to increase the rate. Occasionally in sick sinus syndrome transvenous pacing may be necessary.

(4) Atrial ectopic (premature) beats

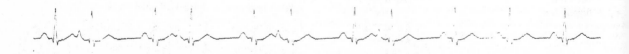

Fig. 4.6

A stimulus for a beat occurs earlier than expected, arising not in the sinoatrial node but in another part of the atrium. The distance between the previous beat and the ectopic beat is much shorter than normal and it may be followed by a longer than normal interval before the next beat occurs ('compensatory pause').

Aetiology. These beats are often present in the normal heart but may be induced by stimulants, such as caffeine, nicotine, and stress. They may occur pathologically as a result of infections, ischaemia, electrolyte imbalance, underlying heart disease, and drug toxicity, such as theophylline and digoxin.

Treatment. Only indicated in the healthy person, if the ectopic beats are symptomatic or precipitate atrial tachycardia. Avoidance of recognized provoking factors is usually sufficient. Digoxin or beta blockers may be used if symptomatic.

(5) Supraventricular tachycardia (SVT)

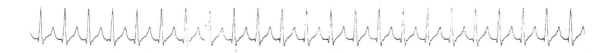

Fig. 4.7

A rapid, regular rhythm with a rate of between 140 and 250 bpm, usually of sudden onset. P waves may be present but abnormal or obscured by the rapid rate QRS complex. There may be difficulty distinguishing SVT with aberrant ventricular conduction from a ventricular tachycardia. Carotid sinus massage (see below) or IV adenosine (initially 3–6 mg followed by 12 mg if no effect in 1–2 minutes) can slow the rate sufficiently to allow diagnosis of the tachycardia.

Aetiology. SVT can occur in patients with healthy hearts but may also occur in heart disease and WPW syndrome. It is distinguished from sinus tachycardia by its sudden onset or cessation.

Treatment. A supraventricular tachycardia is treated with IV amiodarone (300 mg over 15 minutes followed by an infusion of 10–20 mg/kg/24 h). Verapamil (5–10 mg bolus) may be used, although it should be given with great care to patients in heart failure and those receiving beta blockers as severe hypotension and bradycardia may result.

(6) Atrial flutter

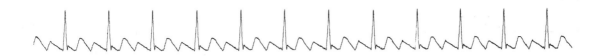

Fig. 4.8

Atrial flutter is an ectopic atrial rhythm which produces characteristic 'sawtooth' or 'picket fence' P waves. The atrial rate is usually between 250 and 300 bpm. The ventricular rate is variable depending on the degree of AV nodal block. If 1 QRS occurs to every 2 P waves then the ventricular rate is 125–150 bpm. If 1 QRS occurs to every 3 P waves then the ventricular rate is 75–100 beats per min. The QRS is normal unless there is aberrant conduction.

Aetiology. Usually, there is underlying heart disease, such as ischaemic or rheumatic heart disease.

Treatment. If there is haemodynamic compromise or a very fast ventricular rate then synchronized DC cardioversion should be carried out. If the rate is acceptable and the patient stable then IV amiodarone (dose as above), verapamil (dose as above), or digoxin (loading dose 0.5 mg–1.5 mg IV given as periodic infusions of 0.5 mg, followed by 0.25 mg daily until the ventricular rate is slowed to 60–100 bpm). The dose may then have to be reduced further) can be used.

(7) Atrial fibrillation

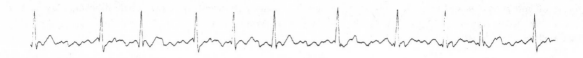

Fig. 4.9

An irregular QRS pattern with no discernible P waves. The QRS width is usually normal. The atria are fibrillating at a rate of about 400–600 bpm. The QRS rate is usually greater than 100 bpm.

Aetiology. Chronic atrial fibrillation can occur as a result of heart disease and paroxysmal atrial fibrillation occurs as a result of a variety of acute disorders as well as WPW syndrome. Digitalis toxicity may cause atrial fibrillation and should be suspected if the ventricular rate is slow, there is evidence of A–V block, and ventricular ectopics are associated.

Treatment. In chronic atrial fibrillation, the aim is to control the ventricular rate with digoxin. In paroxysmal atrial fibrillation, the aim is to restore sinus rhythm following treatment of the primary cause. If there is haemodynamic compromise, cardioversion may be required. Amiodarone IV (dose as above) can be used to restore sinus rhythm or digoxin IV (dose as above).

(8) A–V junctional (nodal) premature beats (ectopics)

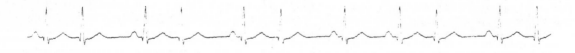

Fig. 4.10

A premature stimulus occurs arising from the atrioventricular node. This is conducted simultaneously through the ventricle and retrogradely through the atria. The QRS is usually normal.

Aetiology. A–V junctional ectopics may occur in the normal person but are most commonly associated with heart disease. They can be a sign of digitalis toxicity.

Treatment. Management is similar to atrial ectopics.

(9) Junctional (nodal) tachycardia

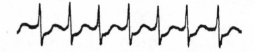

Fig. 4.11

A rapid regular rhythm originating in the atrioventricular node. There are no upright P waves but inverted P waves may be visible. QRS waves are normal unless there is aberrant conduction. Rate is up to 140 bpm. Differentiation between atrial and junctional tachycardia may be difficult at fast rates.

Aetiology. Paroxysmal junctional tachycardia is classified and treated as SVT. A non-paroxysmal or accelerated junctional rhythm is caused by digitalis toxicity. It may also occur with myocardial infarction, rheumatic fever, and myocarditis.

Treatment. As for SVT if paroxysmal.

Accelerated junctional rhythm caused by digitalis toxicity is treated by discontinuing digoxin. Correction of any underlying physiological disturbance may be sufficient to terminate the arrhythmia.

(10) Junctional (nodal rhythm)

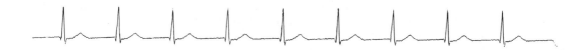

Fig. 4.12

Failure of the SA node to generate impulses will result in the AV node taking over as pacemaker. There are no discernible P waves. The QRS is normal unless there is aberrant conduction. The intrinsic rate is slower (40–70 bpm) and the rhythm is regular.

Aetiology. Junctional rhythm can occur in the normal person. It is usually associated with myocardial infarc-tion or increased vagal tone. Occasionally seen in digi-talis toxicity.

Treatment. Discontinue digoxin if toxicity is suspected. Treatment is usually only necessary if there are symp-toms or haemodynamic compromise. Atropine 0.3 mg IV can be given if excessive vagal tone is suspected.

(11) Sick sinus syndrome

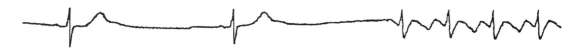

Fig. 4.13

A variety of disruptions to rhythm occur including, SA node bradycardia, SA node arrest, wandering pacemaker (the origin of the impulse occurs in different parts of the atria), and atrial ectopic beats. These are accompanied by episodes of rapid atrial arrhythmias, such as atrial fibrillation, flutter, and SVT.

Aetiology. Intrinsic disease of the sinoatrial node and conducting system produces symptoms of palpitations and episode of fainting (Stokes–Adams attacks). These may be idiopathic in the elderly but can be associated with infarction affecting the atria, rheumatic heart dis-ease, and pericarditis.

Treatment. Permanent pacing is often required with pharmacological control of tachyarrhythmias if necessary.

(12) Ventricular premature contractions (ectopics)

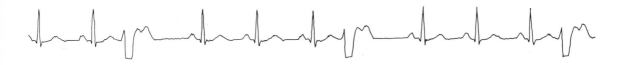

Fig. 4.14

A stimulus arises earlier than expected from the Purkinje fibre network in the ventricles. There is no P wave present prior to the beat, although an inverted P wave from retrograde conduction may be seen after the beat.

The QRS is widened and bizarre in shape with a notch and increased amplitude. A compensatory pause may follow the beat.

Bigeminy occurs when each normal beat is accompanied by an ectopic beat. Trigeminy occurs when every second normal beat is followed by an ectopic beat.

Multifocal ectopic beats appear as different shaped QRS complexes and arise from different areas within the ventricle.

Aetiology. A common arrhythmia that can occur in any age at any time. They are common in myocardial disease or as a result of increased myocardial irritability (e.g. hypoxia, hypokalaemia, digitalis intoxication). Ectopic beats are associated with heart disease in the over-40s, if they are frequent, occur in runs, and are multifocal.

Treatment: Occasional ventricular premature contractions require no treatment. If they are multifocal, occur in runs, frequent (> 5/min) or occur very close to the apex of the T wave of the previous beat then they may require treatment if the patient is symptomatic. Correction of underlying disorders, such as hypokalaemia, digitalis intoxication, and hypoxia, is essential. Lignocaine IV 50–100 mg bolus followed by an infusion at 4 mg/min for the first half hour tailing down to 1 mg/min according to patient response, is frequently used.

(13) Ventricular tachycardia

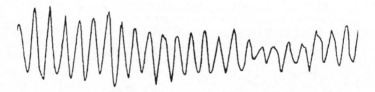

Fig. 4.15

A ventricular ectopic focus stimulates a series of rapid and regular beats. There are no P waves present and the QRS complex is bizarrely shaped and widened. The rate is between 100 and 220 bpm.

Aetiology: Occurs commonly following myocardial infarction or as a result of digitalis intoxication. The stimulus arises in the Purkinje fibres and it is thought to continue as a re-entry mechanism (see later). The fast rate and the loss of co-ordinated atrial contraction into

the ventricles produces a severe drop in cardiac output which may require cardiopulmonary resuscitation (CPR).

Treatment: Defibrillation is the treatment of choice if there is haemodynamic deterioration. If the patient is stable, lignocaine or amiodarone IV (dose as above) should be given. Potassium and magnesium levels should be checked, and other underlying physiological disorders corrected.

(14) Torsades de Pointes

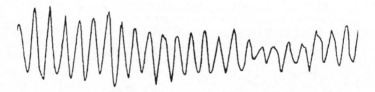

Fig. 4.16

This is a specific variety of ventricular tachycardia — Torsades de Pointes means 'twisting of the points'. The QRS complex is ventricular in origin and broadened but the axis changes from positive to negative and back again. It appears to be a transitional rhythm between

ventricular tachycardia and fibrillation. It is associated with a prolonged Q–T interval.

Aetiology: Development of Torsades de Pointes is more likely with a prolonged Q–T interval (> 0.44 seconds). Conditions, such as hypokalaemia, hypocalcaemia, and hypomagnesaemia; or antiarrhythmic agents, such as disopyramide and quinidine, will increase the Q–T interval. Prolonged Q–T has also been reported with tricyclic antidepressants and phenothiazines as well as insecticide poisoning.

Treatment: It is important that the rhythm is recognized and treated accordingly as conventional treatment for ventricular tachycardia (lignocaine) will cause the condition to worsen.

Correction of any underlying electrolyte imbalance and discontinuation of any pharmacological cause is the first step. Isoprenaline, adrenaline, and dopamine IV have been used to treat Torsades de Pointes but IV magnesium is now considered the treatment of choice.

(15) Ventricular fibrillation

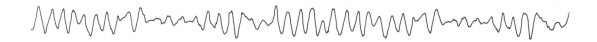

Fig. 4.17

Rapid, chaotic, and ineffectual contractions of the ventricle. It is always accompanied by complete loss of cardiac output and unless CPR is carried out immediately the patient will die.

Aetiology: Associated with ischaemic heart disease, hypoxia, metabolic disturbances, following electrocution; and as a result of drug toxicity (e.g. digoxin, tricyclic antidepressant overdose).

Treatment: Immediate defibrillation is the only treatment of ventricular fibrillation (see Chapter 6). Following successful defibrillation the patient is treated with lignocaine or amiodarone (dose as above).

Disorders of impulse conduction

(16) First degree heart block

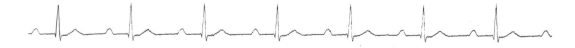

Fig. 4.18

Delay in impulse conduction occurs at the AV node. The PR interval is greater than 0.20 s.

Aetiology: First degree block can occur in normal or diseased hearts. It may be a precursor to second or third degree block.

Treatment: First degree block does not require treatment and is only significant if it precedes second or third degree block.

(17) Second degree heart block

There are two types of second degree heart block: Mobitz type I (Wenkebach) and Mobitz type II.

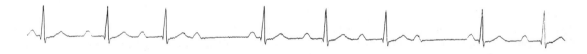

Fig. 4.19 Mobitz type I.

In Mobitz type I (Wenkebach) a delay at the AV node gradually increases through a series of beats until conduction of the impulse does not occur. The whole process is then repeated. The QRS complex is normal.

Aetiology: Mobitz type I is usually associated with acute reversible conditions and is relatively benign.

Treatment: Treatment is only necessary if there is haemodynamic compromise associated with the block.

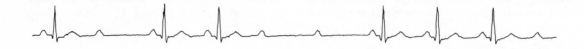

Fig. 4.20 Mobitz type II.

In Mobitz type II, a varying ratio of QRS to P waves are conducted through the A–V node (e.g. 2 P:1 QRS or 3P:1QRS, etc.). The PR interval in conducted beats remains constant.

Aetiology: Mobitz type II block indicates more severe impairment of A–V conduction and is associated with

myocardial infarction. It may precede complete heart block.

Treatment: Monitoring is essential but treatment depends on the cardiac output. If this is compromised or the ventricular rate is very slow then treatment is indicated. Isoprenaline or atropine IV may be used. Alternatively, transvenous pacing may be required.

(18) Third degree (complete) heart block

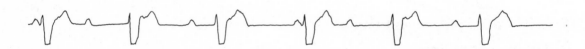

Fig. 4.21

There is a complete block of conduction between atria and ventricles at the A–V node. The atrial rate continues at a normal or slightly faster rate but the QRS rate will be slower. There is no relationship between the P and the QRS complexes. If the QRS originates in the A–V node then the rate will be between 50 and 60 bpm and the QRS will be normal. If the QRS originates in the ventricles then the rate will be between 30 and 40 bpm and the QRS will be widened and enlarged.

Aetiology: The commonest causes are acute myocardial infarction and idiopathic degeneration of the conducting system with age. It can occur following cardiac surgery particularly on the mitral or aortic valves.

Treatment: In anterior myocardial infarction treatment is urgent and occurrence of complete heart block is associated with more extensive infarction. In other patients, treatment will depend on symptoms and haemodynamic compromise. The definitive treatment is transvenous pacing, although external cardiac pacing

(see Chapter 6) can be used for short periods to maintain cardiac output. If this is not available IV atropine or isoprenaline infusion can be tried.

(19) Wolff–Parkinson–White (WPW) syndrome

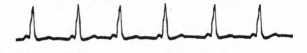

Fig. 4.22

This syndrome consists of episodes of paroxysmal tachyarrhythmia characterized by a shortened PR interval and a widened QRS complex. In the non-tachyarrhythmic state the QRS complex has a notch known as the delta (δ) wave which is indicative of early ventricular stimulation via the accessory conduction pathway which bypasses the A–V node.

The PR interval is shortened due to rapid conduction through the accessory pathway which unlike the A–V node does not slow conduction.

Aetiology: There is a faulty embryonic development of the AV ring of fibrous tissue whereby strands of myocardial tissue act as a bridge of conducting tissue across the non-conducting A–V ring. This conduction pathway is known as the bundle of Kent.

The accessory pathway is capable of supporting arrhythmias, most commonly atrial fibrillation (AF) and paroxysmal supraventricular tachycardias (PVST).

Treatment: If haemodynamically unstable in AF or PSVT, cardioversion is carried out.

Amiodarone IV is the treatment of choice. Digoxin should be avoided as it lengthens A–V nodal block and may increase conduction via the aberrant pathway.

Mechanisms of tachyarrhythmias

Re-entry tachycardias
Re-entry is thought to occur in the following circumstances:

  (i) there is more than one available route for conduction of an impulse,

 (ii) circumstances such as ischaemia, high potassium levels, and blockage of the Purkinje system produce an area of depressed conduction such that stimuli can be conducted in only one direction in one of the available routes,

(iii) conduction is slow so that the normally functioning route is repolarized and available for a second depolarization.

A stimulus is therefore conducted down the normal conduction route but blocked through the depressed area in that direction. The impulse is then slowly propagated retrogradely through the depressed area in the opposite direction and then re-stimulates the normal route which has by now repolarized. Re-entry tachycardias can occur in any area of the conduction system and are probably the cause of various supraventricular and ventricular tachycardias.

Monitoring the Q–T interval

The normal value for the Q–T interval depends on the heart rate. As it increases, the Q–T interval shortens and as it decreases the Q–T interval lengthens. The formula for correcting the Q–T interval for heart rate is:

$$Q\text{–}Tc = Q\text{–}T \, / \, \sqrt{R\text{–}R}$$

Q–T = interval measured from beginning of QRS to end of T wave.

$\sqrt{R\text{–}R}$ = square root of time between two successive R waves.

The Q–Tc is prolonged if it exceeds 0.44 s.

A prolonged Q–T interval is associated with hypokalamia, hypocalcaemia, hypomagnesaemia, and tricyclic drugs. It can lead to Torsades de Pointes.

The 12-lead ECG

This is performed in order to:

1. Make a clinical diagnosis.

2. Monitor cardiac progress.

The frequency of recording a 12-lead ECG will depend on the patient's clinical condition and diagnosis. In the absence of cardiac problems this may be on a daily or alternate day basis but those who have undergone cardiac surgery or have cardiac dysfunction (e.g. myocardial infarction, unstable angina) may require more frequent recordings.

The 12-lead ECG records the flow of current in several planes so that a more comprehensive view of the heart's electrical activity can be obtained. This is achieved by placing one electrode on each limb and six electrodes on the chest wall. The electrode placed on the right leg acts as an earth and is not an electrical lead.

The electrodes should be placed over positions of least muscle mass to avoid interference from skeletal muscle (i.e. the inside of the wrist and the inner aspect of the ankle). Ideally, the electrodes should be in the same position for each serial ECG.

The standard leads (limb leads)

Three major planes of electrical activity can be viewed using the limb heads which record the differences in electrical forces between each of the limb electrodes. The three limb leads are termed I, II, and III (see Table 4.6).

These views form a hypothetical triangle with the heart at the centre. Electrical current flows between a negative and a positive pole. When current flows towards a positive pole the ECG shows an upward (positive) deflection. When current flows away from a positive pole the ECG shows a downward (negative) deflection. The positions of the positive and negative electrodes in leads I, II, and III are shown in Fig. 4.1.

Table 4.6 The 12-lead ECG

Lead	Electrode 1 (Neg.)	Electrode 2 (Pos.)
I	RA	LA
II	RA	LL
III	LA	LL
VR	RA	LA and LL
VL	LA	RA and LL
VF	LL	RA and LA

RA, right arm; LA, left arm; LL, left leg.

The complete 12-lead ECG consists of:

- 3 limb leads: I, II, and III,
- 3 augmented (modified) limb leads termed:
- aVL [augmented view left]
- aVR [augmented view right]
- aVF [augmented view foot or left leg],
- 6 chest leads: V1, V2, V3, V4, V5, and V6.

Electrodes recording the limb and augmented limb leads

These show the direction of viewing the heart (from electrode 1 to electrode 2), thus each lead will have characteristic upward and downward deflections.

The chest leads

The positions of the chest leads are:

V1: 4th intercostal space to the right of the sternum,
V2: 4th intercostal space to the left of the sternum,
V3: midway between V2 and V4,
V4: 5th intercostal space mid-clavicular line,
V5: anterior axillary line at same level as V4,
V6: mid-axillary line at same level as V4.

All 12 leads will show different electrocardiographic patterns due to the different positions of the electrodes. The direction of deflection depends on the view of the heart in that particular electrical lead. Some waves may change polarity (a normally negative deflection becomes a positive one) due to disease. Figure 4.23 shows a 12-lead ECG taken from a patient with a normal heart.

The ECG should be analysed for rate, rhythm, axis, P wave, PR interval, QRS complex, QT interval, ST segment, and T wave to enable diagnosis of:

- abnormal rhythms and conduction,
- changes secondary to ischaemic heart disease,
- changes secondary to pericardial disease,
- changes secondary to metabolic and other diseases,
- ventricular hypertrophy.

Axis

This is the sum of the ventricular electrical forces during depolarization. Figure 4.24 shows the orientation of the

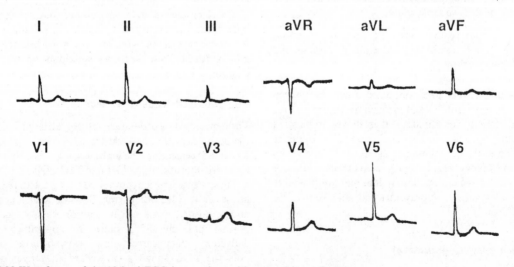

Fig. 4.23 Waveforms of the 12-lead ECG in a patient with normal heart function.

limb leads. The normal axis of the heart lies between $-30°$ and $90°$ (i.e. towards the left as the left ventricular mass is greater than the right). If the axis lies outside $-30°$ this is termed left axis deviation and if greater than $+90°$ right axis deviation. The axis is determined by determining the vector of the forces between lead I ($0°$) and lead aVF ($+90°$) (see Fig. 4.25).

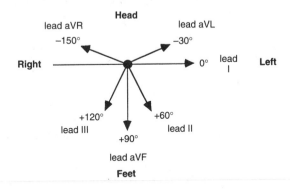

Fig. 4.24 Orientation of limb leads.

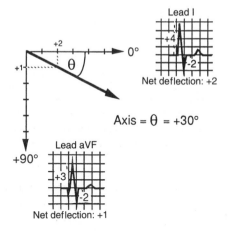

Fig. 4.25 Calculation of the axis.

Analysis of 12-lead ECG

A variety of disease processes can be assessed from 12-lead ECG analysis.

Changes secondary to ischaemic heart disease

The area of the heart affected by injury, ischaemia, or infarction can be determined by observing which leads show abnormal changes as shown in Table 4.7

Table 4.7 Changes secondary to ischaemic heart disease

ST segment depression	Myocardial injury/ischaemia
ST segment elevation (convex)	Myocardial injury/ischaemia If prolonged: suggestive of aneurysm
Pathological Q wave	Myocardial infarction
T wave inversion	Myocardial injury/ischaemia/ infarction

- Changes in the anteroseptal area are indicated by leads V1–V4.

- Changes in the anterolateral area are indicated by leads I, aVL, V5, V6.

- Changes in the inferior area are indicated by leads II, III, and aVF.

- Changes in the posterior area are indicated by a mirror-image (i.e. upside-down changes) seen in leads V1 and V2.

Changes secondary to pericardial disease

Concave ST segment elevation and tachycardia may be seen in acute pericarditis while low voltages (and, occasionally, alternating QRS complexes) may be seen with a large pericardial effusion.

Changes due to ventricular and atrial hypertrophy

Large QRS complexes are suggestive of hypertrophy this finding may be normal in adults under 35 years old. Left ventricular hypertrophy is present when the sum of the R wave in V5 or V6 plus the S wave in V1 exceeds 35 mm. In right ventricular hypertrophy a 'dominant' R wave is seen in Lead V1 (i.e. a large R wave relative to the S wave) but a normal-width QRS complex.

A 'strain pattern' is seen when ST depression and T wave inversion coexist in the appropriate leads and is suggestive of ischaemia in the hypertrophied ventricle.

Changes due to other diseases

ECG changes of pulmonary embolism are those of acute right heart strain and include:

- sinus tachycardia,

- right axis deviation,

- 'S1-Q3-T3' — deep S wave in lead I, pathological Q wave and inverted T wave in lead III,

- right ventricular strain,

- partial right bundle branch block (i.e. M-shaped QRS complex but width <0.12 s),

- peaked P waves,

- atrial fibrillation.

Pulse oximetry

Pulse oximetry is used to monitor continuously the oxygen saturation of arterial blood (S_aO_2). It provides immediate detection of hypoxaemic episodes without the discomfort and hazards of repeated arterial puncture.

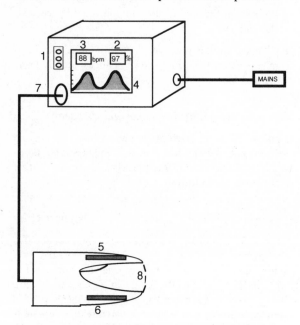

Fig. 4.26 The pulse oximeter. 1 = on/off, alarm settings; 2 = S_aO_2 display; 3 = heart rate display; 4 = pulse waveform display; 5 = light-emitting diodes; 6 = photodetector; 7 = patient cable; 8 = patient's digit.

A probe is attached to the patient. Various types of probe are available but they must be placed over a pulsating arteriolar bed (e.g. the finger or earlobe). The probe is connected to a monitor which will give a continuous digital display of the oxygen saturation. Some monitors will also show the heart rate and a pulsatile waveform (see Fig. 4.26).

Pulse oximetry works by measuring the variations in light absorption across the vascular bed. The calculation of oxygen saturation is based on the principles of Beer's law.

Beer's law states that the concentration of an unknown solute dissolved in a solvent can be determined by light absorption (Lynne *et al.*, 1990). The intensity of light transmitted through a substance depends on the amount of incident light, the concentration of the substance (in this case haemoglobin), and the distance that the light travels.

The probe

The probe consists of two light-emitting diodes which emit light at two specific wavelengths; 660 nm (red) and 940 (infrared). At these wavelengths the absorption characteristics of reduced haemoglobin and oxyhaemoglobin are quite different (Lynne *et al.*, 1990). The light passes through the tissue and is sensed by a photodetector at the base of the probe (see Fig. 4.26). During its passage, the majority of light is absorbed by skin, bone, connective tissue, pigmentation and venous vessels and this amount is constant with time (the baseline measurement). The only relevant fluctuations in absorption are caused by the increase in blood flow during systole. The peaks and troughs of the pulsatile and baseline absorptions for each wavelength are detected by the photodetector and the ratios of each are compared. There is, however, no mathematical correlation between these ratios and the oxygen saturation. The oxygen saturation is calculated by a microprocessor using a calibration curve obtained from experimental data.

Dedicated probes are used for each site. The digit (finger or toe) is the most common position, but alternative sites are the nasal bridge, above the eyebrow in the adult, or the arch of the foot in the neonate.

There may be potential problems of pressure on the skin from the probe and for this reason the probe site should be changed at least every 8 hours in the adult and 4-hourly in the neonate.

Accuracy of the pulse oximeter

The oxygen saturation displayed by the pulse oximeter does not give an indication of the oxygen content of the blood as this is determined by the oxygen-carrying capacity of the blood (i.e. how much haemoglobin is present to carry oxygen). Therefore, if the patient is anaemic the oxygen saturation may read 100%, since all the available haemoglobin is fully saturated, but in fact the oxygen content of the blood may be markedly low. In severe anaemia (< 5 g/dl) a 'low perfusion' alarm may be displayed.

Although the pulse oximeter is generally accurate if the oxygen saturation is in the range 70–100% there are specific conditions that will make the readings inaccurate. These are described below.

1 The presence of dysfunctional haemoglobins

The light source in the probe uses only two wavelengths of light and can therefore only determine the concentrations of two substances (reduced haemoglobin and oxyhaemoglobin). The oxygen saturation calculated by the pulse oximeter is termed the 'functional' saturation of haemoglobin. In order to take into account the concentration of other types of haemoglobins additional wavelengths must be used. A Co-oximeter (spectrophotometric hemoximeter) is a more accurate method of measuring oxygen saturation as it uses four or more wavelengths of light and is therefore able to identify the concentration of additional haemoglobins, such as methaemoglobin and carboxyhaemoglobin. The oxygen saturation calculated in this way is termed the 'fractional' oxygen saturation of haemoglobin (Lynne *et al.* 1990).

Pulse oximeter

$$\text{'Functional' saturation} = \frac{\text{Oxyhaemoglobin}}{\text{oxy} + \text{deoxyhaemoglobin}}$$

Co-oximeter

$$\text{'Fractional' saturation} = \frac{\text{Oxyhaemoglobin}}{\text{Oxy} + \text{Deoxy} + \text{Dysfunctional haemoglobin}}$$

Thus, in the following situations, oxygen saturation measured by pulse oximetry may therefore be inaccurate:

- Smoke inhalation. This raises carboxyhaemoglobin levels. The pulse oximeter interprets carboxyhaemoglobin as oxyhaemoglobin because the absorption coefficients of both are very similar. Therefore, in the presence of carboxyhaemoglobin the pulse oximeter will give false high readings compared to measurements by a Co-oximeter (Baker, 1987).

- The administration of drugs that cause methaemoglobinaemia. These include lignocaine, nitrates, and metoclopramide. Normal cellular mechanisms usually prevent the accumulation of methaemoglobin (formed when the iron in haemoglobin is oxidized from the ferrous state to the ferric state), but significant levels may be induced by these drugs (Smith and Olson 1989).

- The administration of certain dyes and pigments. These include methylene blue, indigo carmine, and indocyanine green. Methylene blue absorbs light at a similar frequency to reduced haemoglobin and the pulse oximeter may give false low readings of oxygen saturation (Sidi *et al.* 1987). There are contradictory data on the effect on pulse oximetry readings in patients with hyperbilirubinaemia (Lynne *et al.*, 1990), and if there is any uncertainty the readings should be checked on a Co-oximeter.

2. Low perfusion

If there is poor perfusion to the vascular bed over which the probe is placed it will be difficult for the photodetector to distinguish the pulsatile and baseline absorptions. Often the monitor will flash a 'low perfusion' alarm but false low readings may be displayed. The probe should be moved to a different site and low readings checked by aterial puncture and Co-oximeter calculation.

Poor perfusion may be due to hypovolaemic states, hypotension, septicaemia or peripheral vascular disease. The digits and earlobe sites are most commonly affected in these conditions.

3. Other conditions to avoid

- Avoid application of the probe distal to blood pressure cuffs, venous, or arterial catheters and intravenous lines as any increased venous or arterial pulsations can affect the readings.

- Nail varnish must be removed from fingers and toes.

- Do not use restrictive tape at the probe site.

- Light interference should be minimized from surgical lamps, direct sunlight, infrared warming lamps, and phototherapy lamps. These may cause light to be sensed by the photodetector without first passing through the tissue. If necessary, the probe may be covered with an opaque material.

Specific nursing interventions

- High and low alarm limits should be set according to the patients' clinical condition.

- The probe site should be rotated regularly and the area checked for pressure or irritation.

- The probe must be securely attached.

- Pulse oximetry should be used as a continuous guide to arterial oxygen saturation and not for its absolute values. Abnormal readings should be checked by arterial blood gas analysis/co-oximetry.

End tidal carbon dioxide monitoring (ETCO$_2$)

Peak end tidal carbon dioxide concentrations can be measured at the end of expiration and be continually displayed as a waveform or digital reading. This can be used as a guide to arterial CO_2 tension.

Measurement is achieved by placing a sensor between the patient's endotracheal tube and the ventilator tubing. A transducer detects the amount of infrared radiation that is absorbed by the expired gas and the ETCO$_2$ is derived from the level of radiation absorbed by carbon dioxide.

Alveolar CO_2 levels, in the presence of normal ventilation/perfusion relationships, can accurately reflect the adequacy of alveolar ventilation and a good correlation is seen between arterial and alveolar CO_2 levels. It is less accurate when ventilation/perfusion mismatch occurs or if there is significant air trapping (e.g. in asthma).

This technique is particularly useful as a guide to CO_2 elimination in patients who do not have arterial access for blood gas analysis. It can also be used to verify the correct placement of an endotracheal tube in the trachea at intubation.

Blood pressure (BP)

The technique for recording blood pressure using a sphygmomanometer and cuff will not be discussed as this should be more than familiar. However, several points may need emphasis.

Cuff size

To ensure accurate blood pressure recording the correct size of cuff is important. If the cuff is too narrow or applied too loosely the BP will be falsely high and if it is too wide it will under-read. The bladder width should ideally be 40–50% of the upper arm circumference. The bladder length should encircle 80% of the arm. The cuff should also be at the level of the heart to maintain a true zero level.

Comparing blood pressure recorded by different techniques

There are occasions when a BP recorded by one method may need to be verified using a different method. It must be remembered that each are methodologically different and measure different phenomena. Direct intra-arterial measurements record pressure impulses and indirect measurements record volume displacement (oscillometry) or flow detection (Doppler). Values obtained by auscultation may be lower than those obtained by direct measurement, since blood flow begins before sound is heard and the sound may also be absorbed by the surrounding tissues. Even with accurate techniques direct intra-arterial pressure can be expected to be 5–20 mmHg greater than by indirect measurement. Potential inaccuracies can occur in all techniques and this makes direct comparisons difficult even when the BP is recorded simultaneously. Such inaccuracies in indirect measurements include wrong cuff size and placement, personal variations, lack of stethoscope sensitivity, poor technique, and instrument errors.

Oscillometry

A more reliable method for measuring BP non-invasively is by oscillometry. An automated machine uses a cuff to compress the limb and measures BP by sensing the arterial pulsations (oscillations) as a function of cuff pressure. The sensor on the cuff is placed in the correct position (an arrow on the cuff indicates its placement over an artery) and the cuff is automatically inflated. As the cuff deflates the arterial pressure becomes equal to the cuff occluding pressure and blood begins to flow through the artery. The oscillations in the artery wall are small but as the cuff continues to deflate flow is increased and the amplitude of the oscillations reaches a maximum. As the cuff completely deflates the oscillations in the arterial wall lessen due to the reducing resistance to flow as the cuff occluding pressure is less than the diastolic pressure. The rapid increases and decreases in oscillations correspond to the systolic and diastolic pressures and the mean pressure is the lowest cuff pressure with the greatest oscillations.

Oscillometry may be less useful when used on severely hypotensive patients as the oscillation amplitude may be too small to be accurate.

Gastrointestinal tonometry

Gut tonometry is used to calculate the intramucosal pH (pHi) of either the stomach or (less commonly) the sigmoid colon. This has been shown to reflect oxygen delivery to the mucosa and a low level is said to be indicative of splanchnic ischaemia.

There is evidence that the blood supply to the gut is the first to be affected when oxygen delivery is reduced for whatever reason (e.g. myocardial dysfunction, haemorrhage, hypoxaemia). If this can be detected then effective treatment strategies can be instituted early in the hope of preventing subsequent organ failure.

The technique

The gastric tonometer is a modified nasogastric tube which, by the addition of an extra lumen, allows gastric aspiration, enteral feeding, and pHi measurement. At the tip of the tube is a silicone balloon that is permeable to carbon dioxide.

To make a measurement the tubing and balloon are primed with 0.9% sodium chloride to remove any air. The balloon is then filled with 2.5 ml of sodium chloride and left *in situ* for at least 20 minutes to allow equilibration to occur. The solution is then aspirated (the first ml is discarded as this has been in the tubing) and the remaining 1.5 ml is passed through a blood gas analyser to determine the PCO_2. An arterial blood gas is drawn at the same time for measurement of bicarbonate. The saline CO_2 and the arterial bicarbonate (assumed to be the same as the bicarbonate level in the gastric mucosa) are placed in a modified Henderson–Hasselbach equation to enable calculation of pHi:

$$pH_i = 6.1 + \log_{10} \frac{(HCO_3^-)}{(PCO_2 \times K \times 0.03)}$$

where

6.1 = pK for HCO_3^-/CO_2 system in plasma (i.e. pH value where concentrations of bicarbonate and carbonic acid are equal).
HCO_3^- = actual arterial bicarbonate concentration.
PCO_2 = CO_2 tension in tonometer saline.
K = equilibration period correction factor
0.03 = solubility of CO_2 in plasma at 37 °C.

The theory

The principle underlying this technique is that in low oxygen delivery states, anaerobic respiration will occur and CO_2 will be produced. The PCO_2 of the saline in the balloon will reflect the PCO_2 level in the gastric mucosa which, in turn, reflects the CO_2 tension in the capillaries supplying the mucosa. Therefore, if the pHi falls, indicating an acidotic state with a surplus of CO_2, it may be assumed that blood supply to the gastric mucosa is inadequate for tissue oxygen requirements.

There are two consequences of this which may have clinical significance. First, the patient may initially compensate for a low perfusion state and there may be no other detectable signs of reduced tissue oxygen delivery. Secondly, the gut can be rendered 'leaky' if allowed to become ischaemic, resulting in translocation of bacteria and endotoxins into the surrounding structures. However, this has not yet been shown in humans (see Chapter 10).

A number of drawbacks are present, for example, if gastric acid is present in the lumen of the stomach this may react with alkaline bile refluxing back through the pylorus and produce CO_2. This would invalidate the tonometer measurement of PCO_2 as a measure of gut mucosal CO_2. A H_2-antagonist (e.g. ranitidine) or a proton pump inhibitor (e.g. omeprazole) must then be administered to block gastric acid production. The effect of enteral nutrition in the stomach remains unknown. There are also a number of assumptions inherent in the technique, e.g. arterial bicarbonate is used as a substitute for gut mucosal bicarbonate and any metabolic acidosis present in the blood will automatically produce a low pHi. Thus, the most effective use of the tonometer should be when a low pHi is present despite a normal arterial blood pH. However, the cost of the tonometer makes routine usage prohibitive and waiting for clinical deterioration to occur before inserting a tonometer may well negate much of its utility.

Doppler techniques

Doppler ultrasound can be used to measure blood flow in a variety of vessels. An ultrasonic transducer transmits a single frequency ultrasound at the blood vessel. The same or another transducer (depending on the type of ultrasound used) picks up the ultrasound waves reflected back off the moving blood corpuscles. These waves have shifted in frequency according to the velocity of the moving blood. These Doppler frequency shifts can be converted into audible signals or, after computer analysis, displayed on a monitor as velocity–time waveforms.

To calculate the flow volume, the cross-sectional area of the vessel must be measured ([e.g. by echocardiography]) or approximated. The following equation is then applied:

Flow volume =
    Mean velocity × Cross-sectional area of vessel

Cardiac output can be measured in this way by placing a Doppler probe in the suprasternal notch to record the mean velocity of blood flowing in the ascending aorta. A drawback of this approach is the inability to hold the probe in place, thereby preventing continuous measurement. A new approach via the oesophagus can also be used to measure blood flow continuously in the descending thoracic aorta. An estimate of cardiac output to some 85–90% accuracy can be provided using a nomogram incorporating the patient's age, height, and weight. This approach does make a number of assumptions about flow going to the head and neck and the aortic cross-sectional area but appears to be generally reliable in clinical practice.

Doppler probes can also be used by the nurse at the bedside to check for the presence of pulsatile flow in ischaemic limbs, particularly following distal vascular surgery. In these cases, they are used to check primarily that there is blood flow (a pulse that can be heard) rather than to calculate flow volume and can be extremely useful in detecting a pulse that is difficult to palpate.

Invasive monitoring

Invasive methods of monitoring are now commonplace on the ICU but the potential value of such techniques must be carefully considered prior to insertion. They can be potentially hazardous for the patient due to complications that can arise either from their insertion or by remaining *in situ*. However, they can also provide invaluable information for the monitoring of disease processes and manipulation of treatment strategies.

The nurse must be fully aware of the operating techniques and the potential hazards and complications of the equipment used in order to minimize risk to the patient.

Each device will have its associated complications but the very fact that it is an invasive procedure means infection is a potential problem.

Local policies and practices should be followed for dressing changes and changes of cannulae and tubing (including transducers). Routine infection control measures should be instituted. These should include:

- effective handwashing,

- the use of a strict aseptic technique when inserting or redressing cannulae,

- clear semi-permeable dressings over cannula sites to allow regular inspection,

- minimal disturbance of the dressing; redress as necessary rather than routinely,

- minimal use of 3-way taps to limit potential entry for infection,

- labelling of lines and transducers with the date and time that they were last changed.

Most invasive lines will be sutured in position and these should be well secured to prevent accidental removal by the patient. Some devices, such as pulmonary artery catheters (with associated cardiac output leads), are quite heavy and the weight will need to be supported by securing these to the pillow or bedding.

Pressure monitoring

Most patient monitors have the facility to display pressures continuously from invasive monitoring. These can include systemic arterial, pulmonary artery, and central venous pressures.

Transducers are needed in the monitoring circuit to measure and transmit the pressure recorded within the heart or blood vessel to the monitor. Transducers come in varying shapes and forms depending on the manufacturer and the type of monitor used. These can be obtained already assembled with all the patient tubing attached and are very easy to prepare (see Fig. 4.27). Some older equipment may still require each part of the transducer to be connected separately with individual sterile domes and separate tubing and taps.

In general, transducers are small, fluid-filled devices. Tubing from the patient cannula is connected to one side of the transducer and from the other side a giving set is connected to a bag of heparinized crystalloid solution. This solution must be kept under continuous pressure (usually 300 mmHg for arterial lines but can be less for venous lines) to prevent a back-flow of blood from the patient into the circuit. Adjacent to the transducer is a flushing device which ensures the continuous delivery of fluid (3 ml/h) through the patient's cannula and allows the tubing to be manually flushed at any time (such as after taking blood samples). The flushing device keeps the cannula patent.

Pressure is transmitted from the cannula through the fluid-filled pressure tubing to the transducer. From here it is relayed via an electrical cable to the monitor where it is usually displayed as both a waveform trace and as a digital readout providing systolic, diastolic, and mean pressure measurements.

There are several points to remember to ensure accurate pressure readings:

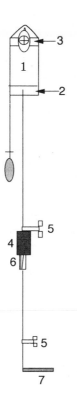

Fig. 4.27 Transduced pressure monitoring system.
1 = infusion fluid 2 = pressure bag; 3 = pressure gauge;
4 = transducer; 5 = 3-way tap; 6 = flush device; 7 = patient
cannula.

- The transducer must always be level with the zero reference point. This is usually the right atrium (mid-axilla) for CVP lines. If the patient is moved, the transducer must be re-aligned.

- The transducer must be calibrated to atmospheric pressure ['zeroed'] before use, intermittently while in use (e.g. at the beginning of each shift), and whenever the patient tubing or transducer is changed. This procedure will vary according to the type of monitor being used but basically entails turning the 3-way tap in the circuit 'off' to the patient, thus exposing the transducer to atmospheric pressure (air), and pressing a zero button on the monitor. When the monitor shows a zero reading the 3-way tap can be turned back 'on' to the patient and placed at the zero reference point. The transducer will now read an arterial or venous pressure calibrated to atmospheric pressure.

- Only dedicated manometer tubing should be used throughout the system. This is rigid tubing with a low compliance and small diameter. Soft, flexible tubing should not be used as the pressure changes will not be accurately conducted.

- Excessively long tubing or air bubbles in the tubing or transducer may cause a 'dampened' trace with consequent inaccurate readings. The presence of 3-way taps in the circuit will also 'dampen' the trace.

Arterial cannulation

Intra-arterial cannulation can be utilized for optimizing patient management and for rapid reassessment. It allows:

- continuous monitoring of blood pressure,

- frequent blood sampling without patient disturbance and repeated vessel puncture.

The radial, femoral, or dorsalis pedis arteries are the most commonly used. The radial artery is preferred as the hand usually has a good collateral circulation, the artery is near to the skin surface and the cannula site is easily observed. However, in patients with Raynaud's disease or inadequate ulnar circulation, hand ischaemia, skin necrosis, radial nerve damage, and thrombosis can occur. Before insertion of a radial arterial cannula the collateral circulation can be checked by manually occluding the radial and ulnar arteries. The patient is then instructed to flex the fingers which should result in blanching of the hand. The pressure is then released from the ulnar artery and if collateral circulation is good the hand should flush (this is called Allen's test).

The femoral artery is often cannulated in severely hypotensive patients because the femoral pulse is often the most easily palpable and its superficial location makes it easy to access. However, if blood flow to the limb is compromised the patient is exposed to a potentially large area of ischaemia. Regular assessment of pedal pulses and skin temperature should be carried out. Since the groin cannot be continually exposed and therefore observed, unseen haemorrhage at this site can have dire consequences. It is imperative that lower alarm limits are set on the monitor and a clear waveform is visible so that any accidental disconnection is discovered immediately. This is not the preferred cannulation site for diabetic patients (who may have poor wound healing and microcirculation problems) or patients with occlusive vascular disease.

The dorsalis pedis artery can also be used but the vessel is small and often difficult to cannulate, makes mobilization difficult for the patient and it can be difficult to obtain a good waveform. It should be avoided if possible in patients with peripheral vascular disease or diabetes. Collateral circulation should be confirmed (it can be checked against flow in the posterior tibial artery in a method similar to Allen's test described above). Thrombosis can occur and the toes should be observed for ischaemia. Due to the greater distance from the heart and the smaller vessel lumen, the blood pressure recorded from the dorsalis pedis (and the radial artery also) will be higher than that in the femoral artery and may not necessarily reflect the perfusion pressure in other regions.

The brachial artery should not be used except for short term placement when no other cannulation sites are available/accessible. As it is an end-artery, vessel damage/thrombosis at this point may result in loss of the blood supply of the forearm. Haematoma formation at the cannula site can result in median nerve compression. Nerve damage and reduced joint mobility can occur as well as the universal potential complication of embolization. This site is also uncomfortable for the patient as mobility is reduced.

In summary, whichever artery is chosen:

- there should be a good collateral blood supply to the limb,

- it must be easily observable with access for nursing care,

- it should not be located in an area prone to contamination or where a wound exists,

- it should not be sited in limbs that have vascular prostheses.

Complications of intra-arterial cannulation

Specific complications have been mentioned above. In addition to thrombus formation, embolization, infection, and exsanguination due to disconnection, the following are also recognized complications:

- accidental intra-arterial injection of drugs

- air embolus (from air within the flush system)

- arteriovenous fistula

- pain

- aneurysm

- local haematomas

- necrosis of skin and digits.

Removal of the cannula

When the catheter is removed digital pressure must be applied for as long as necessary to achieve haemostasis. Assess the peripheral circulation, as thrombosis can occur after removal.

The arterial waveform

This reflects the pressure generated in the arterial tree following contraction of the left ventricle after electrical activation. Hence, when the arterial waveform is evaluated in conjunction with the ECG the electrical activity will occur before the mechanical activity. It should be stressed that the arterial pressure does not equate with blood flow or cardiac output. For example, a high blood pressure may be produced by the vasoconstricton response to hypovolaemia while a low blood pressure may be associated with a high flow, vasodilated state as seen in sepsis. (See Fig. 4.28.)

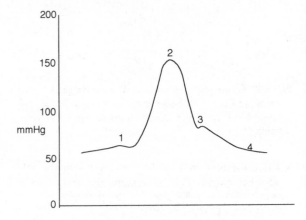

Fig. 4.28 The arterial waveform. 1 = anacrotic notch; 2 = peak systolic pressure; 3 = dicrotic notch; 4 = diastolic pressure.

The anacrotic notch

This is only seen in central aortic pressure monitoring or in some pathological conditions. During the second phase of ventricular systole there is a presystolic rise in pressure which occurs before the opening of the aortic valve. This is the anacrotic notch.

The peak systolic pressure

This is the maximum left ventricular systolic pressure. The sharp upward rise in pressure is generated by the outflow of blood from the ventricle into the arterial system.

The dicrotic notch

The dicrotic notch reflects the closure of the aortic valve caused by a rise in pressure in the aorta. When the pressure in the aorta is greater than in the left ventricle the blood attempts to flow backwards causing the valve to close. On the waveform trace the dicrotic notch marks the end of systole and the onset of diastole. The dicrotic notch wave is markedly elevated in patients with decreased cardiac output and increased peripheral vascular resistance.

The diastolic pressure

The diastolic pressure is related to the degree of vaso-constriction in the arterial system and the diastolic time during the cardiac cycle. During diastole there must be sufficient time for blood to drain into the smaller arteriolar branches. If there is a short diastole, as in a fast heart rate, there is insufficient time for this drainage to occur and, consequently, the diastolic pressure may be higher.

Pulse pressure (PP)

The pulse pressure is the difference between the systolic and diastolic pressure. Factors which may affect this include changes in stroke volume (affects systolic pressure) or changes in vascular compliance (affects diastolic pressure).

Mean arterial pressure (MAP)

Many monitors have the ability to calculate the MAP from the arterial waveform. This value is the average pressure in the arterial system during one complete cycle of systole and diastole. Since at normal heart rates systole usually requires one-third of the cardiac cycle time and diastole two-thirds this is reflected in the equation for calculating MAP:

$$MAP = DBP + \frac{(SBP - DBP)}{3}, \text{ or}$$

$$MAP = \frac{SBP + (DBP \times 2)}{3}$$

where

SBP = systolic pressure.
DBP = diastolic pressure.

Observation of the arterial waveform can also provide information in some clinical conditions.

Atrial fibrillation: the characteristic ECG rate and rhythm irregularity is reflected on the pressure monitor by variable amplitudes of the arterial waveform. This equates to the variable stroke volumes produced as a consequence of altered diastolic filling times during atrial fibrillation. A 12-lead ECG is needed to make a firm diagnosis of atrial fibrillation as multiple supraventricular ectopic beats can mimic the irregular rhythm.

Pulsus alternans: there is a regular alternating of peak systolic pressure amplitude with the patient in sinus rhythm and is classically seen in patients with left ventricular failure.

Aortic stenosis: this may produce a narrow pulse pressure since the systolic pressure is lower and the slowed ventricular ejection through the stenotic valve causes a delayed systolic peak. The dicrotic notch is not well defined because the valve leaflets close abnormally at the onset of diastole.

Aortic regurgitation: this causes a wide pulse pressure and (usually) a higher peak systolic pressure due to the left ventricle receiving more blood as it backflows through the incompetent valve during diastole.

Normal respiration can also cause changes in amplitude of systolic pressure due to changes in intrathoracic pressure. During inspiration in the spontaneously breathing person, intrathoracic pressure is lower (i.e. more negative) thereby causing a pooling of blood in the pulmonary vasculature. This causes less blood to reach the left side of the heart and peak systolic pressure may be 3–10 mmHg lower. At expiration, the blood that had pooled in the pulmonary bed is shunted to the left side of the heart increasing the left ventricular filling volume and causing a higher peak systolic pressure. The opposite is seen with mechanical positive pressure ventilation.

'Pulsus paradoxus' is a term used when the difference in peak systolic pressure is greater than 10 mmHg between inspiration and expiration. This is an accentuation of the normal pattern and an exaggerated swing in systolic pressure over the respiratory cycle in seen on the monitor. Causes of this include pericardial disease (e.g. pericardial tamponade) which impedes ventricular filling, exaggerated inspiration by the patient, or pathological causes that result in gross changes in intrathoracic pressure during respiration (e.g. asthma). Probably the commonest cause of an exaggerated 'respiratory swing' in the critically ill patient is hypovolaemia, particularly when the patient has concurrently high airway pressures.

Specific nursing care

Safety

Accidental disconnection can result in considerable blood loss unless detected immediately. For this reason the cannula site should always be visible (unless the femoral artery is used). Alarm limits (particularly the lower limit) must be set on the monitor if the cannula is transduced; this will allow disconnection to be recognized immediately. If the femoral artery is used this is essential as the site will not be continuously visible.

All connections within the circuit should be Luer locked and firmly connected. A loose connection can cause loss of pressure within the circuit, back-flow of blood from the patient, and blood loss at the connection site.

Inadvertent administration of drugs can have dire consequences and arterial lines must be labelled clearly to avoid confusion with venous lines.

Limb perfusion

Perfusion distal to the cannula site must be observed regularly. Occlusion of the artery by a thrombus or adjacent haematoma can severely reduce blood flow to the area supplied by that vessel. *If the limb becomes cold, white, or painful senior medical staff must be informed immediately.* The cannula should be removed and circulation must be assessed manually by capillary refill or the use of Doppler to identify pulsatile flow. If collateral circulation is good, the limb may be saved but there is a danger, particularly if the brachial artery has been used, that circulation may not be restored.

Arterial spasm can also result in blanching and pain in the limb. This can be caused by very cold and frequent administrations of flush solution or the accidental injection of a drug into the cannula. The cannula should be removed and the limb kept warm. In the case of accidental drug administration into the arterial line the cannula should be flushed vigously using the flushing device. An additional treatment option for persisting arterial spasm is to inject papaverine intra-arterially. (See also Table 4.8.)

Intra-arterial blood gas electrode

A very thin probe containing specialized electrodes can be placed through the cannula into the artery and will continuously measure the arterial PO_2, PCO_2, and pH which are displayed on a monitor. Studies have shown a good correlation between the values derived from arterial samples and the intra-arterial electrodes. The oxygen measurement in particular is prone to drift and thus the sensor requires re-calibration at 12–24-hourly intervals. The probe may also 'dampen' the arterial waveform trace by partially or fully occluding the cannula. It does, however, provide a continuous guide to arterial blood gases allowing direct assesment of the effect of interventions and the early recognition of problems. Potentially spurious results must be confirmed by arterial sampling.

Central venous pressure (CVP) and right atrial pressure

In order to monitor CVP, a catheter is usually inserted into the internal jugular or subclavian veins, though long lines inserted via the femoral or brachial veins can also be used. The tip of the catheter does not need to lie inside the right atrium but can be within one of the larger veins leading to the heart, though it should be within the thoracic cavity. The CVP at this point equals right atrial pressure which, in turn, equals right ventricular end diastolic (filling) pressure. The pressure within the right atrium does not necessarily reflect either intravascular volume status or left heart pressures. It therefore has limitations in the acute stages of critical illness. However, the resultant access to a large vein enables the infusion of hypertonic solutions, solutions that are irritant to peripheral veins and drugs that require a rapid effect.

Single, double, or triple lumen catheters are available. Multiple-lumen catheters are particularly useful as they allow dedicated lumens for inotropes, infusion fluids that should not be mixed with others (such as Total Parenteral Nutrition, sodium bicarbonate) and the bolus administration of drugs without the inadvertent flushing of drug infusions.

The catheter is inserted under sterile conditions, usually by the Seldinger technique. An introducer (a large-bore needle or cannula) is inserted into the vessel, a flexible wire is fed into the vein via the introducer, and the introducer is then withdrawn completely. The catheter is then inserted over the wire to a satisfactory depth (usually 15–20 cm for jugular or subclavian lines) and the wire is then removed.

It is vital that the catheter position is confirmed before drugs or infusion fluids are administered. To verify this there must be an easy withdrawal of blood from the catheter. The catheter can be attached via a giving set to a bag of crystalloid solution which is then placed below the level of the patient; blood should flow back into the giving set if it is in a blood vessel. If there is no return of blood, removal of the catheter should be considered.

Table 4.8 Summary of problems associated with arterial cannulae

Problem	Cause	Action
'Damped' trace leading to underestimated BP (blunt pressure peak, loss of dicrotic notch)	• Loss of pressure or no fluid in the infusion pressure bag	• Inflate pressure bag to 300 mmHg. Check there is sufficient flushing solution
	• Thrombus/fibrin formation at tip of catheter	• Withdraw blood and then flush catheter
	• Air in tubing or transducer	• Disconnect tubing from catheter and flush through to expel air before reconnecting. If necessary, change transducer
	• Too many 3-way taps in the circuit	• Remove excess taps
	• Long length of tubing between catheter and transducer	• Shorten tubing
	• Poor position of limb, tip of catheter against vessel wall, kinked tubing	• Manipulate catheter and/or limb to achieve a better trace
No arterial waveform (straight line)	• Taps turned off to patient or transducer	• Check taps are on to patient and transducer
	• Disconnection of catheter	• Check catheter site — reconnect immediately
	• Disconnection of transducer cable to monitor	• Check connections — reconnect
	• Poor catheter position (tip against vessel wall)	• Manipulate position, flush catheter
	• Asystole	• Institute CPR
Backflow of blood from catheter towards transducer	• Loose tap connection within the circuit	• Check all connections are secure
	• Flush bag pressure too low (below patient's BP)	• Inflate bag to 300 mmHg pressure

This additional test safeguards against the possibility that the catheter is in the pleural space of a patient who has a haemothorax on that side. In this situation, blood may be aspirated from the catheter even though it is outside the vein. A chest X-ray must be performed to verify the catheter position and detect any complications. When the correct position is confirmed a transducer system or giving set can be attached and drugs or infusions administered as necessary.

Potential complications associated with the insertion of a CVP catheter

• Pneumo/haemothorax
This can result from accidental puncture of the pleura during the procedure. The patient's haemodynamic and respiratory status must be monitored closely during and after insertion. The post-insertion chest X-ray should be carefully examined. Not only may the patient be compromised if a pneumothorax is present but if fluids and drugs are infused into the pleural space a potentially disastrous situation can result. The consequent pleural effusion may cause respiratory deterioration and the drugs and infusion fluids given would be ineffective as they have not entered the systemic circulation. The catheter must be removed immediately and pleural aspiration/drainage may be required while supportive respiratory care is given.

• Haematoma caused by trauma to the vein and/or surrounding tissue
Observe site for bleeding, bruising, and swelling. Occasionally, an artery may be accidently punctured by the introducer whilst attempting insertion. If this is known to have occurred, particular attention must be focused on the site to identify bleeding or swelling. Prolonged direct

pressure may be necessary to stop bleeding although this is difficult if the subclavian artery has been punctured.

● Catheter in incorrect position.
Occasionally, the catheter may follow a path away from the heart towards the head or down the arm. This will not give an accurate reading of the CVP and should be repositioned.

● Air embolus
This may occur if the catheter is not properly connected to the appropriate tubing, or if one of the portals or 3-way taps is left 'open to air' and the patient is making spontaneous breathing efforts (negative intrathoracic pressure sucking the air in). The catheter and tubing should always be primed with fluid prior to insertion.

Measuring the CVP

The CVP may be measured using a transducer system (see Fig. 4.27), or manually using a manometer (this method is now less common within the ICU as it is far less accurate). Manual measurement allows only intermittent recordings to be made and requires a fluid-filled manometer tube to be connected to the catheter. The manometer is aligned so that the point on the scale of the manometer that is level with the right atrium of the patient is regarded as zero. The manometer is filled with fluid from a bag of 0.9% sodium chloride or 5% glucose to a level well above the expected CVP. The manometer tap is then turned so that fluid runs down the manometer into the patient. It will come to rest at a level which is the CVP and the reading can be made from an adjoining scale. The fluid in the manometer should gently rise and fall with respiration.

A transduced catheter will give a continuous display of the CVP on a monitor. The waveform on the monitor should show small undulations reflecting the changes in pressure within the right atrium during the cardiac cycle (see Fig. 4.29).

The normal range for CVP measurements is 3–10 mmHg. It must be remembered that any increase in intrathoracic pressure such as positive pressure ventilation or positive end expiratory pressure will increase the CVP measured relative to atmospheric pressure. The juxtacardiac pressure (i.e. CVP minus intrathoracic pressure) may be considerably lower. Hypovolaemia can thus be camouflaged by a seemingly normal or high CVP, especially in the presence of concurrently high intrathoracic pressures.

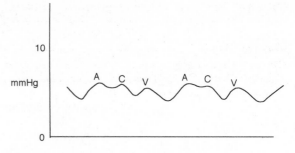

Fig. 4.29 The right atrial pressure waveform (A, C, and V waves).

The right atrial pressure waveform has three characteristic positive deflections corresponding to the electrical events of the ECG.

1. The A wave
This reflects right atrial contraction and follows the P wave on the ECG. The descent after this represents atrial relaxation. An elevated A wave may be associated with right ventricular failure or tricuspid stenosis.

2. The C wave
This represents tricuspid valve closure and follows the QRS on the ECG tracing. The distance A–C should be the same as the P–R interval.

3. The V wave
This represents the pressure generated to the right atrium by the contracting right ventricle despite the tricuspid valve being shut. It corresponds to the latter half of the T wave on the ECG. An elevated V wave is associated with tricuspid insufficiency.

Conditions that affect the CVP (see Table 4.9)

Table 4.9 Conditions affecting the CVP

Increased values	Decreased values
Right ventricular failure	Hypovolaemia
Pericardial tamponade	Peripheral vasodilatation (including sepsis, drugs, regional analgesia, sympathetic dysfunction)
Fluid overload	
Pulmonary hypertension	
Tricuspid regurgitation	
Pulmonary stenosis	
Superior vena caval obstruction	

Removal of the CVP catheter

In order to reduce the risk of an air embolism the patient should lie flat, or if condition allows head tipped down, when the catheter is withdrawn. After removal a sterile, occlusive dressing should be placed over the site.

Pulmonary artery catheterization

In many critically ill patients, particularly those with pulmonary disease or isolated right heart or left heart dysfunction, the measurement of right atrial pressure gives no indication of the function of the left side of the heart. If the determinants of cardiac function (see below) can be known and manipulated, more effective treatment strategies can be instituted. This can be achieved using a pulmonary artery catheter.

The pulmonary artery catheter

The pulmonary artery (PA) catheter is inserted to measure (or derive) a range of intracardiac and pulmonary artery pressures, vascular resistance, and cardiac output.

The standard pulmonary artery catheter consists of three or four lumens, is 110 cm long, and is marked in 10 cm increments to aid placement (see Fig. 4.30). Various modifications exist including:

- extra lumens for drug/fluid administration,

- thermistor and computer connector for cardiac output measurement,

- continuous mixed venous oxygen saturation,

- a pacing wire or external electrodes for temporary pacing,

- right ventricular volume measurements and ejection fractions.

The proximal injectate port

This lumen opens 30 cm from the tip of the catheter, therefore, when the tip of the catheter is in the pulmonary artery the opening of the proximal lumen should lie within the right atrium. It is used to monitor right atrial pressure but can be used for drug/fluid infusions. This port is used to administer the injectate fluid necessary for recording the cardiac output.

The distal lumen

This runs the entire length of the catheter opening at the tip which lies in the pulmonary artery. It is connected to a transducer which continually monitors the pulmonary artery pressure and permits the recording of pulmonary artery wedge pressure. During insertion of the catheter it is used to monitor all intracardiac pressures as it passes through the heart. Blood samples can be withdrawn from this lumen to obtain blood. This is known as mixed venous blood (i.e. where blood from the IVC and SVC are well mixed).

The thermistor connection

This is connected to the monitor cable to enable core and injectate fluid temperatures to be detected.

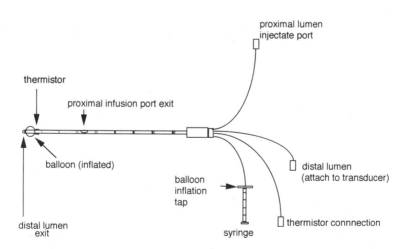

Fig. 4.30 The standard pulmonary artery catheter.

The thermistor
This lies 4 cm from the tip of the catheter and senses blood temperature. Two insulated wires run the length of a lumen to end at the thermistor connection.

Balloon inflation lumen
This lumen is used to inflate and deflate the balloon when recording the pulmonary artery wedge pressure. A 1.5 ml capacity syringe is attached at this point and a tap allows the lumen to be turned off to the syringe when not in use. All catheters for adults will accommodate the full 1.5 ml of air in the balloon and this is inflated only whilst the wedge pressures are taken. Overinflation by injection of extra volumes may result in balloon rupture.

Insertion of the catheter

The most common insertion sites for the pulmonary artery catheter are the internal jugular and subclavian veins, although the external jugular, antecubital, and femoral veins can be also be used. The subclavian vein approach may result in kinking in the catheter due to anatomical reasons and this can cause a dampened waveform.

Before insertion all lumens of the catheter are flushed with a standard $\pm$ heparinized saline solution and the integrity of the balloon is checked by inflating it with 1.5 ml of air. The ballon should be seen to inflate evenly and not remain asymmetric. A sterile sleeve adapter is placed over the catheter before insertion and this allows later manipulation while keeping the enclosed catheter portion sterile.

The catheter is inserted under strict aseptic conditions. Using the Seldinger technique a larger size introducer cannula is first inserted into the vessel and the pulmonary artery catheter is then passed through a self-sealing valve at the top of the introducer into the vessel itself.

The distal lumen of the catheter is connected to the transducer and by observing the monitor during placement the catheter tip location can be determined by the changes in waveform and pressure.

The catheter is advanced with the balloon deflated until it is beyond the end of the introducer cannula; it can then be inflated. If the internal jugular or subclavian veins are used the catheter tip should enter the right atrium at 15–20 cm (femoral vein distance is 30 cm and right antecubital fossa 40 cm). The characteristic waveform of the RA will be seen at this point (see Fig. 4.31).

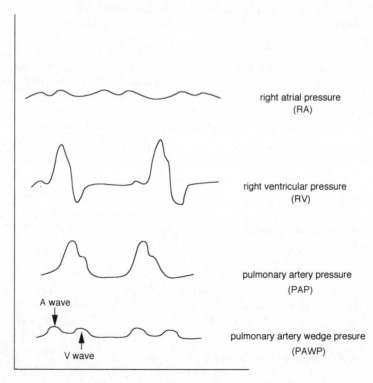

Fig. 4.31 Pressure waveform characteristics during insertion of the pulmonary artery catheter.

The catheter is advanced until a right ventricular waveform is displayed on the monitor and ventricular systolic and diastolic pressures are noted. This should be achieved within 10–15 cm of entering the right atrium. Failing this, the balloon should be deflated, the catheter withdrawn, and the procedure repeated until the right ventricular waveform is seen. If the right ventricle is not entered, the catheter may advance down the vena cava or into the coronary sinus (which may give the impression of a 'wedged' trace (see later) which is achieved well before the expected 50 cm insertion distance).

The catheter is further advanced, through the pulmonary valve into the pulmonary artery where a change in waveform occurs (rise in diastolic pressure). This point will be approximately 40–45 cm from the insertion site if the internal jugular vein is used.

The catheter is then advanced a further 5–10 cm until it is in a 'wedge' or occluded position. If the catheter is not wedged at this length there may have been some coiling in the right ventricle. The balloon should not be left inflated for more than 15 seconds and a clear pulmonary artery waveform should always be seen on the monitor.

Waveform characteristics

Right ventricular pressure

The waveform shows tall upright peaks corresponding to ventricular systole. The baseline corresponds to ventricular diastolic pressure. This is similar to RA pressure due to the low resistance across the tricuspid valve. As the catheter is passed through the ventricle particular attention must be paid to the ECG monitor as ventricular arrythmias can occur (due to irritation of the ventricular wall by the catheter tip). If ventricular ectopics occur continue with the procedure, but if ventricular tachycardia occurs the catheter should be withdrawn from the ventricle.

Pulmonary artery pressure

A rapid ejection of blood from the right ventricle into the PA represents the pulmonary artery systolic pressure. Since the pulmonary valve is open at this point PASP is usually equal to RV systolic pressure. At the end of systole the PA pressure falls and the pulmonary valve closes, creating a dicrotic notch on the waveform. The PADP is usually 5–10 mmHg higher than the RVDP.

Pulmonary artery wedge pressure (PAWP)

When the balloon is inflated in a branch of the pulmonary artery this occludes flow completely. Thus, all influences on pressure measured at the catheter tip resulting from flow from the right side of the heart are removed. The pressure at the tip of the catheter therefore reflects only the pressure ahead of it. Assuming an open circuit through the pulmonary vasculature and into the left heart, the left ventricular end diastolic pressure equals the left atrial pressure, the pulmonary venous pressure and the pulmonary capillary pressure. The pulmonary artery wedge (or occlusion) pressure is thus a good reflection of the LVEDP except in certain circumstances (see later). The PAWP waveform is characteristic of the pressure changes within the left atrium. Small A and V waves can be distinguished which represent left atrial and left ventricular systole. The pressure in the left atrium is usually slightly higher than in the right atrium and slightly less (1–3 mmHg) than the PADP.

The PAWP is measured at the end of the A wave (i.e. at the end of ventricular diastole, and at the end of expiration). At this point, the intrathoracic pressure is closest to barometric pressure against which the pressure transducer is zeroed.

Measuring the PAWP

- Whilst watching the monitor, *slowly* inflate the ballon until the characteristic flattened waveform is seen. The balloon is now occluding blood flow in the vessel and is said to be 'wedged' (Fig. 4.12).

- Stop inflating *as soon as this waveform is seen*.

- Freeze the monitor screen if the monitor has this facility (if not, read the wedge pressure from the monitor display. If the patient is mechanically ventilated, the lowest value should be taken as this corresponds to the PAWP at the end of expiration).

- Deflate the balloon rapidly. The balloon should not be left inflated for more than 15 seconds.

- If a screen freeze facility is available, ascertain the wedge pressure by moving the cursor control on the monitor to the correct position on the waveform (see Fig. 4.32).

- Unfreeze the screen to restore the continuous pulmonary artery waveform.

- Ensure that a pulmonary artery waveform is present.

Special points

- Do not use more than 1.5 ml of air to inflate the balloon or there is a risk of rupture of the balloon or vessel. If less than 1.2 ml of air is required to obtain the wedged waveform the catheter tip is too far advanced. As this also carries an increased risk of pulmonary artery rupture the balloon should be deflated and the catheter withdrawn slightly.

- The catheter is 'overwedged' if the trace rises sharply while the balloon is being inflated. This is due to the high pressure within the over-inflated balloon being transmitted to the transducer (see Fig. 4.12). If this occurs when the balloon is inflated with less than 1.2 ml of air the catheter tip is situated in a small vessel; the ballon should be *immediately* deflated and the catheter withdrawn to a more proximal position.

- Inflation time must be kept to a minimum and the balloon should not remain inflated for more than 15 seconds (approximately 2–3 cycles of respiration).

- Never flush the catheter when the balloon is inflated.

- Never inject fluid into the inflation port.

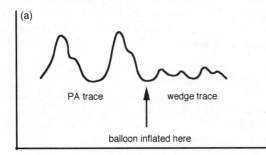

(a)

PA trace   wedge trace

balloon inflated here

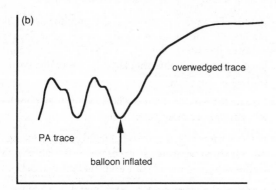

(b)

overwedged trace

PA trace

balloon inflated

Fig. 4.32 The pulmonary artery wedge trace: (a) waveform showing a wedge trace; (b) waveform showing an overwedged trace caused by overinflation of the balloon.

The correct wedge pressure can be easily achieved in a patient who is mechanically ventilated but it is more difficult to gain accurate readings in patients who are breathing spontaneously (with or without ventilatory assistance), particularly if deep breaths are being taken as this may result in large 'respiratory swings' on the monitor.

During spontaneous respiration the PA and PAWP both fall during inspiration (i.e. as the intrathoracic pressure becomes more negative) and rise with expiration. All pressures are recorded at the end of expiration (i.e. closest to atmospheric pressure) therefore this is just before the pressures start to fall on the waveform trace. The opposite occurs in ventilated patients because positive pressure ventilation causes the intrathoracic pressure to increase with inspiration causing an increase in PA and PAWP. As the patient expires the pressures fall. Thus, in the ventilated patient, readings are made just before the trace on the waveform begins to rise (see Fig. 4.33).

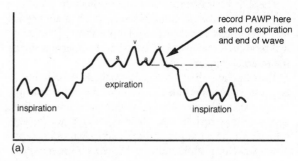

record PAWP here at end of expiration and end of wave

expiration

inspiration   inspiration

(a)

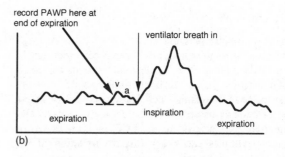

record PAWP here at end of expiration

ventilator breath in

expiration   inspiration   expiration

(b)

Fig. 4.33 Where to measure the PAWP: (a) in a patient breathing spontaneously. (b) in a mechanically ventilated patient.

There are certain conditions where PAWP does not accurately reflect LVEDP:

PAWP > LVEDP

- greatly raised intrathoracic pressure,

- pulmonary venous obstruction,

- mitral stenosis,

- left atrial myxoma.

Catheter position in the pulmonary artery

The catheter tip should be located in a main branch of the pulmonary artery. Catheter tip position changes can cause potential risks to the patient. The catheter may migrate into a more distal branch of the pulmonary artery when the balloon is deflated causing it to be partially or completely wedged. This can be identified by the characteristic wedged tracing on the waveform. The catheter must not remain in this position due to the potential risk of pulmonary artery occlusion or rupture and must be repositioned (usually by withdrawing the catheter by 1–2 cm).

Occasionally, the tip of the catheter may slip back into the right ventricle giving a ventricular waveform tracing. The tip may cause irritability to the ventricle and predispose to ventricular arrythmias (ventricular fibrillation, tachycardia, or ectopics). If this occurs, the balloon should be inflated and refloated into the pulmonary artery.

The catheter tip position in the lung is important for accurate PAWP recordings. The lungs have three physiological ('West') zones of blood flow depending on the interraction of alveolar, pulmonary arterial, and venous pressures (West 1990). In order to reflect left atrial pressure the catheter tip should lie in zone III where flow is continuous (see Fig. 4.34). If it is placed in zones I or II alveolar pressures are reflected and may give a spuriously high indication of LVEDP. These zones are not fixed anatomically and will change gravitationally with body position. Hypovolaemia and positive end expiratory pressure (PEEP) will increase the proportions of zones I and II. Thus, the zone within which the catheter tip is located may change with body posi-

tion, hypovolaemia, or PEEP. Paradoxically, therefore, the wedge pressure may rise with hypovolaemia. The correct position can be identified on a lateral chest X-ray where the tip of the catheter should be below the level of the left atrium. An alternative means of confirming a satisfactory zone III position is to increase the level of PEEP temporarily (e.g. by 5 cmH$_2$O) and see that the wedge pressure does not increase by at least half the increase in PEEP (e.g. 2–3 mmHg).

Zone I. The alveolar pressure is greater than the pulmonary arterial and venous pressure, therefore there is no blood flow from the pulmonary capillary beds.

Zone II. The alveolar pressure is higher than the pulmonary venous pressure but the arterial pressure is high enough to allow some blood flow. PAWP recordings will be less accurate than if the tip is in zone III. PEEP may increase the alveolar pressure causing zone II to be similar to zone I.

Zone III. The pulmonary venous pressure is higher than the alveolar pressure and all pulmonary capillaries are open.

Specific complications of pulmonary artery catheterization

- Pulmonary artery rupture or perforation due to the catheter tip or overinflation of the balloon (particularly in patients with pulmonary hypertension and the elderly — less distensible arteries).

- Air embolism due to rupture of the balloon.

- Ventricular arrythmias — these can occur on insertion or removal of the catheter or if the tip migrates back into the right ventricle.

- Pulmonary artery infarction results from loss of blood supply to a branch of the pulmonary artery due to the catheter spontaneously wedging if the catheter migrates forwards, or to the balloon remaining inflated.

- Valvular damage can occur if the balloon is inflated while the catheter is withdrawn.

- There is a recognized incidence of right-sided valvular vegetations. The proportion leading to clinically significant endocarditis or valve dysfunction is open to question.

See Table 4.10.

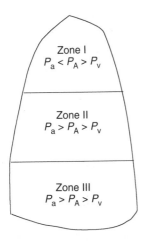

Fig. 4.34 Lung zones as described by West (1990). The tip of the pulmonary artery catheter should lie in zone III to provide accurate recordings of PAWP. P_A = pulmonary alveolar pressure; P_a = pulmonary artery pressure; P_v = pulmonary venous pressure.

Table 4.10   Summary of problems associated with pulmonary artery catheterization

Problem	Potential cause	Action
Unable to obtain wedge when balloon inflated	• Catheter tip not in correct position	Inform medical staff • Catheter needs to be advanced
	• Balloon rupture • Pulmonary hypertension	• Remove catheter • May not obtain wedge, use other readings
Overwedged trace when balloon inflated	• Incorrect position of catheter: tip is advanced too far and lies in a small vessel	Inform medical staff • Catheter needs to be pulled back into larger vessel
Blood in syringe when air removed from balloon	• Rupture of balloon	Inform medical staff • Do not attempt to inflate balloon or an air embolism may result • Turn off stopcock to syringe • Catheter must be removed
Spontaneous wedge (wedge trace seen when balloon not inflated)	• Catheter has migrated into a small vessel	Inform medical staff • Catheter must be withdrawn until PA waveform is seen otherwise there is a risk of pulmonary infarction
RV waveform instead of PA trace	• Catheter has slipped back into the right ventricle	Inform medical staff • Potential for ventricular arrhythmias • Catheter must be repositioned in the PA
'Damped' pressure trace	• Loose connections	Inform medical staff • Check connections are secure
	• Catheter tip against vessel wall	• Reposition catheter
	• Low pressure in pressure bag	• Check pressure bag inflated to 300 mmHg
	• Excessive length of tubing from transducer	• Remove any excess tubing
	• Air bubbles or blood in transducer	• Check transducer: change if necessary
	• Fibrin deposition at tip	• Flush catheter or replace (use a 2ml syringe to aspirate or for a high pressure flush)

Removal of the pulmonary artery catheter

The PA catheter alone can be removed leaving the introducer *in situ*; therefore ascertain if only the catheter or both are to be removed. Infusions via the PA catheter should be transferred to the side arm of the introducer or other infusion sites and any cardiac output equipment should be disconnected.

Emergency equipment for defibrillation and predrawn up IV lignocaine should be at hand as there is a potential risk of ventricular arryhthmias as the catheter passes through the ventricle.

The procedure is carried out aseptically.

Procedure

• Assemble equipment

• Explain procedure to patient

• Lay patient in supine position to reduce the risk of air embolism.

• Ensure the balloon is deflated and a PA waveform is shown on the monitor.

• Unclip the sleeve adapter from the introducer sheath.

• Remove the dressing and cut sutures.

• Remove during expiration in the spontaneously breathing patient or time removal with the inspiratory cycle of the ventilator: this reduces the risk of air embolism.

• While observing the ECG monitor, gently withdraw the catheter. As the catheter tip passes from PA to RA the characteristic change in waveforms will be seen. Particular observation of the ECG is necessary as the tip passes through the RV. If ventricular arrythmias occur, continue withdrawing the catheter as these will often terminate once the catheter is removed.

If there is any difficulty in withdrawing the catheter, discontinue the procedure immediately. On no account use force as this resistance may be due to knotting or kinking of the catheter, or it may be caught on a valve or other structure. Seek senior medical help. If the catheter is in the RV and unable to be withdrawn, and ventricular arrhythmias are occurring, consider inflating the balloon and advancing the catheter forward to hopefully stop the arrhythmias.

• When the PA catheter has been completely removed a haemostatic valve will close over the entrance in the introducer. This should prevent entry of air and exit of blood but can occasionally be damaged by the passage of the catheter. A sterile occlusive cap should therefore be placed over the exit site.

• If the introducer is also to be removed it is easier to remove the PA catheter first and then remove the introducer. Ensure haemostasis by manual pressure and cover with an occlusive dressing.

Cardiac output determination

There are a variety of methods to measure cardiac output. The thermodilution method is practical for the intensive care patient and is relatively simple to perform.

The Fick method

The measurement of cardiac output is based upon the principle of Adolph Fick. The Fick principle states that the amount of substance that is taken up by an organ is equal to the organ's blood flow rate and its arterial — mixed venous oxygen difference. The Fick method uses the lungs as the organ and oxygen as the substrate and cardiac output can be calculated as follows:

$$CO = \frac{\text{Oxygen consumption (ml/min)}}{\text{Oxygen difference}}$$

It is a cumbersome method, and unsuitable for use in critically ill patients as the method demands a steady physiological state. The error in CO measurement by the Fick method is estimated to be approximately 10%.

The dye dilution method

This method involves the injection of a dye into the blood (usually through a central venous catheter) and measuring the subsequent dilution after a designated time. The dilution of the dye will indicate the amount of fluid that it was added to. The usual dye is indocyanine green and its subsequent dilution can be measured by a densitometer downstream of where it was injected. Serial measurements are taken over a period of time and a dye dilution curve is produced. From this, the cardiac output can be calculated.

This method is time-consuming and has been superceded in most situations by thermodilution.

The thermodilution method

This involves the injection of an exact amount of cold fluid into the right atrium via a PA catheter. Its dilution by the blood is calculated by serial changes in pulmonary artery temperature.

Measured amounts (5 or 10 ml) of preferably ice-cold 5% glucose (although glucose at room temperature can also be used) are injected into the proximal lumen of the PA catheter. Greater accuracy is achieved when using 5 ml volumes if it is ice-cold. The injection must be rapid (within 4 seconds), and enters the blood in the right atrium. As the solution mixes with the blood the blood is cooled temporarily. A thermistor at the tip of the PA catheter senses the blood temperature and a time-temperature curve can be plotted. A cardiac output computer is required to compute the output and takes into consideration the injectate volume, blood and injectate temperature, and the specific heat and gravity of the blood and injectate. As the fluid is injected a curve will be displayed on the cardiac ouput monitor. This represents the change from a cooler to warmer temperature and the area under the graph is inversely proportional to the cardiac output.

A closed injectate set is available whereby syringes of injectate can be drawn without disconnecting the circuit. Alternatively, pre-filled syringes can be prepared and used at room or iced temperature.

Injectate temperatures

A computer constant must be fed into the monitor before cardiac output measurements are made. This constant depends on the make and model of catheter, the volume of injectate fluid used, and the temperature of the injectate.

Once selected, the temperature of the injectate must be within a defined range for each set of measurements that are taken (see Table 4.11).

The computer constants are found accompanying the catheter.

Table 4.11 Injectate temperatures

System	Injectate volume (ml)	Temperature range (°C)
Pre-filled syringes	10	0–5 (iced)
Closed injectate system	10	6–12 (iced)
	5	8–16 (iced)
	10	19–25 (room temp.)

Recording the cardiac output
• Enter the computer constant before any recordings are made.

• A good catheter position is necessary so that the thermistor is free-floating

• Concomitant infusions into the proximal tubing should be turned off when the measurements are made.

Making the measurements
• The monitor must be 'ready', the system primed, injectate at the desired temperature, and the computer constant entered. A single flush of injectate is injected through the proximal tubing if cold solution is used in order to prime the tubing with cold fluid. The injectate temperature is displayed on the monitor and should be in the correct range for the system used.

• Press the 'start' button on the monitor and inject immediately. The injection must be smooth and completed within 4 seconds.

• Do not hold the syringe barrel when injecting as this may warm the injectate fluid.

• The cardiac output measurement will be displayed on the monitor after approximately 15 seconds. After 45 seconds, when the monitor states 'ready' a second measurement can be made.

• It is recommended that at least three cardiac output measurements should be made and these are averaged to give a final value. The outputs averaged should be within 10% of each other and selected measurements can be rejected if they are beyond this range. For example, in the following series of cardiac output measurements (l/min) the value 5.2 should be rejected:

> 3.5
> 3.7
> 5.2—REJECT
> 3.4

The timing of measurements should be varied across the inspiratory and expiratory phases.

• The first value of the series is often discarded but this is not necessary unless it falls outside the 10% range.

• Modern computers will signify a poor measurement by displaying 'unsteady trace' or another such message.

For problems encountered when determining cardiac output see Table 4.12.

Table 4.12 Summary of problems associated with measuring cardiac output (CO)

Problem	Potential cause	Action
Difficulty injecting solution through proximal lumen	• Proximal lumen occluded/kinked • Catheter tip against wall of vessel	Inform medical staff • Unkink/replace catheter • Reposition catheter
Blood temperature not displayed	• Faulty thermistor • Fibrin growth on thermistor	• Replace catheter
Injectate temperature not displayed	• Faulty injectate temperature probe	• Replace probe
Wide discrepancies in serial CO recordings	• Inaccurate amounts of injectate drawn up • Poor technique (uneven injection) • Arrhythmias (atrial fibrillation, ventricular ectopics) • Valvular disease (tricuspid insufficiency) causing turbulent flow • Patient movement during recordings • Malfunction of CO computer	• Ensure exact injectate volume is drawn up • Inject evenly and within 4 s • Observe ECG, avoid injection during arryhthmias • Use alternative method for obtaining CO • Limit patient movement during measurements • Replace computer
Inappropriately high values for CO	• Incorrect injectate volume (usually too low or leaking connection) • Injectate temperature too low • Incorrect computer constant • Poor injection technique	• Check correct volume to be used (5 or 10 ml) • Check temperature of injectate • Check computer constant • Inject evenly within 4 s
Inappropriately low values for CO	• Incorrect injectate volume (usually too much) • Injectate temperature too high • Start button pressed after beginning of injection • Incorrect computer constant • Delivery of injectate longer than 4 s • Concomitant infusions at high flow rates (>150 m/h) through distal lumen	• Ensure correct injectate volume • Check temperature of injectate, do not hold barrel of syringe when injecting • Press start button at the same time/ just before beginning the injection • Check computer constant • Ensure injection is within 4 s • If possible, turn off concomitant infusions during measurements

References and bibliography

Barker, S. and Tremper, K. (1987). The effects of carbon monoxide inhalation on pulse oximetry and transcutaneous PO_2. *Anaesthesiology*, **66**, 677–9.

Bone, R. and Balk, R. (1988). Noninvasive respiratory care unit: a cost effective solution for the future. *Chest*, **93**, 390–4.

Brunel, W. and Cohen, N.H. (1988). Evaluation of the accuracy of pulse oximetry in critically ill patients. *Critical Care Medicine* **16**, 432.

Cengiz, M., *et al.* (1983). The effect of ventilation on the accuracy of pulmonary artery and pulmonary capillary wedge pressure measurements. *Critical Care Medicine*, **11**, 502–7.

Drew, B.J. (1993). Bedside electrocardiogram monitoring. *AACN Clinical Issues in Critical Care Nursing*, **4**, 26–33.

Edwards, D. (1988). Principles of oxygen transport. *Care of the Critically II*, **4**, 13–16.

Fiddian-Green, R.G. (1992). Tonometry; theory and applications. *Intensive Care World*, **92**, 60–5.

Hathaway, (1978). R. The Swan–Ganz catheter: a review. *Nurses Clinics of North America*, **13**, 380–407.

Gardner, P. (1993). Pulmonary artery pressure monitoring. *AACN Clinical Issues in Critical Care Nursing*, **41**, 98–118.

Gorney, D.A. (1993). Arterial blood pressure measurement technique. *AACN Clinical Issues in Critical Care Nursing*, **4**, 66–79.

Hanowell, L. (1987). Ambient light affects pulse oximeters. *Anaesthesiology*, **67**, 864–5.

Hartmann, M., Montgomery, A., Jonsson, K., *et al.* (1991). Tissue oxygenation in haemorrhagic shock measured as transcutaneous oxygen tension and gastrointestinal intramucosal pH in pigs. *Critical Care Medicine*, **19**, 205–10.

Headley, J.M. (1989). *Invasive haemodynamic monitoring: physiological principles and clinical applications*. Baxter Healthcare Corporation, Edwards Critical-Care Division, USA.

Kadota, L.T. (1985). Theory and application of thermodilution cardiac output measurement: a review. *Heart and Lung*, **14**, 605–14.

Kaye, W. (1983). Invasive monitoring technique: arterial cannulation, bedside pulmonary artery catheterization, and arterial puncture. *Heart and Lung*, **12**, 395–424.

Kidd, J.F. (1988). Pulse oximeters: basic theory and operation. *Care of the Critically Ill*, **4**, 10–13.

Low, J.M. (1990). Haemodynamic monitoring. In *Intensive care manual*, (ed. T.E. Oh.), (3rd edn), pp. 578–91. Butterworth, London.

Lynne, M., Scnapp, M.D., Neal, H., and Cohen, M.D. (1990). Pulse oximetry: uses and abuses. *Chest*, **98**, 1244–50.

Mackenzie, S.J. (1992). Haemodynamic monitoring in intensive care. In *Intensive care in Britain*, (ed. M. Rennie). Greycoat, London.

Neff, T. (1988). Routine oximetry: a fifth vital sign? *Chest*, **94**, 227.

Oh, T.E. (ed.) (1990). *Intensive care manual*, (3rd edn), Butterworth, Sydney.

Ramsey M. (1991). Blood pressure monitoring: automated oscilloscope devices. *Journal of Clinical Monitoring*, **7**, 56–67.

Rithalia, S.V.S. and Edwards, D. (1992). Intra-arterial oxygen electrode. *British Journal of Intensive Care*, **2**, 29–33.

Sidi, A., Paulus, D., Rush, W., *et al.* (1987). Methylene blue and indocyanine green artificially lower pulse oximetry readings of oxygen saturation: studies in dogs. *Journal of Clinical Monitoring*, **3**, 249–56.

Smith, R. and Olson, M. (1989). Drug induced methaemoglobinaemia on pulse oximetry and mixed venous oximetry. *Anaesethiology*, **70**, 112–17.

Sprafka, J.M., Strickland, D. Gomez-Marin, O., and Prineas, R.J. (1991). The effect of cuff size on blood pressure measurements in adults. *Epidemiology*, **2**, 214–17.

Urban, N. (1991). Haemodynamic clinical profiles. *AACN Clinical Issues in Critical Care Nursing*, **1**, 123–4.

Veyckemans, F., Baele, P., *et al.* (1989). Hyperbilirubinaemia does not interfere with with haemoglobin saturation measured by pulse oximetry. *Anaesthesiology*, **70**, 118–22.

White, K.M. Using continuous S_VO_2 to assess oxygen supply/demand balance in the critically ill patient. *AACN Clinical Issues in Critical Care Nursing*, **4**, 134–145.

West, J.B. (1990). *Respiratory physiology — The essentials*, (4th edn), pp. 41–3. Williams & Wilkins, Baltimore.

Woods, S.L., and Osguthorpe, S. (1993). Cardiac output determination. *AACN Clinical Issues in Critical Care Nursing*, **4**, 81–94.

Appendix

Abbreviations used in the text

Abbreviation	Term	Definition	Normal value
CVP	Central venous pressure	Pressure recorded within vein near to the heart	3–10 mmHg
RA or RAP	Right atrial pressure	Pressure within the right atrium	3–8 mmHg
MRAP	Mean right atrial pressure	Mean pressure of right atrium	4–6 mmHg
RVSP	Right ventricular systolic pressure	Systolic pressure in right ventricle	15–25 mmHg
RVDP	Right ventricular diastolic pressure	Diastolic pressure in right ventricle	3–8 mmHg
PASP	Pulmonary artery systolic pressure	Systolic pressure in pulmonary artery	15–25 mmHg
PADP	Pulmonary artery diastolic pressure	Diastolic pressure in pulmonary artery	8–12 mmHg
PAWP or PAOP or PCWP	Pulmonary artery wedge pressure (also known as PA occlusion pressure or pulmonary capillary wedge pressure)	Closely reflects ventricular filling pressure (or left ventricular end diastolic pressure)	6–12 mmHg
LA or LAP	Left atrial pressure	Pressure in left atrium	6–12 mmHg
MAP	Mean arterial pressure	$\dfrac{SBP + (DBP \times 2)}{3}$	70–105 mmHg
SV	Stroke volume	Volume of blood ejected from the left ventricle per beat: $SV = \dfrac{CO}{HR}$	60–100 ml
CO	Cardiac output	Volume of blood expelled by left ventricle per minute	4–8 l/min
CI	Cardiac index	Cardiac output related to body size: $\dfrac{CO}{BSA}$	2.4–4.0 l/min
EF	Ejection fraction	Stroke volume expressed as a percentage of EDV	60–70%
EDV or LVEDV	End diastolic volume	Amount of blood left in left ventricle at end of diastole	120–150 ml
ESV	End systolic volume	Amount of blood left in left ventricle at end of systole	50–70 ml
SVR	Systemic vascular resistance	Measures resistance to the left ventricle $\dfrac{(MAP - RAP) \times 80}{CO}$	800–1200 dynes.s/cm^5
PVR	Pulmonary vascular resistance	Measures resistance to the right ventricle $\dfrac{(MPAP - PCWP) \times 80}{CO}$	<250 dynes.s/cm^5

5. Cardiovascular problems

Anatomy and physiology

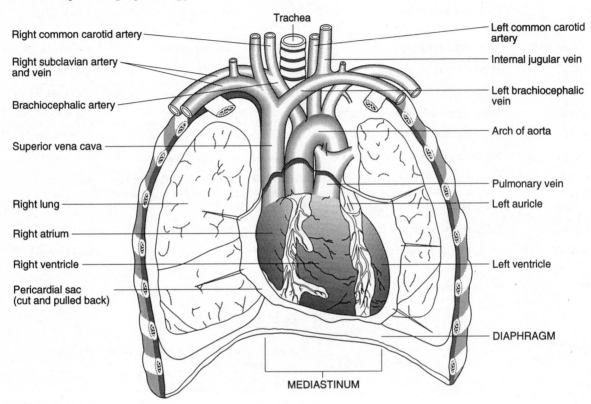

Right common carotid artery
Right subclavian artery and vein
Brachiocephalic artery
Superior vena cava
Right lung
Right atrium
Right ventricle
Pericardial sac (cut and pulled back)

Trachea

Left common carotid artery
Internal jugular vein
Left brachiocephalic vein
Arch of aorta
Pulmonary vein
Left auricle
Left ventricle
DIAPHRAGM

MEDIASTINUM

Fig. 5.1 General view of the heart in the anatomically correct position.

The principal functions of the cardiovascular system are as follows:

(1) carriage of oxygen to the tissues from the lungs,

(2) carriage of carbon dioxide from the tissues to the lungs,

(3) carriage of nutrients from the digestive tract to the tissues,

(4) carriage of metabolic waste from the tissues to the kidneys,

(5) carriage of hormones from endocrine glands and other sources to site of action,

(6) transportation and radiation of excess heat.

The cardiovascular system includes:

1. The pulmonary circulation consisting of the pulmonary artery, pulmonary capillaries, and pulmonary veins. This is supplied by the right ventricle.

2. The systemic circulation consisting of the aorta, arteries, capillaries, and veins of the rest of the body. This is supplied by the left ventricle.

Flow of blood through the heart

Venous blood returns to the right atrium via the inferior and superior venae cavae. The atria act as a top-up system which force extra blood into the respective ventricles immediately prior to ventricular contraction.

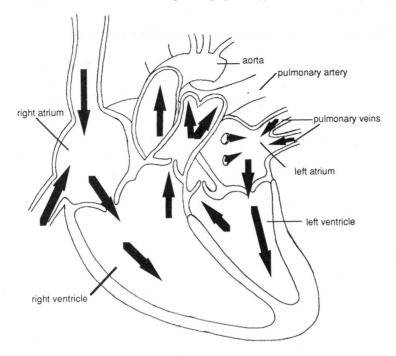

Fig. 5.2 Diagram of a cross-section of the heart showing direction of flow

The pressure created by commencement of ventricular contraction closes the valves between atria and ventricle. Continuing ventricular contraction then forces blood out from the right ventricle into the pulmonary artery and from the left ventricle into the aorta. Due to the disparity of pressures between pulmonary and systemic circulations, the left ventricle is considerably thicker and more muscular than the right. It also has a globular shape as opposed to the half-moon shape of the right ventricle.

Pressure changes during a cardiac cycle

Ventricular pressure changes

(a) left ventricle

- maximum pressure of ≈ 120 mmHg during systole (this pressure rises with age),

- during diastole, the pressure falls to thoracic cavity pressure of ~ 0 mmHg,

- left ventricular pressure changes are therefore 120/0 mmHg.

(b) right ventricle

- maximum pressure of ~ 25 mmHg

  - (same volume of blood as left ventricle but lower pressure),

- during diastole the pressure falls to the thoracic cavity pressure of ≈ 0 mmHg,

- right ventricular pressure changes are therefore 25/0 mmHg.

Aortic pressure changes

- maximum pressure is the same as left ventricular pressure: ≈ 120 mmHg,

- during diastole, aortic pressure is maintained by the elastic recoil of arterial walls and pressure falls to ≈ 80 mmHg,

- aortic pressure changes are therefore 120/80 mmHg.

Pulmonary artery pressure changes

- maximum pressure is the same as right ventricular pressure: ≈ 25 mmHg,

- during diastole, pulmonary artery pressure falls to ≈ 8 mmHg,

- pulmonary artery pressure changes are therefore 25/8 mmHg.

Atrial pressure changes

Pressure changes are much more complex due to bulging of tricuspid and mitral valves during ventricular systole and downward movement of the atrioventricular ring following opening of pulmonary and aortic valves. Return upwards of the atrioventricular ring and filling from venae cavae and pulmonary veins cause increases in atrial pressure until the mitral and tricuspid valves open again and atrial contraction occurs.

Excitation, contraction, and conduction

Features of cardiac muscle

(1) Syncytium

Cardiac muscle is similar to skeletal muscle apart from the lattice-like interconnection of fibres between muscle cells. This is known as a syncytium and forms a complex network which allows almost simultaneous spread of excitation and contraction. The atria form one syncytium, which is divided from the ventricular syncytium by fibrous tissue. The division is important to allow separate atrial and ventricular contraction.

(2) Automatic rhythmicity

Some areas of muscle fibre have the ability to depolarize rhythmically without external stimulation. This occurs because the membrane of the muscle fibre is permeable to sodium allowing a continual leak of sodium ions into the cell. This increases the electrical charge until it hits a 'threshold' level triggering an action potential. After the action potential occurs the membrane is temporarily less permeable to sodium ions but more than normally permeable to potassium ions which leak out recreating a negative charge across the membrane.

The speed of rhythmic depolarisation is determined by the length of time it takes to increase the membrane potential to the 'threshold' level once more. Sinoatrial node fibres have the fastest inherent rhythmicity and thus act as the pacemaker.

(3) Prolonged muscle contraction

The action potential includes a plateau phase which last for almost 0.3 s before returning to baseline due to the slow repolarization of cardiac muscle.

Membrane potential

All cells have an electrical potential across the cell membrane, which is negative inside the cell in resting conditions. The potential is due to the differences between ion composition in intracellular and extracellular fluids. This is maintained by the sodium–potassium pump, which transports sodium ions to the outside of the cell while transporting potassium ions inside. The membrane is very permeable to potassium ions but very impermeable to sodium ions. Potassium ions tend to leak out leaving large negatively charged ions inside the cell which give the cell its relative negative charge.

---

(4) Increased speed of contraction and repolarization with increased cardiac rate

This is partly due to a shortened period of systolic ejection but mostly to a shortened diastolic period. Thus, in prolonged tachycardia, time for muscle rest and coronary blood flow is greatly reduced. The absolute refractory period is protected to prevent tetanic or chaotic excitation.

Table 5.1 Duration in seconds of contraction and repolarization

Event	Duration (s) at rate of 75 bpm	Duration (s) at rate of 200 bpm
Cardiac cycle	0.80	0.30
Systole	0.27	0.16
Action potential	0.25	0.15
Absolute refractory period	0.20	0.13
Relative refractory period	0.05	0.02
Diastole	0.53	0.14

Depolarization

A stimulus alters the polarized cell membrane permeability by inactivating the sodium–potassium pumps and allowing sodium ions to diffuse rapidly into the cell via 'fast sodium channels' in the cell membrane. This results in a reversal of relative electrical charge. When the polarity reduces from the resting potential of -80 mV to -35 mV the 'calcium channels' of the cell membrane are opened. There is an immediate influx of calcium ions which, combined with the continuing sodium ion influx, increases the polarity across the membrane to $+30$ mV. When this threshold point is reached the cells on either side are stimulated and membrane permeability altered, thus depolarization becomes self-propagating. This is known as an action potential and calcium release is triggered to allow muscular contraction (see below). If the critical level of depolarization is not reached then the depolarization will remain local to the cell and calcium release will not be activated.

Repolarization

The first phase of repolarization is the closure of the 'fast sodium channels'. Potassium begins to move out of the cell and there is an influx of calcium and sodium ions into the cell via slow channels. This is the plateau phase of repolarization (phase 2), which is represented on the electrocardiogram the (ECG) as the ST segment. During phase 3, the slow channels close and the influx of calcium and sodium ions is halted. There is increased permeability to potassium ions and further movement of potassium ions out of the cell until the negative polarity of the cell's resting state is restored. This appears as the T wave on the ECG. Finally, phase 4 of repolarization reactivates the sodium–potassium pumps allowing the ratio of sodium to potassium ions inside the cell to be regained.

The refractory period

Cardiac muscle cells will not respond to further stimulation between phase 0 and phase 3 of the action potential and repolarization. This is known as the refractory period. There are two parts:

(1) absolute refractory period, and

(2) relative refractory period.

(a) Absolute

This covers phase 0 to phase 2 of depolarization and repolarization. No stimulus will be able to effect a response during this period. On the ECG, this is seen as the beginning of the QRS complex to just after the beginning of the T wave.

(b) Relative

This covers phase 3 of repolarization when membrane potential is more negative than -50 mV. A relatively strong stimulus will effect a response but conduction is slower than when fibres are fully repolarized. This is seen as the majority of the T wave on the ECG.

The occurrence of an ectopic stimulus during the relative refractory period can initiate life-threatening dysrhythmias. This is known as an 'R on T' ectopic.

Mechanical response to depolarization

Calcium ions are released from the terminal cisterns of the sarcoplasmic reticulum surrounding the sarcomere in response to the stimulus of the action potential. A sarcomere is shown in Fig. 5.3.

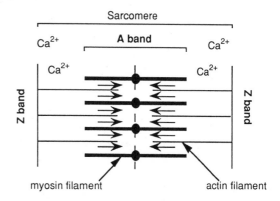

Fig. 5.3 Diagram of a sarcomere ($\leftarrow$ = direction of contraction).

Free calcium ions activate contraction by combining with the protein troponin situated on the actin filaments. Calcium bound troponin acquires a slightly different position on the filament and uncovers binding sites on the actin which interact with the myosin filaments. Release of energy from ATP allows the two filaments to move past each other, shortening the distance between two Z bands. This shortening is the basis of myocardial contraction. Calcium is taken up again by the sarcoplasmic reticulum and contraction ceases as the binding sites are once again covered. The sarcomere lengthens and relaxation occurs.

Conduction

In order for virtually simultaneous contraction to take place throughout individual chambers of the heart, there must be a very fast conduction pathway. Electrical stimulation can be conducted from cell to cell but this is too slow to provide optimal contraction. (The conduction pathways are shown in Fig. 5.4.).

All specialized cells within the conduction pathway possess automaticity but the discharge rate varies. The fastest discharge rate and therefore the normal pacemaker of the heart is the sinoatrial (SA) node. The discharge rate of the SA node is 60–100 bpm.

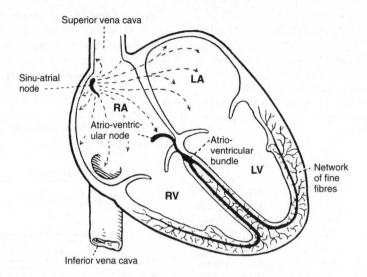

Fig. 5.4 The conduction system of the heart. (From J.S. Ross and K.J.W. Wilson (1973): *Foundations of anatomy and physiology* (3rd edn), p.144, Fig. 120, Churchill Livingstone, Edinburgh, with permission.)

Movement of the action potential through the atria is via a number of tracts. This means that the action potential from different atrial areas will arrive at the atrioventricular (AV) node at different times. The AV node is normally the only electrical pathway between atria and ventricles and thus the action potential is delayed here to allow all action potentials to be conducted to the ventricles at the same time. AV nodal delay is usually approximately 0.1 second. The AV node is continuous with the bundle of His and excitation spreads rapidly down this, the right and left bundle branches, the Purkinje fibres and the rest of the ventricles.

Automatic discharge rate of cardiac tissues	
Sinoatrial (SA) node:	60–100 bpm
Atrioventricular (AV) node:	40–60 bpm
Ventricular tissues:	20–40 bpm

Depolarization starts on the left of the ventricular septum and then passes to the right across the mid-portion. It then moves down to the apex and out to the ventricular walls.

The electrical events of the cardiac cycle can be recorded by the ECG. The ECG records fluctuations in electrical potential from the heart. These fluctuations are conducted by body fluids (the large quantities of electrolytes conduct current) and measured on the body surface (Fig. 5.5). The principles of recording the ECG are detailed in Chapter 4.

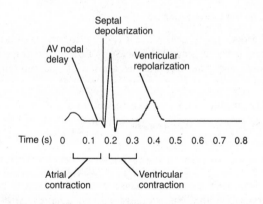

Fig. 5.5 Electrical and mechanical events during the cardiac cycle.

External regulation of the heart rate

The heart rate is influenced by two major external controls:

  (i) autonomic nervous system,

  (ii) catecholamines.

(i) Autonomic influence

Both the SA and the AV nodes are innervated by parasympathetic and sympathetic fibres. Some myocardial fibres are also innervated by sympathetic nerve fibres.

Parasympathetic stimulation via the vagus nerve causes release of acetylcholine near the nodal cells. This causes:

(a) decreased heart rate by delayed depolarization,

(b) decreased force of contraction,

(c) delayed conduction of impulses through the A–V node.

Sympathetic stimulation releases noradrenaline near the nodal cells. This stimulates specific receptor sites known as β_1-adrenergic receptors. This causes:

(a) increased heart rate by an increased rate of nodal depolarization,

(b) increased strength of cardiac contraction,

(c) increased rapidity of cardiac impulse conduction.

(ii) Influence of catecholamines

The release of adrenaline and noradrenaline into the bloodstream by the adrenal medulla will also have a direct effect on the heart in the same way as sympathetic nervous stimulation.

Heart rate and blood pressure

Two reflexes adjust heart rate to blood pressure (BP) via the cardioregulatory centre in the medulla.

1. The aortic reflex

(a) aortic and carotid sinus baroreceptors respond to alterations in systemic blood pressure,

(b) sensory impulses sent to the cardioregulatory centre produce the responses shown in Table 5.2.

2. The Bainbridge effect

Receptors in the venae cavae are stimulated by an alteration in venous return. They send sensory impulses to the cardioregulatory centre. (see Table 5.3).

Table 5.2   The aortic reflex

Alteration in BP	Cardioregulatory centre response	Physiological response
Raised BP	Increase in vagal stimulation or decrease in sympathetic stimulation	Decreased heart rate causes decreased cardiac output and decreased BP
Lowered BP	Increase in sympathetic stimulation or decrease in vagal stimulation	Increased heart rate and force of contraction causes increased cardiac output and increased BP

Table 5.3   The Bainbridge effect

Alteration in venous return	Cardioregulatory response	Physiological response
Increased venous return	Increase in sympathetic stimulation and a decrease in parasympathetic stimulation	Increased heart rate
Decreased venous return	Increase in parasympathetic stimulation and decrease in sympathetic stimulation	Decreased heart rate

Haemodynamics

Under certain physiological conditions the normal heart should compensate to meet demands placed upon it. However, a diseased heart or alterations in the peripheral circulation may mean that attempts to maintain adequate cardiac performance is impaired.

Determinants of cardiac performance can be divided into the following components:

- cardiac output
- preload
- heart rate
- afterload
- stroke volume
- contractility

When assessing the haemodynamic status of the patient the interrelationships of all these factors must be taken into account.

Cardiac output (CO)

The cardiac output (CO) is the amount of blood ejected from the left ventricle in one minute. It is determined by the stroke volume and heart rate, therefore manipulation of either can alter CO:

$$CO = \text{Heart rate} \times \text{Stroke volume}$$
(Usual range = 4–7 l/min)

The CO can be adjusted to body size by dividing by body surface area (BSA). This is termed the cardiac index (CI):

$$CI \ (l/min/m^2) = \frac{CO \ (l/min)}{BSA \ (m^2)}$$

(Normal value = 2.5–4.0 l/min/m².)

Body surface area is determined using a nomogram derived from height and weight. Cardiac output normally decreases after the age of 35 years by about 1% per annum.

Heart rate

Elevated heart rates can compromise cardiac output by:

- Increasing the amount of oxygen consumed by the myocardium

- Reducing the diastolic time which may result in less time for perfusion of the coronary arteries

- Shortening the ventricular filling phase of the cardiac cycle causing a decreased blood volume to be pumped on the next contraction

Decreased heart rates may also be detrimental because:

- A longer filling time may initially increase cardiac output but, if the heart is diseased, the myocardium may be so depressed that that the muscle cannot contract long enough to eject this volume — this will result in a decrease in CO.

A healthy heart should be able to tolerate a range of heart rates from 30 to 170 bpm for relatively prolonged periods; however, if cardiac function is compromised this range may be considerably narrower.

Other factors affecting the heart rate include temperature, psychological state, thyroid function, adrenal function, and arrhythmias.

Stroke volume

Stroke volume (SV) is the amount of blood ejected by the left ventricle during one contraction. It is the difference between the end diastolic volume (EDV: the amount of blood left in the ventricle at the end of diastole) and the end systolic volume (ESV: blood volume left in the ventricle at the end of systole).

The volume of blood ejected by each ventricular contraction (stroke volume) is dependent on:

(i) myocardial muscle contractility,

(ii) preload (the volume of blood filling the ventricle),

(iii) afterload (the resistance to blood flow from the ventricle),

(iv) heart rate (tachycardia reduces the time for diastolic filling).

(Normal range of stroke volume = 60–100 ml.)

The stroke volume can be expressed as a percentage of the end diastolic volume and is then called the ejection fraction (EF). (See Chapter 7 for further details.)

Preload

This refers to the degree of stretch of the muscle fibres at the end of diastole. The larger the volume of blood in the ventricle, the greater the degree of muscle fibre stretch. This is a self-regulatory system allowing force of contraction to equal the volume of blood required to be ejected. Starling's law of the heart states that the force of myocardial contraction is determined by the length of the muscle cell fibres (Fig. 5.6).

The volume of blood in the ventricle at diastole is dictated by venous return (the volume of blood returning to the heart) and the ability of the ventricle to contract.

There is an optimal range of stretch beyond which force of contraction is reduced rather than increased

The hypothesized cause of the endpoint of myocardial stretch is that beyond a certain distance (0.22 μm) there are too few actin–myosin binding sites overlapping to provide adequate contraction.

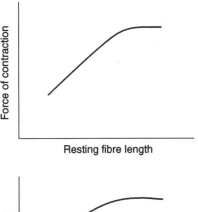

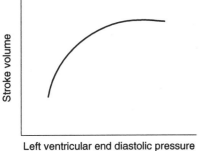

Fig. 5.6 Graph showing Starling's law.

The factors affecting ventricular preload are shown in Table 5.4.

Specific causes of a decreased left ventricular preload include pulmonary embolus and mitral stenosis.

Since preload is difficult to measure at the bedside, the pressures required to fill the ventricles are used as indirect guides to ventricular enddiastolic volume; that is, the right ventricular enddiastolic (filling) pressure (= central venous pressure) for the right ventricle and the left ventricular enddiastolic (filling) pressure (= pulmonary artery wedge pressure) for the left ventricle.

Afterload

Afterload is the resistance to outflow of blood that must be overcome by the ventricles during systole. The most important factor determining this is the vascular resistance. The pulmonary vascular resistance dictates right ventricular afterload and the systemic vascular resistance dictates left ventricular afterload.

Table 5.4 Factors influencing ventricular preload

Decreased	Increased
Volume loss • haemorrhage • vomiting • polyuria	*Volume gain* • renal failure • excess blood products • excess IV fluids
Vasodilatation • pyrexia • drugs (e.g. nitrates) • septicaemia • neurogenic shock • anaphylactic shock	*Vasoconstriction* • hypothermia • drugs (e.g. adrenaline, dopamine — >5 μg/kg/min, noradrenaline) • heart failure • pain, anxiety
Tachycardia (potentially insufficient diastolic filling time)	*Bradycardia*
Impeded venous return (e.g. high intrathoracic pressure, pericardial tamponade)	

The bedside measurement of 'afterload' is the systemic vascular resistance (SVR) for the left ventricle and the pulmonary vascular resistance (PVR) for the right ventricle. The resistance of the vascular system is derived from the cardiac output (CO) and mean arterial pressure (MAP):

$$SVR = \frac{(MAP - RAP) \times 80}{CO} \quad dyn. \ s. \ cm^{-5}$$

(Normal range 800–1200 dyn. s. cm^{-5})

$$PVR = \frac{(MPAP - PAWP) \times 80}{CO} \quad dyn. \ s. \ cm^{-5}$$

(Normal range 50–200 dyn. s. cm^{-5})

where MPAP = mean pulmonary artery pressure
PAWP = pulmonary artery wedge pressure
RAP = right atrial pressure
80 is a conversion factor to present the units of resistance as dyn. s. cm^{-5}.

Afterload has an inverse effect on ventricular function. As the resistance to ejection increases, so does the workload of the ventricle. A dysfunctional ventricle, in particular, may not be able to maintain or increase the stroke volume (the amount of blood ejected from the ventricle in one beat), thus the cardiac output frequently falls in the face of increasing peripheral vasoconstriction.

The opposite is seen with vasodilatation; the heart has less resistance to pump against and cardiac output usually increases as a consequence. This explains why increases in blood pressure may well result in decreases in flow (i.e. cardiac output). A satisfactory blood pressure allowing perfusion of vital organs must be achieved without compromising blood flow (and thus organ perfusion in general) with an excessive afterload.

Factors affecting afterload are shown in Table 5.5.

Table 5.5 Factors affecting afterload

Increased	Decreased
• vasoconstricting drugs (e.g. noradrenaline)	• vasodilatating drugs (e.g. nitrates, hydralazine, sodium nitroprusside)
• anxiety	• anaphylactic shock
• hypovolaemia	• septicaemia
• hypothermia	• hyperthermia
• cardiogenic shock	• neurogenic shock
• atherosclerosis	

Specific causes of increased right ventricular afterload include pulmonary valve disease, pulmonary embolus, and pulmonary hypertension. Specific causes of increased left ventricular afterload include aortic valve disease and systemic hypertension.

Contractility

Contractility refers to the ability to shorten the myocardial muscle fibres without actually altering their length or preload. The force of contraction of myocardial muscle cells alters in response to neural stimuli and levels of circulating catecholamines. Noradrenaline is liberated at sympathetic neuromuscular junctions and binds to β_1-adrenergic myocardial membrane receptors. The mechanism is thought to be mediated by cyclic AMP and produces increases in intracellular levels of calcium and ATP facilitating excitation–contraction coupling (Little and Little 1989).

Factors affecting contractility are shown in Table 5.6.

Blood flow

The heart is responsible for producing the pressure which forces blood into the circulation by pumping a volume of blood into the aorta. However, the actual rate of flow of the blood will depend on the difference between the pressure produced by the heart and the pressure at the end of the vessel.

Table 5.6 Factors affecting contractility

Increased	Decreased
• positive inotropic drugs	• negative inotropic drugs
• endogenous catecholamines	• functional loss of myocardium
• aerobic metabolism	• anaerobic metabolism (intracellular acidosis)
• hypervolaemia	• hypocalcaemia, hypomagnesaemia
• hyperthyroidism	• hypovolaemia
	• hypoxia

Rate of blood flow $\propto$ Pressure difference [difference between mean arterial pressure (MAP) and central venous pressure (CVP)]

Thus, if the pressure in the arterioles is high due to vasoconstriction there will be lower blood flow for the same pressure induced by ventricular contraction. Other factors affecting flow include the diameter of the vessel, the viscosity of the blood, and the vessel length. These form the resistance to blood flow.

Poiseuille's Law states that the ability of blood to flow through any given vessel is:

(i) proportional to the pressure difference between the two ends of the vessel and to the fourth power of the vessel diameter,

(ii) inversely proportional to the vessel length and blood viscosity.

$$\text{Blood flow} = \frac{\text{Pressure} \times (\text{diameter})^4}{\text{Length} \times \text{Viscosity}}$$

Regulation of blood flow

The main regulators of blood flow in different tissues are the arterioles. These are the vessels which produce the greatest decrease in diameter and therefore the highest resistance to flow. Their tiny size and the fact that resistance is inversely proportional to the *fourth power* of their diameter means that any alteration in diameter will result in a major change in blood flow. This alteration in diameter is mediated by the strong muscular wall which can alter diameter by three- to fivefold (Guyton 1985).

The smooth muscle walls respond to two regulatory stimuli. These are:

(i) the local requirements of tissues when nutrient

supply falls below need or exceeds demand — this is autoregulation,

(ii) autonomic signals, particularly sympathetic stimulation.

Autoregulation of blood flow

In the majority of tissues the most powerful stimulus for autoregulation is the need for oxygen. The exceptions are the kidney (concentrations of electrolytes and metabolic waste play a major role in controlling renal blood flow) and the brain (carbon dioxide concentration controls cerebral blood flow). The alteration of flow to match oxygen requirements allows automatic and immediate response to increases in cell activity. If tissue PO_2 falls then arteriolar dilatation occurs producing increased blood flow; conversely, if tissue PO_2 rises then arteriolar constriction occurs and blood flow is reduced. The system allows oxygen delivery to be adjusted according to cellular activity and blood flow to be redirected to areas of need.

Autonomic control of blood flow

Arteries, veins, and particularly arterioles are supplied by sympathetic nerves which moderate the state of vasoconstriction by transmitting a continuous stream of impulses. This maintains vasomotor tone. Vasoconstriction is produced by increased sympathetic impulses and vasodilatation by reduced sympathetic impulses. Autonomic control allows distribution of blood flow to major sections of the body.

Factors altering autonomic control of blood flow:

● Body temperature.

● Exercise.

● Changes in blood volume.

Blood pressure

Arterial pressure is the cardiac output multiplied by the resistance of the blood vessels. Either a change in cardiac output or a change in the vascular resistance will alter blood pressure.

Normal regulation of blood pressure

The mechanisms involved are:

(1) neural control of vasoconstriction and contractility,

(2) capillary fluid shift mechanism altering blood volume,

(3) renal excretory and hormonal mechanisms which alter blood volume and vasoconstriction.

(1) Neural control

The vasomotor centre in the brain stem controls vasomotor tone and heart rate via the sympathetic and parasympathetic nervous systems. Vasomotor tone is primarily controlled by sympathetic nervous outflow. Heart rate and contractility are controlled by the balance of sympathetic and parasympathetic stimulation and inhibition. The vagus nerve is the primary parasympathetic control and stimulation will reduce heart rate and decrease contractility. Sympathetic stimulation will increase heart rate and force of contractility.

Heart rate and contractility

Increased sympathetic stimulation = increased heart rate + increased force of contraction

Decreased sympathetic stimulation = decreased heart rate + decreased force of contraction

Increased parasympathetic stimulation = decreased heart rate + decreased force of contraction

---

Vasomotor tone

Increased sympathetic activity = vasoconstriction: decreased arteriolar diameter, decreased venous reservoirs = increased venous return and blood pressure

Decreased sympathetic activity = vasodilatation: increased arteriolar diameter, increased venous reservoirs = decreased venous return and blood pressure

---

The baroreceptor system. Receptors that are sensitive to the degree of stretch exerted by pressure in the arteries are situated in the aortic arch and the carotid sinuses. They transmit impulses which increase in rate as blood pressure rises. These impulses inhibit the sympathetic outflow of the vasomotor centre so that heart rate and contractility as well as vasomotor tone are reduced.

If there is a fall in blood pressure, the baroreceptor is less stimulated and impulses decrease. The vasomotor centre loses inhibition and increases sympathetic signals to the heart and vessels.

(2) Capillary fluid shift mechanism

This is a longer-term mechanism for blood pressure regulation which is particularly important when blood volume tends to become either too low or too high.

Increased circulating blood volume will raise systemic pressure and hydrostatic pressure within the capillaries. This will increase the shift of fluid across capillary membranes into the interstitial space.

Decreased circulating blood volume will lower capillary hydrostatic pressure and allow oncotic pressure exerted by plasma proteins to pull fluid by osmosis from the interstitial space into the capillaries.

This response takes between 10 minutes and several hours to readjust the arterial pressure back towards normal.

(3) Renal excretory and hormonal mechanisms

The kidneys are highly important in the long-term control of blood pressure and circulatory volume.

Formation of urine by the kidneys is regulated by the pressure in the renal arteries. A fall in blood pressure will produce a fall in renal artery blood flow which will decrease or stop the formation of urine. Alternatively, a rise in blood pressure will produce an increased urinary output.

A secondary hormonal mechanism — the renin-angiotensin system (described fully in Chapter 8) will respond to falls in blood pressure which reduce renal perfusion. Angiotensin II, a hormone produced by this mechanism is a potent vasoconstrictor which increases blood pressure. It also stimulates the adrenal cortex to secrete aldosterone which acts on the distal tubules and collecting ducts of the kidney to increase reabsorption of sodium and water. This results in increased circulating volume which will increase blood pressure.

The vasomotor centre can be stimulated by higher cerebral centres. The limbic system and hypothalamus are thought to mediate emotionally induced alterations in blood pressure such as vasovagal collapse brought on by bad news.

The mid-brain is thought to mediate the initial hypertension associated with severe pain and the later fall in blood pressure following prolonged severe pain.

Elevated intracranial pressure can produce reflex increases in arterial blood pressure due to medullary hypercapnia and hypoxia. The increase in arterial pressure increases medullary perfusion which reduces the hypercapnia and hypoxia.

Diagnostic and investigative procedures

Electrocardiogram monitoring, arrhythmias, and conduction disturbances as well as the 12-lead diagnostic ECG are detailed in Chapter 4.

Echocardiography

Ultrasound waves emitted in pulses by a probe directed at the heart are reflected back to the probe off the different surfaces and interfaces within the heart. A composite picture of these 'echoes' is built up and rebuilt multiple times per second, producing a structural representation of the heart in motion, either in one dimension ('M mode' echo) or two (2D echo). As these can be viewed in real-time, movement of the atrial and ventricular walls, and opening and closing of the valve leaflets through the cardiac cycle can be imaged.

More sophisticated echocardiography machines have a Doppler ultrasound facility incorporated to measure the degree and direction of blood flow within the heart. This is particularly useful for assessing and quantifying valvular regurgitation and stenosis, and septal defects non-invasively. The cardiac output can also be measured by Doppler echocardiography, using the Doppler ultrasound to measure blood flow velocity through either mitral or aortic valves, and the echocardiographic image to measure the valvular cross-sectional area.

The probe can be placed on the skin ('transthoracic') in various locations such as the parasternal, apical (over the apex of the heart), or epigastric regions. The patient can either be resting supine or rolled on to the left hand side. These changes in posture and probe site help to facilitate the view of a particular region of the heart. Signal acquisition is improved by smearing a conducting gel over the probe tip.

As ultrasound travels poorly through air, patients with hyperinflated lungs (e.g. emphysema) or after sternal opening (e.g. post-cardiac surgery) may be difficult to image. Likewise, patients with a thick chest wall may prove awkward. Use of a transoesophageal echocardiography probe overcomes these problems as high quality signals are obtained from behind the heart with minimal artefact. This technique can be performed in conscious, sedated patients but is also being used successfully in mechanically ventilated patients in the operating threatre and ICU environments. However, these probes are very expensive and require considerable expertise.

Uses of Doppler echocardiography

(1) Pericardial disease
   A pericardial effusion or haemopericardium can be imaged and drained

(2) Myocardial disease
   (a) Wall motion abnormalities can be detected. Lack of movement (akinesia) of a region of

ventricle during systole indicates infarction or ischaemia, though the latter is temporary. Reduced movement (hypokinesia) of a ventricular segment may also be seen with ischaemia. Paradoxical movement of a region (i.e. in the wrong direction during systole), indicates a ventricular aneurysm.

(b) The wall thickness can be measured and hypertrophy diagnosed.

(3) Chamber size

The size of the four heart chambers can be estimated and dilatation or underfilling diagnosed. This can be used for therapeutic assessment of drugs and other therapies such as PEEP. The left and right ventricular ejection fraction [i.e. (end diastolic volume − end systolic volume) ÷ (end diastolic volume)] can also be calculated as a guide to contractility.

(4) Valvular defects

Valvular stenosis and regurgitation can be diagnosed by characteristic movement of the valves and by the appearance of abnormal flow jets using colour-flow Doppler which can also be used to quantify the pressure gradient across stenotic valves.

(5) Septal and congenital defects

Atrial and ventricular septal defects, either congenital or acquired (e.g. post-infarction) can be readily imaged. The colour flow facility enables the operator to determine whether a left-to-right or a right-to-left shunt exists, and how significant it is.

(6) Cardiac output estimation

(7) Thrombi, vegetations, and neoplasms

Although a negative result does not exclude the presence of either intramural thrombi or valvular vegetations, echocardiography is a very useful diagnostic technique, especially for larger lesions. The transoesophageal approach is superior in view of the better picture quality obtained. Atrial myxomas can also be readily imaged by this technique.

(8) Aortic aneurysm

The transoesophageal approach is well suited for imaging the aortic root, arch, and descending thoracic aorta for the presence of an aneurysm.

Other diagnostic techniques

Electrocardiography and echocardiography can be performed at the bedside of a critically ill patient whereas other imaging techniques require transfer of the patient to an appropriate facility. As a consequence, other techniques are performed infrequently and occasionally used for diagnosis.

Nuclear scans

Radionuclide ventriculography involves the injection of technetium-99 labelled blood (or albumin). A gamma camera is placed over the heart and 'counts' the amount of radioactivity emitted by the technetium in the heart chambers at different points in the cardiac cycle. This is achieved by connection ('gating') to an electrocardiogram and is known colloquially as a 'MUGA' scan (multiple gated analysis). The difference in counts at the end of diastole and systole can be used to determine the ejection fraction of both left and right ventricles. Regional wall motion abnormalities can also be detected.

Regional myocardial perfusion can be assessed by injection of thallium-201 which is taken up into the muscle. Non-perfused areas of muscle produce a defect on the subsequent scan. This can be permanent after an infarction, or transient in the case of ischaemia which can be produced by exercise, or infusion of dipyridamole or dobutamine.

Technetium pyrophosphate is also not taken up by normal myocardium and can be used as a diagnostic tool for myocardial infarction when either the ECG or cardiac enzyme results are non-conclusive, not available, or non-interpretable.

Angiography

Cardiac catheterization involves insertion of a catheter through either a vein into the right heart (see pulmonary artery catheterization in Chapter 4) or via an artery (usually brachial or femoral) into the left heart under fluoroscopy (X-ray imaging). The latter is usually performed in a specialized laboratory and enables a number of investigations and procedures:

(i) visualization of the coronary arteries by placement of the catheter into the individual coronary artery orifices followed by injection of a radiopaque dye, the path of which is recorded on to cinefilm. The patency of the vessels (including previous bypass grafts) and the degree of collateral flow can be determined.

(ii) assessment of the degree of stenosis or regurgitation of a damaged valve with quantification of the pressure gradient across the valve.

(iii) angioplasty or valvuloplasty (i.e. dilatation of an artery or a stenosed valve) can be performed by inflation of a balloon sited near the tip of the catheter. More recent techniques include recannulation of a stenosed artery by laser.

(iv) diagnosis of a dissecting aortic aneurysm.

(v) diagnosis and assessment of congenital heart disease, shunts, etc., as well as the ability to perform an endomyocardial biopsy (e.g. cardiomyopathy, histological evidence of rejection of transplanted heart).

(vi) sampling of blood for measure of oxygen saturation within the different heart chambers (used in diagnosis and quantification of intracardiac shunts).

As with any invasive procedure, cardiac catheterization does carry a recognized morbidity and mortality, including the potential to arrhythmias, thromboembolism, vessel dissection, and infection.

Pacing

Pacing refers to the technique of stimulating a myocardial contraction using a small current electrical energy delivered to the heart.

Pacing may be either temporary or permanent:

Temporary pacing utilizes a pulse generator external to the body

Permanent pacing utilizes an implanted pulse generator.

There are two types of pacing electrode:

(1) *Unipolar* has only one conducting wire and electrode. Electrical current returns to the pacemaker via body fluids. These are used with permanent pacing systems

(2) *Bipolar* has two conducting wires and two electrodes. The impulse passes down one wire to (usually) the distal electrode. The circuit is then completed via the second electrode and wire back to the pacemaker.

Pacing routes

(1) Transvenous endocardial

The wire passes down a vein (usually the subclavian) to the endocardial surface of the septal region of the right ventricle. It is a bipolar electrode wire to which an inflatable balloon may be incorporated to aid flotation of the catheter during 'blind' placement. Placement of pacing wires without balloons is carried out under X-ray imaging. The wire is advanced through the right atrium into the right ventricle where it is positioned against the ventricular septal wall. Positioning is confirmed using ECG monitoring. Right atrial stimulation produces large P waves and right ventricular stimulation produces large, widened QRS complexes occurring at the rate set on the pacing box. A pacing spike (a deflection of the ECG trace) is seen prior to each stimulated complex. The voltage threshold should then be checked for good electrode placement suggested by a threshold of less than 0.5 V (see later).

(2) Epicardial

Electrodes are sutured on the pericardial surface of the heart during cardiac surgery (see Chapter 7). One or two electrodes may be used. If only one is used, a skin surface electrode is used to complete the circuit.

(3) External (transcutaneous)

Large surface area, adhesive skin electrodes are placed on the patient's chest and back and three ECG electrodes are connected from the external pacer to the usual positions on the patient's chest. Current is passed between the skin electrodes inducing a paced heartbeat (see Chapter 6). This is the method of choice in an emergency as it is rapidly placed and effective, requiring little operator skill

(4) Transoesophageal

A difficult and unreliable method of pacing in an emergency using an electrode placed in the patient's oesophagus.

Modes of pacing

Most temporary pacemakers are only capable of single chamber demand or fixed-rate pacing. More advanced models have the ability to synchronize pacing in dual chambers

Fixed rate

The heart is stimulated at a fixed rate per minute and will not alter in response to any intrinsic activity. This is rarely used unless there is no evidence of any underlying rhythm as arrhythmias may result if the pacing beat occurs close to the patient's intrinsic beat.

(3) Demand

An impulse is initiated if a pre-set interval elapses without an intrinsic stimulation of the ventricle. The interval is determined by the rate at which the pacemaker is set (e.g. a setting of 60 bpm on the pacemaker will only initiate pacing if the patient's own rate falls below 60 bpm.

Synchronous

Electrodes placed in both the right atria and ventricle allow synchronization of the stimulus in both cardiac chambers. For example, a sensing electrode in the atria will sense an atrial contraction and stimulate a ventricular beat via a pacing electrode in the ventricle, this allows atrial contraction to fulfil its role of optimally filling the ventricle.

A–V sequential

Stimulation of both atria and ventricles can be accomplished when necessary with a set interval between atrial and ventricular stimulation.

The Intersociety Commission for Heart Disease (ICHD) Pacemaker Code

Chamber(s) paced (I)	Chamber(s) sensed (II)	Mode of response(s) (III)
0 = none	0 = none	0 = none
A = atrium	A = atrium	T = triggered
V = ventricle	V = ventricle	I = inhibited
D = dual (atria and ventricle)	D = dual (atria and ventricle)	D = dual (triggered and inhibited)

Note. Other categories for programmable and anti-tachycardia functions are also included but are not relevant for temporary pacing in the ICU.

Fixed-rate pacing would be designated V00 or A00 under this code because the atria or the ventricle is the chamber paced but there is no sensing in either chamber and therefore no response to sensing.

Ventricular demand pacing would be designated VVI because the ventricle is the paced chamber, the ventricle is the sensed chamber and the pacemaker is inhibited by the sensed beat.

Atrial synchronized pacing would be designated VAT because the ventricle is the paced chamber, the atria is the sensed chamber and the ventricular pacemaker is triggered by the sensed atrial beat (P wave). (See Table 5.7 for types of pacing.)

Table 5.7 Types of pacing

Types of pacing	Indications
Ventricular demand (VVI)	Emergency situations: life-threatening bradycardias
A–V sequential (DVI)	Impaired A–V conduction with atrial bradycardia
Atrial synchronous ventricular inhibited (VDD)	Normal sinus rhythm with impaired A–V conduction
A–V universal (DDD)	Different functions according to underlying problem

Overdrive pacing for terminating tachycardias

Pacing at rates of 10–15 beats above the spontaneous rate may suppress ventricular or atrial arrhythmias. Arrhythmias suitable for overdrive pacing are paroxysmal supraventricular tachycardias, atrial flutter, and ventricular tachycardia. However, it is not effective in sinus tachycardia and atrial fibrillation.

Care of the patient with a pacemaker

Electrical safety

The pacing wire provides a direct efficient conduction route for electrical current into the heart. This is a particular problem with older forms of temporary pacing generator. Therefore, contact with any poorly insulated source of electrical current could prove dangerous to the patient. Any connections between pacemaker and pacing wire should be securely fixed and if necessary protected with gauze or tape.

Monitoring

In the acute setting, the patient with temporary pacing should be monitored in the ECG lead which gives the clearest picture. The paced rhythm can be clearly seen as a 'spike' either negatively or positively on the ECG. Any failure in pacing will cause an absence of the spike or a spike without a following QRS complex.

Note. Battery failure can be a cause of loss of pacing. Pacing box batteries should always be checked prior to use and if failure is suspected.

Failure to capture

Absence of a QRS complex following a spike is known as 'failure to capture' and can be due to an increase in threshold (see below) or displacement of the pacing electrode. An increase in delivered current may overcome an increase in threshold or the pacing wire may have to be resited or replaced.

Pacing threshold

This is the minimum level of current required to consistently pace the heart. This is measured when the pacemaker is first attached and should be < 1.0 mA. It should then be checked daily or if there is a change in monitored rhythm. Ideally, the pacemaker current should be set at 2–3 mA above the threshold to allow for minor variations and the usual increase in threshold level that occurs over a period of days after pacing is initiated. The threshold increase is thought to be due to fibrosis around the electrode tip.

mA = milliampere

Patient assessment

Assessment of the ICU patient with a cardiac disorder is achieved by using information derived from a variety of sources. These include:

- History.
- Physical assessment.
- ECG.
- Non-invasive and invasive monitoring.
- Serum biochemical and haematological tests.
- Chest X-ray.
- Other diagnostic tests (e.g. echocardiogram, angiography, p.128).

History

Details should include: type of pain, length of history, precipitating factors, relieving factors, social history (smoking, alcohol, drugs, etc.), familial history.

Physical assessment

Full details of physical assessment are given in Chapters 3 and 4. Table 5.8 gives observations that are particularly important in the patient with a cardiac disorder.

Table 5.8 Physical assessment in the patient with a cardiac disorder

	Observation	Note particularly if:
Skin	Colour Touch	Pale, cyanosed, mottled cold, clammy, hot, presence of ankle oedema
Respiration	Rate Depth	tachypnoeic, dyspnoeic, using accessory muscles, orthopnoeic: breathless lying flat
Pulse	Feel Rate	Thready, full volume, bounding tachycardic, irregular
Pain	Site Duration Severity	Associated with respiration, movement, at rest, position, eating
Other		Oliguria, nausea, vomiting, presence of cough possibly due to pulmonary oedema. Anxious, restless

The assessment of pain can be an important diagnostic tool and may help differentiate pain of cardiac origin from that of respiratory, oesophageal, or musculoskeletal disorders.

Characteristic descriptions of chest pain

Stable angina
Typically constricting, retrosternal pain, radiating to the arms (predominantly the left), neck, or jaw. It often occurs in response to stimuli that increase the oxygen demand of the heart (e.g. physical exertion or emotion) and is relieved by resting.

Unstable angina

As in stable angina but the periods of pain are prolonged, may occur at rest and have no precipitating factors.

Myocardial infarction

Typically severe, crushing, retrosternal pain which may extend to the arms, neck, jaw, or back and often lasts > 30 minutes. It is often accompanied by nausea, vomiting, and sweating. The onset of pain is not always associated with exertion and is not relieved by rest. Some patients, however, may have little or no pain, especially the elderly and diabetics.

Pericarditis

The pain is usually sharp and retrosternal and may be more apparent on inspiration. It is often worse when lying flat but is relieved when sitting up and leaning forward.

Pleuritic pain

This is usually a sharp, localized pain, worse on inspiration and coughing.

Pulmonary embolism

The pain is pleuritic in nature and may be associated with haemoptysis and breathlessness.

Oesophageal pain

Oesophageal pain is usually associated with, or eased by, food, and typically worse when lying flat. Oesophageal rupture is usually preceded by vomiting.

Aortic dissection

The patient experiences a 'tearing' pain (as opposed to the crushing pain of myocardial infarction). This pain is typically felt in the back.

Musculoskeletal pain

Pain due to spinal or muscular disorders can usually be identified by the effect of movement and position. Unlike the other conditions, the chest wall is tender to touch at the specific location.

ECG: 12-lead and continuous monitoring

When making a diagnosis the 12-lead ECG must be viewed in conjunction with the patient's history, physical examination, and the results of blood tests. If the ECG shows unequivocal changes then it can be extremely valuable, particularly in confirming a diagnosis of myocardial infarction.

Non-invasive and invasive monitoring

Full details of non-invasive and invasive monitoring are given in Chapter 4. The extent of monitoring will depend on the patient's condition. Increasingly complex regimens (e.g. for the treatment of cardiogenic shock) will require an increased complexity of monitoring.

Treatment stategies should be guided by data gained from invasive monitoring and used in conjunction with the assessment of physical signs (e.g. cool peripheries, pallor, confusion), biochemical tests, chest X-ray, and urine output.

Serum biochemical and haematological tests

Routine blood tests will include:

- cardiac enzymes,

- urea and electrolytes,

- haemoglobin,

- glucose,

- clotting studies (usually only if anticoagulant therapy has been administered),

- cholesterol and triglyceride levels.

    Other biochemical and haematological tests:

- serum urea, electrolytes, glucose, and haemoglobin are taken on admission and thereafter according to the patient's treatment or condition,

- clotting studies are usually only required following thrombolytic therapy,

- arterial blood gas analysis will be indicated if acidosis or hypoxaemia are suspected,

- other specific tests may be indicated (e.g. digoxin levels).

Chest X-ray

Usually taken on admission and thereafter according to the patient's condition. It provides valuable information on heart size, the presence of pulmonary oedema, and aortic dissection.

Priorities of care

The main function of the cardiovascular system is to maintain perfusion of tissues in order to deliver an adequate supply of oxygen and nutrients and to remove carbon dioxide and waste substances. The priority in caring for any critically ill patient is to support the ability of the cardiovascular system to carry out its functions.

(1) Support and maintenance of tissue perfusion and oxygenation — particularly cerebral, cardiac, and renal perfusion.

(2) Prevention or early detection of arrhythmias.

Adequate monitoring is essential to allow assessment of cardiac function. This should include a minimum of ECG monitoring and arterial blood pressure monitoring which is preferably continuous. Central venous pressure, pulmonary artery pressure, and mixed venous oxygen saturation monitoring may also be indicated. Urine output will provide a valuable guide to renal perfusion.

Emergency equipment should be available (see Chapter 2) and familiarity with the use of defibrillators and external pacing systems are important (see Chapter 6).

Oxygenation and oxygen transport

Any patient with a compromised cardiovascular system (either a low output state or a high output state such as sepsis) may have poor tissue perfusion and will require increased levels of tissue oxygenation. This will attempt to redress the oxygen deficit induced when oxygen transport is limited by cardiovascular function or impaired tissue perfusion. Ensuring that tissues are well supplied with oxygen should be a target for treatment in the critically ill in order to prevent tissue hypoxia and subsequent organ dysfunction and failure. The pulmonary artery catheter can be used to determine oxygen delivery and consumption and, if necessary, effective treatment strategies can then be instituted to improve oxygen supply to the tissues.

Oxygen delivery

This is the amount of oxygen that is actually delivered to the tissues by the blood and depends on the blood flow and the amount of oxygen carried in the blood. Blood flow to the tissues is measured by the cardiac output and the amount of oxygen carried in the blood is determined by the haemoglobin concentration and oxygen saturation. Therefore, if the cardiac ouput, the arterial oxygen saturation, and the haemoglobin level are known, the delivery of blood to the tissues can be calculated:

$$\text{Oxygen delivery (DO)} = \text{CO} \times (1.34 \times \text{Hb} \times S_aO_2) \times 10$$

where

CO = cardiac output (l/min)
1.34 = ml O_2 carried by 1 g Hb
Hb = the haemoglobin content of the blood (g/100 ml)
S_aO_2 = % saturation of arterial Hb
10 is used to convert ml of oxygen/100 ml blood to ml/l. (Normal DO_2 for the resting adult is approximately 1000 ml/min.)

When oxygen has been extracted from the blood by the tissues there remains an oxygen reserve in the venous blood. If the demand for oxygen by the tissues increases, the venous oxygen reserve may decrease if the oxygen supply does not improve to meet the increased demand.

Oxygen consumption

This is the amount of oxygen used by the tissues over one minute (VO_2). It can be calculated by measuring the arteriovenous oxygen difference (i.e. the difference in oxygen content between arterial and venous blood). Blood taken from the pulmonary artery is considered true mixed venous blood and the percentage of oxygen saturation of this blood is termed the mixed venous oxygen saturation (S_vO_2). Venous blood is aspirated from the pulmonary artery and a sample is taken from an arterial line. The oxygen saturation of both are measured in a co-oximeter. This can then be used to calculate the oxygen extraction ratio which is the amount of oxygen extracted by the peripheral tissues divided by the amount of oxygen delivered:

$$O_2 \text{ extraction ratio } (O_2ER) = \frac{\text{Arterial} - \text{venous } O_2 \text{ saturation}}{\text{Arterial } O_2 \text{ saturation}}$$

The normal value in an adult is about 25%.
Factors increasing the O_2 extraction ratio are:

• decreased cardiac output,

• increased oxygen consumption (not compensated by improved oxygen delivery),

• anaemia,

• decreased arterial oxygenation.

The venous oxygen reserve is the oxygen content in the venous blood over one minute:

$$\text{Venous oxygen reserve} = CO \times (1.34 \times Hb \times S_vO_2) \times 10$$

Oxygen consumption = oxygen delivery − venous oxygen reserve.

The normal value in an adult is 225–275 ml/min.

DO_2 and VO_2 can be adjusted for the patient's size by dividing by the body surface area to produce DO_2^I and VO_2^I.

The normal range for oxygen consumption index is 125–165 ml O_2/m^2.

Methods of increasing oxygen delivery

Physiological responses

When the body's requirement for oxygen increases (e.g. during exercise), this need stimulates mechanisms in the respiratory and circulatory systems that will effectively increase oxygen delivery to the tissues.

Respiratory system

• respiratory effort is increased in order to increase oxygen intake and CO_2 elimination.

Circulatory system

• Venous return is increased (and thus preload).

• Heart rate is increased (due to adrenergic stimulation).

• Contractility is increased (due to adrenergic stimulation).

All of these mechanisms serve to increase cardiac output.

Clinical interventions

Critically ill patients are often unable to increase oxygen delivery sufficiently by their own physiological mechanisms and, if delivery does not match consumption, specific cardiovascular and respiratory interventions (see Table 5.9) can be instituted.

The technique of measuring oxygen transport is given in Chapter 4.

When oxygen transport is limited by cardiac output (e.g. cardiogenic shock), oxygen consumption by the tissues is maintained by increased oxygen extraction from the blood. Thus, the normal S_vO_2 is 70–75%. However, if increased oxygen extraction occurs it may drop to well below 50%. $S_vO_2 < 40\%$ is associated with a serious disturbance in the oxygen supply – demand relationship.

Table 5.9 Interventions to improve oxygen delivery

Manipulation	Rationale	Intervention
Cardiovascular: • Optimize preload • Reduce afterload (if possible) • Increase contractility • Increase heart rate (if bradycardic)	Blood flow to the tissues will be increased	• Serial fluid challenges until no further increase in SV (Starling curve) • Reduce afterload (e.g. with nitrates) to normalize SVR • Inotropes to increase cardiac output (e.g. dobutamine, dopexamine, adrenaline)
Maintain Hb level within normal values	The oxygen carrying capacity of the blood will be maximized	Transfuse to keep Hb > 10 g/d
Respiratory: • Maintain arterial oxygen saturation >95% • Respiratory support if patient fatigued or hypoxaemic	• The blood reaching the tissues will be adequately oxygenated • The work of breathing may in itself increase oxygen demand	• Increase inspired oxygen to maintain S_aO_2 • Hyperoxygenate prior to suction procedures if necessary

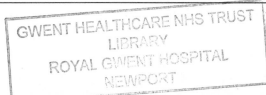

General principles of care

Hypotension

There is no level of blood pressure that can define hypotension as this depends on the clinical condition of the patient and the premorbid state (e.g. history of chronic hypertension). However, it is usually considered to be when the MAP falls to <60 mmHg or is associated with clinical symptoms of organ hypoperfusion. It is important to note that impaired organ perfusion can be present despite a normal or elevated blood pressure.

The aims of treatment of hypotension should be directed at:

- establishing and treating the cause
- maintaining tissue oxygenation where appropriate by increasing cardiac output, haemoglobin, and/or arterial oxygen saturation
- maintaining tissue perfusion pressures by increasing the systemic blood pressure.

Ensure that the blood pressure recording is correct. If a cuff is being used, confirm it is the right size and correctly applied to the arm. Repeat the measurement. If an arterial line is being transduced check for damping of the trace (e.g. air bubbles in the circuit), kinking (e.g. wrist movements), the position of the transducer relative to the left atrium and that it is zeroed correctly. If doubt exists regarding transducer accuracy, confirm a low reading by a cuff measurement.

Causes of hypotension include:

- Hypovolaemia
- Cardiogenic causes:
  - cardiac failure
  - tachy/brady arrhythmias
  - valvular stenosis/incompetence
- Obstructive causes:
  - cardiac tamponade
  - pulmonary embolism
  - tension pneumothorax
- Sepsis/inflammation
- Anaphylactic reactions

Manifestations of organ hypoperfusion

- Kidneys: oliguria
- Skin: pallor, cool peripheries
- Brain: confusion, drowsiness, agitation, syncope
- Metabolic acidosis
- Compensatory tachycardia

Treatment strategies and choice of drugs may vary amongst different intensive care units and will be influenced by the methods of monitoring that are available. However, the underlying principles of managing hypotension will be the same.

Blood pressure should be restored by one or more of the following:

- ensuring circulating volume is adequate before positive inotropic drugs are used,
- administering inotropic drugs to attain adequate cardiac output and organ perfusion,
- administering vasopressor drugs, rather than inotropes, in the hypotensive patient with a high cardiac output and low systemic vascular resistance (e.g. sepsis, anaphylaxis),
- specific treatment where appropriate (e.g. drainage of a tension pneumothorax).

Hypovolaemia as a cause of hypotension (See box)

Hypovolaemia can be caused by:

- haemorrhage (e.g. trauma, dissecting/ruptured aortic aneurysm, bleeding ulcers)
- fluid loss (e.g. vomiting, diarrhoea, burns)
- pooling of fluid in extravascular spaces (e.g. increased capillary permeability secondary to an insult, ileus following bowel surgery)
- inadequate fluid input
- relative vasodilatation and loss of peripheral vascular tone

---

Management of hypovolaemia
The underlying cause must be identified and treated. The usual cardiovascular effects in the hypovolaemic patient are tachycardia, hypotension, oliguria, decreased cardiac

output, and high SVR. However, young, fit patients can compensate by increased vasoconstriction and maintain a normal blood pressure until the hypovolaemia is advanced. It is therefore important not to rely solely on blood pressure as an indicator of shock.

Immediate treatment is the rapid administration of fluid guided by monitored haemodynamic variables. If there is no stroke volume measuring technique *in situ* intravascular fluid status can be guided by CVP measurements. Fluid challenges should be repeated until the CVP rises ⩾3 mmHg; 5–10 minutes after the challenge has been completed. If the CVP rises ⩾3 mmHg and MAP remains <60 mmHg in the presence of oliguria then pulmonary artery catheterization will provide more valuable information. No response in stroke volume to a fluid challenge suggests that positive inotropic support and vasodilators or vasoconstrictors will be necessary. Heart rate, blood pressure, urine output, and level of consciousness/ orientation can also provide a guide to improvement in organ perfusion.

The fluid used to restore intravascular volume will depend on the cause. If hypovolaemia is due to haemorrhage, give colloid until crossmatched blood is available or use group-specific or O rhesus-negative blood if haemorrhage is severe. Administer rapidly, under pressure if necessary, and continue until organ perfusion and blood pressure are maintained at adequate values.

If hypovolaemic hypotension is due to excessive fluid loss from vomiting, nasogastric aspirate, diarrhoea, or pooling of fluid extravascularly then colloid can be given rapidly as a series of fluid challenges. Blood pressure, ± stroke volume, ±CVP, ±PAWP, and urine output should be checked after each challenge. If the CVP, PAWP, and BP remain unchanged and the stroke volume (if measured) continues to rise, colloid challenges should be given repeatedly until adequate pressures and organ perfusion are achieved. Adequate organ perfusion is sometimes achieved at surprisingly low blood pressures. Following resuscitation, the hourly fluid requirements of the patient should be reviewed and a crystalloid solution, such as 0.9% sodium chloride, may need to be given or increased to replace fluid losses.

Cardiogenic causes of hypotension

These include arrhythmias (e.g. tachyarrhythmias, heart block), myocardial pump failure, intracardiac shunts, and valvular dysfunction.

If hypotension is secondary to tachy- or bradyarrhythmias, the arrhythmia must be treated in order to restore blood pressure.

Cardiogenic shock results from failure of the heart to maintain adequate organ perfusion (see p. 146 for full details). Such patients will require intensive monitoring and complex treatment strategies.

The initial treatment for cardiogenic hypotension is with inotropes. However, fluid should be considered as hypovolaemia may coexist. The fluid is administered by colloid challenges (see p. 136 for details).

Treatment of the severely hypotensive patient should not be withheld while a pulmonary artery catheter is being inserted. Empiric 'best guess' therapy may be needed.

Dobutamine or adrenaline are inotropic drugs commonly given and dosages are titrated according to response. If systemic vascular resistance is high, a vasodilator (e.g. glyceryl trinitrate) may be infused and titrated according to SVR. Normalizing a raised SVR is an important way of improving cardiac efficiency since peripheral resistance and hence left ventricular work is decreased. Cardiac overdistension should also be treated by decreasing venous return. Care must be taken to ensure that the intravascular volume is maintained while vasodilators are given otherwise further hypotension may result.

Obstructive causes of hypotension

These include cardiac tamponade, pneumothorax, and pulmonary embolus. The cause must be identified and treated in order to restore blood pressure (Chapters 3 and 11 for further details).

'Inflammatory' causes of hypotension

Infection, or other insults, such as burns, pancreatitis, and trauma, will stimulate a generalized inflammatory response resulting in loss of peripheral vascular tone and increased capillary leak. The resultant vasodilatation and relative hypovolaemia cause hypotension. Full details of the causes and management of hypotension due to infective processes are given in Chapter 14.

The management of sepsis syndrome is aimed at identification of the source of infection, prescribing appropriate antibiotic therapy and maintaining organ perfusion and tissue oxygenation.

Monitoring of vital signs will usually show low central venous, pulmonary artery wedge and systemic arterial pressures, low SVR, tachycardia, pyrexia, and a high cardiac output. These represent a hyperdynamic circulation and are common to such patients. The skin may feel hot to touch and the patient may have a bounding pulse.

A minority of such patients may present with hypotension but are apyrexial with a low cardiac output. This may be due to pre-existing poor cardiac function or to inflammatory mediator-induced myocardial depression.

Fluid resuscitation is usually the first treatment. However, for severe hypotension, empiric therapy with adrenaline or noradrenaline may also be needed while adequate monitoring is being inserted, in order that a minimum satisfactory perfusion pressure is rapidly restored. The choice of fluid is controversial; in Europe, colloids are generally used, whereas in North America, crystalloid solutions are preferred. Although lower volumes of colloid would be needed, no benefit in outcome has been shown between the two solutions.

Fluid restoration has the aim of maximizing stroke volume. Large volumes may be required and infusion should continue until no further improvement in stroke volume is seen. Due to capillary leak, intravascular volume expansion may still be required even if there is evidence of oedema. If respiratory function is severely compromised with coexisting ARDS it may be necessary to institute vasopressors at an earlier stage and to restrict the amount of fluid given.

If the patient remains hypotensive after fluid resuscitation, vasopressors will be required; often high dosages are necessary. Noradrenaline (or high-dose dopamine) are the drugs of choice as they are effective vasoconstrictors. If myocardial dysfunction is present and the SVR is high, dobutamine or adrenaline may be of benefit as they increase myocardial contractility.

Anaphylaxis as a cause of hypotension

The acute reaction to an allergenic substance can cause severe hypotension or even cardiovascular collapse. Severe anaphylactic reactions may require full cardiorespiratory resuscitation. Allergenic substances (e.g. food, blood, drugs, insect stings) can result in degranulation of mast cells. These release histamine and other mediator substances that cause vasodilatation, smooth muscle constriction, and increased capillary permeability. Hypotension is caused by the vasodilatation and loss of fluid from the capillaries resulting in a relative hypovolaemia.

Hypotension and tachycardia may be severe. There may be dyspnoea and cyanosis due to bronchospasm or laryngeal obstruction, skin flushing, urticarial rash, soft tissue swelling, nausea, vomiting, and diarrhoea.

Immediate treatment for anaphylactic hypotension is to provide respiratory support if required, adrenaline and fluid infusion (usually colloid). Adrenaline (0.5–1 mg) is given intramuscularly but may be given intravenously in situations where severe shock may impede absorption. Adrenaline should not be given subcuta-

neously for this reason. An intravenous infusion may also be necessary. Hydrocortisone 200 mg and chlorpheniramine 10 mg are also given intravenously. Colloid should be given rapidly to correct hypovolaemia, ideally guided by CVP or PAWP measurements, but in its absence by blood pressure, heart rate, urine output, and physical assessment.

The causative agent of the reaction should be identified in order to avoid re-exposure. If an anaphylactic reaction occurs during a transfusion of blood or blood products the bag of fluid should be retained and sent back to the haematology department for analysis. A sample of the patient's blood should also be taken for subsequent analysis (see Chapter 12 for further details).

Summary of changes in haemodynamic parameters

Table 5.10 shows common changes seen in many patients but are by no means universal to all (Table 5.15 lists the drugs used for treating hypotension.)

Table 5.10 Hypotension: haemodynamic parameters

Cause of hypotension	CO	PAWP	SVR
Hypovolaemia	↓	↓	↑
Cardiogenic	↓	↑ or ⇄	↑
Inflammatory	↑	↓	↓
Obstructive	↓	↑ or ⇄	↑
Anaphylactic	↑	↓	↓

↑, increased; ↓, decreased; ⇄, unchanged.

Hypertension

Hypertension can be defined as a sustained, raised blood pressure above that which would be considered normal for the patient's age. The 'normal' blood pressure is difficult to quantify because it is a statistical range of values based on the mean of the population, therefore the level of blood pressure at which treatment should be started is not clear-cut. Before diagnosing a patient as hypertensive the blood pressure must be recorded correctly, and be consistently elevated.

Antihypertensive therapy is generally begun if the resting diastolic blood pressure is consistently above 100 mmHg in those under 65 years old or above 105 mmHg in patients over 65 years old (Hope et al. 1992). However, treatment may be started if the diastolic pressure is lower than this if there is evidence of organ damage or the need to keep pressures low (e.g. dissecting aortic aneurysm).

The level of the diastolic pressure is more significant than the systolic pressure because its value is more closely related to an increase in the incidence of complications.

If the cause of the hypertension cannot be identified it is termed 'primary' (or 'essential') hypertension. If there is an identifiable cause it is termed secondary hypertension. Primary hypertension exists in 90–95% of patients with hypertension and is diagnosed by elimination of the identifiable causes of secondary hypertension. Hypertension may be a natural response to pain and stress and this will require the appropriate treatment (e.g. analgesia).

Causes of secondary hypertension

- Endocrine
  - phaeochromocytoma
  - Conn's syndrome (primary hyperaldosteronism)
  - Cushing's syndrome
  - hyperparathyroidism
  - acromegaly

- Renal
  - chronic glomerulonephritis
  - chronic pyelonephritis
  - renal artery stenosis
  - polycystic disease
  - polyarteritis nodosa

- Pregnancy-induced

- Intracranial haemorrhage

- Coarctation of the aorta

- Drug-related (e.g. withdrawal of antihypertensive drugs — clonidine, contraceptive pill; monoamine oxidase inhibitors (MAOI) antidepressants with tyramine-containing foods, e.g. cheese)

Blood pressure is regulated by multiple factors including endocrine, neuronal, humoral, and renal that moderate vasomotor and vasoconstrictor responses (see earlier). However, the mechanisms involved in causing primary hypertension, remain complex and are not fully understood.

Vascular tone is important in maintaining blood pressure and if arterioles become narrowed due to an increase in vascular tone there is an increase in peripheral vascular resistance. This increase in peripheral resistance causes hypertension. In the early stages this can be effectively reversed by vasodilator drugs. However, over a period of time the tunica media (the smooth muscle layer of the arterioles) become permanently hypertrophied due to the chronically raised pressure (medial hypertrophy). The effect of this is a narrowing of the lumen of the vessel which reduces blood flow to the tissue it supplies and can result in ischaemic damage. Any tissues of the body can be affected but since a large portion of the cardiac output flows to the brain, heart, and kidneys these organs are particularly vulnerable in hypertension. Unfortunately, in chronic hypertension, patients are often asymptomatic until there is irreversible damage.

Manifestations of hypertension

- Neurological
  - headache
  - dizziness
  - transient ischaemic attacks
  - focal disturbances
  - confusion
  - fits, coma (hypertensive encephalopathy)
  - strokes

- Cardiovascular
  - palpitations
  - left ventricular failure (causing pulmonary oedema)
  - angina
  - myocardial infarction
  - retinopathy

- Renal
  - renal failure
  - proteinuria

- Other
- retinopathy

Disorders that may cause an acute hypertensive crisis include:

- malignant hypertension

- phaeochromocytoma

- pre-eclampsia/eclampsia

- any cause of raised intracranial pressure (ICP)

- drug-related (withdrawal of clonidine, reaction of MAOI with foods containing pressor amines)

Management of an acute hypertensive crisis

If symptomatic (headaches, confusion, drowsiness, fits, agitation), the aim of treatment is to reduce the blood pressure urgently, but smoothly, and not excessively aiming for a diastolic of 110–120 mmHg. Sudden drops in blood pressure should be avoided. If the cause of the hypertension is raised ICP the blood pressure is usually allowed to remain high to maintain adequate cerebral perfusion pressure.

Intravenous drug therapy will usually be required and continuous blood pressure monitoring is essential. The choice of hypotensive drug will depend on the cause of the hypertension and its urgency of treatment. The most commonly used in the ICU are sodium nitroprusside, which produces a rapid effect and can be finely controlled, glyceryl trinitrate, labetalol, and hydralazine which can all be given by infusion. The drug dosage should always be titrated against response. Nifedipine can be used, although sublingual administration of the fluid contained in the capsule has a variable absorption rate and a variable sometimes abrupt hypotensive effect.

Hypertensive encephalopathy

This can be caused by uncontrolled hypertension of any cause. In addition to systemic organ damage it is characterized by neurological signs that are a result of reduced cerebral blood flow. There may be areas of cerebral infarction, haemorrhage, or transient ischaemia. Symptoms are initially severe headaches and nausea but progress to a deteriorating level of consciousness, *grand mal* seizures, and then coma. If the hypertension is treated early the changes may be reversible but mortality is high.

Malignant hypertension

Malignant hypertension is a distinct pathological condition where there is progressive severe hypertension (diastolic pressure may be > 140 mmHg). Patients can develop severe organ damage; renal failure, heart failure, retinal haemorrhages, papilloedema, and hypertensive encephalopathy. If untreated, mortality is 90% within one year of onset.

Treatment is strict bedrest and antihypertensive drugs (e.g. nitroprusside or labetalol) to reduce the blood pressure slowly but not excessively to a diastolic of 110–120 mmHg. Overaggressive reduction may result in poor perfusion and a stroke.

Specific conditions

Myocardial infarction (MI)

This arises when a region of the myocardium becomes irreversibly necrosed. It is usually due to thromboembolic occlusion of the coronary artery supplying that area of heart muscle, although MI can occasionally follow direct trauma or electrocution.

Each year more than 300 000 people in the United Kingdom suffer acute MI. It is the commonest single cause of death (approximately 25–30% of all deaths, higher in males). Approximately 40% die before arrival in hospital and a further 5–10% will die while in hospital. Recent advances in care, notably the use of thrombolysis, has significantly improved outcome. Numerous large-scale international multicentre trials are being continually undertaken to improve prognosis and function still further.

Risk factors for MI are well recognized, particularly smoking, hypercholesterolaemia, and hypertension. Other factors include obesity, age, diabetes, family history, and geographical and environmental factors (Scotland, Northern Ireland, and Finland have a particularly high incidence, whereas Mediterranean countries have a low incidence). The incidence of MI has dropped considerably in the United States over the last two decades as a direct result of health education and primary prevention programmes, however, the reduction has been far less dramatic in the United Kingdom.

Assessment

Physical

Pain — classically, the patient presents with crushing central chest pain, with or without radiation of pain down the left arm, neck, or jaw. Unless relieved by medication, the pain usually lasts more than 30 minutes and is not eased by posture or food. 'Silent' infarcts, that is without chest pain are not infrequent, especially in elderly or diabetic populations and the pain may occasionally be atypical (e.g. short-lived or epigastric in location).

Skin — the patient may be sweating, pale, grey or cyanosed, and peripherally constricted.

Respiratory — the patient may be tachypnoeic or dyspnoeic and there may be evidence of pulmonary oedema (see Chapter 3).

Other physical signs — nausea and vomiting may occur.

Psychological

Anxiety — the patient usually appears distressed and anxious and may require considerable comfort and reassurance.

Confusion — the patient may appear confused due to hypoxaemia or poor cerebral perfusion.

Physiological

Blood pressure — may be normal, elevated, or depressed.

ECG monitoring — may show tachycardia, and arrhythmias may occur.

Urine output — may be oliguric due to poor renal perfusion.

Blood glucose — may be raised due to sympathetic activity (see later).

Investigations

12-lead ECG

Depending on the time from onset of symptoms, a 12-lead ECG will initially show convex ST elevation and T wave inversion (implying injury and ischaemia) in the leads adjacent to the infarcted area (see p. 95). Leads opposite the area will show inverse changes (e.g. V1, V2 in posterior MI). Pathological Q waves will then develop, although this can vary from minutes to days. Approximately 20% of patients with subsequently proved infarction will present without ST elevation or clearly identifiable Q waves. Occasionally, no Q waves (non-Q wave infarction) or other electrocardiographic evidence will develop despite conclusive proof from other sources (e.g. rise in cardiac enzymes). Coexisting left bundle branch block may also obscure ECG signs of an acute MI. Serial ECGs and cardiac enzyme estimations should be taken over three days to confirm the occurrence of an acute MI and to show its evolution.

Cardiac enzymes

Necrosed myocardium releases enzymes into the blood and measurement of these can assist in the diagnosis of myocardial infarction. Three specific enzymes are measured and the levels of these peak at different times.

Care must be taken in interpreting these results as muscles other than the heart also release these enzymes. If there is doubt as to the origin of the enzyme the measurement of isoenzymes for creatine kinase can identify enzymes released specifically from cardiac muscle as opposed to skeletal muscle or brain.

1. *Creatine kinase* (*CK*). Released up to 3 days post-infarction. Levels peak at 30–60 hours. Skeletal muscle is also rich in CK and false positive results may arise in patients with:

- intramuscular injections,
- recent vigorous exercise,
- trauma
- surgery
- rhabdomyolysis.

If doubt exists the CK-MB isoenzyme can be measured.

2. Aspartate transaminase (AST). Released 1–3 days post infarction. Levels peak at 24–48 hours. Diseases of the liver, brain, kidney, and lung may all give false positives.

3. Lactic dehydrogenase (LDH). Released 2–10 days post-infarction. Peak levels occur at 3 days. Red cells also contain LDH and any cause of haemolysis may produce false positive results.

Cardiac enzymes need to be measured on admission and over the next two days (Fig 5.7). An early rise in creatine kinase (> ×2 normal) in the absence of other causes such as trauma is highly suggestive of MI. A rise in CK to diagnostic levels (×2 normal) may take up to 4–8 hours and, if early doubt persists, a repeat CK level should be performed within hours of the first measurement. None of the cardiac enzymes routinely measured are specific for heart muscle thus the temporal change related to the time of MI is important. In cases of doubt, the cardiac isoenzyme of creatine kinase (CK-MB) can be assayed.

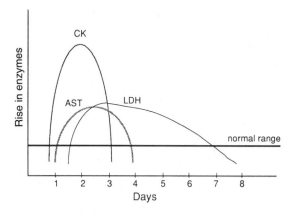

Fig. 5.7 Temporal change in cardiac enzymes (CK, creatine kinase; AST, aspartate transaminase; LDH, lactate dehydrogenase).

The diagnosis of MI is usually made on the strength of at least two likely positives from the history, ECG appearance and evolution, and temporal change in cardiac enzymes.

Causes of central chest pain

Angina	Gastritis and peptic ulceration
Pericarditis	Pancreatitis
Myocarditis	Pneumonia
Oesophagitis	Chest wall — intercostal
Pulmonary	myalgia, costochondritis,
embolism	pre-rash shingles
Pleurisy	Acute aortic dissection

A particular concern is with acute aortic dissection where the pain is usually tearing in nature and radiating through to the back. In this situation, administration of thrombolysis is contraindicated. A good history, in particular noting the duration, character and radiation of the pain, precipitating, temporal and relieving factors, and associated symptoms, in conjunction with a careful examination and appropriate investigations may enable MI to be distinguished from other causes of chest pain. Sometimes, however, definitive diagnosis still proves difficult and the patient may receive treatment purely on a strong presumptive basis. GTN may also relieve the pain of oesophageal spasm and therefore should not be considered diagnostic.

Priorities of care

Intervention should occur promptly while undertaking a rapid assessment of the patient, obtaining a brief but pertinent history and performing appropriate assessment and investigations. The patient's cardiorespiratory status must be adequately evaluated and resuscitative measures commenced as appropriate. If diagnostic doubt exists more time may be spent before instituting certain steps (e.g. administration of thrombolysis).

- High-concentration, high-flow oxygen should be administered.

- 2–4 puffs of GTN spray or one sublingual GTN tablet.

- Continuous ECG and pulse oximetry monitoring, regular BP recording.

- Wide-bore peripheral venous access.

- Intravenous opiate (e.g. diamorphine 2.5–5 mg) and antiemetic if in pain or distress. The opiate dose should be repeated as necessary.

- Appropriate investigations (including 12-lead ECG, cardiac enzymes, potassium, glucose, lipids, and chest-X-ray).

- Thrombolytic agent (unless contraindicated) plus aspirin or heparin (see later).

- Management of complications (cardiac arrest, pulmonary oedema, cardiogenic shock, life-threatening or haemodynamically compromising arrhythmias).

- Relief of patient anxiety and distress using skilled, competent care, and providing information appropriate to the situation is essential.

- Assist patient into a comfortable position and reduce effort and stress.

Principles of care

The patient should then be admitted to a high dependency area, such as a coronary care unit (CCU), although admission to an intensive care unit may be warranted if complications are present. Thrombolysis should ideally not be delayed until the patient is transferred to a CCU. Indeed, some centres give pre-hospital thrombolysis while others admit patients directly to a chest pain unit to prevent unnecessary delays in diagnosis and treatment.

The patient without complications should be on strict bedrest with continuous ECG and regular BP monitoring for the first 24 hours. Both patient and family should be reassured and provided with information about rehabilitation and suggestions in lifestyle alteration. Blood glucose estimations (by BM stix) should be performed regularly as the insult of an MI often results in glucose intolerance and diabetes. This will often settle over the following week, although may occasionally need either short- or long-term insulin or oral hypoglycaemic treatment. A pyrexia is common for the first 2–3 days.

On day 2 the patient may be allowed to mobilize slowly. Discharge to a general ward often takes place after 1–2 days. Most hospitals have their own mobilization regimens with the patient being discharged at approximately 7 days by which time he/she will have climbed a staircase. After hospital discharge the patient will be advised to undertake a slowly increasing exercise regimen and will be followed up in cardiac rehabilitation classes and the outpatient clinic. Return to work is generally delayed for 2–6 months depending on the type of activity involved. Further investigations, such as angiography, may be indicated, particularly in a young person or if complications develop. Surgery or angioplasty may then be recommended if appropriate.

Therapies

1. Thrombolysis

As coronary thromboembolism is the predominant cause of myocardial infarction, administration of a thrombolytic agent to dissolve the clot will, it is hoped, recanalize the occluded coronary artery and re-perfuse the affected region of myocardium. If the area has fully infarcted then little can be achieved by thrombolysis. However, early administration may reverse or at least minimize the amount of permanently necrosed muscle. Large multi-centre trials have conclusively shown benefit with mortality reduced from approximately 13% to 8%; ideally the thrombolytic agent should be given as soon as possible, preferably within 4–6 hours from the onset of symptoms, however, treatment has been shown to be effective for up to 24 hours.

Two choices are available — either naturally occurring thrombolytics, such as streptokinase (or occasionally urokinase), or agents produced by recombinant therapy, namely tissue plasminogen activator (rTPA) or anisoylated plasminogen streptokinase activator complex (APSAC). Although the last two are specific for newly formed clot and less likely to cause allergic or anaphylactic reactions (especially rTPA), they are considerably more expensive and have a much shorter half-life, necessitating the use of intravenous heparin for a few days to prevent re-occlusion of the vessel. Streptokinase is, therefore, the current first-line therapy unless the patient has any contraindications (see box). If this is the case, rTPA should be used.

Contraindications to the use of streptokinase
  (i)   previous reaction
  (ii) previously treated with streptokinase within the previous 5 days to 54 months
  (iii) recent streptococcal infection (<1 month)
  (iv) imminent surgical or invasive procedure anticipated

Some centres consider rTPA as first-line therapy in young patients (<45 years), in large anterior MI presenting early (<4 hours), and in cardiogenic shock. However, rTPA should not be used more than 6 hours after the onset of symptoms (except when streptokinase has been previously given), in patients over 75 years old (greater risk of cerebrovascular accidents), and in the absence of diagnostic ECG changes.

Little difference has been seen in terms of clinical benefit between the different fibrinolytic agents although the GUSTO study (Global Utilization of Streptokinase and tPA for occluded coronary arteries) suggested that an increased risk of stroke exists with rTPA (3–4/1000), especially in old and/or hypertensive patients, which offsets any small mortality reduction advantage.

Contraindications to thrombolysis are shown in Table 5.11 and may either be absolute or relative. Thrombolysis may be given even when relative contraindications exist when the mortality risk from the MI (e.g. with associated hypotension) outweighs the risk of bleeding.

Table 5.11 Contraindications to thrombolysis

Absolute contraindications	Relative contraindications
Active gastrointestinal bleeding	Traumatic or prolonged CPR
Aortic dissection	Recent obstetric delivery
Neurosurgery/head injury/ cerebrovascular accidents within 2 months	Prior organ biopsy
Intracranial neoplasm/ aneurysm	Bleeding diathesis
Proliferative diabetic retinopathy	Recent puncture of major vessel
Serious trauma, major surgery within 10 days	
Systolic BP >200 mmHg	

Drug doses of thrombolytic agents
Streptokinase: 1.5 million units in 100 ml 0.9% saline IV over 1 hour
rTPA: 100 mg IV over 90 min (15 mg bolus, 50 mg/30 min, 35 mg/60 min)
APSAC: 30 units IV over 5 minutes

Arterial and/or central venous cannulation should not be delayed following commencement of thrombolysis if clinically indicated. Cannulation should be performed by an experienced operator, avoiding the subclavian route.

If considerable haemorrhage does occur from either attempted cannula insertion or other causes (e.g. peptic ulcer), this can be often reversed by stopping the infusion, giving fresh frozen plasma and either: (i) aprotinin 500 000 units over 10 minutes, then 200 000 units over 4 hours; or (ii) tranexamic acid 10 mg/kg repeated after 6–8 hours.

Revascularization arrhythmias are common post-thrombolysis. Of these, over 90% are benign and do not require treatment. If these occur during infusion, temporary cessation may be all that is necessary. Allergic or anaphylactic reactions to thrombolytic therapy (e.g. hypotension and rash) are relatively rare and should be treated by stopping the streptokinase infusion and giving hydrocortisone 200 mg IV, chlorpheniramine 10mg IV, and ranitidine 50 mg IV. The circulation should be supported if necessary with the aim of restarting thrombolytic therapy; rTPA may be given instead.

2. Aspirin/heparin
Unless there is a known contraindication, the patient should be given aspirin 150–325 mg once daily as soon as possible after MI, preferably by the GP who first sees the patient or in the casualty department. Aspirin is given for its antiplatelet aggregation effect. Unless the patient has received a short-acting thrombolytic, such as rTPa, there is no added benefit to aspirin by giving heparin.

3. Beta blockers
The early large multi-centre studies that pre-dated thrombolytic therapy concentrated on the effects of beta blockers. Although benefit was shown, particularly when an early IV dose was given, and they proved generally safe, a major effect on outcome was not seen with mortality being reduced by only 1% (i.e. an extra 1 hospital survivor per 100 hospital admissions). Most hospitals have developed their own post-infarction treatment protocol which often includes beta blocker therapy.

4. Other agents
(a) Angiotensin-converting enzyme (ACE) inhibitors have been shown to improve outcome in patients with chronic heart failure and a number of large-scale trials have been undertaken to assess their efficacy post-infarction. Apart from reducing cardiac work by their afterload-lowering properties, they also appear to reduce wall stress within the heart thereby limiting infarct expansion and excessive ventricular dilatation. The ISIS-4 study of 58 000 patients from 1000 hospitals in 30 countries showed a small but significant improvement in survival with captopril, while the AIRE study using ramipril confirmed long-term efficacy.

(b) Despite early reports suggesting benefit from intravenous magnesium, both meta-analysis and the recent ISIS-4 study demonstrated no effect.

(c) Although small-scale trials and meta-analyses suggested that oral nitrate therapy may be of use, the ISIS-4 study failed to reveal an overall improvement in survival.

(d) Lipid lowering agents will obviously not have any effect on short-term survival, although whether long-term benefit exists remains controversial.

Complications
- arrhythmias (see p.85–92),

- heart failure/cardiogenic shock (see p.146)

- hypertension/(see p.138),

- post-infarction angina, (see p.145)

- pericarditis, (see p.150)

- rupture of papillary muscle, ventricular septal defect, LV aneurysm formation,

- cardiac rupture.

Table 5.12 Summary of benefits of therapy

Agent	Benefit at 1 month	Groups that particularly benefit
Aspirin	20–30 lives/ 1000	All suspected MI or unstable angina Continue after hospital discharge
Thrombolytic therapy	30+ lives/ 1000	All suspected MI with ST elevation or bundle branch block within 24 hours of onset (ideally within 4–6 hours)
ACE inhibitors	5 lives/1000 (10 lives/ 1000 in high-risk groups)	Anterior or previous MI, or if developing heart failure. Start early, continue long-term
Heparin, magnesium, oral nitrates	Minimal	

Hypertension may occur for a variety of reasons after myocardial infarction. Pain and anxiety are two causes, although excessive vasoconstriction, perhaps due to inappropriate use of diuretics, may also contribute. If treatment is necessary, this should aim to bring about a gradual rather than precipitate reduction. Hypotension post-infarction may also be due to hypovolaemia secondary to inappropriate diuretic usage or be drug-related (e.g. β-blockade, ACE inhibition) and it should not be automatically assumed that the cause is pump failure.

Post-infarction angina has to be treated aggressively (see later) and is one of the indications for angiography with a view to either angioplasty or bypass surgery. This pain can usually be distinguished from pericarditis which may either occur within a few days of the infarct or after a lag period of 2–6 weeks. This latter situation, known as Dressler's syndrome, is thought to be related to formation of autoantibodies against the myocardium. Other causes and management of pericarditis are described later.

Papillary muscle rupture results in disruption of the mitral valve. It usually presents with acute pulmonary oedema; echocardiography will reveal severe mitral regurgitation and the damaged valve. The patient should be treated as for severe heart failure and also referred for urgent cardiac surgery.

A ventricular septal defect may occur after septal infarction. It usually presents several days after the MI as acute heart failure. Colour-flow Doppler echocardiography will reveal the abnormal flow jet across the defect while sampling of blood from right atrium and right ventricle will reveal a 'step-up' in oxygen saturation due to the left-to-right shunt. Again, the patient should be treated for heart failure and also considered for urgent cardiac surgery.

Ventricular aneurysm formation usually develops over weeks to months after the infarction. Clues are persistent elevation of ST segments on electrocardiography and a bulge in the cardiac contour on chest X-ray. Echocardiography or angiography will reveal the abnormal and often paradoxical movement of the aneurysmal area during the cardiac cycle and possibly an associated mural thrombus. Complications that may develop include arrhythmias, heart failure, and systemic embolization. Cardiac rupture is recognized, although is invariably a terminal event. Treatment depends on the size and the degree of compromise or complications caused; it may either be conservative or surgical (aneurysmectomy).

Angina pectoris

The usual cause is critical narrowing of one or more coronary arteries leading to a myocardial oxygen debt and ischaemia during periods of increased demand such as exercise. Angina at rest or on minimal exertion indicates severe stenosis of the artery and is a recognized major risk factor for infarction. Approximately 20% of patients with unstable angina will die within one year if left untreated. Prinzmetal angina is chest pain occurring at rest and is due to coronary artery spasm. Other rarer causes of angina include aortic stenosis or hypertrophic obstructive cardiomyopathy where both aortic and coronary blood flow may be severely compromised, and severe anaemia where the oxygen-carrying capacity of the blood is significantly reduced. Significant arrhythmias may also compromise cardiac output leading to the development of angina.

Assessment

Physical

Pain — ischaemia of the myocardium results in a build-up of lactic acid and the development of pain which is classically crushing and retrosternal. This pain may radiate down the left arm or both arms, or up to the neck or jaw. Occasionally, chest pain may be absent. The pain generally lasts less than 30 minutes and is usually exertion-related but may also be precipitated by cold weather, anxiety, or during a meal. The pain is not eased by posture or food but is usually relieved by either rest and/or sublingual glyceryl trinitrate. Development of anginal pain at rest, or of increasing severity on minimal exertion is termed 'unstable angina'.

Skin — the patient may sweat and appear pale, grey, or cyanosed. There may be peripheral vasoconstriction and the patient will feel clammy.

Respiratory — the patient may become dyspnoeic or tachypnoeic.

Other symptoms — the patient may complain of nausea or actually vomit.

Investigations

A 12-lead ECG may reveal ST segment elevation and T wave flattening or depression. It may be normal outside an attack but should be repeated if possible during pain to confirm electrocardiographic changes of myocardial ischaemia. Cardiac enzyme estimation over several days will show no serial rise. Further tests include stress (usually treadmill, cycle, dipyridamole, or dobutamine), electrocardiography, and thallium radionuclide scanning. An angiogram may be necessary, especially if the diagnosis is uncertain.

Priorities of care

- Administration of high-flow, high-concentration oxygen.

- Pain relief by administering sublingual GTN tablet or spray, repeated as necessary. Diamorphine may be necessary in severe pain.

Principles of care

Rest

If the pain does not resolve quickly, occurs with much greater frequency than normal, is brought on by minimal exertion or occurs at rest, this is termed 'unstable' (or 'crescendo') angina and warrants hospital admission, bedrest, aggressive medical treatment, and investigation with a view to a coronary revascularization procedure (angioplasty or bypass surgery).

Relief of anxiety

The patient will require reassurance in the form of competent and skilled nursing care, appropriate, information and empathetic listening.

Drug therapy

Unless a certain drug type is specifically contraindicated, medical treatment of unstable angina consists of intravenous nitrates, beta blockade, a calcium channel blocker, such as nifedipine or diltiazem, full heparinization, and aspirin. Thrombolysis is of no benefit. If the symptoms do not resolve quickly with this aggressive pharmacological therapy, angiography should be performed urgently and treatment continued accordingly. If the pain does settle and does not recur for a number of days, despite gradual mobilization, the patient may be discharged home and be investigated as an out-patient.

Therapies

Interventional therapy depends on the angiographic findings. Left main stem coronary artery disease and triple vessel coronary artery disease are indications for which bypass surgery has been shown to improve outcome. In other cases, symptoms will usually improve after bypass grafting although will often recur after a number of years. A newer technique is balloon angioplasty whereby a balloon, on the end of a catheter inserted percutaneously into an artery, is placed under X-ray control at the stenotic site. The balloon is then inflated to widen the lumen and a stent may be inserted afterwards to help keep the artery patent. The recurrence of symptoms is greater than after surgery, necessitating either repeat angioplasty or bypass grafting. It is therefore essential to have cardiac surgical back-up if angioplasty is carried out.

Heart failure

The commonest cause of acute heart failure is pump failure due to ischaemia or infarction. However, other causes should be considered as many have specific treatments (Table 5.13). Some pathologies will result in high output cardiac failure (e.g. thyrotoxic crisis).

The body's response to a fall in cardiac output is sympathetic induction of vasoconstriction and tachycardia. Paradoxically, this will increase the workload and thereby exacerbate the strain on a damaged heart. The blood pressure will thus be initially maintained in the face of a falling cardiac output and may camouflage a barely adequate (or inadequate) cardiac output. Indeed, there may be an exaggerated vasoconstrictor response which, with coexisting anxiety, may cause an initial elevation in blood pressure, a further increase in LV afterload, and a greater reduction in cardiac output. Only when this vasoconstrictor reflex response fails will the blood pressure fall; when organ hypoperfusion coexists, this is recognized as cardiogenic shock.

Table 5.13 Heart failure: causes and treatment

Cause	Specific treatment
Myocardial infarction	Thrombolysis: consider early surgical revascularization
Drugs (e.g. beta-blockers, verapamil)	Specific 'antagonists' (e.g. β-agonists, calcium)
Dysrhythmias	Appropriate antidysrhythmic agents or pacemaker insertion
Valve dysfunction	Valve replacement, valvuloplasty (NB antibiotics for endocarditis)
Ventricular septal defect	Surgery
Pericardial tamponade	Drainage
Constrictive pericarditis (e.g. TB)	Surgery
Haemorrhage and anaemia	Resuscitation and transfusion, correction of cause
Pulmonary embolus	Thrombolytics, embolectomy
Cardiomyopathy, myocarditis	Specific (e.g. immunosuppression)
Hypertension	Antihypertensives, treat cause if found
Thyrotoxic crisis	Iodine, propranolol, steroids, carbimazole
Wet beri-beri (i.e. Vitamin B deficiency resulting in heart failure)	Vitamin B replacement

The consequences of an inadequate cardiac output are clinically manifested through inadequacies of forward blood flow and increased retrograde venous congestion. Left-sided retrograde congestion results in an increase in left atrial and pulmonary venous pressures and increasing hydrostatic pressures within the lung thereby forcing water from intravascular to interstitial compartments. When the lymphatics' absorptive capacity is exceeded pulmonary oedema with resulting dyspnoea and orthopnoea ensues. Gas exchange is impaired with resulting hypoxaemia. Right-sided retrograde congestion causes a raised CVP, hepatic congestion with elevated liver enzymes and bilirubin and, eventually, progression to dependent oedema.

The combination of hypoxaemia, lactic acidosis, increased extravascular lung water, and anxiety will cause tachypnoea and an increase in the work of breathing, accounting for up to 30% of total body oxygen consumption. Either the left and/or right heart may be affected by the disease process. A worsening of lung disease may cause acute right ventricular decompensation. Myocardial ischaemia/infarction may affect predominantly one ventricle. The normal co-relationship between ventricular filling pressures no longer holds, for example, with right ventricular infarction there may be high right-sided pressures (CVP) but low left filling pressures (PAWP).

Ventricular compliance will be affected; this falls due to a variety of factors including myocardial ischaemia, increased afterload, and fluid overload. As a consequence, the ventricle becomes stiffer, altering the intraventricular pressure–volume relationship such that a higher filling pressure is required to achieve the same end diastolic volume (LVEDV). For the same filling pressure the LVEDV will thus be smaller and the stroke volume may fall. Monitoring the patient on filling pressures (i.e. CVP and PAWP) alone is thus unhelpful.

Finally, the patient's fluid balance status in acute heart failure is often misjudged. The clinical or radiological presence of pulmonary oedema does not imply total body fluid overload. By the time of arrival in hospital the patient in acute pulmonary oedema may well be in negative fluid balance through a combination of sweating, mouth breathing, and inadequate fluid intake. The fluid is thus in the wrong compartment and requires redistribution rather than removal. The fall in cardiac output and intravascular volume leads to a drop in renal blood flow, stimulating the renin–angiotensin–aldosterone system to produce still more vasoconstriction and oliguria.

With time, secondary hyperaldosteronism will promote fluid retention and an increase in circulating blood volume. The threshold of lymphatic drainage of pulmonary interstitial fluid will be raised and higher pulmonary arterial hydrostatic pressures will be tolerated. However, in the acute phase, the intravascular compartment is often contracted, a situation which may be further aggravated by fluid restriction and diuretic usage.

Assessment

Physical
Skin — cyanosis, pallor, and sweating may all be apparent. Inadequate forward blood flow resulting in organ hypoperfusion produces cold, shut-down peripheries. Peripheral oedema (leg or sacral) may be seen with right-sided heart failure.

Respiration — the patient may be tachypnoeic, and producing blood-stained frothy sputum as a result of pulmonary oedema. Wheeze ('cardiac asthma') may be a presenting feature.

General — the patient may show signs of generalized weakness and fatigue.

Auscultation — the apex beat of the patient's heart is often displaced, and a gallop rhythm (due to a 3rd and/or 4th heart sound) may be heard on auscultation. In left heart failure end-inspiratory crepitations at the lung bases may be heard.

Physiological
CVP — will be high with right-sided heart failure, PAWP will be high with left-sided heart failure.

Blood pressure — may be low or high.

Heart rate — tachycardia will be evident unless bradycardia is the primary cause of failure.

Renal function — urine output may be reduced and renal dysfunction evident from blood urea and creatinine levels.

Lactic acidosis is produced through insufficient tissue oxygen delivery and impaired hepatic uptake.

Neurological/psychological
The patient may exhibit anxiety and distress. Mental obtundation may be seen as drowsiness, confusion, or agitation as a result of poor cardiac output and cerebral hypoperfusion.

Investigations

Urgent investigations include 12-lead ECG, chest X-ray, echocardiography (if indicated, e.g. for suspected valve dysfunction or pericardial tamponade) and appropriate blood investigations such as urea and electrolytes, haemoglobin, glucose, and cardiac enzymes.

Chest X-ray — LVF has a characteristic chest X-ray appearance with upper lobe blood diversion, increased fluid in the lymphatics (Kerley B lines) and the lung fissures, pleural effusions, and cardiomegaly. A 'bat's wing' appearance may be seen at the pulmonary hilum.

Echocardiography may show regions of the ventricular wall that either move poorly, irregularly, or not at all, or other causes such as pericardial tamponade or valvular dysfunction.

Priorities of care

- Basic resuscitation measures are aimed at restoration of an adequate circulation as quickly as possible.

- Administration of high-flow, high concentration oxygen.

- Preload and afterload reduction (by vasodilators, diuretics, opiates).

- Anxiolysis (opiates, e.g. diamorphine 2.5 mg IV repeated when required), reassurance, information, and comfort.

- If required, augmentation of cardiac output by inotropes.

- Failure to respond promptly may warrant urgent mechanical ventilation and/or intra-aortic balloon pulsation (IABP).

- After initial stabilization of the patient, further monitoring and investigations should be instituted.

Principles of care

Monitoring
This depends on the severity of the failure and usually consists of a minimum of continuous ECG monitoring, pulse oximetry, and frequent blood pressure monitoring. In progressively more severe cases, invasive arterial pressure monitoring, central venous pressure monitoring, and pulmonary artery catheterization with monitoring of cardiac output, mixed venous saturation, and wedge pressure will be required. Once adequate monitoring is in place, treatment can be titrated precisely to achieve adequate organ perfusion.

Rest
The heart can be 'rested' by reducing excessive degrees of preload and afterload, by removing the work of breathing through mechanical ventilation, and by insertion of an IABP.

Optimizing intravascular fluid volume
The PAWP provides a rough guide to left ventricular filling. Abnormal elevations in PAWP (> 18–20 mmHg) are seen in left heart failure and usually indicate the need for preload reduction. However, patients with chronic heart failure will often run a high PAWP in the non-acute

situation, sometimes > 30 mmHg. Likewise, treatment with vasoconstrictors will increase peripheral tone and reduce ventricular compliance, thereby elevating the PAWP for the same end diastolic volume. Thus, rather than routinely aiming for a target figure of 14–18 mmHg, the PAWP should be used for dynamic challenges to optimize stroke volume. Because of potential alterations in ventricular compliance, and vasoconstriction induced by coexisting hypovolaemia (e.g. excessive diuretics), a fluid challenge should be contemplated even when the PAWP is 'normal' or even raised. No rise in stroke volume and a rise in PAWP > 3 mmHg following a challenge suggests that optimal filling of the intravascular compartment has been achieved. The patient is very unlikely to decompensate with a single fluid challenge and the circulating volume should be optimized before introducing other drugs. A fall in blood pressure on a low vasodilator infusion dose suggests underfilling of the left ventricle. Even in patients with poor gas exchange a fluid challenge should not be withheld as the patient will generally die from organ hypoperfusion rather than hypoxaemia.

Support of cardiac output
Failing the above measures, the heart can also be 'driven' by inotropes although this should not be more than absolutely necessary to maintain adequate organ perfusion. No target figure of cardiac output exists. In general, the cardiac index (output indexed for body surface area) should exceed 2.2 l/min/m^2 (approx 3.5 l/min) but this is a rough guide. More relevant is the worsening or improvement in base deficit and lactic acidaemia, the production of adequate urine, good cerebration, etc. The mixed venous oxygen saturation (S_vO_2) is a sensitive guide to the ability of the cardiorespiratory system to meet whole body oxygen demands. In low output states the tissues compensate for the decrease in oxygen delivery by extracting more oxygen and the S_vO_2 falls. In severe heart failure this can drop below 30%, indicating virtually maximal extraction with very little reserve held. Other than in sepsis, where a defect in tissue oxygen extraction often exists, the S_vO_2 is a sensitive indicator of the adequacy of tissue oxygen delivery. A mixed venous saturation of 60% is a useful goal in haemodynamic management.

Reducing systemic vascular resistance (SVR)
SVR is usually raised in heart failure and thus cardiac workload is increased. Reducing LV afterload will reduce cardiac work. The cardiac output is usually augmented by vasodilatation although further filling may be found necessary. Likewise for right ventricular failure, manipulation of the pulmonary vascular resistance will allow optimization of right ventricular output.

Therapies

The standard textbook approach is of oxygen, low-dose opiates, diuretics, and nitrates. These may preceded or followed by inotropes depending on the presence or persistence of a low cardiac output/low blood pressure state. Diuretics are traditionally believed to cause an initial vasodilatation followed, 20–30 minutes later, by a diuresis. Although the vasodilatation is beneficial, the diuresis is not if the patient is not fluid overloaded. Falls in cardiac output following diuretic treatment of heart failure are well documented. Although symptomatic relief is quickly afforded, the diuresis may result in significant hypovolaemia leading to a metabolic acidosis with compensatory tachypnoea and oliguria. The tachypnoea and oliguria may be mistaken for worsening pump failure resulting in the administration of additional, and larger, doses of diuretic which compound the problem further.

Diuretic therapy should not be totally discounted. It does have a role in certain situations, notably total body fluid overload as is often found with chronic heart failure. Furthermore, patients on long-term diuretic therapy will often require diuretics to maintain an adequate diuresis and discontinuation, if indicated, should be gradual. For those patients not on diuretics an effective diuresis may frequently be achieved by small doses (i.e. 10–20 mg).

Nitrates can be given rapidly either by oral nitrolingual spray or sublingually while an infusion is being prepared. They have both preload and afterload reducing properties which are dose-dependent although tolerance will develop by 24 hours, necessitating a higher dose to achieve a similar effect. A drop in blood pressure on low-dose infusion is suggestive of hypovolaemia. Once stabilized, the patient can be commenced on increasing doses of an ACE inhibitor.

No drug used to increase cardiac contractility is a pure inotrope — all have additional vasodilator or vasoconstrictor properties to greater or lesser degrees. Falls in blood pressure are occasionally seen with dobutamine and, more commonly, with the phosphodiesterase inhibitor inodilators such as enoximone and milrinone. Reductions in dose, or fluid challenges, may be required to restore systemic blood pressure to satisfactory levels. The advantage of dobutamine over the currently available phosphodiesterase inhibitors is its much shorter half-life. Adrenaline, dopamine, and noradrenaline all possess vasoconstrictor properties. A balance has to be achieved between adequate vasoconstriction to maintain a reasonable coronary perfusion pressure, and excessive vasoconstriction which will increase cardiac work, and myocardial

oxygen consumption, possibly resulting in a fall in cardiac output. As noradrenaline and higher doses of dopamine have more of a vasoconstrictor effect than adrenaline, they should be generally used in heart failure states only in combination with dobutamine or a vasodilator.

Table 5.14 Directed management of heart failure

Physiological derangement	Directed management
(i) SVR elevated $\geqslant 1300$ dyn. sec. cm^{-5}	*PAWP low*? Colloid challenges to optimal stroke volume *PAWP high*? Increase nitrate infusion
(ii) SVR remains elevated despite optimizing fluid/nitrates as (i) above	Commence dobutamine (or inodilator) Consider: • intra-aortic balloon pump • mechanical ventilation
(iii) $S_vO_2 \leqslant 60\% \pm$ signs of inadequate organ perfusion persisting despite optimization of ventricular filling and attempted normalization of afterload	Inotropes $\pm$ inodilators $\pm$ mechanical ventilation $\pm$ intra-aortic balloon pump $\pm$ ventricular assist device
(iv) Low blood pressure	Exclude hypovolaemia Commence dobutamine (but BP may fall) or adrenaline $\pm$ mechanical ventilation $\pm$ intra-aortic balloon pump $\pm$ ventricular assist device
(v) Total body fluid overload	Diuretics • initially low doses. • increase as necessary Poor response to diuretics? • haemofiltration
(vi) Poor urine output	Exclude hypovolaemia Treat low output state as above Commence low-dose dopamine Consider further elevation in mean systemic BP Has an ACE inhibitor been administered? If so, consider stopping because of renovascular disease Consider diuretics (initially at low doses) or haemofiltration

Other drugs that may be useful in the short-term management of heart failure include digoxin which has inotropic in addition to antiarrhythmic properties. The effects are not immediate as the patient has to be 'loaded' over a number of hours to achieve adequate therapeutic levels.

Mechanical ventilation with or without the addition of positive end expiratory pressure (PEEP) reduces the work of breathing, allows the use of heavy sedation, reduces right and left ventricular preload, and left ventricular afterload. In an overfilled state, cardiac output will be augmented, however, when the intravascular compartment is contracted, a fall in output may be seen. CPAP may be considered as a good intermediate step, decreasing venous return, augmenting cardiac output, and improving gas exchange.

Intra-aortic balloon counterpulsation and ventricular assist devices (see Chapter 7) can also be considered although their availability tends to be restricted to specialist centres. (See Table 5.14, for the management of heart failure.)

Indications for surgery are few. Some centres in the United States and Germany have shown significant improvements in outcome for post-infarction ventricular failure by salvaging ischaemic but not yet necrosed myocardium through either immediate angioplasty or surgery. A permanently damaged myocardium will not improve following revascularization. Other surgically remediable causes include papillary leaflet rupture of the mitral valve, aortic stenosis, and ventricular septal defect. Surgery may be required for rarer pathologies such as constrictive pericarditis and hypertrophic obstructive cardiomyopathy.

Pericarditis

Inflammation of the pericardium due to a variety of causes (see box).

Causes of pericarditis
Infection (e.g. viruses: coxsackie, echo; TB)
Myocardial infarction: either within 1–2 days, or Dressler's syndrome (see p. 144)
Malignancy
Radiotherapy
Trauma (including cardiac surgery)
Uraemia
Connective tissue disorders (e.g. SLE)

Assessment

Physical
Pain — usually presents as a sharp, constant central chest pain eased by sitting forward and worsened by deep inspiration or coughing. It may radiate to the neck, arm, shoulder, or occasionally abdomen. It is not related to food nor eased by GTN.

Auscultation — may reveal a pericardial friction rub: a scratchy noise heard throughout the cardiac cycle caused by rubbing together of the inflamed surfaces.

Pulsus paradoxus, a raised JVP, and muffled heart sounds may be present with severe constrictive pericarditis or a significant effusion.

Physiological
ECG — reveals concave-upwards ST segment elevation in all leads with no reciprocal changes in the opposite leads.

Heart rate — tachycardia may be evident.

Pyrexia — may be present.

Pericardial tamponade may present with signs of heart failure (although no pulmonary oedema) or with cardiac arrest.

Investigations

Chest X-ray usually reveals no abnormality unless a pericardial effusion, constrictive pericarditis, or associated myocarditis is present. A significant pericardial effusion produces a globular cardiac contour on X-ray.

Echocardiography usually reveals no abnormality unless a pericardial effusion, constrictive pericarditis, or associated myocarditis is present. Fluid in the pericardial space may be visualized by echo. In the case of constrictive pericarditis, small heart chambers and restricted filling are seen on echo. Calcification may be visible in longstanding tuberculous pericarditis.

Principles of care
• Bedrest

• Anti-inflammatory agents such as indomethacin,

• Treatment of the cause wherever possible.

Steroids are rarely indicated. Occasionally, surgery is needed when constrictive pericarditis causes haemodynamic compromise.

Pericardial tamponade

Significant pericardial effusions may require drainage (pericardiocentesis), either percutaneously or by open surgical drainage. The percutaneous approach is often done under echocardiography, fluoroscopic screening, or may be performed 'blind'. In this case, the ECG V lead is usually attached to the needle to detect whether the myocardium is being penetrated (ST segment changes or multiple ventricular ectopics are often seen). The patient is laid resting semi-supine and after cleansing of the site and injection of local anaesthetic, a long, 18-gauge catheter connected to a syringe is introduced by the side of the xiphisternum under the costal margin and advanced in the direction of the scapula. When fluid is aspirated the catheter should be advanced no further. At this stage, a three-way tap can be attached and total drainage performed. Alternatively, a guide wire may be advanced through the cannula into the pericardial space, the cannula removed, and a pigtail catheter placed over the guide wire. Specimens should be sent for culture and cytology where appropriate. Blood may be aspirated from the space (haemopericardium), particularly after trauma, cardiac surgery, or malignancy. This differs from blood aspirated from within the heart chamber as it does not clot. If in doubt, the catheter may be transduced to see whether a characteristic right ventricular pressure waveform is seen. Further details on tamponade are in Chapter 11.

Complications of needle pericardiocentesis include damage to the ventricle or a coronary artery, arrhythmias, or pneumothorax.

Infective endocarditis

Previously known as subacute bacterial endocarditis, this is an infection of the heart valves with or without vegetations which may lead to destruction of the valve. Any bacteraemia may cause colonization of a heart valve. Recognized precipitating causes include dental manipulation, venous cannulation (iatrogenic or drug addicts), and surgery. Abnormal or prosthetic valves are more prone to colonization but half of all cases occur on previously normal valves. Left-sided heart valves are more commonly affected except in intravenous drug abusers who usually have right-sided heart valve lesions, particularly tricuspid. The commonest infecting organism is *Streptococcus viridans*, although others include enterococci (e.g. *Strep. faecalis*), *Staph. aureus*, other bacteria, *Coxiella burnetti* ('Q fever'), fungi, and chlamydia.

Assessment

Physical
The patient may demonstrate the physical features of acute heart failure (see earlier) or may present with embolic phenomena such as stroke.

Vasculitis may also occur.

There may be signs of chronic illness and infection (e.g. clubbing, splenomegaly, and weight loss).

Auscultation may reveal heart murmurs.

Physiological

- Pyrexia is usually present.

- Chest X-ray is usually normal.

- ECG is usually normal

Endocarditis affecting chronically damaged or congenitally abnormal valves, or long-term implanted prosthetic valves have a more insidious presentation with non-specific signs such as fever, malaise, weight loss, night sweats, and splenomegaly.

Investigations

Repeated blood cultures should be taken.

Echocardiography may reveal vegetations on the affected valves, however, these have to be large enough to be visualized (usually >3mm). Transoesophageal echocardiography is a more sensitive technique for detection of vegetations. Bacterial and histological examination of any removed emboli may also aid diagnosis.

Priorities of care
- Treatment as for heart failure (see p. 146)

Principles of care
- Treatment of any complication, such as heart failure or emboli, should be carried out on conventional grounds.

- Antibiotic treatment has to be aggressive and prolonged (at least 4–6 weeks). Depending on sensitivities, intravenous benzylpenicillin and gentamicin are usually given initially for streptococcal and enterococcal infections, whereas flucloxacillin and gentamicin are given for staphylococcal infections. Careful monitoring of drug levels must be performed. Other causative organisms, such as fungi or coxiella, should be treated with the appropriate antibiotics.

- Surgical removal of the damaged valve may be necessary though, if possible, this should be delayed until a course of antibiotics have been given.

- Rest is an important part of the patient's management

- Education of the patient and information about the

disease and preventive measures are important. Prophylaxis is very important in patients with known
abnormal or prosthetic valves undergoing surgical or
dental procedures.

Valvular heart disease: Stenosis

Valvular stenosis predominantly affects the aortic and
mitral valves.

Assessment

Aortic stenosis (AS) may present with angina, symptoms
of heart failure, low output (including syncope —
'Stokes–Adams' attacks') or sudden death. Mitral stenosis (MS) usually presents with symptoms of heart
failure including fatigue and breathlessness. Atrial fibrillation may also be a presenting feature of MS.

Investigations

Characteristic murmurs are heard for AS (ejection systolic murmur) and for MS (mid-diastolic rumbling
murmur); their absence or prolongation may indicate
increasing severity. The pulse pressure is usually narrow
with AS. In MS, the chest X-ray may show an enlarged
left atrium and radiological signs of pulmonary oedema
and a bifid P wave (P mitrale) may be seen on ECG. The
definitive investigation for both valves is echocardiography where both the orifice area and the pressure gradient
across the stenosed valve can be estimated non-invasively. Mural thrombi may also be seen, especially in
cases of atrial fibrillation. Angiography may be needed,
especially for AS where the coronary arteries may also be
narrowed at their origin.

Principles of care

Heart failure is treated in conventional fashion, although
digoxin and anticoagulation therapies are often used in
concurrent atrial fibrillation for control of rate and
prophylaxis against emboli. Valvotomy or balloon valvuloplasty may be attempted if the valve is still pliant,
otherwise prosthetic replacement may be needed. Antibiotic prophylaxis against SBE should be taken for
dental and surgical procedures.

Valvular heart disease: incompetence

Valvular incompetence may be due to either direct valve
damage (e.g. endocarditis) or secondary to dilatation of
the ventricle. Regurgitant flow occurs, either back into
the atria during systole with mitral and tricuspid incompetence, or back into the left ventricle during diastole
with aortic incompetence.

Assessment

Incompetence results in a decrease in forward flow with
symptoms of low output (e.g. fatigue) and an increase in
retrograde congestion which may result in breathlessness
from pulmonary oedema for left-sided lesions and hepatic congestion and peripheral oedema for right-sided
lesions.

Investigations

Characteristic murmurs are heard for AR (high-pitched
early diastolic murmur), MR (pan-systolic murmur), and
TR (pan-systolic murmur louder on inspiration). The chest
X-ray may show cardiomegaly. A wide pulse pressure with
a collapsing pulse is present with AR and a pulsatile liver
with TR. Doppler echocardiography is again diagnostic.

Causes of valvular incompetence		
Aortic incompetence	*Mitral incompetence*	*Tricuspid incompetence*
Rheumatic heart disease	Rheumatic heart disease	Rheumatic heart disease
Endocarditis	Mitral valve prolapse	Functional (due to dilated ventricle)
Ankylosing spondylitis, Marfan's syndrome	Ruptured chordae tendinae or papillary muscle (after MI or trauma)	Endocarditis (especially drug abusers)
Aortic dissection	Functional (due to dilated ventricle)	
Syphilis	Endocarditis Cardiomyopathy	

Principles of care

Heart failure is treated in conventional fashion, although the valve should ideally be replaced before significant dysfunction has occurred. Antibiotic prophylaxis against SBE should also be given.

Cardiomyopathy/Myocarditis

Cardiomyopathy is idiopathic heart muscle disease not related to ischaemia. There are three types:

(1) congestive,

(2) hypertrophic (obstructed) — HOCM,

(3) restrictive.

Causes of congestive and hypertrophic cardiomyopathy are unknown, although many cases of HOCM are congenital. Restrictive cardiomyopathy is due to stiffening of the endomyocardium; in the tropics it is due to idiopathic fibrosis while amyloid is the commonest cause in the United Kingdom.

Assessment

Physical

- Signs of heart failure (congestive).

- Simulating constrictive pericarditis (restrictive).

- Angina (HOCM).

- Syncope (HOCM).

- Palpitations may be experienced and a late systolic murmur may be heard due to obstruction of the left ventricular outflow tract (HOCM).

- Dyspnoea (HOCM).

Sudden death is a not uncommon presenting feature of HOCM.

Physiological
Heart rate — the pulse is jerky with a double apex beat (HOCM)

Investigations

Echocardiography — definitive diagnosis is usually made by echocardiography.

Principles of care

- Treatment as for heart failure.

- Angina may require β-blockade and amiodarone may be needed for arrhythmias.

- Surgery (e.g. myomectomy) or transplantation may be necessary.

- Patients will require counselling and education regarding the disease and its prognosis

Other types of heart muscle disease

The symptoms are usually those of congestive cardiomyopathy with signs and symptoms of heart failure.

Causes of other types of heart muscle disease	
• Hypertension	• Haemochromatosis
• Alcohol	• Sarcoidosis
• Postpartum	• Friedrich's ataxia
• Diabetes	• Myotonic dystrophy
• Hyper- and hypothyroidism	• Radiation and cytotoxic drugs such as adriamycin

Myocarditis

The commonest cause of an acute myocarditis is viral, especially coxsackie. Other infections (e.g. diphtheria), rheumatic fever, connective tissue diseases (e.g. SLE), and drugs (e.g. cocaine) are also recognized.

The patient usually presents with symptoms of heart failure, angina, or dysrhythmias. Acute and chronic phase viral serology should be taken. Echocardiography usually shows dilated, poorly functioning ventricles.

Treatment is bedrest, and treatment of heart failure or angina, if present. As arrhythmias are not infrequent the patient should be continuously monitored. Patients usually recover spontaneously but may progress to severe irreversible heart failure requiring cardiac transplantation.

Aortic aneurysm

A tear in the intimal lining of the aortic vessel wall allows blood to track into the media. The blood may track along the media dissection, — either up or down the aorta, occluding branch vessels. Alternatively, rupture may occur through the outer adventitial layer. Atheroma is the commonest underlying pathology and this may be accelerated by hypertension and hyperlipidaemia. Congenital conditions such as Marfan's syndrome and other connective tissue disorders are also recognized. A major cause is trauma (see Chapter 11).

Assessment

Physical

- Sudden cardiovascular collapse

- *Pain* — an abrupt onset tearing pain in the chest or upper abdomen radiating through to the back is the classical mode of presentation.

- *Neurological symptoms* — syncope, headache, stroke, or paraplegia

- *Pulses* — one or more of the major pulses may be absent or asymmetric.

- Signs of acute aortic incompetence, if the ascending aorta is involved. This may be with or without anginal symptoms due to occlusion of the origins of one or more coronary arteries.

Physiological

- *Blood pressure* — there may be a discrepancy in systolic pressure between right and left arms of more than 15 mmHg.

Investigations

Chest X-ray may reveal mediastinal widening.

ECG is usually unremarkable although ischaemic changes may be present.

Echocardiogram (particular from the transoesophageal approach) may be diagnostic although the definitive diagnosis is usually made by either:

- CT scan, or

- angiography — this will delineate the extent of the aneurysm (see Fig. 5.8)

Priorities of care
- Urgent resuscitation if there is cardiovascular compromise, including immediate transfer to the operating theatre if necessary

- Pain relief (opiates are usually given)

- High-flow, high-concentration oxygen

- If hypertensive, blood pressure should be reduced using an infusion of either sodium nitroprusside or labetalol commenced with the aim of reducing systolic blood pressure to 100–120 mmHg.

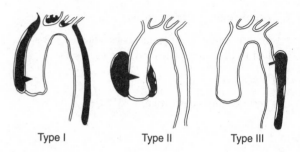

Type I   Type II   Type III

Fig. 5.8 Classification of thoracic aortic aneurysms.

Principles of care

- Arterial cannula — for continuous blood pressure monitoring.

- Bladder catheter — to measure urine output. Oliguria suggests that the lowering of blood pressure may be excessive while anuria is suggestive of aneurysmal involvement of the renal arteries.

- It is important to reassure the patient and prevent unnecessary agitation.

The regional cardiac unit should be contacted if a thoracic aortic aneurysm is suspected and the patient transferred promptly for any further investigations and surgery if necessary. Ascending aortic aneurysms usually require surgery while those involving the descending aorta are often managed conservatively in the first instance.

Pulmonary embolus

Detachment of part or all of a thrombus, usually from the deep veins of the legs or pelvis, passes into the pulmonary vasculature, blocking forward blood flow. The extent of flow obstruction depends on the size of the clot giving rise to signs and symptoms of major (massive) or minor pulmonary embolism (PE). The patient may have recently undergone surgery or a prolonged period of immobilization; there may be signs and symptoms of deep venous thrombosis.

Assessment

Physical
Major embolism

- Respiration — the patient will have acute dyspnoea

- Cardiovascular collapse

- Syncope

- Cyanosis

Minor embolism

- Pain — the patient will experience pleuritic pain

- Respiration — dyspnoea and haemoptysis will occur

Physiological
Major embolism

- Blood pressure — hypotension

- Heart rate — tachycardia

- CVP — raised

Investigations

Chest X-ray: pulmonary oligaemia (reduced blood vessel markings) may be seen in one of the lung fields

ECG may show signs of right ventricular strain (S_1, Q_3, T_3, right axis deviation, partial right bundle branch block, tachycardia).

Arterial blood gas analysis may show a low P_aO_2, a low P_aCO_2, and a metabolic acidosis. None of the above may be present with minor embolism, however, one or more wedge-shaped pulmonary infarcts may be seen on chest X-ray.

A radioisotope ventilation/perfusion (V/Q) scan will provide an indication of the likelihood of PE by showing an area of lung (or multiple areas if multiple emboli are present) being ventilated but not perfused. However, spiral CT scan with contrast or pulmonary angiography may be necessary for definitive diagnosis, especially if surgery is being contemplated. A normal plasma D-dimer level has been recently shown to be a good means of excluding pulmonary embolus.

Priorities of care
- Resuscitation if cardiovascular collapse has occurred; fluid loading is the important first step in circulatory management, even though the CVP is usually elevated.

- High-flow, high-concentration oxygen

- Inotropes — fluid should be given before inotropes (adrenaline or dobutamine)

Principles of care
- Mechanical ventilation — may be necessary but gas exchange may worsen because of loss of preferential shunting of blood.

- Early thrombolytic therapy is important for massive embolism — no comparative trials have studied large bolus doses of streptokinase. Thrombolysis with rTPA followed by heparin anticoagulation has been shown to be superior to heparin alone.

- Positioning — the patient may prefer to lie flat to improve symptoms of dyspnoea.

- Surgery — the role is controversial; embolectomy may be of benefit for single, centrally placed, massive clots.

- Heparin infusion — if the patient survives the acute episode the prognosis is generally good. Heparin infusion should be continued until the patient is fully warfarinized (usually 2–3 days).

Antiarrhythmic drugs

Only those antiarrhythmic drugs particularly relevant to the critically ill patient will be detailed in this chapter. Further reading may be found in Opie (1991).

Antiarrhythmic drugs are categorized into four classes (I-IV) determined by their action on the electrophysiological mechanisms of the myocardial cell.

Class I

Class IA drugs lengthen the effective refractory period by: (1) inhibiting the fast sodium current and thus the speed of action potential; (2) prolonging the action potential duration (e.g. *disopyramide, quinidine*).

Class IB drugs inhibit the fast sodium current while shortening the action potential duration. This action is selective on diseased or ischaemic tissue and is thought to promote conduction block thereby interrupting re-entry (e.g. *lignocaine, mexiletine, phenytoin*).

Class IC drugs possess three major electrophysiological effects: (1) powerful inhibition of His–Purkinje conduction with QRS widening; (2) marked inhibition of fast sodium channel with depression of speed of action potential; (3) shortened action potential in the Purkinje fibres only, leaving surrounding myocardium unaltered (e.g. *flecainide, propafenone*).

Class II

These agents include β-adrenergic antagonists. They also act on the β-receptors in the myocardium and block their effect (e.g. *atenolol, labetalol, propanolol*).

Class III

These agents lengthen the action potential duration and hence the effective refractory period; they also homogenize the action potential pattern throughout the myocardium. There is little or no negative inotropic effect (e.g. *amiodarone, sotalol, bretylium*).

Class IV

These inhibit slow channel-dependent conduction through the AV node (e.g. *adenosine, diltiazem, verapamil*).

Amiodarone

This is a complex antiarrhythmic drug sharing at least some of the electrophysiological properties of all four classes of antiarrhythmics. Amiodarone lengthens the effective refractory period by prolonging the duration of the action potential. It also has a powerful class I effect, inhibiting inactivated sodium channels. It noncompetitively blocks α- and β-adrenergic receptors and a calcium antagonist effect may be responsible for the bradycardia and AV nodal inhibition sometimes associated with its use.

Indications
Control of life-threatening ventricular tachyarrhythmias, recurrence of paroxysmal atrial fibrillation or flutter, paroxysmal supraventricular tachycardias, and WPW arrhythmias.

Dosage
In life-threatening arrhythmias, amiodarone 300 mg IV may be given over 10–15 min (Leak 1986) followed by an infusion of 10–20 mg/kg/24h. The loading dose is essential because of the slow onset of full action.

Side-effects
In higher doses, pneumonitis may occur potentially leading to pulmonary fibrosis. Torsades de Pointes may result from QT prolongation plus hypokalaemia. Amiodarone has a complex effect on the metabolism of thyroid hormones, the main action being inhibition of peripheral conversion of T_4 to T_3.

Nausea can occur in 50% of patients with cardiac failure.

Precautions
A proarrhythmic effect may occur if given with other drugs prolonging the Q–T interval. Amiodarone will prolong prothrombin time and may cause bleeding in patients on warfarin.

Lignocaine

This is a class IB agent that acts preferentially on the ischaemic myocardium and is more effective in the presence of a high plasma potassium level.

Indications
Emergency treatment of ventricular arrhythmias. Suppression of ventricular arrhythmias associated with myocardial infarction and cardiac surgery.

Dosage
An initial loading dose of 100 mg IV is given followed by an infusion of 1–4 mg/min. This is gradually decreased after 24–30 hours. The dose should be decreased in the elderly where lignocaine toxicity develops rapidly.

Side-effects
Relatively few side-effects are seen although high infusion rates may result in drowsiness, speech disturbances, and dizziness.

If toxicity develops there may be convulsions, agitation, disorientation, and coma.

Precautions
Clearance of lignocaine via the liver may be reduced if the patient is receiving cimetidine, propanolol, or halothane. Lignocaine metabolites circulate in high concentrations and may contribute to toxic and therapeutic actions (Opie 1991). Drugs that induce hepatic enzymes, such as barbiturates, phenytoin, and rifampicin, may increase the dosage requirements.

Adenosine

This has multiple cellular effects which include opening of potassium channels and inhibition of sinoatrial and atrioventricular nodes. Opening of potassium channels produces an indirect calcium antagonist effect due to the change in polarity away from that required to open the slow calcium channel.

Indications

It is chiefly used in paroxysmal supraventricular tachycardia and is particularly effective if these are re-entrant tachycardias via the AV node.

It is used as a useful diagnostic test to distinguish between VT or SVT with aberrant conduction. If it is effective in slowing the tachycardia then the arrhythmia is usually SVT with aberrant conduction. Occasionally, adenosine is effective in some types of VT.

Dosage

A rapid IV bolus of 3–6 mg is given initially; if not effective within 1–2 min a further IV bolus of 12 mg is given. The 12-mg dose may be repeated once. The effect is almost instantaneous but will last no longer than 10–30 s.

Side-effects

These are principally dyspnoea due to bronchoconstriction, flushing, and headache due to vasodilatory effects. Transient new arrhythmias may occur at the time of chemical cardioversion. Very occasionally, the induced heart block may be prolonged.

Precautions

Adenosine should not be used in patients with asthma, 2nd or 3rd degree heart block or sick sinus syndrome. The dose should be reduced if the patient is on dipyridamole therapy due to the inhibitory effect of dipyridamole on adenosine breakdown. Caffeine and theophylline will competitively antagonize adenosine.

Verapamil

This inhibits the action potential of the upper and middle nodal regions where depolarization is calcium-mediated. It is therefore able to terminate tachycardias of re-entry origin believed to be the cause of most paroxysmal supraventricular tachycardias. It increases AV nodal block as well as the effective refractory period of the AV node and will reduce the ventricular rate in atrial fibrillation or flutter.

Indications

It is used in supraventricular tachycardias and chronic atrial fibrillation or flutter where myocardial depression is not a problem.

Dosage

A slow bolus of 5–10 mg IV over at least 1 min can be repeated 10 min later if necessary. Calcium gluconate or chloride (5–10 ml, 10% solution) should be available for rapid administration (or pre-treatment) if there is a negative inotropic effect associated with the verapamil bolus.

Side-effects

These include hypotension and bradycardia. Vasodilatory effects produce flushing, headaches, and dizziness. Rarely, there may be facial, epigastric and gingival pain, hepatotoxicity, and transient mental confusion.

Precautions

Verapamil should not be give to patients with AV nodal disease, sick sinus syndrome, or myocardial depression. It should be given only with extreme caution if the patient has been treated with β-adrenergic blockers, digoxin, disopyramide, or quinidine.

Disopyramide

This antiarrhythmic drug lengthens the effective refractory period by inhibiting the fast sodium channel and thus the upstroke of the action potential and prolonging the action potential duration which prolongs repolarization time.

Indications

It is used to terminate or prevent ventricular arrhythmias, supraventricular tachycardias, and atrial arrhythmias associated with WPW syndrome.

Dosage

Initial slow IV injection of 0.5 mg/kg over 5 minutes can be repeated after 5 minutes up to three times. A further infusion of 1 mg/kg/h from 0 h to 3 h, followed by 0.4 mg/kg/h from 3 h to 18 h can be given.

Side-effects

There may be severe negative inotropic effects and anticholinergic activity (it is an inhibitor of muscarinic receptors) producing urinary retention, worsening glaucoma, and constipation. Excessive Q–T prolongation may increase the risk of Torsade de Pointes and there may be occasional hypoglycaemia and cholestatic jaundice.

Precautions

The drug should only be administered IV under ECG monitoring and the drug should be discontinued if there is development of 2nd or 3rd degree block, uni- or bifascicular block.

Administration in patients already receiving negative inotropes, such as beta blockers or verapamil, will substantially reduce cardiac output. Similarly, it should not be given in combination with other drugs likely to depress nodal tissue or conduction such as digoxin.

Magnesium sulphate

It is hypothesized that a low serum magnesium or a low intracellular magnesium content in the presence of acute myocardial infarct (AMI) is associated with tachyarrhythmias (Zwerling 1987). A study by Rasmussen *et al.* (1986) found a significantly reduced arrhythmia rate in a group of 56 patients given infusions of magnesium following AMI as opposed to a control group of 74 who received placebo.

The actual mechanism by which it works has not yet been identified but could either be direct inhibition of the efflux of potassium from the cell, alteration of cellular calcium metabolism, decreasing peripheral vascular resistance, or stimulating a membrane-stabilizing enzyme (Zwerling 1987).

Indications
Recurrent ventricular arrhythmias (Iseri *et al.* 1975; Allen *et al.* 1989) have been terminated with the intravenous administration of magnesium sulphate. It is also used as a preventative measure in patients following AMI (Schechter *et al.* 1990) and in patients with heart failure (Sueta *et al.* 1994).

However, use of magnesium is considered a relatively safe intervention which may be used when other antiarrhythmic agents have failed or when there is reason to suspect magnesium depletion.

Dosage
The optimal dosage and frequency has still not been fully determined. The usual dose is 10–20 mmol immediately, followed by up to 20 mmol given over 5–10 hours.

Side-effects
Flushing, sweating and a sensation of heat may occur with rapid IV injection.

Precautions
Serum magnesium levels should be monitored and kept below 2.7 mmol/l as these levels are associated with bradycardia, prolonged PR intervals and AV block.

Clinical studies have provided evidence that mortality is decreased in patients with an acute myocardial infarction if magnesium sulphate is infused in the first 24 hours (Teo 1991; Woods *et al.* 1992). The ISIS-4 study (1995) did not, however, confirm this. The mechanism respon-

sible is still unclear. Magnesium has been postulated as having several cardioprotective actions which have been confirmed in experimental studies but have not been supported in clinical trials to date.

Possible mechanisms for the beneficial effect of magnesium in acute myocardial infarction include the following:

Coronary and systemic vasodilatation. Magnesium reduces peripheral vascular resistance and dilates the coronary arteries. During the first few days following myocardial infarction magnesium levels tend to fall (Rasmussen *et al.* 1986) and there may be raised local levels of vasoconstrictors such as angiotensin, noradrenaline, and serotonin. These increase coronary artery tone and potentiate myocardial necrosis. An infusion of magnesium at this time may protect against ischaemic injury or the progression from ischaemic to infarcted tissue (Teo *et al.* 1991; Woods *et al.* 1992).

Platelet inhibition. Animal studies have shown that magnesium inhibits platelet function and therefore may have a role to play in the prevention of thrombus formation. This has not been confirmed in clinical trials (Woods *et al.* 1992).

Antiarrhythmic effects. Magnesium has been shown to increase the excitation level of myocardial cells (Ghani *et al.* 1977) and may suppress abnormal foci of excitation near ischaemic or infarcted tissue. Following an acute myocardial infarction patients are at particular risk of serious arrythmias including ventricular fibrillation, and prophylactic infusion of magnesium may be beneficial in the immediate post-infarction period when magnesium levels tend to fall. Several studies have shown a decrease in the incidence of arrhythmias in patients who have been given magnesium post-infarction. However, at present none have proven statistically conclusive (Teo *et al.* 1991; Woods *et al.* 1992).

Treatment regimens, dosage, and time spans vary ranging from 30–90 mmol of magnesium given over periods of 24–48 hours. Magnesium sulphate should be administered as a loading dose (over 10–15 minutes) followed by a continuous infusion over 24 h.

There are few side-effects. Transient flushing and nausea can be experienced by the patient when the loading dose is given but is usually related to the speed of administration. Sinus bradycardia has been associated with treatment with magnesium and is irrespective of the site of the infarction. Atrium bundle of His conduction can also be slowed and heart block is a potential risk. Since magnesium is excreted via the kidneys, magnesium levels should be closely monitored in patients with renal impairment.

Drugs commonly used in the treatment of hypotension

Inotropic drugs can be termed either positive or negative in their effect on heart muscle. Positive inotropes increase the contractility of the myocardium and hence the stroke volume (e.g. adrenaline). Negative inotropes decrease the contractility of cardiac muscle (e.g beta-blockers). Chronotropic drugs are those that increase the heart rate (e.g. atropine).

The effect of the drugs used depends on their specific receptor activity. There are two types of adrenergic receptors — alpha(α) and beta(β).

Alpha-receptors

There are two types of alpha-receptor: α_1 and α_2. The principal effect of α-receptors is to cause the vasoconstriction of vascular smooth muscle.

- α_1-receptors are the postjunctional receptors of vascular smooth muscle

- α_2-receptors are found in the vascular smooth muscle of the skin and are also the prejunctional receptors of nerve fibres. They inhibit the release of noradrenaline.

Beta-receptors

The are two types of beta-receptor. β_1 and β_2. The principal effects of β-receptors are to cause vasodilatation and an increase in the rate of the heart and its contractility.

- β_1-receptors are found in the sinoatrial node and myocardium and influence contractility and heart rate

- β_2-receptors are found in the arterioles of heart, liver, and skeletal muscle and in the smooth muscle of the bronchioles and cause vasodilatation.

Beta blockers should be given with caution to patients with asthma or a history of obstructive airways disease, unless no alternative treatment is available, since there is a risk of inducing bronchospasm. The use of beta blockers may also mask the compensatory physiological responses to hypoglycaemia and sudden haemorrhage (tachycardia and vasoconstriction) so particular care should be paid to diabetics and patients with blood loss. Beta blockers may also compromise blood flow in patients with peripheral vascular disease.

β_2-Adrenergic agonists (e.g. salbutamol) depress plasma potassium and raise glucose levels, therefore these should always be monitored in patients receiving such drugs.

The dosages of drugs should be titrated according to the patient's response and will require frequent or continuous monitoring of cardiovascular variables. In general, begin at the lowest dose and increase gradually in increments according to their effect. Observe for side-effects, particularly arrhythmias and tachycardias.

The infusions of these drugs should not be discontinued abruptly but the dose gradually decreased, observing for any deleterious effects.

Dopamine

The cardiovascular effects of dopamine depend on the dosage infused. It is used at low dosage mainly to improve or maintain urine output and at higher dosages for its positive inotropic effect.

At low doses (1–3 µg/kg/min — often called the 'renal' dose), it acts on specific dopaminergic receptors causing vasodilation of the splanchnic circulation. The renal vascular resistance decreases and renal blood flow increases. It also has β-adrenergic effects causing an increase in cardiac output, contractility, and coronary blood flow. At this dose, however, it has little effect on heart rate and the blood pressure may in fact fall slightly due to the decrease in systemic vascular resistance. At a dosage of 5–10 µg/kg/min it stimulates mainly β-receptors but at higher doses (> 10 µg/kg/min) α-adrenergic effects predominate. There is increased peripheral vasoconstriction which causes an increase in venous return and systolic blood pressure. These doses are approximate; some patients will react to much lower doses.

Dopamine is administered as a continuous intravenous infusion via a flow-regulated pump. It should always be administered through a central vein due to its peripheral vasoconstrictive action. If extravasation occurs it can cause ischaemic tissue necrosis and skin sloughing.

Side-effects include tachycardia, arrhythmias, angina, nausea, and vomiting.

Dobutamine hydrochloride

Dobutamine is a positive inotrope and a mild chronotrope. It is used to increase cardiac output in patients with low output cardiac failure (e.g. myocardial infarction, cardiogenic shock, following cardiac surgery).

It directly stimulates the β_1-cardiac-receptors increasing heart rate and stroke volume. Systemic vascular resistance and left ventricular end diastolic pressure also decrease as it has some vasodilator properties (β_2).

It must be administered as a continuous intravenous infusion (due to its short half-life of approximately 2 minutes), ideally centrally, but can be given via a peripheral vein if necessary.

Dosage is 2.5–40 µg/kg/min titrated according to response.

Side-effects are dose-related and include tachycardia, arrhythmias, headache, and chest pain.

Dobutamine increases A–V conduction especially if hypovolaemic, and patients with atrial fibrillation may develop rapid ventricular responses. Use with care in patients with myocardial infarction as an increased heart rate may precipitate angina and intensify ischaemia.

Some patients may become tolerant of dobutamine and in continuous infusions of longer than 72 hours larger doses may be required to maintain the same effect.

Dopexamine hydrochloride

Dopexamine is an arterial vasodilator, a positive inotrope, and also causes splanchnic vasodilation. It is used to increase cardiac output in patients who have a raised systemic vascular resistance.

It stimulates β_2-adrenergic and peripheral dopamine receptors, increasing cardiac output, heart rate, and reducing afterload.

The vascular smooth muscle of the renal and mesenteric beds are also dilated, increasing blood flow to these areas. It is not, therefore, necessary to give a 'renal' dose dopamine infusion to patients who are being given dopexamine as both have the same effect on renal blood flow.

Dopexamine is administered by continuous infusion, via a flow regulated pump, into a central or large peripheral vein. Its half-life is 6–11 minutes.

Dosage is 0.5–6 µg/kg/min. Start at 0.5 µg/kg/min and increase in increments of 0.5–1 µg/kg/min at intervals of not less than 15 minutes.

Side-effects include tachycardia (dose-related), nausea, vomiting, tremor, and headaches. An increase in heart rate is the most common side-effect and may precipitate angina or intensify cardiac ischaemia.

Adrenaline

Adrenaline is a positive inotrope and affects both α- and β-receptors. It is the most potent α-receptor activator. Low doses produce predominantly beta effects and higher doses produce more alpha effects.

It increases heart rate, cardiac output, systolic blood pressure, and myocardial oxygen consumption.

When administered as a bolus intravenously it causes a rapid rise in systolic blood pressure by increasing the strength of ventricular contraction, increasing heart rate, and the constriction of the arterioles of the skin, mucosa, and splanchnic areas of circulation. However, when administered as an infusion there is often a decrease in peripheral resistance due to the action of adrenaline on the β-receptors of skeletal muscle. This vasodilator effect may predominate and any increase in blood pressure is a result of cardiac stimulation and increase in cardiac output. Peripheral resistance may rise or be unaltered owing to a greater ratio of alpha-to-beta activity in different vascular areas.

Although splanchnic blood flow is increased, renal blood flow can be decreased by up to 40%.

Adrenaline causes a raised blood glucose because it decreases insulin secretion and increases glucagon secretion and the rate of glycogenolysis. It is also a bronchodilator but tends to increase the viscosity of secretions.

When administered as an infusion it should be given via a central vein. Dosage is titrated according to response starting at 0.01 µg/kg/min by continuous infusion or 0.05–1mg for bolus doses.

Side-effects include tachycardia, palpitations, myocardial ischaemia, and headache.

Noradrenaline

Noradrenaline acts predominantly on α-receptors and increases blood pressure by increasing the peripheral resistance. Cardiac output usually falls as a result.

Hepatic, renal and splanchnic circulation is decreased but coronary blood flow is increased due to the increase in diastolic pressure.

It decreases insulin secretion leading to a raised blood glucose.

Noradrenaline is administered by continuous intravenous infusion via a flow-regulated pump. It should only be infused into a central vein.

Dosage is titrated according to response starting at 0.01 µg/kg/min.

Side-effects include arrhythmias, chest pain, and headache.

Intravenous hypotensive drugs

Sodium nitroprusside

Sodium nitroprusside acts directly on vascular smooth muscle causing predominantly arteriolar vasodilation. It has an immediate effect but short duration of action, therefore is administered by continuous infusion.

Table 5.15 Summary of drugs used in hypotension.

Drug	Primary action	CVS effect
Dopamine	Positive inotrope Vasoconstrictor (high dose) Vasodilator (low dose)	↑ Cardiac output SVR (high dose) ↓ SVR (low dose)
Dobutamine	Positive inotrope (*Note.* may vasodilate)	↑ Stroke volume Cardiac output (heart rate) ↓ SVR
Dopexamine	Vasodilator Positive inotrope	↑ Cardiac output ↓ SVR
Adrenaline	Positive inotrope Vasoconstrictor	↑ Cardiac output
Noradrenaline	Vasoconstrictor Some inotropic properties	↑ SVR

↑, increased; ↓, decreased.

It should be administered via a flow-regulated pump and through a dedicated vein.

Intra-arterial pressure monitoring is considered essential as sodium nitroprusside can cause profound hypotension.

Cardiac output usually increases due to the decrease in systemic vascular resistance.

The drug causes cerebral vasodilation and may increase intracranial pressure in normocapnic patients.

Dosage is 0.5–1.5μg/kg/min initially and then adjusted according to response. The usual range is 0.5–8 μg/kg/min.

Side-effects include headache, dizziness, nausea, palpitations, and retrosternal pain.

When sodium nitroprusside is metabolized it forms cyanide ions and has the potential to produce cyanide toxicity. This is related more to the rate of the infusion rather than the total dose given and the rate should not exceed 8 μg/kg/min. Ideally, it should not be given for more than 24–36 hours. A rising, and unexplained metabolic acidosis may be due to cyanide accumulation.

The solution must be protected from the light.

The drug is excreted renally but is removed by haemodialysis.

Glyceryl trinitrate and isosorbide dinitrate

Nitrates act by causing vasodilation of veins at lower doses but at higher doses, both arteries and veins are vasodilated; and can allow a smooth reduction in blood pressure. They will cause cerebral vasodilatation and may raise intracranial pressure. Duration of action is 2–5 minutes for the intravenous form.

They should be administered via a volumetric pump and can be given into a peripheral vein.

Dosage is:

• Glyceryl trinitrate: 5–200 μg/min.

• Isosorbide dinitrate: 2–83 μg/min.

Side-effects include headache, tachycardia, and nausea.

Tolerance ('tachyphylaxis') will develop within 24 hours requiring increasing doses to achieve the same effect.

Hydralazine

Hydralazine acts on vascular smooth muscle, predominantly arteriolar, causing peripheral vasodilation. It decreases systemic vascular resistance and can cause a compensatory tachycardia with an increased cardiac output. This tachycardia may precipitate pre-existing angina. A β-adrenergic blocking drug is often given in combination with hydralazine to counteract this.

It can be given as a repeated, slow bolus injection, or a continuous infusion via a volumetric pump.

Dosage is 20–40 mg when given as a bolus intravenously (and repeated as necessary), or as a continuous infusion at 200–300 μg/min initially and then 50–150 μg/min.

It is incompatible with dextrose solutions as the contact with glucose causes hydralazine to be rapidly broken down.

Side-effects include nausea, vomiting, headache, tachycardia, palpitations, and flushing.

Phentolamine

Phentolamine acts by blocking α-adrenergic receptors. This causes vasodilation and a reflex tachycardia. It increases respiratory tract secretions, salivation, insulin secretion, and gut motility.

Phentolamine is particularly useful when hypertension is due to a phaeochromocytoma, reaction between foods containing pressor amines and monoamine oxidase inhibitors or clonidine withdrawal.

It can be given as a slow bolus injection or continuous infusion via a volumetric pump.

Dosage is 5–10 mg when given as a bolus intravenously (and repeated as necessary) or as a continuous infusion at a rate of 5–60 mg over 10–30 minutes, and thereafter at 0.1–2 mg/min.

Side-effects include tachycardia, arrhythmias, dizziness, nausea, vomiting, and diarrhoea.

Labetalol

Labetalol acts by blocking both α- and β-adrenoceptors, although β-blockade predominates.

It blocks the α-adrenoceptors in the peripheral arterioles and therefore lowers systemic vascular resistance.

The concurrent β-blockade protects the heart from the reflex sympathetic drive that can be induced by this vasodilation.

There is little change in cardiac output.

It can be administered as a repeated, slow bolus injection or as a continuous infusion via a volumetric pump. In a hypertensive crisis when the blood pressure needs to be reduced urgently 50 mg may be given as an intravenous bolus over at least 1 minute. This may be repeated at 5-minute intervals but not exceeding 200 mg in total. By intravenous infusion the rate is variable according to the cause of the hypertension and can be up to 160 mg/hour.

Side-effects include headache, rashes, difficulty in micturition, nausea, and vomiting. It can cause severe postural hypotension.

There may be a small decrease in heart rate but severe bradycardia is unusual.

Propanolol

Propanolol is a β-adrenoceptor antagonist. It is a negative inotrope, reduces heart rate, and increases peripheral resistance.

It is administered as a slow bolus injection of 1–10 mg, repeated as necessary. Side-effects include bradycardia and bronchospasm. It may also block the sympathetic response to hypoglycaemia by impairing the gluconeogenetic response. Heart failure and heart block may be precipitated and peripheral vascular disease exacerbated.

Esmolol

Esmolol acts by β-adrenoceptor blockade but has a very short half-life (9 minutes). It decreases cardiac output and heart rate.

It is administered by continuous infusion, via a volumetric pump, at a rate of 50–150 µg/kg/min.

Side-effects include bronchospasm, nausea and vomiting, and bradycardia.

Captopril

Captopril is an angiotensin-converting enzyme (ACE) inhibitor. ACE inhibitors act on the angiotensin–renin–aldosterone system causing mixed venous and arteriolar vasodilation.

Captopril lowers blood pressure by several mechanisms:

- inhibiting the conversion of angiotensin I to the powerful vasoconstrictor angiotensin II,

- inducing a natriuresis by reducing the secretion of aldosterone and increasing renal vasodilation,

- increasing peripheral vasodilation by stimulating the synthesis and release of prostaglandins.

Captopril can cause severe hypotension, particularly in patients with high renin states such as renal artery stenosis, hyponatraemia, or following vigorous diuretic therapy (e.g. in congestive heart failure). An initial test dose of 6.25–12.5 mg is usually given for this reason and its effect on blood pressure should be assessed prior to a regular prescription. After absorption from the stomach a response can occur within 15 minutes.

In hypertension, treatment is titrated according to the patient's needs and should be the lowest effective dose. The range is usually 12.5–50 mg twice daily. In the treatment of heart failure captopril is often given (in conjunction with a diuretic), up to a maximum dosage of 150 mg per day.

Renal function must be carefully monitored as the drug is excreted via the kidneys. It is effectively removed by haemodialysis.

Side-effects include hyperkalaemia, angioedema, cough (due to increased sensitivity of the cough reflex), and altered immune function (neutropenia, skin rashes).

References

Abraham, A.S., Rosenmann, D., Kramer M., Balkin, J., Zion, M.M., Farbstien, H., and Eylath, U. (1987). Magnesium in the prevention of lethal arrhythmias in acute myocardial infarction. *Archives of Internal Medicine*, **147**, 753–5.

Allen, B.J., Brodsky, M.A., Capparelli, E.V., Luckett, O.R., and Iseri, L.T. (1989). Magnesium sulfate therapy for sustained monomorphic ventricular tachycardia. *American Journal of Cardiology*, **64**, 1202–4.

Armstrong, R.F., Bullen, C., Cohen, S.L., Singer, M and Webb, A.R. (1991). *Critical care algorithms*. Oxford University Press, Oxford.

Chatterjee, K., Swan, H.J.C., Kaushik V.S. *et al.* (1976) Effects of vasodilator therapy for severe pump failure in acute myocardial infarction on short-term and late prognosis. *Circulation*, **53**, 797.

Des Jardins, T.R. (1988). *Cardiopulmonary anatomy and physiology: essentials for respiratory care.* Delmar Publishers, New York.

DeSanctis, R.W., Doroghazi, R.M., Arsten, W.G., and Buckley, M.J. (1987). Aortic dissection. *New England Journal of Medicine*, **317**, 1060.

Editorial (1992). Thrombolysis for pulmonary embolus. *Lancet*, **340**, 21.

Forrester, J.S., Diamond, G. McHugh, T., Swan, H.J.C. (1971) Filling pressures in the right and left sides of the heart in acute myocardial infarction. A reappraisal of central venous pressure monitoring. *New England Journal of Medicine*, **285**, 190.

Ghani, M.F. and Rabah, M. (1977). Effect of magnesium chloride on electrical stability of the heart. *American Heart Journal*, **94**, 600–2.

Goldhaber, S.Z., Haire, W.D., Feldstein, M.L. *et al.* (1993). Alteplase versus heparin in acute pulmonary embolism: randomised trial assessing right ventricular function and pulmonary perfusion. *Lancet*, **341**, 507.

Goldhaber, S.Z., Simons, G.R., Elliott, G., *et al.* (1993) Quantitative plasma D-Dimer levels among patients undergoing pulmonary angiography for suspected pulmonary embolism. *Journal of the American Medical Association*, 2819.

Gruppo Italiano per lo studio della streptochinasi nell'infarcto miocardico. GISSI-2 (1990). A factorial randomised trial of alteplase versus streptokinase and heparin versus no heparin among 12490 patients with acute myocardial infarction. *Lancet*, **336**, 65.

Hampton, J.R. (1986). *The ECG in practice*, (3rd edn). Churchill Livingstone, London.

Hope, R.A., Longmore, S.M., Moss, P.A.U. and Warrens, A.N. (1992). *Oxford handbook of clinical medicine*, (2nd edn). Oxford University Press, Oxford.

Iseri, L.T., Freed, J., and Bures, A.R., (1975). Magnesium Deficiency and Cardiac Disorders. *American Journal of Medicine*, **58**, 837–46.

ISIS-2 (1988). Randomised trial of intravenous streptokinase, oral aspirin, both, or neither among 17187 cases of suspected acute myocardial infarction: ISIS-2. *Lancet*, **ii**, 349.

ISIS-4 (1995). A randomised factorial trial assessing early captopril, oral mononitrate, and intravenous magnesium sulphate in 58,050 patients with suspected acute myocardial infarction. *Lancet*, **345**, 669–85.

Leak, D. (1986). Intravenous amiodarone in the treatment of refractory life-threatening cardiac arrhythmias in the critically ill patient. *American Heart Journal*, **111**, 456–62.

Levick, J.R. (1991). *An introduction to cardiovascular physiology.* Butterworths, London.

Nelson, G.I.C., Ahuja, R.C., Silke, B., Hussain, M., and Taylor, S.H. (1983) Haemodynamic advantages of isosorbide dinitrate over frusemide in acute heart failure following myocardial infarction. *Lancet*, **i**, 730.

Opie, L.H. (1991). *Drugs for the heart*, (3rd edn). W.B. Saunders, Philadelphia.

Rasmussen, H.S., Aurup, P., Hojberg, S., Jensen, E.K., and McNair, P. (1986). Magnesium and acute myocardial infarction: transient hypomagnesaemia not induced by renal magnesium loss in patients with acute myocardial infarction. *Archives of Internal Medicine*, **146**, 872–4.

Rasmussen, H.S., Norregard, P., Lindeneg, O., McNair, P., Vacker, V., and Balslev, S. (1986). Intravenous magnesium in acute myocardial infarction. *Lancet*, 234–6.

Sasada, M.P. and Smith, S.P. (1990). *Drugs in anaesthesia and intensive care.* Castle House Publications, Tunbridge Wells.

Shechter, M. Hod, H., Marks, N. Behar, S., Kaplinsky, E. Rabinowitz, B. (1990). Beneficial effect of magnesium sulfate in acute myocardial infarction. *American Journal of Cardiology*, **66**, 271–4.

Singer, M. (1993) The management of acute heart failure: an iconoclastic view. *Care of the Critically Ill*, **9**, 11.

Stein, P.D., Hull, R.D., Saltzman, H.A., and Pineo, G. (1993). Strategy for diagnosis of patients with suspected acute pulmonary embolism. *Chest*, **103**, 1553.

Sueta, C.A., Clarke, S.W., Dunlap, S.H., Jensen, L., Blauwet, M.B., Koch, G., Petterson, J.H., and Adams, K.F. (1994). Effect of acute magnesium administration on the frequency of ventricular arrhythmia in patients with heart failure. *Circulation*, **89**, 660–6.

Swedberg, K., Held, P. *et al.* (1992) Effects of the early administration of enalapril on mortality in patients with acute myocardial infarction. Results of the cooperative new Scandinavian enalapril survival study II (CONSENSUS II). *New England Journal of Medicine*, **327**, 678.

Teo, K.K., Yusuf, S., Collins, R., Held, P.H., and Peto, R. (1991). Effects of intravenous magnesium in suspected acute myocardial infarction: overview of randomised trials. *British Medical Journal*, **303** (Dec. 14), 1499–1503.

The GUSTO Investigators (1993). An international randomised trial comparing four thrombolytic strategies for acute myocardial infarction. *New England Journal of Medicine*, **329**, 673.

Timmis, A.D. (1985). *Cardiology.* Gower Medical Publishing, London.

Woods, K.L., Fletcher, S., Roffe, C., and Haider, Y. (1992). Intravenous magnesium sulphate in suspected acute myocardial infarction: results of the second Leicester Intravenous Magnesium Intervention Trial [LIMIT-2]. *Lancet*, **339**, 1553–8

Woods, K.L. (1993). Hypomagnesaemia and the myocardium. *Lancet*, **341**, 155.

Zwerling, H.K. (1987). Does exogenous magnesium suppress myocardial irritability and tachyarrhythmias in the nondigitalized patient? *American Heart Journal*, **113**, 1046–53.

6. Cardiac arrest and cardiopulmonary resuscitation

Introduction

Approximately 45% of hospital patients who have a cardiac arrest are initially resuscitated but only 15% survive to be discharged home. Successful resuscitation is more likely in accident and emergency departments and specialist areas such as coronary care units (BRE-SUS study 1992). Cardiac arrests are less common within general ICUs, with an average of about 5% of total hospital arrests occurring per year. This is possibly due to a combination of close observation, timely intervention, the type of patients admitted to the ICU and the expertise associated with dealing with the critically ill. However, there is no doubt that personnel working in the ICU should be familiar with and skilled in cardiopulmonary resuscitation (CPR). Training should include aspects pertinent to resuscitation in the ICU, such as the use of monitoring to give more information, or dealing with the ventilated patient who has a cardiac arrest.

It should be stressed at this point that the skills of basic life support are essentially practical ones which must be learnt and practised regularly using resuscitation training manikins in order to ensure retention. Research into proficiency in CPR has shown that up to 57% of qualified nurses were completely ineffective in performing basic life support (Wynne and Marteau 1987). Although this work was carried out among general ward nurses, similar studies in junior doctors have echoed this result (Skinner *et al.* 1985) and the need for continuous updating and practice of these skills cannot be overemphasized. This chapter will outline the pathophysiology associated with cardiac arrest, discuss the overall management, and examine in detail the techniques and drugs used for CPR. Finally, the care of the patient and his family following successful and unsuccessful resuscitation will be discussed.

Definition

Cardiac arrest is defined as the absence or severe reduction of cardiac output resulting in inadequate perfusion of vital organs and causing cerebral and myocardial ischaemic damage. This is associated with the following arrhythmias:

- Ventricular fibrillation (VF).
- Ventricular tachycardia (VT).
- Asystole.
- Electromechanical dissociation (EMD).

Other arrhythmias (see Table 6.1 and Chapter 5), may also produce a severe reduction or absence of cardiac output and in this instance should be treated as cardiac arrest.

(Note. Ventricular tachycardia is not always associated with a severe reduction or loss of cardiac output, see Chapter 5).

Pathophysiology

The events following cardiac arrest consist of:

(1) Loss of oxygen supply due to loss of blood flow.

(2) Rapid depletion of high energy phosphates, such as ATP, in the myocardial cells. These are not replenished due to the lack of oxygen supply and absence of aerobic metabolism.

(3) Failure of pacemaker activity, impulse conduction, and myocardial contractility due to lack of ATP.

(4) Complete loss of electrical activity. It is possible for electrical dysfunction to be the primary event in which case the order of events will commence with (4).

Ventricular fibrillation occurs early in most cardiac arrests unless the primary cause is electrical dysfunction. The ventricular fibrillation will rapidly degenerate into a small amplitude waveform (the so-called 'fine' VF) and finally to electrical standstill (asystole).

In spite of what may appear to be good pulse volume and blood pressure the actual cardiac output associated with external cardiac massage (ECM) is only 20–30% of

Table 6.1 Arrhythmias associated with cardiac arrest

Feature:	Ventricular fibrillation (VF)	Pulseless ventricular tachycardia (VT)	Asystole	Electromechanical dissociation (EMD)
Definition:	Sudden loss of co-ordinated electrical activity leading to random contraction of individual myocardial fibres	A repetitive electrical discharge from a ventricular ectopic focus	Complete absence of electrical activity	Organized electrical activity but no effective myocardial contraction takes place
ECG trace:	Rapid irregular activity without rate or recognizable shape	Rapid, wide QRS complexes (rate 150–220 bpm)	No recognizable activity although occasional agonal (dying) beats may be seen	QRS complexes are present
Arterial pressure waveform	None	None or very low	None	None or very low pressure

normal (Peters and Ihle 1990). This is because pressure does not directly equate with blood flow. The 'pulse' felt during CPR is more likely to be a pulse pressure wave transmitted down the arteries from chest compression. It is therefore more readily felt in atherosclerotic arteries which are less elastic and therefore likely to transmit the pressure to a greater extent. Thus, the pulse cannot be relied upon as a marker of adequacy of CPR.

These marginal levels of cardiac output produced by ECM mean that inadequately oxygenated tissues will convert to anaerobic glycolysis with the production of lactic acid and the development of metabolic acidosis. This is compounded by the respiratory acidosis which may have built up from the period without ventilation. Once adequate ventilation occurs the arterial pH returns to normal but the venous pH remains low due to high mixed venous CO_2 levels associated with poor pulmonary perfusion (Weil *et al.* 1986).

The peripheral blood vessels are initially vasoconstricted by the release of high levels of catecholamines (up to 300 times normal levels). This is followed by a fall in systemic vascular resistance (SVR) due to loss of blood flow and vasodilatation due to hypoxia, lactic acidosis, hypercapnia, and ischaemia.

There is then thought to be a down-regulation of response to catecholamines by α-receptors in the vasculature due to overstimulation from the high initial endogenous catecholamine release (Lindner 1991). Further response may then be limited to high levels of catecholamines and to α_2-receptors. This vasodilatation produces a rapid equilibration of arterial and venous pressures.

Table 6.2 Factors associated with sudden ventricular dysrhythmias

Drug toxicity	Electrolyte disturbance	External factors
Digoxin (often precipitated by hypokalaemia and hypomagnesaemia) Amphetamines Tricyclic antidepressants Adrenergic drugs Cocaine	Hypokalaemia Hypomagnesaemia Hypercalcaemia	Unsynchronized cardioversion attempt Exacerbating factors of myocardial ischaemia (hypoxaemia, carbon monoxide poisoning, hypoperfusion due to hypovolaemia, ventricular failure, rapid tachycardia) Electrocution

Assessment

The clinical signs of cardiac arrest are:

- Absence of pulse — this should be felt for at least 5 seconds (usually the femoral or carotid, as central pulses are less likely to be affected by vasoconstriction and are most easily felt).

- Loss of consciousness.

- Minimal or absent respirations.

- ECG exhibiting any of the above traces accompanied by loss of the arterial waveform.

Recognition of cardiac arrest in the ICU is facilitated by ECG and haemodynamic monitoring which is usually already in place on the patient. Alarms will alert the nurse immediately and intervention can be swift.

(*Note.* Monitors are not infallible; if the patient is otherwise well and has a palpable pulse, check for disconnection of leads or damping/kinking/blockage of the arterial cannula or tubing.)

Although some authorities have previously recommended assessing the pupillary response to light, this is not a reliable method of determining loss of cardiac output. It takes between 45 seconds to 1 minute for pupils to become fixed and dilated and they can be affected by other drugs commonly used in the ICU such as opiates (pupillary constriction in high doses), and atropine or adrenaline (pupillary dilatation).

Aims of treatment

(i) Establish and maintain an airway.

(ii) Provide adequate ventilation with 100% oxygen or as near as possible.

(iii) Support organ perfusion with external cardiac massage until spontaneous cardiac output is restored.

(iv) Restore spontaneous cardiac output and stabilize the patient.

The overall aim of intervention is the return of an adequate spontaneous circulation with minimal cerebral dysfunction. Resuscitation can only really be considered successful if the patient is able to return home with intact cerebral function. The probability of an unsuccessful outcome increases with the length of time taken to restore cardiac output.

Factors likely to affect outcome following cardiac arrest	
Negative	*Positive*
Asystole on ECG trace	Witnessed arrest
Lengthy resuscitation period	Early defibrillation
Severe underlying disease	

Basic life support techniques

These are based on the guidelines of the Resuscitation Council (UK, 1994), but are specifically applied to the ICU situation.

Confirm cardiac arrest

In the previously conscious patient, the first step to achieving this is by shouting the patient's name or 'Are you all right?' and shaking them. In many cases in the ICU this is unnecessary or inappropriate, either because ECG and arterial blood pressure monitoring make cardiac arrest obvious or because the patient is unresponsive for other reasons such as sedation.

Summon assistance

This is the next most important step. There should be no hesitation in using the cardiac arrest buzzer or shouting loudly even if the exact situation is uncertain. Commencing basic life support without ensuring there is the back up of advanced life support is only likely to decrease the chances of resuscitation.

Precordial thump

If ECG monitoring indicates VF, VT, or asystole and immediate defibrillation is not available, a precordial thump should be attempted.

This should be taught and practised during resuscitation training. It is essentially a blow on the lower third of the patient's sternum using the lateral aspect of a closed fist. The degree of force should not be excessive; about that obtained using the weight of a swing from the elbow. The sudden blow of mechanical energy acts like the electrical energy associated with a defibrillatory shock and dissipates the chaotic electrical system in ventricular fibrillation sufficiently for sinus rhythm or some other pacemaker activity to return. It has also been shown to be effective in pulseless ventricular tachycardia. There is a small risk of exacerbating a ventricular arrhythmia, in particular deteriorating a ventricular tachycardia to asystole (Bossaert and Koster 1992) but this is outweighed by the potential benefit of terminating the arrhythmia swiftly.

Debrillation

> The faster ventricular fibrillation is terminated the better the outcome for the patient.

Although this does not form part of basic life support it is a priority which should be considered immediately in the intensive care unit. The chances of successful defibrillation are optimal within the first 90 seconds before global hypoxia has occurred [Resuscitation Council (UK) 1994]. If defibrillation is successful within this time there is also an increased likelihood of long term survival. In most ICUs, access to a defibrillator is not a problem and defibrillation should be the first response if the patient is in ventricular fibrillation. Nurses remain in a difficult position in some hospitals where defibrillation is not considered part of the nursing role. However, if nurses are adequately trained to defibrillate there is no reason why they should not carry this out. Immediate defibrillation can save valuable time and may influence the patient's ultimate outcome. If defibrillation cannot be carried out immediately then basic life support should be commenced. The ability of the heart to respond to resuscitative measures and the consequent survival rate deteriorate with delay in initiating cardiac compression. The number of joules (units of energy) and technique of defibrillation will be discussed in detail later in the chapter.

Airway control

Non-intubated patients

If there is no artificial airway of any kind then the patient's own airway must be assessed for patency and kept open. The suggested manoeuvre for opening the airway is the use of the head tilt and chin lift (Fig. 6.1), which should pull the base of the tongue away from the back of the throat.

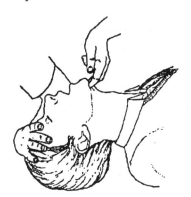

Fig. 6.1 Opening the airway. Reproduced with permission from *Advanced life support manual*, (2nd edn 1994), (ed. A.J. Handley and A. Swain). Resuscitation Council, UK.

This means placing two fingers of one hand under the point of the chin and the other hand over the forehead. The head is then tipped back pulling the chin upwards. The airway should be cleared of any obvious obstruction using a Yankauer sucker. Well-fitting dentures should be left in place to improve the seal around the mouth for ventilation but loose-fitting or broken dentures should be removed. An oropharyngeal airway, such as a Guedel airway, is useful in maintaining the patient's airway and can be inserted once the airway is clear.

An alternative airway is the laryngeal mask airway (LMA). This is a conventional endotracheal tube at one end, which has an inflatable elliptical cuff at the other. The LMA is placed through the patient's mouth into the pharynx until the cuff is at the level of the larynx. When inflated, this cuff forms an airtight seal around the posterior perimeter of the larynx allowing ventilation of the patient. The technique of insertion is more easily taught than endotracheal intubation but it may not be as effective in preventing aspiration and its place in resuscitation has yet to be established.

Intubated patients

These are patients with endotracheal tubes and tracheostomies.

> If there is any doubt about the patency of the endotracheal tube a suction catheter should be inserted to check for and, if possible, remove any occlusion

If there is an immovable obstruction or doubts about the position of the tube in the trachea it should be removed as a matter of urgency. This should only be done by nurses in the unlikely event that there are no medical staff available. The patient should be re-intubated as quickly as possible but may be maintained in the short term by bag and mask ventilation.

If the tube is patent, the patient should be ventilated on 100% O_2 during the arrest and until stabilization is achieved

---

Breathing

If the patient is not intubated, there are a number of ways that ventilation can be carried out. The most basic is mouth-to-mouth ventilation which requires no equipment but will only deliver expired air to the patient. This has an oxygen concentration of only 16% which will provide little in the way of oxygen to meet the needs of the patient even if it is delivered properly. In the cardiac arrest situation *the patient should be ventilated with as near to 100% oxygen* as possible in order to maximize arterial PO_2.

In the ICU, 100% oxygen is readily available and the patient should be ventilated via a bag and tight-fitting anaesthetic mask. The manual resuscitation bag (MRB) used for ventilation should not be a rebreathing bag as this will increase P_aCO_2 if used for any length of time. A bag with a one-way valve, such as an Ambu bag with a reservoir attached, is more suitable for resuscitation. Bag–mask ventilation is a skill that requires considerable practice on training manikins and it can be done very poorly by novices. If there is no one who can effectively ventilate with the bag and mask then mouth-to-mask ventilation using a facemask with a supplemental oxygen port (such as the Laerdal facemask) is recommended by the Resuscitation Council (UK).

Positioning of the patient's head and neck is important. When maintaining the airway without intubation the patient should have no pillow under the head and the neck should be flexed with the head tipped back (see Fig. 6.1). While ventilating the patient via the mask, the head tilt is maintained by lifting the lower jaw forward at the angle using the thumb while the fingers secure the seal of the mask to the face.

When the anaesthetist is ready to intubate a pillow can be placed under the patient's shoulders to facilitate placement of the tube in the trachea.

Whichever method of ventilation is used the patient should initially be given two slow breaths sufficient to cause the chest to rise. It is vital that chest movement is observed as it is the only indicator that the airway is patent and that tidal volume is sufficient. The volume of air used to inflate the lungs should be sufficient to cause the chest to rise.

Each of the initial breaths should last for 1–1.5 seconds (Melker 1985) so that the chest is seen to rise and fall between breaths. If breaths are given too rapidly there is an increased likelihood of inflation of the stomach with possible regurgitation and aspiration of stomach contents.

If the patient is already intubated and ventilated then either the ventilator can be turned to 100% oxygen or the patient can be manually ventilated on 100% oxygen using the manual resuscitation bag (MRB). If there is any doubt at all about the efficacy of the ventilator then it is safest to switch to the MRB and investigate any problems of ventilation. However, if high airway pressures are required to inflate the lungs then mechanical ventilation is generally more effective than manual efforts, providing settings are appropriate and correct position of the tube is assured.

Pneumothorax should be considered if airway pressures have increased acutely in the ventilated patient who has a cardiac arrest

---

Circulation

It is very unlikely that there will only be a single person resuscitating in the ICU so it is probable that external cardiac massage (ECM) will be started at the same time as the airway clearance and ventilation is being carried out. Therefore, single-person resuscitation will be discussed only briefly.

The technique of ECM must be carried out with the patient flat on his/her back and on a firm surface. If the patient is in a chair, the floor is the nearest and easiest place. If the patient is on a special pressure support bed the nurse responsible for his/her care should be familiar with the emergency button to flatten or harden the bed.

Compressions are carried out using the heel of one hand placed on the lower third of the sternum in the midline, with the other hand placed on top. Location of the correct position is by placing the middle finger of one hand on the xiphisternum, the index finger above this, and then the heel of the other hand next to the index finger. The arms should be straight and the shoulders above the patient's sternum (see Fig. 6.2).

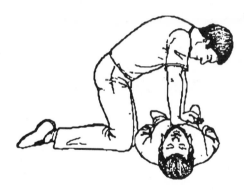

Fig. 6.2 Position for chest compression. Reproduced with permission from *Advanced life support manual*, (2nd edn 1994), (ed. A.J. Handley and A. Swain), Resuscitation Council, UK.

The sternum should be depressed 4–5 cm (1.5–2 inches) in the adult. The compressions can be synchronized with ventilations if the patient is intubated because the ET tube cuff will prevent the force of compression expelling the breath and inflating the stomach.

> The ratio is 5 compressions to 1 breath with more than one resuscitator and 15 compressions to 2 breaths with a single resuscitator

The reason for the difference is that although 5:1 is probably nearer the physiological norm it is very ineffective for a single resuscitator who would spend more time moving from one position to the other than actually carrying out CPR.

It is helpful if the person carrying out ECM counts aloud so that synchronization with ventilation in the non-intubated patient is possible and to assure the team leader that ECM is being carried out. If ECM is discontinued for any reason the count should continue with the word 'off' interposed between each number (i.e. 'One–off, two–off, three–off, four–off', etc.). This reminds the team leader that the patient has no circulatory support during this time.

Advanced life support techniques

Properly performed basic life support will keep the patient alive for up to 20–30 minutes but will not reverse the problem causing the initial arrest. Advanced life support includes the use of defibrillation, drugs, and other supportive measures to increase the efficacy of basic life support and to deal with the problem causing cardiac arrest (see Fig. 6.3).

Points to remember (see Fig. 6.3)

1. Adrenaline should be given as 10 ml of 1 in 10 000 dilution (= 1 mg). The volume of fluid ensures that most of the adrenaline will enter the circulation even without a flush whereas 1 mg in only 1 ml fluid (1 in 1000 dilution) is likely to remain within the IV cannula.

2. ECM should continue immediately following any intervention except between each of the grouped DC shocks in the repeated cycles. The first three DC shocks should be given within 30–45 seconds. Otherwise ECM should not be interrupted for more than 30 seconds as the maximum achievable perfusion pressure will take some time to re-establish.

3. Between administration of each drug, ECM should continue for at least 2 mins to ensure adequate circulation of the drug.

4. If IV access is impossible then endotracheal administration of twice the recommended doses of adrenaline, lignocaine or atropine should be carried out as appropriate.

5. If IV access is peripheral, a large volume of flush (at least 20 ml) should be administered following administration of drugs and the limb should be massaged towards the trunk to assist the returning circulation.

6. The reason for suggesting DC shock for asystole is that in some cases it is possible for 'fine' ventricular fibrillation to look like asystole; if there is any doubt defibrillation should be carried out. The gain on the monitor should be checked and the monitor setting should be on paddles or ECG leads as appropriate. The monitor itself should be checked if necessary.

7. External temporary pacing can be used in asystole. This is an easy and fast method of pacing without the accompanying problems of transvenous or oesophageal systems. It is a system of pacing via electrode pads which are placed anteriorly over the precordium and posteriorly just below the scapula and to the left of the vertebrae. These pads allow excellent conduction of electrical current with an even dispersion over a wide area. This reduces the

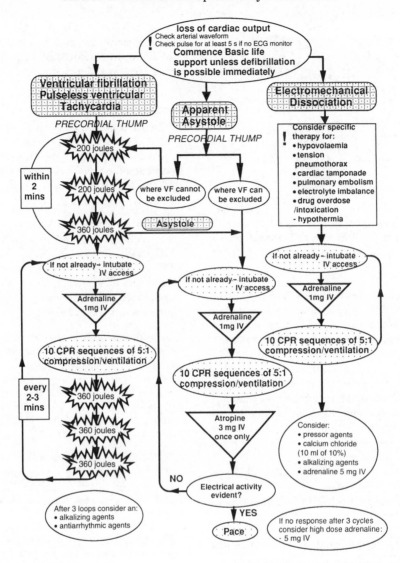

Fig. 6.3 Advanced life support algorithm based on Resuscitation Council (UK) guidelines.

discomfort associated with the electrical stimulus. The pacemaker is connected and set at 80 to 100 beats on 100 mA current. This level may alter according to the pacemaker in use and to the patient's pacing threshold. To find the patient's threshold the level of current is adjusted upwards until QRS beats accompanied by a pulse are obtained (pacing capture) or the maximum is reached. Once capture is achieved the current level is then set to 10–20 mA higher than the patient's threshold. The patient should be paced at a fixed rate while ECM continues to avoid interference. ECM is only discontinued when there is a palpable pulse with pacing.

Defibrillation

All qualified and appropriately trained nursing and medical personnel working in intensive care should be able to defibrillate a patient. The improved resuscitation success rate with fast response defibrillation of VF means that it is now essential that all nursing and medical personnel responsible for acutely ill patients are trained and able to defibrillate (Chamberlain 1989; Resuscitation Council, UK 1994).

Defibrillation

Defibrillation is the passage of a current of electricity through the fibrillating heart. This will depolarize the cells and allow them to repolarize uniformly to organized contractions using standard conduction pathways.

The defibrillator

The defibrillator stores and delivers pre-set amounts of direct current electrical energy via two paddles placed on the patient's chest. The energy is measured in joules. In older models the number of joules displayed refers to the energy stored in the defibrillator and in newer models to the energy delivered to the patient. The guidelines for treating ventricular fibrillation all refer to delivered amounts of energy. Most newer defibrillators have paddles which will also allow monitoring of the ECG (the so-called 'quick-look' paddles).

> In order to monitor ECG via the paddles some defibrillators require setting to 'paddles' while others automatically monitor via paddles until altered to an ECG lead

Safety aspects

The electrical energy delivered by defibrillation is potentially lethal if it strikes a bystander so a number of precautions are essential prior to defibrillation.

> The person defibrillating is responsible for the safety of others

- A warning to stand clear should be clearly stated prior to defibrillation.

- Ensure no other person is in contact with the patient or any conducting surfaces such as the metal frame of the bed just before defibrillation.

- Pressure should be applied to the paddles when placed firmly against the skin to avoid possible arcing (passage of current from paddle-to-paddle, or paddle-to-patient's skin, through air).

- Electrode gel or pads are highly effective electrical conductors and are used to provide an efficient conduction path to the patient. This directs the path of the electrical current and reduces the risk of current passing through less efficient conduction pathways such as air or bare skin. Care should be taken when applying electrode gel and any excess should be wiped off otherwise current may be conducted directly across

the gel or to the person applying the defibrillator paddles. Gel conduction pads should preferably be used. These pads should be changed after every 2–3 shocks to prevent drying out.

- Remove any metal or foil objects on the patient's chest or upper body. They will preferentially conduct the electrical current and, in so doing, will become very hot causing burns to the patient. The patient will also receive a reduced amount of charge. Glyceryl trinitrate patches should also be removed because of their explosive capability.

Defibrillation technique

If the patient is not already monitored, place gel conduction pads or electrode gel in the positions shown in Fig. 6.4 and apply the defibrillator paddles to the chest. Ascertain the patient's heart rhythm and unless it is certain asystole or electromechanical dissociation charge the defibrillator to 200 joules. Press firmly on the paddles, warn all personnel to stand clear (check this visually), confirm VF (or VT) again on the monitor and depress the paddle buttons to discharge the shock. If the defibrillator is a fast charging model then immediately recharge and repeat defibrillation at 200 joules providing the patient remains in VF/VT. If this is not possible, or the patient is no longer in VF/VT then cardiac massage should be recommenced while the defibrillator is recharging or the patient is assessed for alternative interventions.

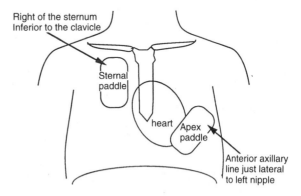

Right of the sternum
Inferior to the clavicle

Sternal paddle

heart

Apex paddle

Anterior axillary line just lateral to left nipple

Fig. 6.4 Paddle positions for defibrillation.

If the patient is still in VF/VT the shock should be immediately repeated, followed by a 360-joule shock if this is unsuccessful. Further management should then follow the advanced life support algorithm (Fig. 6.3).

Transthoracic impedance or the resistance of the chest to conduction of the electrical current is an important and variable factor in delivering the peak amount of current to the myocardium. Bone is a very poor conductor of electricity and should be avoided. Reduction of impedance will assist the delivery of peak current and all possible steps should be taken to do so.

Factors which will reduce impedance

- Firm pressure of approx. 11.25 kg (25 lb) per paddle

- Use of conducting gel or pads

- Multiple shocks (i.e. more than 2 and less than 5 in succession with a short time interval between discharges)

- Increased delivered energy

- Increased paddle surface area

- Application of shocks during the end expiratory phase of respiration

---

An alternative paddle position, which may be useful in the obese patient who has increased transthoracic impedance, is the anterior-posterior position. For this, the patient is rolled on to his/her side and one paddle is placed over the left precordium next to the base of the sternum while the other is placed in the same position posteriorly to the left of the spine.

Factors affecting the success of defibrillation

- Acidosis

- Hypoxia

- Electrolyte imbalance

- Hypothermia

- Drug toxicity

Mechanism of external cardiac massage (ECM)

The cardiac output produced by good external cardiac massage is only 25% of normal ($\sim$ 1.2 l/min) and the cerebral blood flow is only 15% of normal if CPR is carried out immediately the arrest occurs. Cerebral blood flow during CPR diminishes with the time taken to commence ECM. This is obviously a fairly inefficient method of maintaining circulation and there is a great need to find ways to improve it.

The mechanism of ECM is important for two reasons. (1) Depending on the method of blood flow either the rate of ECM or the duration of each compression will have an effect on the cardiac output. (2) Methods of improving the blood flow generated will differ according to the mechanism.

There are two proposed mechanisms by which blood flow is generated during ECM. The first is the 'cardiac pump' theory, which was proposed by Kouwenhaven *et al.* (1960) when they first described external cardiac massage (Fig. 6.5). This theory suggests that ECM produces compression of the heart itself between the lowered sternum anteriorly and the vertebrae posteriorly. The compression increases pressure inside the heart and blood is forced out through the aorta and pulmonary artery. Back-flow through the venae cavae and the pulmonary veins is prevented by the presence of intracardiac and venous valves. Atrioventricular filling would then take place during relaxation as the drop in pressure would draw blood back into the heart. Again, retrograde flow would be prevented by venous valves. If this theory is correct then an increased rate of CPR will improve cardiac output as each compression will only deliver a set amount of blood (i.e. that contained within the heart itself).

The second mechanism is the 'thoracic pump' theory, which suggests that the whole thorax acts as a pump during ECM (Fig. 6.6). The compression raises intrathoracic pressure resulting in blood flow from the lungs (which act as a large capacity reservoir) into the left side of the heart. This forces blood already in the heart out through the aorta. Retrograde flow from the lungs is prevented by partial closure of the pulmonary valve, venae cavae valves, and by collapse of the veins themselves which are then resistant to flow. Atrioventricular filling then takes place during relaxation as the release of pressure in the intrathoracic space would draw blood mainly from the superior vena cava through the right side of the heart to fill the pulmonary vessels. If this theory is correct then increased depth and time of compression and increased intrathoracic pressure is likely to increase the cardiac output because an increased volume of blood will be squeezed from the lungs. This would also explain the improvement in cardiac output seen with asynchronized ventilation and compression.

In both mechanisms, the cause of flow is increased pressure with cardiac and venous valves ensuring one-way flow. The normal arterial resistance to flow is not

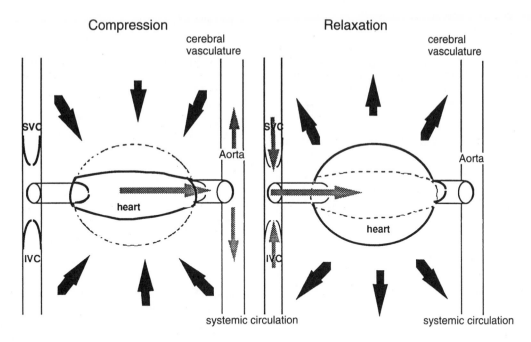

Fig. 6.5 Model of the 'cardiac pump' theory.

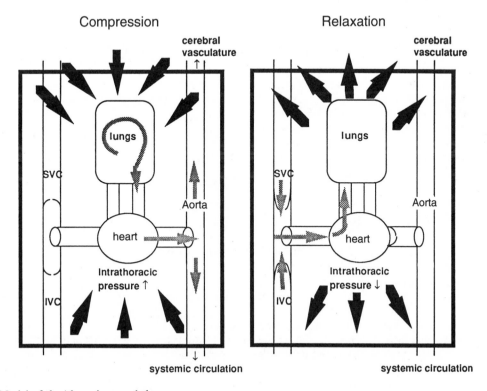

Fig. 6.6 Model of the 'thoracic pump' theory.

present due to the loss of vasoactive peripheral tone during hypoxia, ischaemia, and acidosis (see above). Arterial and venous pressures rapidly equilibrate and forward blood flow (arterial to venous) must therefore be generated by a pressure differential between the mean aortic and the mean right atrial pressure.

Most research supports the 'thoracic pump' theory because:

(i) The tricuspid and mitral valves are open during ECM.

(ii) During chest compression with a flail segment (see Chapter 11), the arterial pressure does not increase until the segment is stabilized (by intermittent positive pressure ventilation).

(iii) Consciousness during VF can be maintained by encouraging repeated coughing which also increases intrathoracic pressure and can maintain an arterial pressure of up to 100 mmHg.

Rate and duty cycle

Duty cycle refers to the duration of compression as a fraction of the total compression/relaxation movement in ECM.

Research into the length of the duty cycle and rate of compressions has shown that maximum systolic flow is obtained with a compression rate of around 100/min and a 50% duty cycle. Unfortunately, this can be subject to other variables such as blood volume and distribution, vascular resistance, force of chest compression, and drugs. A rate of 100/min is extremely difficult for a single resuscitator to maintain and as there is not a vast difference between the output produced by 80 bpm and that produced by 100 bpm the recommendations in Europe remain at 80 compressions per minute.

Management of cardiac arrest

The high stress and need for immediate response associated with cardiac arrest make it one of the most potentially disorganized situations liable to occur within the ICU. In order to avoid the ineffective chaos that can ensue, all personnel should be trained in advanced cardiac life support and management of the arrest should follow structured lines. Training should include simulated cardiac arrests with feedback and debriefing managed in a constructive way.

One person *only* should be designated 'team leader' at a cardiac arrest. Decisions on interventions should be made by this person and all information pertaining to the situation should be passed to them. They should not take a practical role (unless it is essential) but, if possible, remain slightly detached with an overview of all that is going on. Management of cardiac arrest requires an optimum number of people. Too many will increase the confusion and may physically impede necessary personnel reaching the patient. Too few will mean unnecessary delays in instituting interventions. It has been shown that survival decreases with increasing numbers of personnel attending the arrest (BRESUS study 1992).

Most authorities suggest between three and five people. The Royal College of Physicians recommends a minimum of two doctors, usually a medical registrar and an anaesthetist, as well as one other member who may be a technician, or another doctor. In most cases, a nurse who has specialist knowledge or training is included on the team. In the ICU this will generally be the nurse caring for the patient, who will form the all-important link between knowledge of the patient and his/her condition and the specialist knowledge provided by the team. A back-up nurse can provide assistance as necessary. This back-up should reflect the experience and skills of the nurse assigned to the patient. A junior nurse will require experienced back-up, while an experienced nurse can be assisted by a junior who can learn from the experience. The nurse-in-charge should be fully aware of the situation but may not necessarily need to remain with the patient provided the back-up is appropriate.

Causes of cardiac arrest in the ICU patient

- Hypovolaemia
- Myocardial infarction
- Hypoxaemia
- Myocardial ischaemia
- Pneumothorax
- Intrinsic cardiac instability (arrhythmias)
- Brainstem CVA
- Hypothermia ($< 28\ °C$)
- Drugs (e.g. verapamil)
- Anaphylaxis
- Iatrogenic (e.g. disconnection from or failure of the ventilator)
- Metabolic imbalance (e.g. calcium, magnesium, potassium, phosphate)

Roles during cardiac arrest

Nurse 1 (the nurse caring for the patient)
Diagnose cardiac arrest, alert other team members, initiate CPR, inform other team members of the history and preceding events, record events and interventions, protect the patient's dignity and rights where possible, speak to the family with the doctor.

Nurse 2 (back-up)
Bring emergency equipment, prepare defibrillator and defibrillate if appropriate, draw up drugs and infusions, record events and interventions, take over CPR from nurse 1 when required.

Team leader
(The senior doctor attached to the ICU, otherwise the duty medical registrar or, if no medical staff are present, the nurse-in-charge.)
Re-affirm arrest diagnosis and arrhythmia, direct overall resuscitation, decide on interventions, assess response, may defibrillate if appropriate, may obtain central venous access if appropriate, prescribe drugs, ensure CPR is being done correctly and that ECM is rotated so that fatigue is not a problem, call in outside help if necessary, decide on end-point if resuscitation is unsuccessful, speak to the family.

Anaesthetist
Intubate, secure airway, obtain central venous access, ventilate or attach to ventilator and, if necessary, assist with ECM.

Agents used in resuscitation

Oxygen

The poor levels of cardiac output produced by ECM mean that anything less than 100% oxygen saturation of haemoglobin will limit the amount of oxygen delivered to the tissues. In order to ensure full saturation, 100% oxygen should be given as soon as possible and 100% oxygen saturation should be maintained following successful resuscitation to help the patient to clear the tissue oxygen debt that will have built up during CPR.

Vasopressors (α-receptor agonists)

The principal drug used to support CPR is adrenaline. It has mixed α- and β-receptor actions (see Chapter 5) but it is predominantly the α-effects which are responsible for supporting resuscitation. The α-effect consists primarily of vasoconstriction which increases aortic diastolic blood pressure and coronary and cerebral perfusion. The β-receptor action has chronotropic and inotropic effects on the myocardium and a vasodilator effect on the coronary arteries.

Disadvantages associated with its use are:

- Increase in myocardial oxygen demand in VF (probably related to increased frequency and amplitude of fibrillatory contractions).

- Impairment of subendocardial blood flow (probably by increasing the muscular tension which compresses coronary vessels).

The recommended dose is 1 mg IV (10 ml of 1:10 000 solution) every 5 min (14 µg/kg/5 min). Current research suggests a dose of 5 mg every 5 min (70 µg/kg/5 min) may be more effective in increasing aortic diastolic pressure and improving initial resuscitation success. However, this has not as yet been shown to make any difference to hospital discharge rates (Lindner 1991). It is recommended in the Resuscitation Council (UK) guidelines for use in unresponsive asystole and electromechanical dissociation.

Atropine

Atropine effectively blocks vagal influence on the heart at the level of the sinoatrial nodal pacemaker. It enhances the rate of discharge of the sinus node and decreases atrioventricular conduction time. It is most effective in cases of asystole caused by toxic effects of choline esters (e.g. methacholine, carbachol), anticholinesterases (e.g. neostigmine, pyridostigmine), or other parasympathomimetic drugs (e.g. pilocarpine). It has not been established whether it has any effect in other causes of asystole.

- There are no known disadvantages associated with its use in the asystolic arrest.

The recommended dose is 3 mg IV given once only.

Lignocaine

Lignocaine is a membrane-stabilizing antidysrhythmic. It primarily inhibits retrograde conduction and re-entry mechanisms by equalizing the action potential duration of individual cells so that they are less likely to depolarize before the myocardium as a whole (see Chapter 5). It may alter the defibrillatory threshold by stabilizing the arrhythmia thereby making defibrillation more difficult.

A disadvantage associated with its use is:

● Potential increase in the defibrillatory threshold.

The recommended dose is 100 mg IV bolus. This is given either as 10 ml 1% lignocaine or 5 ml 2% lignocaine.

It is not recommended in the algorithm for VF/VT (Fig. 6.3) by the Resuscitation Council (UK) but should be considered if no response has been obtained after 3 loops of defibrillation and adrenaline.

The initial bolus dose is only effective for approximately 10 minutes and should be followed by a further bolus dose or an infusion. Following successful resuscitation from VF or VT, a lignocaine infusion of 2–4 mg/min may be commenced.

Bretylium

Bretylium prolongs the ventricular action potential and the refractory period. It also causes early release of noradrenaline with a positive inotropic response, but this is followed by a decrease in SVR and hypotension may ensue. It is thought to raise the threshold for ventricular fibrillation without decreasing the defibrillation threshold.

It is no longer specifically recommended by the Resuscitation Council (UK) as a second-line antiarrhythmic drug in refractory VF but should be considered along with amiodarone and lignocaine if a response has not been obtained after 3 loops of maximum defibrillation and adrenaline.

Disadvantages associated with its use are:

● Onset of antiarrhythmic action is slow (up to 20 minutes).

● Initial catecholamine release may exacerbate ventricular irritability.

● Decrease in SVR may lower aortic diastolic pressure during CPR.

The dose is 5 mg/kg IV with further boluses of up to 10 mg/kg at 15–30 minute intervals to a cumulative maximum of 30 mg/kg. Further prolonged defibrillation attempts for up to 20 minutes should be carried out after each bolus.

Sodium bicarbonate

Sodium bicarbonate was originally used during CPR to reverse metabolic acidosis. It was given as a first-line response to cardiac arrest but is now regarded as a second-line drug to be considered in arrests lasting longer than 10–15 minutes. Research has shown an increase in venous CO_2 levels following administration of sodium bicarbonate ($NaHCO_3$) and it may actually exacerbate intracellular and respiratory acidosis. In the blood, bicarbonate (HCO_3^-) combines with hydrogen ions (H^+) to form H_2CO_3 which dissociates into H_2O and CO_2. This CO_2 diffuses rapidly into cells and combines with H_2O to form H_2CO_3 (carbonic acid). The HCO_3^- does not diffuse into the cell as rapidly and therefore cannot buffer the intracellular acid. Paradoxical intracellular acidosis is thereby increased despite a decrease in extracellular acidosis. This is particularly apparent in the CSF due to the free diffusibility of CO_2 through the blood–brain barrier where increased acidosis has marked impairment on cerebral blood flow

Other problems associated with sodium bicarbonate are:

● Increased plasma osmolality following infusion and the ensuing cerebral damage related to serum osmolality of greater than 350 mOsm/l

● Arterial alkalosis causing a shift in the oxyhaemoglobin dissociation curve to the left resulting in decreased availability of oxygen to the tissues.

● Arterial alkalosis may also increase cerebral vascular resistance thus reducing cerebral blood flow.

● Arterial alkalosis may reduce the effectiveness of vasopressors.

Its use is correctly restricted to prolonged arrests (> 10–15 minutes) where the acidosis is severe, and in hyperkalaemia or anaphylaxis with bronchoconstriction where adrenaline may be potentially ineffective because of marked acidosis.

The dose is 50 mmol (50 ml of 8.4% solution) which can be repeated as necessary.

Calcium

Calcium is essential in myocardial excitation–contraction coupling, in increasing contractility and in enhancing ventricular automaticity during asystole. In the past, calcium was administered in the arrest situation for the above effects but evidence to support this is lacking. Unfortunately, there are other effects associated with calcium which are potentially more deleterious to outcome, namely:

● Prevention of reperfusion of ischaemic areas of the brain and heart due to vascular spasm related to intracellular calcium overload and impairment of oxidative phosphorylation of the mitochondria.

- Cytoplasmic calcium accumulation is associated with cell death.

- Inhibition of calcium accumulation following an ischaemic episode preserves myocardial function.

There is some experimental evidence that cerebral blood flow and neurological recovery following global ischaemia may be promoted by calcium antagonists but this has yet to be confirmed.

Calcium is recommended for use only in highly specific circumstances where hypocalcaemia or blockage of calcium channels may be the cause of the arrest. This includes hypocalcaemia, hyperkalaemia, hypermagnesaemia, and untoward reaction to calcium channel blockers such as verapamil.

The dose is 10 ml of 10% calcium chloride. Calcium chloride is used in preference to calcium gluconate because the number of free calcium ions produced is three times greater for the same volume of drug (2.25 mmol in 10 ml 10% Calcium gluconate to 6.8 mmol in 10 ml 10% calcium chloride).

Magnesium

Magnesium has been shown to suppress myocardial irritability and prevent tachyarrhythmias *in vitro* but clinical evidence of this remains inconclusive. The actual mechanism by which it works has not yet been identified but could either be by direct inhibition of the efflux of potassium from the cell, alteration of cellular calcium metabolism, decreasing peripheral vascular resistance, or stimulating a membrane-stabilizing enzyme (Zwerling 1987).

However, use of magnesium is considered a relatively safe intervention which may be used when other antiarrhythmic agents have failed or when there is reason to suspect magnesium depletion.

The usual dose is 10–20 mmol immediately, followed by 20–40 mmol given over 5–10 hours.

Amiodarone

Amiodarone is a potent ventricular and supraventricular antiarrhythmic. It works by prolonging the duration of the action potential, equalizing the length of repolarization in all myocardial cells, and increasing the effective refractory period. It is used for atrial fibrillation and flutter, prevention of ventricular fibrillation and tachycardia, and for arrhythmias in Wolff–Parkinson–White syndrome. During resuscitation it can be used as a stabilizing agent following defibrillation.

The dose is 300 mg or 5 mg/kg IV given over 10–15 minutes followed by an infusion of 10–20 mg/kg/ 24 h.

Intravenous fluids

It is usual to set up a crystalloid solution, such as 0.9% sodium chloride, to provide a flush for IV drugs and dilution if necessary. If hypovolaemia is suspected then colloid or O rhesus-negative blood (for severe blood loss) may be infused.

Care should be taken to ensure that drugs are actually reaching the circulation and if there is any doubt an alternative IV access should be used. Ideally, there should be central venous access as poor peripheral circulation makes it unlikely that drugs given peripherally will have a chance to circulate.

Note. The intracardiac route for drugs is no longer recommended as there is little advantage to it. The high level of complications and the difficulty of insertion make it a dangerous proposition without real added benefit.

Care of the successfully resuscitated patient

It is usual for patients in the post-arrest period to be admitted to the ICU. The exceptions may be the patient in the coronary care unit whose ventricular fibrillation responds immediately to defibrillation or the patient who has an end-stage disease where intensive care is not appropriate. Immediately post-arrest, the patient remains unstable and extremely vulnerable to further problems. The decision to transfer to intensive care should be made by the team leader in consultation with the ICU staff and the medical staff responsible for the patient.

Even with the most effective cardiopulmonary resuscitation, the patient will have suffered a period of relative ischaemia which will have the greatest effect on those organs most dependent on a continuous supply of oxygen. The cerebral tissues are particularly susceptible due to their high energy requirements and the minimal substrate reserves for anaerobic metabolism. There is, therefore, a high risk of cerebral damage which is exacerbated by hyperglycaemia and acidosis. Certain interventions will protect the cerebral tissues from further injury related to the return of blood flow (reperfusion injury — see Chapter 9) and may reduce the damage already present.

Treatment following resuscitation

1. Mechanical ventilation to achieve normocapnia. Some authorities recommend short-term hyperventilation to reduce PCO_2 (usually to 3.5–4.0 kPa). This causes cerebral vasoconstriction and reduces cerebral blood volume which may help to limit any increase in intracranial pressure, but may also increase cerebral ischaemia. Its use remains controversial.

2. Maintenance of an adequate cardiac output and normotension to avoid further ischaemia and preserve cerebral perfusion pressure (see Chapter 9).

3. Adequate oxygenation to avoid hypoxaemia

Following the return of spontaneous circulation

The nurse should:

1. Check the patient's ventilation is adequate and that there is air entry to both lungs.

2. Attach a pulse oximeter if this is not already in place and confirm that the patient is ventilated on 100% oxygen.

3. Check the blood pressure either with a sphygmomanometer or using the arterial trace.

4. Obtain an arterial blood gas sample and measure blood gases, electrolytes, blood glucose, and haemoglobin.

5. Confirm with medical staff whether the patient is to be kept ventilated and administer sedation as prescribed if necessary.

6. Obtain a chest X-ray to check for: fractured ribs, pneumothorax, possible aspiration, position of ET tube, NG tube, and central venous lines.

7. Take a 12-lead ECG.

8. Measure CVP and urine output.

More specific responses (e.g. insertion of a pulmonary artery catheter) will be necessary according to the individual patient's needs and treatment will probably have to be changed frequently at first to accommodate changes in the patient's condition.

When the patient is stable, intravenous catheters placed during the cardiac arrest should be assessed and replacement considered in view of the non-sterile circumstances in which they were inserted.

Once the patient is stable, full attention can be turned to the patient's family. Although they should have been updated during the cardiac arrest they will still require a full explanation of what has happened. If the patient arrested on the ward and has been transferred to the ICU then the family will require details of what this entails. It is often helpful to have a nurse from the ward who knows the patient's family present to provide a known point of contact for them. A senior member of the medical staff and a nurse should explain what has occurred, giving as much information as the family can absorb. Much of it will require repetition due to the distressed state they are in and care must be taken to avoid jargon and emotive terms such as 'shocked out of VF'.

Complications of resuscitation

The technique of ECM can produce some complications and an awareness of this possibility should be maintained when assessing the patient post-resuscitation. These include fractured ribs, flail chest and pneumothorax, all of which should be excluded on chest X-ray and examination.

Ethics of resuscitation

The main concern for all those associated with resuscitating patients is that inappropriate cardiopulmonary resuscitation will simply prolong the act of dying rather than offering a chance of survival. Resuscitation attempts do not allow a peaceful and dignified death. They invariably remove the family and loved ones from the scene and guarantee a technical, intervention-dominated approach to what may be the patient's final minutes. Resuscitation is a valued and appropriate response if the patient has a chance of recovery and there is no end-stage terminal disease underlying the arrest but if it is carried out in the wrong circumstances then it has little benefit for the patient or family.

There are two situations where assessment is difficult. The first is the resuscitation of 'out of hospital' victims whose medical history and circumstances are unknown to the team. In this case, resuscitation is always attempted. The second is the hospital inpatient who has an end-stage chronic disease or malignancy but who has not been assessed by the medical team for a 'do not resuscitate' (DNR) decision in spite of clearly being unsuitable for resuscitation. Resuscitation will still be initiated by junior staff who do not have the seniority to make any other decision. Following resuscitation, the patient may then require intensive care and unless senior medical staff are called in to assess the patient, they may be admitted inappropriately to the ICU.

There is little that can be done about the first situation but the frequency of the second situation can be limited by the awareness and responsibility of senior medical staff. Discussion of prognosis and DNR orders at an appropriate stage in the patient's terminal illness, either with the patient and/or their family as well is important. Advance directives or 'living wills' may also be brought into the discussion as they can provide a clear record of the patient's wishes (Institute of Medical Ethics Working Party 1993). All regular members of the caring team should also be involved in the discussion. An informed decision which is communicated to all personnel caring for the patient will prevent inappropriate resuscitation.

Resuscitation can produce four results:

- Complete recovery.

- Partial recovery.

- Prolonged survival.

- Death.

The two extremes do not involve the moral problems associated with the grey areas of partial recovery and prolonged survival. Patients who are still decorticate, decerebrate, or flaccid and unresponsive to stimulation 24 hours after arrest have only a 7% chance of wakening. No patient with these findings on the third or fourth day after arrest survived (Snyder and Tabbaa 1987, cited in Abramson 1990). The worst possible scenario is to leave a patient in the so-called 'persistent vegetative state' where all higher neurological function is lost and the patient remains alive and functioning purely on brainstem reflexes (see Chapter 9). These patients may end up in the ICU post-arrest and the problem of how far to continue treatment then ensues. Assessment of neurological function is extremely difficult with no clearly identifiable marker of neurological dysfunction at this level. There is no simple formula that can be applied and each patient has to be assessed as an individual by the team as a whole. It is also appropriate to discuss the situation with the family. However, they should never be made to feel that withdrawal of treatment is their decision, due to the enormous potential for guilt that this could evoke. Ultimately, the decision must be made by the ICU consultant in conjunction with the patient's own consultant and the intensive care team.

References and bibliography

Abramson, N.S. (1990). Cardiac arrest and the brain. In *Update in intensive care and emergency medicine*, (ed. J.L. Vincent), Vol 10, pp. 603–11. Springer, Berlin.

Anderson, F.D. (1988). Issues in the postresuscitation period. *Critical Care Nursing Quarterly*, **10**, 51–61.

Baskett, P.J.F. (1986). The ethics of resuscitation. *British Medical Journal*, **293**, 189–90.

Bossaert, L. and Koster, R. (1992). Defibrillation: methods and strategies. *Resuscitation*, **24**, 211–25.

BRESUS Study (Tunstall Pedoe, H., Bailey, L., Chamberlain, D.A., Marsden, A.K., Ward, M.E., and Zideman, D.A.) (1992). Survey of 3765 cardiopulmonary resuscitations in British hospitals: methods and overall results. *British Medical Journal*, **304**, 1347–51.

Chamberlain, D.A. (1989). Advanced life support. *British Medical Journal*, **299**, 446–8.

Cheney, R. (1988) Defibrillation. *Critical Care Nursing Quarterly*, **10**, 9–15.

Gervais, H.W. and Dick, W.F. (1990). Modern drug therapy during cardiopulmonary resuscitation. In *Update in intensive care and emergency medicine*, (ed. J.L. Vincent), Vol. 10, pp. 593–602. Springer, Berlin.

Institute of Medical Ethics Working Party (1993). Advance directives: partnership and practicalities. *British Journal of General Practice*, **43**, 169–71.

Iseri, L.T., Freed, J., and Bures, A.R. (1975). Magnesium deficiency and cardiac disorders. *American Journal of Medicine*, **58**, 837–46.

Jowett, N.I. and Thompson, D.R. (1988). Advanced cardiac life support: current perspectives. *Intensive Care Nursing*, **4**, 71–81.

Kouwenhoven, W.B., Jude, J.R., and Knickerbocker, G.G. (1960). Closed chest cardiac massage. *Journal of the American Medical Association*, **173**, 94–7

Lindner, K.H. (1991). Vasopressor therapy in cardiopulmonary resuscitation. In *Update in intensive care and emergency medicine*, (ed. J.L. Vincent), Vol. 10, pp. 18–24. Springer, Berlin.

Marsden, A.K. (1989). Basic life support. *British Medical Journal*, **299**, 442–5.

Melker, R.J. (1985) Recommendations for ventilation during cardiopulmonary resuscitation: time for a change? *Critical Care Medicine*, **13** 882–3.

Newbold, D. (1987). The physiology of cardiac massage. *Nursing Times*, **83**, 59–62.

Pepe, P.E. (1990). Current standards and future directions of basic and advanced cardiopulmonary resuscitation. In *Update in intensive care and emergency medicine*, (ed. J.L. Vincent), pp. 565–85. Springer, Berlin.

Peters, J. and Ihle, P. (1990). Mechanics of the circulation during cardiopulmonary resuscitation. Pathophysiology and techniques (Parts I and II). *Intensive Care Medicine*, **16**, 11–27.

Planta, I., Weil, M.H., Planta, M., Gazmuri, R., and Duggal, C. (1991). Hypercarbic acidosis reduces cardiac resuscitability. *Critical Care Medicine*, **19**, 1177–81.

Royal College of Nursing (RCN) (1992). *Resuscitation: right or wrong*. RCN, London.

Redmond, A.D. (1986). Post resuscitation care. *British Medical Journal*, **292**, 1444–6.

Resuscitation Council (UK) (1994). *Advanced life support manual*, (ed. A.J. Handley and A. Swain), (2nd edn). Resuscitation Council (UK), London.

Royal College of Physicians (RCP) (1987). *Resuscitation from cardiopulmonary arrest. training and organisation.* RCP, London.

Saunders, J. (1992). Who's for CPR? *Journal of the Royal College of Physicians*, **26**, 254–7.

Schleien, C.L., Berkowitz, I.D., Traystman, R., and Rogers, M.C. (1989). Controversial issues in cardiopulmonary resuscitation. *Anesthesiology*, **71**, 133–49.

Skinner, D.V., Camm, A.I., and Miles, S. (1985). CPR skills of preregistration house officers. *British Medical Journal*, **290**, 1549.

Weil, M.H., Rackow, E.C., Trevino, R., Grundler, W., Falk, J.L., and Griffel, M.I. (1986). Difference in acid–base state between venous and arterial blood during cardiopulmonary resuscitation. *New England Journal of Medicine*, **315**, 153–6.

Wynne, G. (1990). Revised guidelines for life support. *Nursing Times*, **86**, 70–5.

Wynne, G. and Marteau, T. (1987) Race against time. *Nursing Times*, **83**, 16–17.

Zwerling, H.K. (1987). Does exogenous magnesium suppress myocardial irritability and tachyarrhythmias in the nondigitalized patient? *American Heart Journal*, **113**, 1046–53.

7. Cardiac surgery

Introduction

This chapter is intended to give an overview of the care of patients undergoing cardiac surgery from an intensive care perspective. Cardiac transplantation will be covered briefly. It will concentrate on:

- The physiological consequences of cardiopulmonary bypass.
- Surgical procedures.
- Care of the patient following surgery.
- Complications following cardiac surgery.
- Mechanical cardiac assist devices.

Preparation of the patient prior to surgery

The work of Hayward (1975) and Wilson-Barnett (1984) have illustrated the influence that patient preparation and teaching can have on the response to hospitalization and surgery. It has been shown to reduce anxiety prior to operation and moderate physiological responses to post-operative stress. This is particularly important in the preparation of patients for cardiac surgery where anxiety may already be increased due to the perceived high-risk nature of the operation.

Preparation and provision of information should start from the time of the surgeon's decision that surgery is required. The patient is informed of the risks involved as well as the likely benefits. Preadmission information has been shown to be significantly more effective for retention of knowledge, positive patient mood and improved response to regaining independence post-operatively (Cupples 1991). Many patients visit the cardiac surgery unit a couple of weeks prior to surgery for the pre-operative work-up. This is an ideal opportunity to prepare them and provide information in the form of booklets, videos and one to one counselling sessions.

Elements of pre-operative preparation (see also Table 7.1):
1. Patients and family are seen by a nurse from intensive care who will explain:

- what happens to the patient during the course of their stay and the likely time span,
- what sensations they may feel and what they may hear and see,
- how the presence of the endotracheal tube will affect them and including alternative forms of communication,
- the role of the intensive care nurse,
- the function of the intensive care equipment,
- visiting arrangements and direct line telephone number.

(All this information should be backed up by written details which will allow the patient to refer back to any point requiring clarification or reminder.)

2. Patients and family are offered the opportunity to visit the ICU and become more familiar with the environment.

3. Assessment of the patient's and family's understanding of the operation.

4. Assessment of the patient's physical and psychological status and identification of any problems likely to have an affect in the post-operative phase.

Table 7.1 Guidelines for giving pre-operative information

Establish the patient's understanding

Patient will wake in the ICU:
- he/she may hear before being able to move or respond

Endotracheal tube:
- inability to talk
- need for suctioning and associated sensations
- suggested methods of communicating
- length of time it will be in place

Ventilator:
- what it does
- what it feels like
- the importance of relaxing and letting it do the work

Alarms and buzzers:
- what they mean
- what they sound like

Pain:
- where it will be
- what it will feel like
- what can be done for it (positioning, support, analgesia)
- how to let the nurse know the patient has pain

ICU nurse:
- always nearby: watching and monitoring progress

Physiotherapy:
- pain relief will be given prior to any physiotherapy
- the patient to inform the nurse if this is insufficient
- need for deep breathing and coughing after extubation
- need for leg exercises while in bed
- early mobility

Chest drains:
- what they are
- what they do
- when they will be removed (pain relief prior to removal)

Check the patient has understood. Ask if he/she has any other questions

Anatomy and physiology

Figure 7.1 shows the heart and coronary arteries. Figure 7.2 is a cross-section of the heart showing the valves.

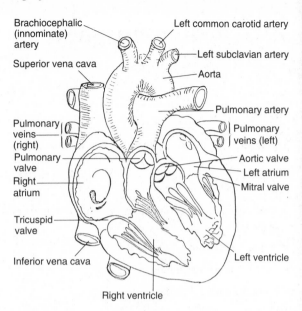

Fig. 7.2 Cross-section of the heart showing the valves and major vessels.

Surgical procedures

Coronary artery bypass graft

Coronary artery disease is a major cause of morbidity and mortality in the Western world with the highest world-wide incidence occurring in Scotland. Numerous

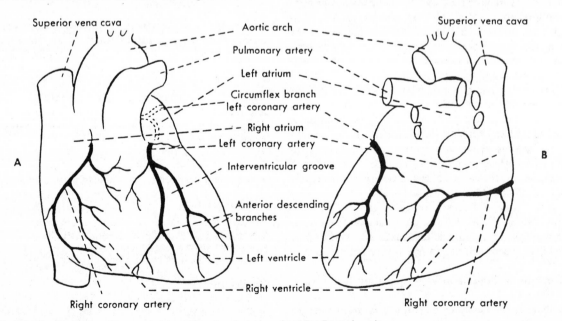

Fig. 7.1 The heart, showing coronary arteries. A = Anterior view; B = Posterior view.

factors are involved in the development of ischaemic heart disease and prevention through health education is obviously the most important health care intervention. Until these initiatives improve the incidence of coronary artery disease, it is likely that demand for coronary artery surgery will remain high. In some types of atherosclerotic narrowing angioplasty is providing an alternative (see below).

By far the most common type of cardiac surgery performed is coronary artery bypass grafting. The aim of this surgery is to relieve ischaemic pain and other symptoms associated with atherosclerotic narrowing of the coronary arteries (ischaemic heart disease). This usually involves grafting of either a piece of saphenous vein from the leg or the internal mammary artery, to a point on the coronary artery below the atherosclerotic occlusion.

Factors associated with risk of heart disease

- Cigarette smoking

- Hypercholesterolaemia

- Obesity

- Hypertension

- Sedentary lifestyle

- Familial history

- Personality type 'A' (competitive, forceful, difficulty in relaxing)

- Diabetes mellitus

- High sugar or fat diet

- In women: oral contraceptives and the menopause

Surgery is established therapy for patients with left main stem (Sang 1991) and proximal triple vessel (left, right, and circumflex coronary arteries) disease. It is also indicated for narrowing of any proximal coronary artery if symptoms are present and persist despite drug therapy.

Indications for emergency coronary artery surgery
1. Continued crescendo angina with maximum medical treatment
2. Failed angioplasty with acute symptoms

Surgery is considered for any patient who does not respond symptomatically to maximal medical therapy or who has unstable angina (angina at rest) which does not settle with optimal conservative treatment. The benefits in terms of prolonging survival are less certain except in cases of left main stem disease and patients who have already sustained damage to the heart muscle from previous heart attacks.

Surgery will not cure atherosclerotic disease; there is a recognized high incidence of graft occlusion and continuing coronary artery atheroma. However, surgery has been shown to improve quality of life.

Improvement in quality of life associated with coronary artery surgery

- Greater relief from angina

- Less limitation of activity

- Better exercise tolerance

- Less need for beta blockers and nitrates

The severity of symptoms is not always a reflection of severity of disease and assessment via coronary angiography is the best method of determining suitability for surgery.

Assessment by coronary angiography establishes
1. Location and severity of coronary occlusion(s)
2. Rate of flow through vessel distal to lesion(s)
3. The functional status of the left ventricle

Poor candidates have diffuse atherosclerotic disease with narrowed vessels and poor flow distal to the lesions. Those with poor left ventricular function (ejection fraction $<40\%$) have an increased risk of mortality.

Ejection fraction = Percentage of ventricular end diastolic volume ejected during systole (normal = $67\% \pm 8\%$)

Surgical technique

The vessel forming the graft may be either a vein (usually the long saphenous vein) or the internal mammary artery (IMA). If the vein is used it must be carefully harvested from the leg (below the knee is better as it is closer to the diameter of a coronary artery) and tested for patency by filling with normal saline or heparinized blood. Care must be taken to ensure that the vein is 'the right way round' and that any valves do not obstruct the flow of blood.

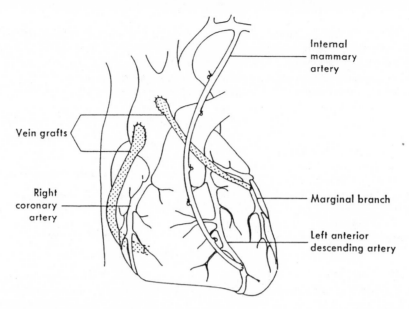

Fig. 7.3 Grafts to the heart including internal mammary artery (IMA) pedicle graft.

The proximal end of the vein graft is attached to the aorta and the distal end to a point on the coronary artery below the occlusive lesion. Grafts can be simple with end-to-side anastomosis (end of vessel to side of aorta or coronary artery), or sequential with a side-to-side anastomosis (side of vessel to side of coronary artery) followed by an end-to-side anastomosis to another artery.

If the IMA is used, it must be dissected and mobilized as a pedicled graft (i.e. the proximal end remains attached to the subclavian artery) to the coronary artery. This involves opening the pleura, freeing the IMA, and cauterizing off the intercostal artery branches. IMA grafts can also be either simple or sequential and can be either left (to the left coronary artery) or right (to the right or circumflex coronary artery).

The IMA has been shown to be superior in terms of long-term patency and degree of atherosclerosis compared with saphenous grafts.

Valve replacement

Valve replacement is usually carried out only for moderate or severe degrees of dysfunction (Table 7.2) because of the risk involved (between 1–4% mortality depending on the valve and pathology). Risk to the individual with endocarditis or a re-operation on the valve is greatly

increased. Although valve disease and dysfunction can involve any intracardiac valve, the lower pressures in the right side of the heart usually mean that tricuspid and pulmonary valve dysfunction are less significant. Surgery is more commonly performed on mitral and aortic valves, less frequently on the tricuspid valve, and rarely on the pulmonary valve. Mitral stenosis is sometimes repaired by valvotomy particularly in the child where replacement at an early age will require larger valves as the child grows. This carries a lower long-term risk than replacement.

Surgical technique

The technique of valve replacement utilizes cardiopulmonary bypass in the same way and for the same reasons as coronary artery bypass grafts. A median sternotomy incision is made. The approach to the mitral valve is through the left atrium and the approach to the aortic valve is via the ascending aorta. The dysfunctioning valve is removed and the annulus measured. A prosthetic valve of the appropriate size is sutured to the annulus and bypass is gradually discontinued as with coronary artery bypass grafts.

The degree of cardiac and other organ dysfunction is often greater in patients requiring mitral valve replacement and the mortality is correspondingly high.

Table 7.2 Clinical effects of valve dysfunction

Disorders requiring valve surgery	Causes	Dysfunction	Effects
Mitral stenosis	Rheumatic heart disease, bacterial endocarditis, calcification	Forward flow through the valve is impeded by fibrosed and contracted valve leaflets, commissures and chordae tendinae	*High left atrial pressures* produce left atrial dilatation, pulmonary hypertension, and right heart failure *Poor left ventricular filling* produces low cardiac output and systemic blood flow
Mitral regurgitation	*Acute*: endocarditis, chest trauma, myocardial infarction *Chronic*: rheumatic heart disease, calcification, myxomatous degeneration, left ventricular dilatation	*Chronic*: retrograde flow from ineffective valve closure is due to disease process causing thickening and contracture of cusps preventing closure. Ventricular dilatation stretches the valve so that the cusps do not meet *Acute*: retrograde flow is due to erosion or perforation of cusps or chordae by infection, and rupture of papillary muscle or chordae by trauma or myocardial infarction	*Chronic*: *high left atrial pressures* produce left atrial dilatation and, late on in the disease, pulmonary hypertension, and right heart failure *Regurgitation of ventricular outflow* produces low cardiac output with ventricular hypertrophy and dilatation *Acute*: insufficient time for compensatory mechanisms means that cardiac output falls dramatically, pulmonary oedema develops rapidly, and shock ensues
Aortic stenosis	Rheumatic fever, calcification of bicuspid valve (a common congenital cause)	Forward flow through the valve is impeded by fibrous contractures and commissure fusion as a result of disease process	*Impeded ventricular outflow* produces low cardiac output and decreased coronary perfusion *Ventricular hypertrophy* increases ventricular volume and pressure. This is reflected backwards and increases left atrial pressures with eventual pulmonary hypertension and right heart failure *Angina due to myocardial ischaemia* occurs as a result of poor coronary perfusion and increased myocardial oxygen demand from ventricular hypertrophy *Syncope* (fainting) occurs when cardiac output cannot increase to meet increased bodily demands (e.g. exercise) and cerebral perfusion is compromised
Aortic regurgitation	*Chronic*: rheumatic fever, aneurysm of the ascending aorta *Acute*: blunt chest trauma, ruptured ascending aortic aneurysm, infective endocarditis	*Chronic*: aneurysm causes annular dilatation so cusps are unable to meet, disease process thickens and retracts cusps, thus retrograde flow of blood occurs during systole *Acute*: ruptured ascending aortic aneurysm dilates and damages the valve. Infection erodes and ruptures the cusps	*Chronic*: *cardiac output decreases* and left ventricular volume and pressure increase *Blood regurgitates* back from the aortic root during diastole leading to widened pulse pressure *Left ventricular hypertrophy and dilatation* occur and eventual increases in left atrial pressure and pulmonary pressures lead to right heart failure *Acute*: *left ventricular failure* develops rapidly with acute development of pulmonary oedema

Cardiopulmonary bypass

In order for complex surgery on the heart to take place, myocardial contractions must cease. Circulatory flow and oxygenation must then be supported by an alternative mechanism. This mechanism is cardiopulmonary bypass (Fig. 7.4). The cardiopulmonary bypass machine consists of one or more pumps, an oxygenator, a bubble trap, reservoir, and filter.

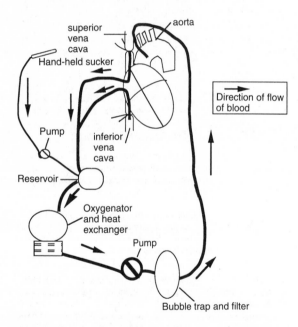

Fig. 7.4 Diagram showing the cardiopulmonary bypass circuit.

Oxygenators

The oxygenator is probably the part of the circuit most likely to cause complications or problems. The two main types of oxygenators in use are the bubble and the membrane oxygenator.

Bubble oxygenator

A high flow of oxygen is forced into a volume of blood producing bubbles which provide a high surface area and blood — gas interface across which gas exchange can take place. The movement of gas is from areas of high partial pressure to those of low partial pressure (see Chapter 3 for details). The bubbles are then removed by exposure to surface active silicone polymer which raises the surface tension of the bubbles causing them to collapse. Filtration and settling of the blood also contribute to clearance of the bubbles and oxygenated blood can then be returned to the patient.

Membrane oxygenator

Gas-permeable microporous polypropylene or silicone membranes separate the blood flow from gas flow. Venous blood is filtered and pumped through the sheets or hollow fibres of the membrane. Movement of gas across the membrane is governed by partial pressures and the solubility of the gas. Alteration of the concentration of oxygen in the gas flow will alter arterial oxygen tension and variation of rate of flow is used to regulate carbon dioxide levels.

Pump mechanisms

There are two types of pump, both of which maintain a constant output (i.e. non-pulsatile flow) and are non-occlusive to avoid direct damage to the blood. Pulsatile flow is more physiological with lower catecholamine release meaning reduced vasoconstriction and less fluid shifts; however, current mechanisms available are complex, costly and carry higher risks of blood damage.

The *roller pump* uses a head which almost occludes a flexible silicone portion of the bypass circuit in a circular motion thus compressing it and forcing blood forwards. This is the most frequently used type of pump in the United Kingdom.

The *centrifugal pump* uses the centrifugal force generated by a rapidly spinning head to suck blood through a circuit. It is thought to cause less damage to red blood cells and platelets but this has not as yet been proven.

Priming

The bypass circuit is primed with a 1–2l volume of balanced electrolyte solution such as Ringer's lactate solution. This produces a reduction in viscosity of the patient's blood which decreases intracapillary sludging related to the non-pulsatile low rate of flow. Complement activation is also decreased. The high added volume of fluid required to maintain a satisfactory circulation via the pump may mean considerable fluid retention by the patient. This is usually eliminated by the patient within 48 hours post-operatively, but can be the source of a number of fluid management problems if the patient has poor renal, pulmonary, or ventricular function.

Before attachment to the patient, the venous and arterial ends of the circuit are connected to form a closed system and the priming fluid is pumped round. This allows any adherent bubbles to be dislodged and gives time for the heat exchanger to raise the priming solution to a uniform temperature of 35–37 °C.

Initiating bypass

Prior to initiation, the patient is anticoagulated to an activated clotting time (ACT) of about 400 seconds using 300–400 iu/kg of heparin. The arterial cannula is then placed in the aorta (most commonly) and the arterial side of the bypass circuit is attached. Venous cannulae are then inserted either into the superior and inferior vena cava or into the right atrium. All venous blood is then siphoned slowly into the bypass circuit and the arterial pump is started to return oxygenated blood to the aorta.

At the same time the patient is cooled to 24–32 °C using the heat exchanger. Once the patient reaches the desired temperature, the ascending aorta is clamped and fibrillatory arrest is induced. In longer procedures cold cardioplegic arrest may be used. Cold cardioplegia is a hyperkalaemic electrolyte solution cooled to 4 °C and infused directly into the coronary arteries. It will cause immediate asystole lasting approximately 30 minutes and protect the myocardium during the ischaemic period of aortic cross-clamping. Infusion will need to be repeated if there is any sign of returning electrical activity or in any case every 15–30 minutes. Cardioplegic arrest of up to 60 minutes is usually well tolerated but prolongation will cause tissue acidosis, subendocardial necrosis, and compromised cardiac performance.

Withdrawal from cardiopulmonary bypass

Once surgery is completed, the patient is re-warmed to 37 °C using the heat exchanger. Air is vented from the heart chambers and aortic root and the aortic cross-clamp is removed. The coronary arteries are perfused and the myocardium is warmed by the circulating blood. A cardiac rhythm may resume spontaneously or ventricular fibrillation may occur which requires defibrillation. Occasionally, pacing may be necessary to initiate an effective rhythm. Pulmonary ventilation is re-started and the rate of cardiopulmonary bypass is reduced. There is a period when blood is passing through the pulmonary circulation and the bypass circuit and the patient's response is assessed. If the cardiac function is adequate bypass is discontinued and the cannulae removed. Heparinization is then reversed with protamine sulphate and the chest is closed.

Protective mechanisms employed during bypass
1. *Hypothermia* — decreases tissue oxygen demand and allows lower rates of flow for bypass, protects cerebral tissue, localized myocardial cooling protects during cross-clamp time.

2. *Anticoagulation* — prevents extravascular coagulation from foreign surface contact.

3. *Haemodilution* — avoidance of extreme intravascular–interstitial fluid shifts during bypass due to almost isotonic perfusate, reduction in blood viscosity reduces peripheral vascular resistance and improves capillary perfusion particularly during hypothermia, reduces sludging of blood components around the bypass circuit and decreases the likelihood of microemboli.

Table 7.3 shows the physiological effects on the patient of cardiopulmonary bypass intervention.

Bypass flow rates
2.4l/min/m^2 to maintain oxygenation at 37 °C
1.2l/min/m^2 to maintain oxygenation at 25 °C

These are the minimum rates and there is uncertainty regarding optimal local blood flow, in particular, cerebral

---

Closure of the chest and completion of surgery

If pacing is thought to be required post-operatively, epicardial pacing wires will be placed on the ventricle and brought out through the chest wall conventionally to the left of the sternal incision. If atrial pacing wires are also required these will be placed on the epicardial surface of the atria and brought out to the right of the sternal incision.

The pericardium is usually left open to help drainage and reduce the risk of cardiac tamponade.

Chest drains are placed in the pericardial space and under the mediastinum. They are brought out through separate incisions at the base of the sternal incision.

Table 7.3 Functional physiological differences during cardiopulmonary bypass and their effects on the patient

Function	Effect	Patient problem
Non-pulsatile low pressure flow	Activates baroreceptors invoking release of ADH and the renin–angiotensin response	Fluid retention Movement of blood from venous reservoirs such as the splanchnic bed
	Increased circulating catecholamines and increased SVR	Peripheral vasoconstriction, increased likelihood of hypertension post-operatively
	Altered glucose transport across cell membrane	Mild hyperglycaemia
Blood contact with foreign surfaces: tubing, oxygenator, filters, and roller pumps	Complement activation and release of other vasoactive substances leading to increased vascular permeability	Fluid shift into interstitial space, loss of circulating blood volume
	Platelet activation of intrinsic clotting pathway and release of vasoactive substances	Risk of microemboli
	Platelet damage with induced thrombocytopenia and altered function	Reduction in platelet coagulability and decrease by 50–70% of platelet numbers Increased risk of post-operative bleeding
Hypothermia	Increased SVR	Peripheral vasoconstriction
	Decrease of normal tissue oxygen requirements Increased blood viscosity but compensated for by haemodilution	
	Impairment of cellular transport mechanisms and pancreatic islet cell release of insulin	Hyperglycaemia
	Possible mild depression of cardiac output and a transient sinus bradycardia	A reduced cardiac output and a slower heart rate may occur which corrects as the patient warms There may be oliguria due to decreased renal perfusion
Haemodilution	Improved capillary flow during hypothermia due to decreased viscosity and decreased shear rates for red blood cells	Reduced haemoglobin and haematocrit
	Increased fluid load, much of which may move into the interstitium due to the effects of vasoactive substances (see above)	Patient may remain fluid-overloaded post-operatively Polyuria post-operatively
Absence or reduction of pulmonary ventilation	Reduced alveolar distension is insufficient to activate surfactant	Increased risk of atelectasis
Absence of pulmonary perfusion	Sequestration of blood in pulmonary microcirculation and breakdown of capillary walls	Increased risk of microthrombi, pulmonary shunting, and interstitial oedema

A pleural drain or drains may be necessary if the pleural space is entered during the procedure.

Haemostasis is achieved and sternal closure using stainless steel wires or sutures is carried out. The skin is closed and dressings applied.

Care of the patient following surgery

During closure of the chest and transfer from theatre the patient may have become less stable. A degree of urgency is therefore necessary in ensuring that the patient is attached to the ventilator, baseline observations and assessment are carried out, and any haemodynamic or respiratory problems are dealt with promptly.

Preparation of bed space for receiving the patient
1. Carry out safety checks and equip bedspace (see Chapter 2)
2. Blood scales and colloid such as hetastarch, gelofusine, etc.
3. Labels for drains, drain bottles, and infusions
4. Ready access to drugs including: sedatives, analgesics, vasodilators, inotropes, potassium, frusemide

---

Immediate interventions

(Note. These are usually performed by two nurses to allow speedy assessment of the patient.)

1. Connect or transfer from portable monitoring — priorities are ECG, arterial line, CVP (check readings and inform medical staff immediately if any problems).

2. Attach the patient to the ventilator after checking the patient's tidal volume, respiratory rate and F_iO_2 settings with the anaesthetist.

3. Auscultate the patient's chest for air entry (see Chapter 3) to assess ET tube placement, evidence of pneumothorax, lung collapse, and possible build-up of secretions.

4. Label chest drains and bottles, mark level of drainage, and check suction on prevacuumed bottles, or attach to suction.

5. Measure urine meter contents and discard into collection bag.

6. Attach maintenance fluid (usually 5% glucose) and check existing drug infusions for dilution and rate.

7. Insert rectal or other core temperature probe and adjust bed clothing to ensure adequate covering for re-warming. Use may be made of warming blankets such as the Bairhugger or space blankets.

8. Attach peripheral temperature probe.

9. Assess the patient for conscious level and signs of pain (see Chapter 9).

10. Check arterial blood gas, electrolytes, and haemoglobin at about 10–15 min after patient is attached to ventilator, unless the patient's condition requires earlier measurement.

11. Perform-12 lead ECG and request chest X-ray.

Complications following cardiac surgery

Patients are usually transferred directly to the ICU following surgery where they are closely monitored and ensuing problems can be dealt with promptly. This is a period of stabilization and rapid recognition of any problems with immediate intervention will often prevent major complications arising.

Goals of post-cardiac surgery care
- Maintain good levels of oxygenation and carbon dioxide
- Haemodynamic stability and adequate organ perfusion
- Maintain haemostasis
- Re-warming without significant problems
- Prevent/reduce atelectasis
- Prevent/reduce cerebral dysfunction
- Provide adequate analgesia
- Maintain fluid and electrolyte balance
- Appropriate and problem-free extubation

Haemodynamic instability

Problem

Hypotension due to either hypovolaemia, arrhythmias, poor left ventricular contractility, or tamponade. Iatrogenic hypotension due to drugs such as vasodilators, beta blockers, or sedatives may also occur.

Goal: generally, the aim is to maintain a systolic pressure >90 mmHg but this may be altered by the individual patient's operative course. If the patient has had saphenous vein grafts, low perfusion pressures during diastole may allow collapse of the non-muscular vein wall and this may cause occlusion if prolonged. More importantly, low mean arterial pressures will reduce vital organ perfusion, such as to brain and kidneys, increasing the risk of cerebral and renal damage.

Management

If CVP or PA pressures are low, rapid volume replacement is given usually as a bolus of fluid. The pressures are rechecked and according to patient response, more fluid is given as necessary.

If CVP or PA pressures are normal or raised following fluid replacement, and hypotension continues, intervention is aimed at improving myocardial contractility with inotropes (see Chapter 5 for details).

If the patient has concurrent arrhythmias intervention is aimed at treating these (see below).

Cardiac tamponade is discussed as a separate problem.

Problem

Hypertension due to:- previous history of hypertension, increased catecholamine release following cardiopulmonary bypass (see above for details), pain and anxiety, hypothermia, or unknown aetiology. Hypertension is a common problem in those suffering from atherosclerotic disease and can be serious postoperatively. High systolic pressures may cause leakage and bleeding at suture sites and even rupture of graft anastomoses.

Goal: maintain the systolic pressure <140 mmHg although this may need to be lower in patients with bleeding problems or friable graft tissue. Different surgeons may stipulate different upper limits of systolic pressure.

Management

It is important to rule out causes, such as pain or anxiety, before using vasodilator therapy. Patient comfort and level of analgesia should be assessed regularly and pain relieved as per unit policy. Hypovolaemia should be corrected prior to the use of vasodilators and adjusted while vasodilatation takes place.

Glyceryl trinitrate (GTN) is usually the first choice for reducing blood pressure but in some circumstances sodium nitroprusside is preferred. Both drugs are delivered as an intravenous infusion which is titrated to maintain systolic blood pressure between 100 and 140 mmHg.

Unless there is a previous history, hypertension is usually short-lived and vasodilators can be weaned off by the following day. In some cases, oral drugs, such as nifedipine or hydralazine, may be necessary to control blood pressure for a longer period.

Arrhythmias

A number of factors contribute to an increased likelihood of arrhythmias in the post-operative period. These are:

(1) the myocardium is more irritable due to handling and surgical trauma,

(2) electrolyte imbalances (especially potassium and magnesium) induced by cardioplegia, fluid shifts, and renal dysfunction,

(3) conduction defects are more common in aortic valve surgery and VSD closure due to the proximity of surgery to the conduction system and atrial fibrillation is common in mitral valve disease

(4) the heart is less able to cope with added stress due to the underlying pathology.

Management

The causes and management of specific arrhythmias are outlined in Table 7.4.

Cardiac tamponade

Compression of the myocardium occurs when blood (or other fluid) accumulates around the heart. This impedes venous return and reduces contractility by restricting ventricular filling, thus reducing stroke volume and cardiac output. Stroke volume is dependent on preload, afterload, and myocardial contractility (this is discussed fully in Chapter 6).

Following cardiac surgery, tamponade is most likely to occur as a result of pericardial chest drain blockage through clotting. If drains are patent and recent brisk bleeding has not suddenly ceased then tamponade is unlikely. Most patients have their pericardium left open

Table 7.4 Causes and management of specific arrhythmias

Sinus tachycardia

Causes: hypovolaemia, catecholamine release (from surgery, from pain and anxiety), possible side-effect of inotropic drugs

Problems: decreased ventricular diastolic filling time compromises cardiac output, increased myocardial oxygen demand increases cardiac work, decreased coronary artery perfusion time reduces coronary artery flow

Management: first, correction of any underlying cause (i.e. give fluid if hypovolaemic, analgesia if in pain, etc.) Review any inotropic support if necessary

Ventricular ectopics

Causes: electrolyte imbalance (principally potassium), hypoxia, surgical trauma, myocardial ischaemia, catecholamine release, occasionally mechanical irritation from chest drains or pulmonary artery catheter if used

Problems: increased risk of ventricular arrhythmias, reduced cardiac output due to poor filling time for premature beat

Management: correct any underlying cause. Keep the serum potassium above 4.5 mmol/l. If ectopics are frequent or close to previous complexes then magnesium, lignocaine, or amiodarone (if there is depressed myocardial function) may be considered

Ventricular tachycardia and fibrillation

Causes: hypoxia, myocardial ischaemia, electrolyte imbalance, myocardial irritability from surgical trauma

Problems: loss of cardiac output

Management: immediate defibrillation with DC shock of 200 J externally or 5–10 J internally

Supraventricular tachycardias (SVT)

Causes: myocardial irritability post-surgical trauma, myocardial ischaemia, possible side-effect of inotropic drugs

Problems: decreased ventricular diastolic filling time with reduced cardiac output, increased myocardial oxygen demand increases cardiac workload, decreased coronary artery perfusion time reduces coronary artery flow

Management: correct any underlying cause. Keep the serum potassium above 4.5 mmol/l. Amiodarone, verapamil, adenosine, magnesium, and DC cardioversion may all be considered

Atrial fibrillation and flutter

Causes: in patients following valve surgery long-standing atrial dilatation and stretching induces atrial fibrillation, hypoxia, poor coronary perfusion and myocardial ischaemia

Problems: loss of 'atrial kick' (top-up filling of the ventricle during atrial systole), if the ventricular rate is also rapid then problems as for SVT

Management: amidarone and digoxin. Keep the serum potassium above 4.5 mmol/l. DC cardioversion if the ventricular rate is rapid and blood pressure is compromised

Bradyarrhythmias (junctional rhythm, atrioventricular blocks and bundle branch blocks)

Causes: depression of the conduction system cells by cardioplegia, myocardial ischaemia, injury to nodes and conduction pathways by surgical intervention, sutures, or oedema. More common in valve surgery due to the proximity of the aortic and mitral valves to the conduction system

Problems: possible decreased cardiac output, increased ventricular filling which may overload the compromised ventricle

Management: atropine bolus and isoprenaline infusion if cardiac output is decreased. If an epicardial pacing wire is *in situ* pacing would initially be used. A transvenous pacing wire may be inserted if necessary.

Sinus bradycardia

Causes: pre-operative use of beta blockers, increased vagal tone

Problems: as above

Management: if the cardiac output is compromised then management is as above. However, isoprenaline may be used prior to atropine unless the cause is increased vagal tone to decrease the risk of tamponade. (See Fig. 7.5 for the effects of cardiac tamponade.)

Management

Support of cardiac output using fluid resuscitation with or without inotropes is necessary until surgical intervention has decompressed the heart. In the acute tamponade, surgery will be carried out at once at the patient's bedside (see below for details). However, if time allows, patients are less likely to suffer complications if they are returned to theatre.

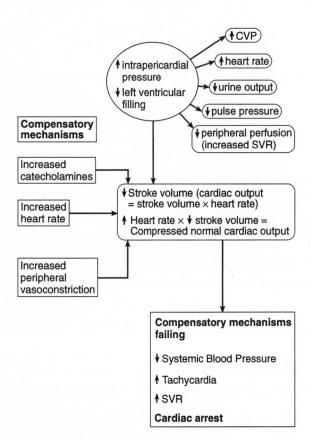

Fig. 7.5 The effects of cardiac tamponade.

Alteration in fluid and electrolyte balance

The total body fluid increases during cardiopulmonary bypass due to pump priming fluid, haemodilution, increased ADH secretion, and activation of the renin–angiotensin–aldosterone response to low perfusion.

However, much of this fluid is actually interstitial rather than intravascular due to alterations in capillary membrane permeability by vasoactive substances. These are released possibly as a response to contact with the foreign surfaces of the bypass circuit or to organ hypoperfusion. There may also be a reduction in colloid osmotic (oncotic) pressure due to haemodilution which will contribute to loss of fluid into the extravascular spaces. The patient may have a positive fluid balance of up to 5 litres and as much as 20% of this may be extracellular. In spite of this excess, it is still possible for the patient to have an intravascular volume deficit which must be corrected in order to prevent a decreased cardiac output and hypotension. This deficit can be further affected by vasodilatation during warming and blood loss.

Sodium levels may be raised due to the effect of the renin–angiotensin–aldosterone response (see Chapter 8) during bypass and it is usual to give only dextrose 5% as crystalloid replacement fluid.

Hypokalaemia is a frequent problem due to haemodilution, use of diuretics, and the renin–angiotensin–aldosterone response (see Chapter 8).

Occasionally, hyperkalaemia is a problem if the patient develops acute renal failure or receives large amounts of cardioplegia

In some units, magnesium is given routinely as there may be significant loss due to diuresis and levels may fall due to haemodilution.

Management

Intravascular fluid volume is maintained using colloid or blood according to the level of the patient's haemoglobin. In most units, haemoglobin is maintained at 10 g/dl however some units allow it to drop to 8.5 g/dl before giving blood.

Crystalloid infusions are generally kept to a maintenance level to avoid further extravascular fluid load.

The CVP or PA wedge pressures are used to monitor intravascular volume status and colloid/blood is given to maintain blood pressure and urine output as required.

Sodium and potassium levels are monitored regularly and potassium is given via central venous access to maintain levels of 4.0–4.5 mmol/l.

Bleeding

Bleeding post-operatively occurs as a result of either incomplete surgical haemostasis or coagulopathy. The main causes of a post cardiopulmonary bypass coagulopathy are:

(i) Inadequate heparin reversal

The heparin antagonist protamine sulphate is usually administered at the end of cardiopulmonary bypass. The dose given is based on the activated clotting time (ACT). This may be inaccurate or insufficient in view of 'heparin rebound'

(ii) The phenomenon of 'heparin rebound'

Heparin that has been sequestrated in the tissues during CPB is mobilized during warming and vasodilatation. This has a delayed anticoagulant effect and further protamine may be necessary.

(iii) Consumption of clotting factors and platelets during bypass

CPB can cause mechanical destruction of platelets due to activation from foreign surface contact. Normally, the platelet count falls to 50–70% of baseline on initiation of CPB but returns to normal within 24 hours due to release of platelets from the spleen into the circulation. Consumption of clotting factors is also a problem on bypass and this can be accentuated by haemodilution post-bypass.

(iv) Platelet dysfunction

Circulating platelets may be damaged due to the effects of passage through roller pumps and filters. Pre-operative use of platelet inhibitory drugs, such as aspirin and dipyridamole, may add to the effect. Post-operative platelet counts are usually low but are not usually replaced unless the patient is actively bleeding or they fall below 50 000/mm^3.

Management

Protamine is given in the first instance if the ACT is prolonged (> 160 s). Tranexamic acid (an antifibrinolytic agent) is also used to support clotting. Clotting factors in the form of fresh frozen plasma are given to replace those consumed.

If the platelet count is low (< 50 000/mm^3), if there is active bleeding, or if the patient has recently been taking non-steroidal anti-inflammatory drugs, platelets are transfused.

Hypertension is controlled (see above).

Some advocate that positive end expiratory pressure (PEEP) of between 10 and 15 cmH$_2$O should be added. The theory behind this is that increasing intrathoracic pressure will: (a) tamponade small oozing blood vessels if this is the cause; and (b) decrease venous return in hypertensive patients thus reducing blood pressure. Its efficacy has not been fully established and it is not the practice in many units.

If bleeding continues at > 150 ml/h for 3 hours or > 400 ml over 1 hour then the patient is usually taken back to theatre for re-exploration.

Pulmonary dysfunction

Post-operative pulmonary complications tend to occur in patients with a prior history of dysfunction. It is therefore important to ascertain any risk factors during pre-operative assessment. Arterial blood gases are not routinely taken pre-operatively but provide a useful baseline in the high-risk patient. Patients who smoke are more likely to have thick, tenacious sputum, and atelectasis and therefore require more physiotherapy, humidification, and suction over the post-operative period. The period of apnoea during bypass can cause alveolar collapse and retention of secretions. This is partly due to the period without ventilation and partly due to the decreased release of surfactant which is activated by alveolar distension. The sequestration of blood in the pulmonary microcapillaries can cause microthrombi and potential shunting. It may also contribute to interstitial oedema which occurs as a result of bypass complement activation causing capillary leak.

Management

It is usual to ventilate patients for a period of time postoperatively to allow the high levels of narcotic analgesia and anaesthesia to wear off and to promote re-expansion of alveoli. Some fit patients can be extubated immediately without ill-effect; however, the majority of patients appear to benefit from a period of ventilation. This allows adequate levels of analgesia to be given without fear of compromising respiration and reduces cardiac work during optimalization of the circulation and re-warming.

Some units recommend the use of 5 cmH$_2$O PEEP during this period.

Once the patient is awake and co-operative, weaning on to a T-piece is carried out and the patient's ability to breathe spontaneously is assessed. Clinical assessment of respiratory function and arterial blood gases give the best guidance and once these are within normal limits the patient is extubated. Following extubation, it is essential that the patient continues to breath deeply and cough in order to prevent collapse of the lung bases and sputum retention. Adequate analgesia should be given to permit this and to allow turning and movement. The patient should be encouraged to hold his chest on either side of the sternal incision with his hands to give support during coughing.

Alternatively, splinting with a pillow may be of benefit. Frequent intervention by nursing staff in encouraging deep breathing and coughing is a vital part of postoperative support as is chest physiotherapy.

Cerebral dysfunction

Protection of cerebral function during the low perfusion pressures of CPB is promoted by hypothermia (reduction of cerebral O_2 requirements) and haemodilution (improved capillary flow at low temperatures). However, post-operative neurological sequelae include short-term memory loss, poor concentration, focal deficits, confusion, cerebrovascular accident, and acute psychosis.

In general, cerebral dysfunction is related to two factors: (1) inadequate perfusion; (2) embolism of air or particulate matter.

The risk of cerebral dysfunction increases with: (1) increasing age: (2) prolonged bypass time, (3) pre-existing carotid or cerebrovascular atherosclerotic disease; (4) valve disease, when calcified material may break loose during manipulation, especially with atrial fibrillation (atrial clots are common because of sluggish blood flow).

Management

Identification of those at risk and frequent neurological assessment will allow early detection of neurological dysfunction. Early intervention to maintain blood pressure and oxygenation to ensure cerebral perfusion and tissue oxygenation is an important part of nursing observation.

Renal dysfunction

There is an increased risk of renal failure associated with CPB. This is due to decreased renal blood flow during bypass, hypotension, hypoperfusion, and free haemoglobin resulting from red blood cell damage and cellular debris damaging the tubules. Increased risk factors include bypass time and pre-existing renal dysfunction. Haemolysis of red blood cells may occur during bypass and haematuria may be seen.

Patients may be polyuric post-operatively as the excess fluid associated with the pump priming is removed. Oliguria can also occur as a result of high levels of antidiuretic hormone (ADH) secreted in response to the low perfusion pressure and non-pulsatile flow of CPB. The renal vasoconstrictive effect is potentiated by high catecholamine levels and renin-angiotensin–aldosterone release. Hypovolaemia, hypotension, and low cardiac output in the peri-operative period may all contribute to oliguria.

Management

Correction of contributory factors, such as hypovolaemia, hypotension, and poor cardiac output, is the first step. Dopamine is usually infused at the 'renal' dose of up to 2.5 µg/kg/min to promote renal perfusion (see Chapter 8). Once the contributory factors are corrected and dopamine has been started if the patient remains oliguric then small doses of diuretic, such as frusemide (10–20 mg), may be required to stimulate urine output.

Pain and anxiety

Pain is an individual and subjective experience and the level of pain perceived by patients following cardiac surgery will vary according to understanding, culture, pain threshold, and perception of the pain experience. Factors that affect perception of the pain experience include anxiety and fatigue. Whatever the level, all patients will experience some pain following surgery related to either the sternal incision and rib spreading, the chest drains, or the leg wound if they have a saphenous vein graft. Patients who have an internal mammary artery graft may experience increased pain and discomfort due to the need for further incisions into the parietal pleura and greater stretching of the intercostal muscles (Mailis et al. 1989).

Pain following surgical incision should be differentiated from ischaemic chest pain.

Pain is an important factor in initiating the sympathetic response of increased catecholamine production, vasoconstriction, raised blood pressure, and tachycardia. Vasoconstriction and tachycardia will increase cardiac work and decrease coronary artery perfusion time neither of which are ideal for the post-operative recovery of cardiac function. Pain relief is therefore an important (as well as humane) intervention and should be a major priority of nursing care.

Management

Physiological indicators of pain and distress, such as raised blood pressure, tachycardia, and sweating, are the criteria used to assess pain levels when the patient first returns from theatre. Later, as the anaesthetic wears off, patients may be able to respond sufficiently to indicate whether they have pain or not. Once the patient is able to respond, the use of a visual analogue is helpful so that patients can rate their pain and efficacy of analgesia can be evaluated.

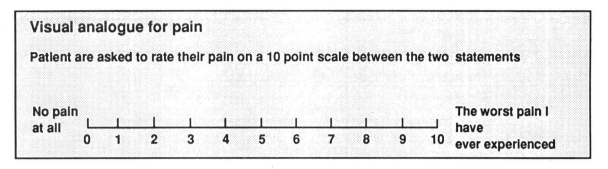

Visual analogue for pain

Patient are asked to rate their pain on a 10 point scale between the two statements

No pain at all | 0 1 2 3 4 5 6 7 8 9 10 | The worst pain I have ever experienced

Intervention

Opiates are the analgesia of choice in the immediate post-operative phase. The secondary effect of suppression of respiratory drive may aid mechanical ventilation until patients are stable and ready to be weaned.

Following extubation, oral analgesia is then preferred as there is less risk of respiratory depression. However, intravenous opiates are still required prior to chest drain removal (Carson *et al.* 1994). Usually, patients are able to take oral analgesia as soon as they can comfortably drink following extubation. The choice of analgesic depends on individual unit policy.

Patient-controlled analgesia is a method used in some units of ensuring patients receive the levels of analgesia they require, when they wish and can be of benefit in the post-operative period. Some recent work suggests that the use of relaxation techniques and music therapy may relieve anxiety which can affect patients' perception of their pain (Barnason *et al.* 1995).

Evaluation

One of the most important and often the most neglected nursing aspect of pain relief is the need to evaluate the effectiveness of analgesia (Tittle and McMillan 1994; Puntillo 1994; Gujol 1994). Again, this is best done using a visual analogue scale and asking the patient to rate their pain. Unless they are obviously asleep and comfortable, further questioning of the intubated patient once analgesia has had time to take effect will indicate whether pain has been relieved.

Psychological disturbance and intellectual dysfunction

Symptoms range from short-term memory loss and poor concentration to anxiety and depression. In the extreme situation, postcardiotomy psychosis may occur. This has been described as a range of behaviour in the post-operative period varying from confusion and disorienta-

tion to visual and auditory hallucinations, delusions, and paranoia (Quinless *et al.* 1985).

Most patients will only experience these symptoms temporarily and may be fully functional by 6 to 8 weeks after surgery (North 1988).

Some factors, such as length of perfusion time, hypotension, and prolonged anaesthesia, have been associated with an increased incidence of postcardiotomy psychosis.

Management

One of the most important aspects of management is giving the patient pre-operative information about the phenomenon so that they are able to recognize and cope with the problems involved. The transient nature of these phenomena should be emphasized. The patient's family should also be warned about this and the possibility of depression and anxiety in the post-operative period. In the true psychotic state, patients do not have insight into their perception of reality and management requires sedation and re-orientation over a prolonged period.

Emergency re-opening of the chest

This procedure is carried out for the following reasons:

(i) the patient deteriorates and does not respond to fluid challenge and inotropes,

(ii) there is a sudden substantial blood loss ($\geqslant$ 500 ml drained in minutes).

If possible, the patient is returned to theatre but even a short journey can be hazardous for an unstable patient.

Sudden loss of cardiac output will also require chest opening and internal (manual) cardiac compression. This is because differentiation between left ventricular dysfunction and cardiac tamponade can be difficult as both cause reduced cardiac output and systemic blood pressure with increased heart rate and central venous pressure. Pulmonary artery wedge pressure and left atrial pressure are also raised.

Chest re-opening may be necessary to determine whether the problem is tamponade or ventricular dysfunction. External cardiac compression is fairly inefficient in the patient with a sternal split and it is difficult to maintain adequate tissue perfusion in the presence of cardiac tamponade. There may also be added trauma caused by the force of massage leading to disruption of suture lines or possible damage to grafts or valves themselves.

Indications for emergency chest re-opening

- Cardiac tamponade

- Cardiac arrest

- Left ventricular dysfunction

- Overwhelming bleeding from disruption of suture lines

Sudden arterial bleeding may occur from suture-line leakage or complete rupture of the anastomosis. If the rate of bleeding exceeds the capacity of the drains then tamponade will add to the hypovolaemic low output problem.

Management

In the first instance, the patient's cardiac function should be supported with colloid blood infusion ±inotropes as appropriate.

Any other contributory factors should be excluded or corrected. These include, hypoxia due to hypoventilation, pneumothorax, or inadequate oxygen delivery and acidosis due to the above or poor cardiac function. Chest drains should be milked or irrigated to make sure they are clear.

Chest re-opening in the ICU

Although this is an emergency, it is important that the atmosphere remains calm. Initially, the equipment necessary for the procedure should be brought to the patient's bedside (Table 7.5).

Havng made the decision to re-open the patient's chest in the ICU, the surgeon will start to scrub up. The necessary equipment is brought to the bedside and the area cleared as far as possible. If necessary, patients in adjoining bed areas may be moved over to allow sufficient space at the bedside. The area should be effectively screened.

Table 7.5   Equipment for re-opening the chest in the ICU

- Thoracotomy set (including wire cutters)
- Theatre light
- Extra suction
- Diathermy
- Defibrillator
- Internal paddles for defibrillator
- Gowns, gloves, masks, hats
- Skin preparation such as povidone-iodine or chlorhexidine
- Drains and drainage bottles
- Sutures, sternal wires, epicardial pacing wires
- Emergency drugs: adrenaline, atropine, isoprenaline, calcium, lignocaine

Procedure

The surgeon may attempt to relieve tamponade immediately by opening the sternal incision at the base of the xiphoid process and dissecting the substernal space up to the edge of the pericardium with his finger. It may be possible to release the pressure by drainage of a collection of blood in this area sufficient to stabilize the patient for return to theatre. If this is not possible, or the patient does not respond, then re-entry to the chest must be carried out in the ICU.

The skin and soft tissue sutures are divided and the sternal wires cut with wire cutters. The ribs can then be spread using a retractor and the heart exposed. If the pericardium was closed during surgery it is re-opened. Access to the heart for internal cardiac compression is then possible and the circulation can be well supported while a bleeding point is located.

Internal cardiac compression is far more efficient for maintaining coronary perfusion, cerebral blood flow, and mean systemic arterial pressure than external cardiac massage (Grishkin 1988).

Causes of ventricular dysfunction

Mechanical

- kinked or occluded bypass grafts

- malfunctioning valve prosthesis

Functional

- coronary vasospasm

- ischaemic mitral regurgitation

Metabolic

- hypoxaemia

- acidosis

The patient may have to go back on cardiopulmonary bypass in order to correct the problem. This will either occur in theatre with the surgeon supporting the circulation by internal cardiac compression on the way or, rarely, in the ICU.

Once the problem has been corrected the patient may require an intra-aortic balloon pump or left ventricular assist support until his/her cardiac function recovers from the insult.

Survival following chest re-opening is related to the underlying cause. Fairman and Edmunds (1981) found that 60% of patients who had chest re-opening performed for bleeding or tamponade survived whereas those who required chest re-opening for circulatory support for ventricular dysfunction did not.

Disadvantages of chest re-opening in the ICU

- Increased risk of wound infection

- Poor lighting and limited equipment

- Often performed in emergency by junior surgeons

- Absence of trained theatre staff to assist

The technique of internal (manual) cardiac compression

1. The ventricles are compressed between the palms of the hands.
2. The heart is compressed between the palm of one hand and the undersurface of the sternum (left anterior thoracotomy approach only)

The heart should be kept in its anatomical position to avoid kinking of the venae cavae and arteries

---

Mechanical cardiac assist devices

Intra-aortic balloon pump (IABP)

The intra-aortic balloon pump was first introduced clinically in 1967 by Kantrowitz and associates. It is designed to improve coronary artery perfusion by inflating during diastole and to reduce left ventricular afterload by deflating during systole.

Description

A central catheter with a 40 ml polyurethane balloon, approximately 25 cm (10 inches) long, is inserted into the femoral artery, either percutaneously or directly

during cardiac surgery and advanced into the descending thoracic aorta. Positioning of the balloon in the thoracic aorta is important. Optimal positioning is approximately 2 cm below the left subclavian artery and as high above the femoral bifurcation as is possible. The bottom of the balloon is then proximal to the renal arteries.

The catheter of the balloon is attached via a luer lock fitting to the console of the pump. This shuttles helium (or carbon dioxide) under pressure through the catheter into the balloon which is inflated. The helium is then sucked out of the balloon by the creation of a vacuum by the pump. This mechanism allows for a very fast response to triggers for inflation and deflation. Some types of balloon also have a central lumen which allows monitoring of aortic pressures from the tip of the balloon.

Triggers for the pump cycle

(1) The standard trigger mechanism is the R wave of the patient's ECG. This will cue inflation of the balloon following systole. Timing of inflation and deflation requires adjustment and will be discussed below.

(2) Systolic arterial pressure may be used if the R wave is unable to trigger properly.

(3) Pacing spikes may also be used to trigger inflation.

(4) Some pumps have an automatic facility for use during cardiac arrest or to provide pulsatile flow during cardiopulmonary bypass.

Components of the IABP

- Intra-aortic ballon

- Monitoring system

- Trigger mechanism

- Gas drive system

Indications for use of the IABP

The two most common uses for the IABP are support of the failing heart in cardiogenic shock and weaning from cardiopulmonary bypass.

The role of the IABP is to provide short-term support allowing the heart to recover from the myocardial infarction, cardiac surgery, or coronary angioplasty. It cannot be considered as a long-term solution although there are cases of use for as long as 46 days (Lazar *et al.* 1992).

Indications for use of the IABP
1. Cardiogenic shock
2. Weaning from cardiopulmonary bypass
3. Refractory ventricular failure
4. Septic shock
5. Unstable refractory angina
6. Impending infarction
7. Mechanical complications due to acute myocardial infarction (i.e. ventricular septal defect, mitrial regurgitation or papillary muscle rupture)
8. Ischaemia related to intractable ventricular arrhythmias
9. Cardiac support for high-risk general surgical patients
10. Support and stabilization during coronary angiography and angioplasty
11. Intra-operative pulsatile flow generation

Contraindications for use of the IABP

(1) Aortic valve incompetence
The most obvious contraindication to the IABP is an incompetent aortic valve. If the aortic valve allows regurgitation of blood flow, this will be compounded by balloon inflation during diastole adding to ventricular work.

(2) Aortic aneurysm
The movement of the balloon in the aorta would be likely to dislodge aneurysmal debris leading to emboli and possibly cause rupture of the aneurysm

(3) Previous aortofemoral or aortoiliac bypass grafts
Insertion of the balloon would be impossible.

(4) Severe peripheral vascular disease
Insertion of the balloon would be difficult and there would be an increased risk of occlusion of the vessel and dislodgement of emboli.

Underlying physiology

In the failing heart, maintenance of cardiac output requires an increased myocardial oxygen demand. This increased demand cannot be met by coronary artery perfusion and tissue hypoxia occurs. Tissue hypoxia is particularly apparent in the myocardial tissues due to the low level of oxygen extraction reserve. The normal level of oxygen saturation in the coronary sinus (venous blood drained from the heart) is 30–40% which leaves little room for increasing oxygen extraction as a method of compensation. Cardiac output continues to fall and a degenerative spiral of cardiogenic shock develops.

The main goals of therapy for a failing left ventricle are to:

(1) decrease left ventricular workload,

(2) improve coronary artery perfusion.

Both of these goals can be achieved mechanically using the intra-aortic balloon pump (IABP).

Decreased left ventricular workload

A major determinant of left ventricular workload is afterload. Afterload is defined as the amount of wall tension which must be generated by the ventricle to raise intraventricular pressure sufficiently to overcome impedance to ejection. Production of the force required to overcome afterload consumes the greatest amount of oxygen during the cardiac cycle. Thus, decreasing impedance will reduce left ventricular workload and myocardial oxygen consumption.

Impedance to ejection is generated by the aortic valve, the aortic end diastolic pressure, and vascular resistance. The aortic valve provides a fairly constant beat to beat impedance to ejection and cannot be manipulated. The aortic end diastolic pressure and the vascular resistance can be manipulated to decrease afterload.

The IABP decreases aortic end diastolic pressure by deflating the aortic balloon immediately prior to systole. This lowers aortic end diastolic pressure and therefore reduces impedance to left ventricular ejection. Left ventricular workload is reduced, left ventricular emptying is increased and myocardial oxygen consumption is decreased. (See Fig. 7.6.)

Improved coronary artery perfusion

Coronary artery perfusion pressure is the difference between aortic diastolic pressure and myocardial wall tension. Myocardial wall tension is greatly reduced during diastole and 80% of coronary blood flow occurs at this time. Reduction of afterload allows increased left ventricular emptying which means that myocardial wall tension during diastole is reduced allowing increased coronary flow.

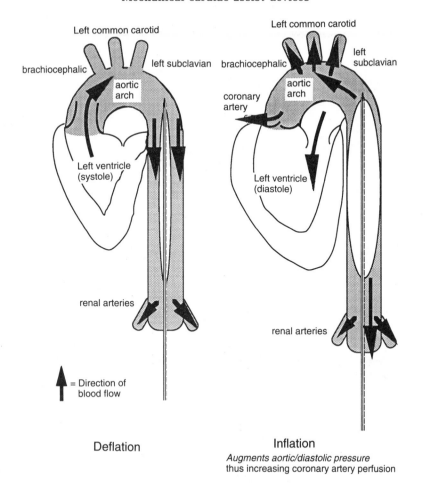

Deflation

Inflation
Augments aortic/diastolic pressure
thus increasing coronary artery perfusion

Fig. 7.6 IABP effects of inflation and deflation.

Coronary artery perfusion pressure = Aortic diastolic pressure − myocardial wall tension

The IABP increases coronary artery perfusion by inflating the aortic balloon during diastole. This increases aortic end diastolic pressure and therefore increases coronary artery perfusion.

Timing

The precise timing of inflation and deflation is an important factor in optimizing the help that the IABP can give. If inflation occurs too early then it will cause impedance to aortic blood flow, if it occurs too late it will reduce the amount of augmentation. If deflation occurs too early then augmentation will be limited and if it occurs too late it will act as an additional impedance to aortic blood flow.

Timing of inflation and deflation is judged from the arterial pressure waveform (see Fig. 7.7).

Inflation should occur at the closure of the aortic valve which is seen on the arterial waveform as the dicrotic notch.

Deflation should occur just before the aortic valve opens or during isovolumetric contraction of the ventricle.

Timing errors

Errors which cause the most harm are *early inflation* and *late deflation*. These actually increase myocardial oxygen consumption and workload adding to the limitations of the failing heart.

Early inflation

The balloon inflates before aortic valve closure acting as an impedance to blood flow and increasing afterload.

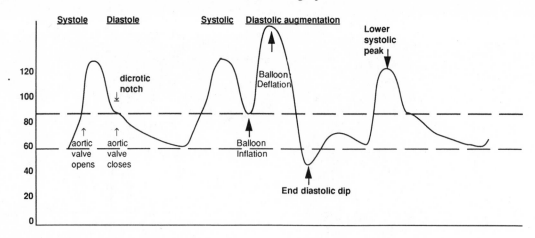

Fig. 7.7 Timing inflation and deflation from the arterial pressure waveform. (Arterial or aortic waveform with IABP on 1:2 assist.)

Arterial or aortic waveform analysis. In order to obtain a clear comparison of augmented and unaugmented pressures the IABP cycle should be set to 1:2 and the frame either frozen or a recording obtained. The patient can then continue on 1:1 while the waveform is analysed.

- Identify the dicrotic notch — inflation should occur at this point on the augmented waveform producing a sharp V shape. This denotes optimal inflation timing of augmentation producing maximal augmented volume.
- Compare systolic and augmented diastolic upstroke — the upstrokes should be parallel to each other and steeply inclined. This gives an indication of the speed of increase in aortic root pressure and thus the effectiveness of increased coronary artery perfusion.
- Compare systolic and augmented diastolic peaks — the augmented peak should be equal to or higher than the systolic. The greater the peak in diastolic pressure the greater the increase in aortic root pressure
- Check the end-diastolic dip — this should fall swiftly with a decreased end diastolic pressure. Correct timing of deflation immediately prior to systole produces a steep drop in end diastolic pressure and reduction of the impedance to the next systolic ejection. This represents the degree of afterload reduction.
- Review the following systolic peak — this should be lower than the unassisted systolic peak. This is because less work is required to overcome resistance to ejection. However, this may not be the case in non-compliant (atherosclerotic) vasculature.

The augmentation upstroke will occur before the dicrotic notch and very close to the systolic peak.

Late inflation
The balloon inflates after the dicrotic notch limiting the diastolic augmentation and reducing assistance to coronary artery perfusion. The waveform between systole and augmented diastole may lose its sharp V shape and look more like a U.

Early deflation
The balloon deflates before diastole is finished thereby producing a steep fall following diastolic augmentation. Augmentation falls sharply and reduction in afterload is less evident leading to increased ventricular work.

Late deflation
The balloon remains inflated acting as an impedance to ventricular ejection and increasing ventricular work. The waveform may appear widened following diastolic augmentation and there is no evidence of the end diastolic dip.

Problem-solving

1. Decreased augmentation

Due to:

(i) Balloon leak or need for balloon refill (evident by decreased augmentation pressure and loss of end diastolic dip). The need for balloon refill is due to the gradual diffusion of helium through the balloon membrane and leakage at tubing connections.

(ii) A change in patient dynamics.

Management

● Check automatic balloon refill programme (if present) is functioning. The balloon is automatically refilled every 2 hours.

● Manually refill the balloon if necessary.

● If a balloon leak has occurred a loss in effectiveness will be evident and return of blood back up the catheter may be seen. Medical staff should be informed at once as the balloon will need removal.

● If the patient has a tachycardia > 120 bpm or decreased intravascular volume, balloon augmentation and effectiveness will be reduced. Switching the timing of assist to 1:2 beats may improve augmentation with a tachycardia. Decreased intravascular volume should be corrected.

2. Dampened waveform

Due to:

(i) Air in the transducer or system.

(ii) An excessive length of pressure monitoring line.

(iii) Build-up of clot at the tip of the monitoring cannula.

Management

● Check transducer and flush system, removing any obvious air bubbles and reducing the length of the pressure line to the minimum required for safety.

● Fast flush the line for several seconds.

3. Deterioration in haemodynamic status

Due to:

(i) The patient. Tachycardia, decreased intravascular volume, decreased systemic vascular resistance, or any other factor liable to affect normal functioning haemodynamic status.

(ii) The IABP. Balloon leak or need for refill, inappropriate timing for any change in cardiac rhythm. The balloon loses approximately 1–2 ml of gas per hour by diffusion across the membrane.

Management

● Correct patient-related problems as per usual protocols.

● Manually refill the balloon and check tubing between balloon and console for any signs of blood leakage (this will occur if there is a leak in the balloon). (See below for management of balloon leak.)

4. Balloon leak

Due to:

(i) Friction with atheromatous plaque in the aorta.

(ii) Faulty balloon. There will be a reduction in the effectiveness of the balloon and eventually blood may leak into the catheter and track back to the connecting tubing.

Management

● Decrease balloon inflation frequency to a minimum and notify the medical staff immediately. There is a risk of gas embolus; the severity of which depends on the gas used to inflate the balloon. Carbon dioxide is much more soluble than helium and therefore less likely to be a serious problem unless the leak is very large. The balloon will have to be replaced as soon as possible.

5. Malpositioning of the balloon
The balloon may become displaced during patient movement and the efficiency of augmentation may be decreased. If displacement is upwards it is possible for the left subclavian artery to become occluded. If displacement is downwards it is possible for the renal arteries to become obstructed.

Management

● The left radial artery should be palpated hourly and the colour and temperature or the limb checked to ensure adequate circulation.

● Any acute loss of urine output may indicate displacement of the balloon.

● The position of the balloon should be confirmed on X-ray and checked by the doctor. If necessary, repositioning should be carried out.

Problems related to the patient with an IABP

1. Potential impairment of peripheral circulation
The presence of the balloon catheter in the femoral artery

will cause a reduction in blood flow to the limb. In some cases, thrombosis of the vessel has occurred and emergency embolectomy has been required.

Management

- The patient's lower limbs should be examined hourly and compared for colour, temperature, and peripheral pulses.

- It is usual for the patient to be prescribed an intravenous heparin infusion to maintain the ACT > 150 seconds throughout the period of balloon insertion.

- Avoidance of hip flexion in the cannulated leg will reduce the risk of blood flow obstruction.

- Inflation and deflation should continue unless the balloon is about to be removed. Total balloon immobility will increase the likelihood of thrombus formation and should never last longer than 30 minutes (Joseph and Bates 1990). If necessary, the balloon can be maintained on minimum augmentation until it can be removed.

2. Restricted movement contributing to atelectasis and pressure area problems
The patient's position is restricted by the need to avoid hip flexion which may obstruct the gas supply to the balloon or the blood flow round the catheter to the patient's leg. His/her mobility is restricted by attachment to the balloon catheter and other cannulae.

Management

- The patient can turn from side-to-side as well as lie supine and should be encouraged to do so. The limiting factor is keeping the degree of hip flexion to a minimum.

- The patient can sit up to an approximate 30 degree angle and this should be encouraged to allow deep breathing and expansion of the lower lobes of the lung.

- The patient is highly susceptible to pressure area problems requiring as much support as necessary to reduce the risk of skin breakdown as well as 2-hourly position changes.

3. Bleeding and coagulopathy
The need for heparinization to avoid thrombus formation around the balloon and in the patient's leg distal to the balloon catheter means that bleeding may become a problem.

Management

- The ACT should be checked regularly, usually 2–4-hourly, unless there are major problems obtaining

anticoagulation when bolus doses of heparin may be used and ACT should be checked shortly after administration. The patient should be observed for any sign of coagulopathy such as bleeding around cannulae sites, mucosa, gums, and evidence of petechiae.

4. Fear of dependency and possible disconnection
Patients may be aware of the presence of the balloon pump and require information from the nursing and medical staff about its role and the length of time it will remain in place. This is a stressful situation and information will require repetition and simplification if it is to be taken in. The patient may develop a dependence on the balloon pump and require frequent reassurance when being weaned from it.

5. Infection
The patient is vulnerable to further infection due to his illness and the number of invasive cannulae which bypass the normal body defence mechanisms.

Management

- Careful asepsis is essential as with all critically ill patients.

- Catheter and cannulae sites should be checked for redness and swelling.

- Dressings which are non-occlusive should be changed if they become wet or soiled.

- Semi-occlusive transparent membrane dressings should be dressed as necessary.
(For further details see Chapter 2.)

Weaning from the IABP

Prior to attempted weaning of the balloon pump the patient should be stable and requiring only low levels of vasopressor or inotropic support. Ideally, they should show evidence of adequate cardiac function, good peripheral perfusion, and adequate urine output.

Weaning can be commenced either by reducing the ratio of assisted beats or reducing the augmentation of the balloon (the volume of inflation/deflation). The ratio of assist is usually reduced initially to 1:2 then 1:3 and so on providing the patient remains stable with adequate cardiac function, peripheral perfusion, and urine output. Where possible, cardiac output measurement will provide optimum monitoring of the response to weaning. The minimum amount of time between each reduction should be 30 minutes although it is usually longer.

The balloon augmentation is usually reduced by 10–20% using the same criteria for patient tolerance.

Removal of the IABP

Depending on whether the balloon was placed surgically or percutaneously the patient will either return to theatre or have the balloon removed in the ICU. Heparinization is discontinued before balloon removal but bleeding may be prolonged from the percutaneous insertion site. This will require manual pressure for up to 30 minutes and a high pressure dressing following this. In some centres a Fogarty catheter is passed proximal to the aortic bifurcation and distal to the popliteal artery to clear any clot that may be present and to prevent emboli.

Following balloon removal the site should be inspected hourly for signs of further bleeding and the peripheral circulation assessed for signs of occlusion.

Ventricular assist devices

These are mechanical devices which work in conjunction with the patient's own ventricle although they are capable of providing total cardiac output if necessary. They can support either or both ventricles.

Indications

The majority of these devices are used as a temporary bridge to allow time to set up cardiac transplantation. However, some are used to support patients who cannot be weaned from cardiopulmonary bypass after surgery and patients in cardiogenic shock following myocardial infarction.

Description

The assist device consists of:

 (i) a blood sac which acts as a prosthetic ventricle,

 (ii) valves to provide unidirectional flow, and

 (iii) a power source to provide the blood flow. This is usually pneumatic for short-term devices, requiring bulky lines and a compressor which limit patient movement. Long-term devices which are implantable currently use electrical power from a rechargeable battery.

Haemodynamic inclusion criteria (from Ruzevich 1991)

MAP	< 60 mmHg
LA and/or RA pressure	> 20 mmHg
Urine output	< 20 ml/h
Cardiac index	< 2.0 l/min/m^2

This is despite maximum drug support, optimal preload, and IABP if appropriate

---

Haemodynamic exclusion criteria (from Ruzevich 1991)

1. Significant complicating illness (other than cardiovascular problem)

 • Chronic renal failure or post-operative renal failure

 • Severe cerebrovascular disease

 • Metastatic disease

 • Severe hepatic disease

 • Significant blood dyscrasia

 • Severe pulmonary disease

2. Uncontrollable haemorrhage
3. Massive air embolization
4. Massive haemolysis
5. Transfusion reaction
6. Technically unsuccessful operation

 • Immediate paravalvular leak

 • Left ventricular outflow obstruction

 • Residual atrioventricular valve

 • Regurgitation

7. Acute cerebral damage resulting in either or both, fixed pupils and a flat electroencephalogram

---

Insertion

Cannulation of the appropriate side of the heart is required. These are usually standard cardiopulmonary bypass cannulae which are placed in the right atrium and pulmonary artery for right ventricular assist and in the left atrium and aorta for left ventricular assist. Biventricular assistance is possible with cannulation of both sides of the heart.

Implantable devices

These devices are limited to left ventricular support and are generally used as a bridge to transplantation.

The pump is placed in the patient's abdomen with a conduit made from Dacron inserted into the left ventricular apex for inflow and another Dacron conduit inserted into the aorta for outflow. External connections for power and drive control are still necessary but are considerably less bulky than the pneumatic drive lines necessary for non-implantable devices.

Advantages:
  (i) decreased risk of infection,

  (ii) decreased risk of thrombus formation,

  (iii) increased patient mobility.

Disadvantages:
  (i) cost,

  (ii) supports single ventricle only,

  (iii) difficult to insert,

  (iv) requires apex cannulation.

Artificial hearts

These have rarely been used in the United Kingdom and most experience is from the United States and France.

The total artificial heart (e.g. Jorvik) is designed to replace the patient's own heart. The patient's own heart is removed and the prosthetic ventricles are attached to the atrial cuff remnants on the inflow. The aorta and pulmonary artery are attached to the ventricular outflow.

Indications

Artificial hearts are occasionally used for temporary support following rejection of a cardiac transplant. They may also be indicated in left ventricular tumour or massive thrombus.

Problems associated with the patient on a ventricular assist device

Bleeding and coagulopathy
Heparin is used to prevent coagulation in the short-term. In the long-term, aspirin and dipyridamole are used. Bleeding may occur as a result of coagulopathy or due to use of cardiopulmonary bypass prior to use of the device. Use of centrifugal pumps and the haemopump device may cause haemolysis.

Infection
Sources may be systemic or via the drive lines from the skin. The patient is highly vulnerable due to his critical state and transplantation cannot occur until clear of systemic infection.

Mechanical failure
With improvement in device reliability this is rarely a problem.

The best survival rates are for the use of left ventricular assist devices (69% survived to transplant and 54% survived overall).

Cardiac transplantation

Since the first human-to-human transplantation was carried out in 1967 the overall survival rate has increased to 80–90% for 1 year and to 50% at 5 years. A major factor in this has been the use of immunosuppressive agents, particularly cyclosporin to prevent rejection.

Indications

The majority of adult patients who receive a cardiac transplant have either ischaemic heart disease or end-stage cardiomyopathy. Only 14% are women and the average age of recipient is 44 years (Large and Schofield 1991).

Indications for cardiac transplant

- End-stage cardiomyopathy

- Severe coronary vessel disease

- Valvular heart disease

- Cardiac tumours

Selection of recipient

This is usually undertaken using experience of absolute and relative contraindications, relative need, and matching with the donor.

Absolute contraindications

(1) *High* (> 15 mmHg) *transpulmonary pressure gradient* (difference between the mean pulmonary artery pressure and the mean left atrial pressure). High pulmonary vascular resistance increases right ventricular afterload causing a risk of right ventricular failure in the donated heart.

(2) *Active systemic infection.* Immunosuppression post-organ donation will drastically reduce any resistance and mortality will greatly increase.

(3) *Malignancy.* Immunosuppression will allow rapid spread of any pre-existing malignancy.

(4) *Irreversible hepatic and renal failure.* There is increased morbidity and cyclosporin is both hepato- and nephrotoxic.

(5) *Peptic ulceration.* Corticosteroids used in immunosuppression will exacerbate the problem.

(6) *Advanced peripheral or cerebral vascular disease.* Increased morbidity may limit the benefit of a transplant.

(7) *Psychologically unstable and socially unsupported,* with or without dependence on alcohol or drugs.

Factors, such as age and diabetes, are relative contraindications and each patient should be assessed on an individual basis.

Donor selection

Full details of preparation for organ donation can be found in Chapter 9.

Once criteria are fulfilled the donor is taken to theatre for organ removal. The heart is preserved by infusion of cold cardioplegia solution and placed in cold normal saline surrounded by ice. Total ischaemic time should be less than 4 hours.

Care of the patient post-cardiac transplantation

On the whole, care is similar to that described for any patient following cardiac surgery, however there are a few differences.

Important changes in the patient following cardiac transplantation include:

(1) *Denervation.* The donor heart has the nerve supply severed so control by the autonomic nervous system is lost. Loss of vagal influence means that resting heart rate is higher than normal (> 100 bpm) and variations due to respiration are not present. Similarly, manoeuvres used to influence the heart via vagal stimulation, such as carotid sinus massage or the valsalva manoeuvre, will have no effect.

The heart has an atypical response to metabolic demands thus tachycardia may not appear as an immediate response to hypovolaemia and exercise initiates only a slow response in cardiac output. In the same way, the heart is slow to respond to discontinuation of these demands and tachycardia may continue for some time. Orthostatic hypotension may also occur as a result of this.

Atropine is ineffective as a treatment for bradycardia and isoprenaline is used because it stimulates the myocardial β-receptors directly.

Pain in response to myocardial ischaemia is no longer transmitted to the brain and the patient will not experience angina. It is therefore necessary to have regular stress testing and angiography.

(2) *Presence of two sinoatrial nodes.* The posterior walls of the right and left atria remain *in situ* including the sinoatrial node. The transplanted heart also has a sinoatrial node and two P waves are visible on the ECG.

(3) *Immunosuppression and infection.* Rejection is a major problem following transplantation. The main immunosuppressants used are cyclosporin, azathioprine, and corticosteroids. These are started in the pre-operative period and, with the exception of corticosteroids, will continue throughout the patient's life.

Infection is thus a major problem for transplant patients and asepsis must be scrupulous for all interventions. Patients are nursed in protective isolation during their initial recovery.

References and bibliography

Allen, J.K. (1990). Physical and psychosocial outcomes after coronary artery bypass graft surgery: review of the literature. *Heart and Lung*, **19**, 49–54.

Barnason, S., Qimmerman, L., and Nieveen, J. (1995). The effect of music interventions on anxiety in the patient after coronary artery bypass grafting. *Heart and Lung*, **24**, 124–32.

Butchart, E.G. (1990). Surgery for heart valve disease. *Hospital Update*, **15**, 963–76.

Carson, M.M., Barton, D.M., Morrison, C.G., and Tribble, C.G. (1994). Managing pain during mediastinal chest tube removal. *Heart and Lung*, **23**, 500–5.

Cupples, S.A. (1991). Effects of timing and reinforcement of preoperative education on knowledge and recovery of patients having coronary artery bypass graft surgery. *Heart and Lung*, **20**, 654–60.

Fairman, R.M. and Edmunds, L.H. (1981). Emergency thoracotomy in the surgical intensive care unit after open cardiac operation. *Annals of Thoracic Surgery*, **32**, 386–91.

Girling, D.K. (1990a). Cardiopulmonary bypass: part 1. *Hospital Update*, **15**, 799–804.

Girling, D.K. (1990b). Cardiopulmonary bypass: part 2. *Hospital Update*, **15**, 875–81.

Grishkin, B.A. (1988). Open-chest resuscitation. *Critical Care Nursing Quarterly*, **10**, 17–24.

Gujol, M.C. (1994). A survey of pain assesment and management practices among critical Care nurses. *American Journal of Critical Care*, **3**, 123–8.

Hayward, J. (1975). *Information: A prescription against pain.* Royal College of Nursing, London.

Joseph, D.L. and Bates, S. (1990). Intra-aortic balloon pumping: how to stay on course. *American Journal of Nursing*, **90**, 42–7.

Large, S.R. and Schofield, P.M. (1991). Heart transplantation. *Hospital Update*, **16**, 808–16.

Lazar, J.M., Ziady, G.M., Dummer, J., Thompson, M., and Ruffner, R.J. (1992). Outcome and complications of prolonged intraaortic balloon counterpulsation in cardiac patients. *American Journal of Cardiology*, **69**, 955–8.

Ley, S.J., Miller, K. Skov, P. and Preisig, P. (1990). Crystalloid versus colloid fluid therapy after cardiac surgery. *Heart and Lung*, **19**, 31–40.

Mailis, A., Chan, J., Basinski, A., Feindel, C., Vanderlinden, G., Taylor, A., *et al.* (1989). Chest wall pain after aortocoronary bypass surgery using internal mammary artery graft: A new pain syndrome? *Heart and Lung*, **18**, 553–8.

Meighan Rimar, J. and Rubin, A. (1988). Emergency reopening of a median sternotomy for pericardial decompression and cardiac massage. *Critical Care Nurse*, **8**, 92–101.

North, N. (1988). Psychosocial aspects of coronary artery bypass surgery. *Nursing Times*, **84**, 26–9.

Puntillo, K.A. (1994). Dimensions of procedural pain and its analgesic management in critically ill surgical patients. *American Journal of Critical Care*, **3**, 116–22.

Quinless, F.W., Cassese, M., and Atherton, N. (1985). The effect of selected pre-operative, intraoperative, and post-operative variables on the development of postcardiotomy psychosis in patients undergoing open heart surgery. *Heart and Lung*, **14**, 334–41.

Raymond, M., Conklin, C., Schaeffer, J., Newstadt, G., Matloff, J.M., and Gray, R.J. (1984). Coping with transient intellectual dysfunction after coronary bypass surgery. *Heart and Lung*, **13**, 531–9.

Ruzevich, S. (1991). Heart assist devices: state of the art. *Critical Care Nursing Clinics of North America*, **3**, 723–32.

Sang, C.T.M. (1991). Routine coronary surgery. *Hospital Update*, **16** 28–36.

Tittle, M. and McMillan, S.C. (1994). Pain and pain-related side effects in an ICU and on a surgical unit: Nurses' management. *American Journal of Critical Care*, **3**, 25–30.

Weber, K.M. (1990). Cardiac surgery and heart transplantation. In *Critical care nursing: A holistic approach*, (ed. C.M. Hudak, B.M. Gallo, and J.J. Benz), pp.259–85. Lippincott, Philadelphia.

Weiland, A.P. and Walker, W.E. (1986). Physiologic principles and clinical sequelae of cardiopulmonary bypass. *Heart and Lung*, **15**, 34–9.

Wilson-Barnett, J. (1984). Alleviating stress for hospitalised patients. *International Review of Applied Psychology*, **33**, 493–503.

8. Renal problems

Introduction

The kidney performs a wide variety of physiological functions. It plays a crucial role in the maintenance of acid–base, electrolyte and fluid balance, and in the excretion of metabolic waste products. The physiological consequences of renal dysfunction can be widespread and devastating.

While some patients admitted to the intensive care unit (ICU) with renal problems are already in established renal failure, others can also be at high risk of development of renal failure following admission. This may occur as a result of direct renal trauma (including urological surgery), inadequate perfusion states, such as heart failure and massive haemorrhage, or as a consequence of multi-system disease involvement, such as systemic lupus erythematosus. The preservation of renal function and the early detection of dysfunction is integral to the care of any ICU patient.

Functional anatomy and physiology

The main functions of the kidneys are shown in Table 8.1. The kidney achieves these functions by filtration, reabsorbtion, and secretion. Additionally, there are two other homeostatic mechanisms which are integral to kidney function, namely the renin–angiotensin–aldosterone (RAA) and antidiuretic hormone (ADH) pathways.

Table 8.1 Functions of the kidney

- Production of urine
- Excretion of waste products
- Control and maintenance of fluid balance
- Maintenance of acid–base balance
- Control and maintenance of electrolyte balance
- Renin production
- Erythropoietin production
- Control of calcium reabsorption and vitamin D hydroxylation

The nephron

The functional unit of the kidney is the nephron of which there are approximately one million per kidney.

Nephrons can be further defined as being either cortical, with their glomeruli in the cortex and short loops of Henlé, or juxtamedullary, with glomeruli in the juxtamedullary region and long loops of Henlé reaching down into the medulla.

Each nephron consists of a glomerulus, a glomerular capsule, a proximal convoluted tubule, a loop of Henlè (descending and ascending limbs), a distal convoluted tubule, a collecting duct, and the accompanying vasculature (Fig. 8.1).

Blood supply

Blood enters the kidney via the renal arteries which are branches of the aorta. Each kidney receives approximately 625 ml/min of blood; this constitutes, in total, 25% of the cardiac output. The renal arteries divide into the interlobar arteries which further divide into arcuate arteries, then into interlobular arteries, and finally into afferent arterioles. Blood flow in the renal cortex is greater than in the renal medulla.

The glomerulus

The afferent arterioles feed the glomerulus which is enclosed within the glomerular capsule. The glomerulus is often described as a 'tuft' of capillaries, this arrangement allows a large surface area to be available for filtration. The capsule is double walled; the outer wall is known as the parietal layer and the inner as the visceral layer. The two are separated by the capsular space. The visceral layer of the capsule and the endothelial layer of the glomerulus constitute the endothelial-capsular membrane, which rests on a layer of contractile mesangial cells.

Modified cells, known as juxtaglomerular cells, are situated around the afferent and efferent arterioles. Parts of the distal tubules lie in close proximity to their originating arterioles; these tubule cells are known collectively as the macula densa. The juxtaglomerular cells and macula densa together form the juxtaglomerular apparatus which secretes renin.

Blood entering the glomerulus from the afferent arteriole is filtered by the endothelial-capsular membrane. The membrane is impermeable to molecules greater than 4 nm in size (molecular weight of 70 000 daltons).

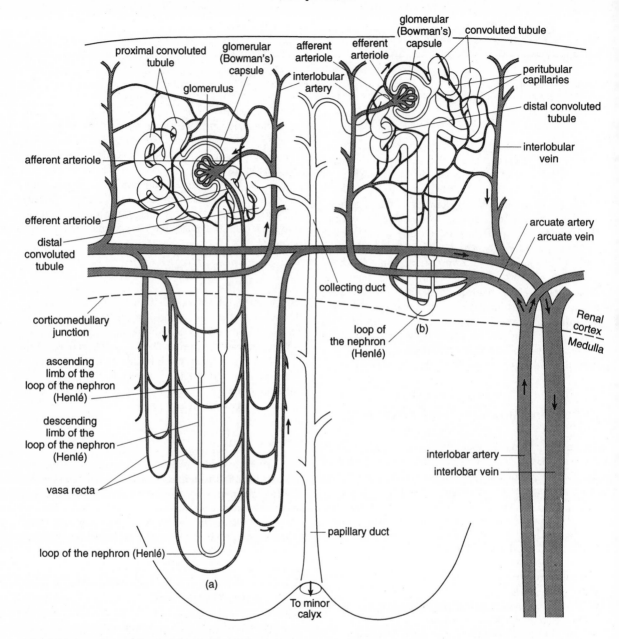

Fig. 8.1 The nephron, showing glomerulus, and proximal, distal, and collecting tubules with blood supply.

Filtration also depends on the molecular shape, electrostatic charge, and opposing pressures within the glomerulus and capsule.

The blood in the glomerulus creates a hydrostatic pressure (~ 60 mmHg) which tends to force fluid out of the afferent vessels. This hydrostatic pressure is opposed by the pressure within the capsular space (~ 20 mmHg) and the osmotic pressure exerted by the blood in the glomerulus (~ 30 mmHg). The filtration pressure is therefore equal to:

$$60 \text{ mmHg } - 30 \text{ mmHg } - 30 \text{ mmHg } = 10 \text{ mmHg}$$

If the glomerular pressure should fall (e.g. during haemorrhage) to a level where it is equal to the sum of the capsular pressure and the osmotic pressure no filtration will occur. Additionally, in the event of a decrease in glomerular filtration rate (GFR), chloride reabsorption by the macula densa cells of the distal tubules is increased, resulting in dilatation of the afferent arterioles and an increase in blood flow and thus GFR. The presence of reabsorbed chloride can promote renin secretion which will cause efferent arteriolar constriction, thus increasing glomerular pressure and hence GFR (Fig. 8.2).

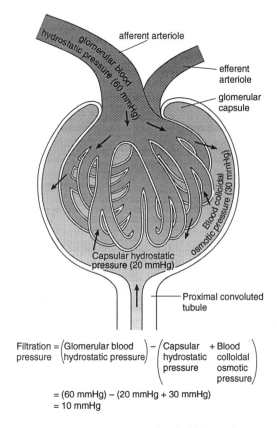

Filtration = (Glomerular blood) − (Capsular + Blood
pressure (hydrostatic pressure) (hydrostatic colloidal
 pressure osmotic
 pressure)

= (60 mmHg) − (20 mmHg + 30 mmHg)

= 10 mmHg

Fig. 8.2 Bowman's capsule, showing fluid dynamics producing filtration pressure.

Blood which is not filtered through the membrane leaves the glomerulus via the efferent arterioles. The efferent arterioles in the cortical region of the kidney divide to form peritubular capillaries around the convoluted tubules. The juxtaglomerular efferent arterioles also form peritubular capillaries but, in addition, form a network of thin-walled vessels known as the vasa recta which reach down into the renal medulla. The peritubular capillaries and the vasa recta eventually join to form

the interlobar veins and, finally, the renal veins. Fluid which is filtered across the endothelial-capsular membrane is known as filtrate and enters the next part of the nephron, the proximal convoluted tubule. The filtrate at this stage possesses an osmolality of 300 mOsmol/l.

> Osmolality is the osmotic pressure of a solution expressed in Osmoles or milliOsmoles per kilogram of water

In the proximal tubule various solutes are reabsorbed (both actively and passively) into the surrounding peritubular capillaries, reducing the filtrate by some 75–80%.

As sodium (a positively charged ion) is reabsorbed, leaving the tubules and moving into the peritubular capillaries, the blood within those capillaries becomes positively charged. Chloride (a negatively charged ion) follows, moving from the filtrate into the capillaries to achieve an electrostatic balance. The presence of sodium and chloride in the peritubular capillary blood increases its osmolality. Water then moves from the filtrate in the proximal tubule into the blood by osmosis (Table 8.2).

Table 8.2 Solutes reabsorbed in the proximal tubule

Sodium (80%)	Water (80%)
Phosphate	Chloride
Glucose	Bicarbonate
Potassium	Sulphate (100%)
Amino acids	Low molecular weight proteins

> **Osmosis** is the movement of a pure solvent (e.g. water) through a semi-permeable membrane from a solution that has a lower solute concentration to one that has a higher solute concentration

> **Diffusion** is the process by which particulate matter in a fluid moves from an area of higher concentration to an area of lower concentration resulting in an even distribution of particles

The proximal tubule is always permeable to water and therefore has no control over water moving out of the tubule. This is referred to as obligatory reabsorption. Water reabsorption, 80 per cent of which occurs in the proximal tubule, is therefore controlled by sodium movement.

After leaving the proximal tubule the filtrate enters the loop of Henlé where more sodium, chloride, bicarbonate, and glucose are reabsorbed into the peritubular blood. The ascending limb of the loop is impermeable to water. Chloride ions are actively reabsorbed, moving from the filtrate into the interstitial fluid and then into the peritubular capillaries. The blood in the capillaries becomes negatively charged and, in order to equalize this, sodium follows chloride passively. This results in the filtrate becoming less concentrated, its osmolality now being approximately 100 mOsmol/l. Conversely, the interstitium surrounding the loop becomes hyperosmolar, in the region of 1200 mOsmol/l.

The filtrate then enters the distal convoluted tubule where further solute reabsorption occurs, making the filtrate even more dilute. Various substances, including creatinine and drugs, are secreted by the distal tubules into the filtrate for excretion. The final part of the nephron is the collecting duct, running through the renal medulla, which takes the filtrate, now called urine, to the ureters.

The distal tubules and the collecting ducts are sites of action for both the RAA and ADH mechanisms (Figs 8.3, and 8.4). The RAA pathway controls sodium reabsorption from the distal tubules and collecting ducts. Sodium reabsorption is dependent on its concentration in the extracellular fluid. Because water accompanies sodium, extracellular volume is also affected. The RAA mechanism can therefore manipulate sodium levels and blood volume. Although 80 per cent of water reabsorption is obligatory via osmosis from the proximal tubule, ADH can control reabsorption of water from the distal tubules and collecting ducts.

Concentrating abilities of the kidney

In the process of reabsorbing solutes, the filtrate becomes progressively more dilute during its passage through the nephron. The impermeability of the ascending limb of the loop of Henlé to water and the control over water reabsorption by ADH in the distal tubules and collecting ducts further ensures a dilute filtrate by the end of the nephron. The reabsorption of solutes results in the interstitium becoming more concentrated, particularly in the medulla of the kidney. However, there are physiological circumstances, such as dehydration, where excretion of waste products in a dilute urine is not desirable. This concentrating ability depends upon the maintenance of a hyperosmolar medullary interstitium.

As previously mentioned, chloride and sodium reabsorption in the ascending limb of the loop of Henle increases the solute concentration in the interstitium

Decreased renal arterial pressure

Stimulates

Juxtaglomerular apparatus to secrete renin

Stimulates conversion of

Angiotensinogen to angiotensin I

Converted to

Angiotensin II (causes arterial vasoconstriction and increases filtration pressure)

Stimulates

Adrenal cortex to increase aldosterone secretion

Stimulates

Increased sodium reabsorption from distal tubules and collecting ducts

Results in

Increased blood volume and restoration renal arterial pressure

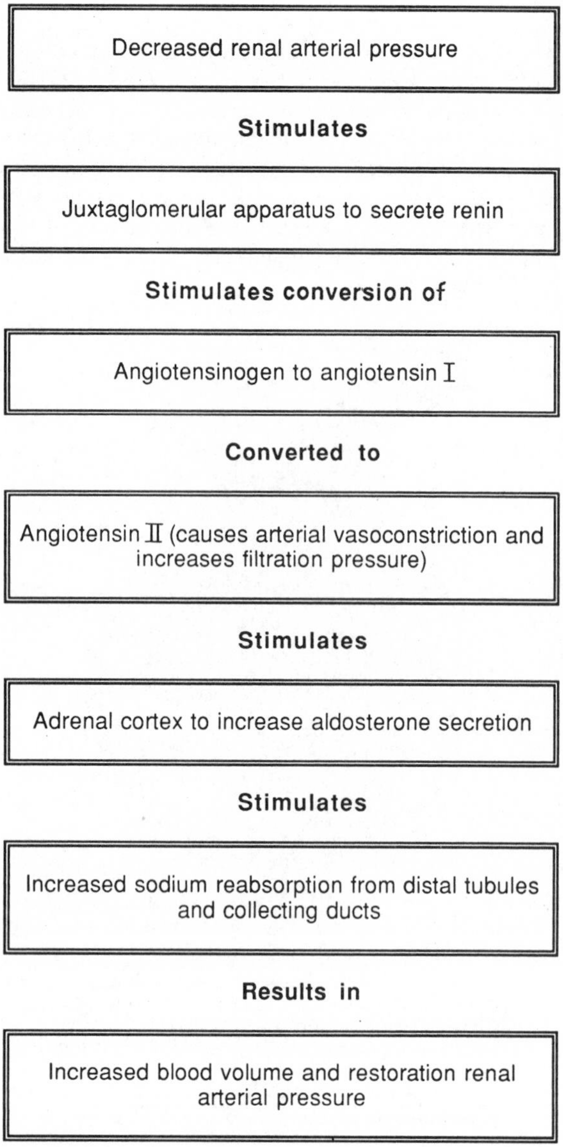

Fig. 8.3 The renin–angiotensin–aldosterone (RAA) mechanism.

which is carried down into the medulla by blood flow in the vasa recta. The osmolality of the medulla is further increased by the movement of sodium and chloride out of the collecting ducts. ADH can promote the movement of water out of the collecting ducts. This results in a high urea concentration within the ducts. Urea then moves, by diffusion, out of the ducts and into the surrounding interstitium. The concentration of urea in the interstitium is greater than in the loop of the nephron and so

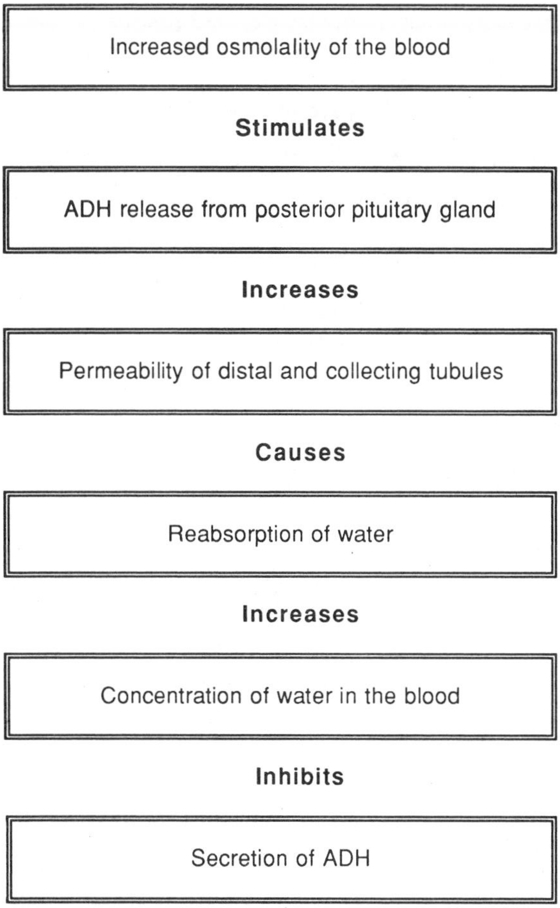

Fig. 8.4 Antidiuretic hormone (ADH) mechanism.

urea moves into the loop, again by diffusion. When the filtrate (containing the diffused urea) reaches the ascending limb of the loop and the distal tubule, water but not urea is removed under the control of ADH, resulting in further concentration of urea in the collecting ducts.

The counter-current mechanism also maintains medullary osmolality. In practical terms, the loop of Henlé consists of two parallel tubes with fluid flowing in opposite directions — 'counter-current flow'.

The descending limb, being impermeable to solutes and permeable to water, allows the movement of water by osmosis into the relatively more concentrated interstitium, thus increasing the concentration of the filtrate. This pattern continues and accumulates through the descending limb, reaching an osmolality of 1200 mosmol/l. Sodium and chloride move from the ascending limb into the interstitium of the medulla. As this part of the loop of Henlé is impermeable to water, the filtrate

becomes progressively less concentrated, being 200 mOsmol/l at the cortex. The accompanying vasa recta are similar to the loop in that there are ascending and descending limbs. Indeed, it is partly this arrangement that keeps the medulla concentrated. As blood moves (within the vasa recta) towards the medulla, solutes enter the blood from the interstitium.

When the now concentrated blood moves into the ascending vasa recta and moves back towards the cortex, the solutes diffuse back into the interstitium. The counter-current mechanism partly depends on a sluggish blood flow within the vasa recta. If that flow increases (e.g. during haemodilution or volume expansion), the medullary osmolality is disrupted, decreasing water absorption and resulting in a dilute urine.

Acid–base balance

An acid is a substance that can provide hydrogen ions (H^+) and a base (an alkali) can accept hydrogen ions. Even in extremely acidic solutions, the concentration of H^+ ions is small and therefore relative values are inconvenient to use. The pH scale is a measurement of the H^+ ion concentration and is a negative logarithm of the H^+ concentration. A change of one pH unit represents a 10-fold change in the H^+ concentration.

The pH of blood is maintained between the narrow limits of 7.36–7.44 and is done so by buffers available in the blood, the lungs (see Chapter 3) and the kidneys. An increase in the blood pH above 7.43 constitutes an alkalosis and a pH below 7.37 an acidosis. The alkalosis or acidosis can be respiratory, metabolic, or mixed in origin. (Table 8.3) (See also Chapter 3 for respiratory alkalosis–acidosis.)

Table 8.3 Causes of metabolic acidosis and alkalosis

Metabolic acidosis	Metabolic alkalosis
Acute and chronic renal failure	Excessive sodium bicarbonate infusion
Ingestion of acids (e.g. salicylates)	Excessive ingestion of alkalis
Severe loss of intestinal (small bowel) secretions	Vomiting with loss of gastric acid
Cardiac arrest, hypoperfusion/ hypovolaemic states (with production of lactate)	Gastrointestinal tract fistula
	Infusion of excessive citrate in stored blood
Diabetic ketoacidosis	Liver failure

In addition to the changes in pH, abnormal bicarbonate values also accompany metabolic acidosis (<21 mmol/l) and metabolic alkalosis (>26 mmol/l).

Blood buffers

Blood buffers can exercise a rapid response to changes in pH but their effects last for a relatively short time. The most important buffer in the extracellular fluid is bicarbonate (HCO_3^-) buffering hydrogen ions to form carbonic acid (H_2CO_3). Carbonic acid easily dissociates into water (H_2O) and carbon dioxide (CO_2). The carbon dioxide can then be eliminated by the lungs.

$$HCO_3^- + H^+ \rightleftharpoons H_2CO_3 \rightleftharpoons H_2O + CO_2$$

Plasma proteins can also act as buffers but this contribution is relatively small compared to the bicarbonate system. Haemoglobin is important as it is present in erythrocytes which are prime sites for carbonic acid formation and is thus immediately available to buffer hydrogen ions from carbonic acid.

Renal system

A low blood pH will stimulate the tubular cells to secrete hydrogen ions into the filtrate. To maintain electrostatic balance, sodium (Na^+) diffuses from the filtrate into the tubular cells where it combines with bicarbonate to produce sodium bicarbonate ($NaHCO_3$). This bicarbonate is then absorbed into the blood and acts as a systemic buffer. In conjunction with the excretion of excess hydrogen ions, the kidney thus attempts to counteract acidosis. Similar processes occur with ammonia and phosphate (see Fig. 8.5).

Acute renal failure

Acute renal failure in the ICU is usually associated with the failure of other organs or body systems (Wendon *et al.* 1989), commonly the respiratory system (Smithies and Cameron 1992). Cameron (1986) stated that the mortality rate for isolated renal failure can be as low as 8 per cent rising to 80 per cent when combined with respiratory failure and to 100 per cent if a constituent of three–system failure.

The role of sepsis in the development and subsequent course of acute renal failure has been extremely well documented; indeed, one study demonstrated that sepsis was the major cause of death in 52 per cent of patients with acute renal failure (Beaman and Adu 1992). These daunting figures serve to emphasize the need for awareness of the precipitating causes of acute renal failure and, thereafter, early detection and treatment.

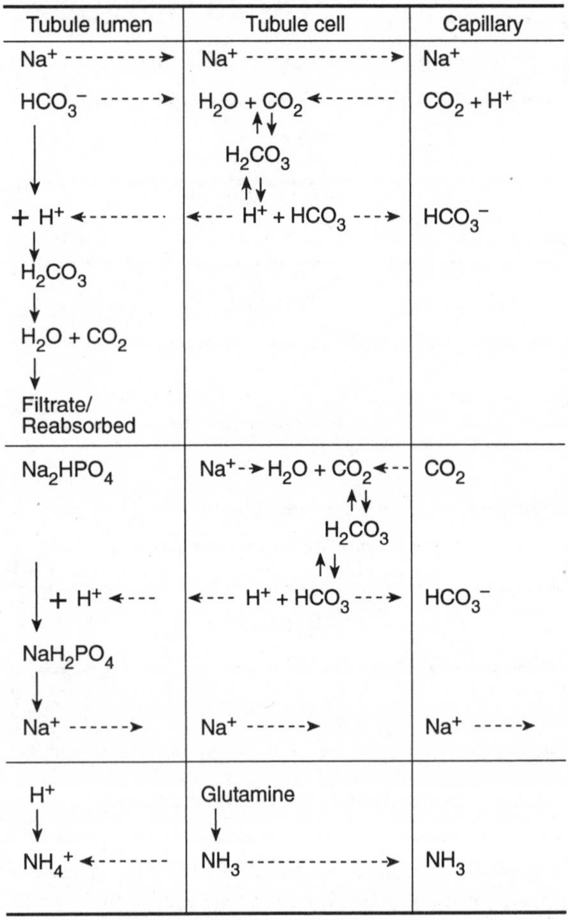

Fig. 8.5 Diagrammatic representation of renal control of acid–base balance.

Definitions

The terminology surrounding acute renal failure can be quite confusing and the following should help clarification.

- *Acute renal failure*
  The sudden development of renal insufficiency, leading to uraemia and loss of electrolyte control in a previously well patient.

- *Oliguria*
  A urine volume of less than 0.5 ml/kg/h in an adult.

- *Pre-renal acute renal failure*
  This is also termed 'reversible renal hypoperfusion' which arises as a result of renal hypoperfusion from hypovolaemia and/or a low cardiac output and/or a low perfusion pressure. It is reversible on restoration of renal blood flow and/or systemic blood pressure, thus possibly preventing the development of established renal failure.

- *Acute tubular necrosis*
  A term frequently used in the clinical setting to describe a form of acute reversible renal failure. This definition often inaccurately reflects histological findings.

- *Non-oliguric acute renal failure*
  Acute tubular necrosis where there is uraemia and loss of electrolyte control though no coexisting oliguria.

Causes of acute renal failure

Frequently, the cause of acute renal failure is multifactorial. However, it is useful to classify the causes into three main groups (see also Tables 8.4, 8.5, and 8.6).

1. Pre-renal

2. Renal (intrinsic)

3. Post-renal

Table 8.4 Pre-renal causes of acute renal failure

Hypovolaemia	Reduced cardiac output
- Burns	- Myocardial infarction
- Haemorrhage	- Cardiac dysrhythmias
- Gastrointestinal losses	- Congestive cardiac failure
- Renal losses	
- Third space losses (e.g. pancreatitis, ascites, peritonitis)	- Pericarditis
	- Cardiac tamponade
	- Pulmonary embolism
- Hypoalbuminaemia	- Acute cardiac valvular dysfunction
- Peripheral dilatation (e.g. sepsis, anaphylaxis)	

Mechanisms of acute renal failure

The most common cause of acute renal failure in the ICU is renal ischaemia secondary to renal hypoperfusion (Smithies and Cameron 1992). A fall in renal blood flow leads to a fall in glomerular filtration rate (GFR) resulting in a reduction in urine output and a decrease in urea and creatinine clearance.

Table 8.5 Intrinsic causes of acute renal failure

Acute tubular necrosis	Cortical necrosis
- Sepsis	- Snake venom
- Unrelieved pre-renal causes	**Nephrotic syndrome**
- Acute haemorrhage	**Renal artery occlusion/ Emboli**
- Haemoglobin/myoglobin	**Renal vein thrombosis**
- Pancreatitis	**Disseminated intravascular coagulation**
- Hepatic failure	
- Septic abortion	**Acute pyelonephritis**
- Eclampsia	**Hepatorenal syndrome**
- Post-operative	**Glomerulonephritis**
- Cardiogenic shock	- Polyarteritis
- Burns	- Post-streptococcal infection
- Nephrotoxins (e.g. radiographic contrasts, heavy metals, organic solvents, aminoglycosides, amphotericin	- Goodpasture's syndrome
	- Wegener's granulomatosis
	- Infective endocarditis
	- Idiopathic
- Systemic lupus erythematosus	- Henoch–Schönlein purpura

Acute interstitial nephritis
- Penicillins: methicillin, ampicillin, benzylpenicillin
- Cephalosporins: cephalexin
- Sulphonamides
- Rifampicin
- Diuretics: thiazides, frusemide
- Non-steroidal anti-inflammatory drugs: indomethacin, naproxen
- Mefenamic acid, ibuprofen, diclofenac
- Cimetidine
- Phenytoin

At this stage, because tubular function and concentrating ability are maintained, rises of urine osmolality, urea, and creatinine and a fall in urinary sodium are seen. If renal perfusion is restored at this point established renal failure can be avoided. However, if renal perfusion is not restored, the GFR further decreases, along with the urine output, with progressive tubular damage. Concentrating ability is lost with a resulting loss of sodium reabsorption.

Table 8.6 Post-renal causes of acute renal failure

Intra-ureteral	Extra-ureteral
• Calculi	• Retroperitoneal fibrosis
• Papillary necrosis	• Tumour
• Crystals (e.g. uric acid)	• Aneurysm
• Tumour	
• Blood clot	

Bladder obstruction	Urethral obstruction
• Prostatic hypertrophy	• Stricture
• Bladder tumour	• Meatal stenosis
• Blood clot	• Phimosis
• Calculi	
• Functional neuropathy	

Despite a decrease in renal perfusion and GFR, there are some patients who present with 'non-oliguric renal failure', maintaining an adequate urine output. The reasons for this remain unclear, however it has been postulated that improved fluid therapy and the increased use of high-dose loop diuretics may contribute. The prognosis is improved for non-oliguric renal failure when compared to oliguric renal failure (Beaman and Adu 1992).

There are a number of theories to explain the events occurring at nephron level following an ischaemic insult to the kidney. Some or all of the following may coexist in acute renal failure.

1. Tubuloglomerular feedback

During periods of renal hypoperfusion, cortical blood flow is proportionally reduced in relation to medullary blood flow; this is felt to be a protective mechanism for the medulla which normally operates on the verge of hypoxia. This action will also decrease the oxygen demand necessary for solute reabsorption as the GFR drops. If this mechanism fails, medullary ischaemia occurs and the solute reaching the macula densa will activate the tubuloglomerular feedback mechanism. Chloride ions in particular are thought to play an activating role. A further consequence of this is vasoconstriction which, in turn, further reduces GFR (Schrier *et al.* 1990).

2. Reduced glomerular permeability

Local stimuli (including angiotensin II, thromboxane, and histamine) cause glomerular mesangial cell contrac-

tion which serves to reduce the area available for filtration and permeability.

3. 'No reflow' phenonemon

Endothelial cell swelling resulting from the ischaemic injury prevents reperfusion of the microcirculation despite the restoration of renal blood flow.

The efferent arterioles of the cortical glomeruli supply blood to the medulla. These arterioles divide and form the vasae rectae, which in themselves are resistance vessels with the ability to control medullary blood flow. The ascending vessels have very thin walls and are susceptible to compression by local swollen tubules.

4. Tubular obstruction

Obstruction of the tubules by debris causes a rise in intratubular pressure until glomerular filtration stops.

5. Filtrate 'back-leak'

The damaged tubular basement membrane allows filtrate to escape and the GFR is further reduced.

The role of mediators produced in the kidney is becoming increasingly recognized. It is known that some prostaglandins (PGI_2 and PGE_2) will act beneficially by promoting vasodilatation, mesangial cell relaxation and inhibiting platelet aggregation. Conversely, thromboxane (TxA_2) will cause vasoconstriction, glomerular cell contraction (reducing filtration surface area), and will promote platelet aggregation (Schieppati and Remuzzi 1990).

Nitric oxide (NO), formerly known as endothelium-derived relaxant factor (EDRF), has been shown to co-ordinate blood flow in resistance vessels (including the vasa recta) to promote vasodilatation. The antagonists to NO are the endothelins which promote vasoconstriction. In response to ischaemia the endothelins are thought to cause mesangial cell contraction (Neild 1990).

The effects of reperfusion of previously ischaemic tissue are increasingly understood. The restoration of oxygen delivery, the accumulation of calcium and the correction of acidosis promotes phospholipid activity and oxygen radical formation. This results in cell membrane damage, a rise in intracellular calcium, a reduction in ATP synthesis, and a reduction in mitochondrial respiration, all of which contribute to cell death. This may also in part explain a continuing deterioration in renal function despite restoration of renal blood flow.

Investigation and diagnosis of acute renal failure

Any investigation or diagnostic method should in the first instance concentrate on distinguishing the cause of the renal failure (pre-renal, intrinsic, or post-renal) to enable prompt and appropriate treatment. The patient may present with pre-renal failure which, with rapid detection and treatment, could prevent the progression to established renal failure. (Table 8.7)

Table 8.7 Investigations of acute renal failure

Urine	Blood
• Urinalysis	• Full blood count
• Urine microscopy, culture, and sensitivity	• Coagulation screen
• Creatinine clearance	• Electrolytes, urea, creatinine, calcium, phosphate, magnesium, glucose
• Electrolytes, osmolality, urea, and creatinine	• Arterial gases
• Urine/plasma ratios of urea, sodium, and osmolality	• Liver function tests
• Myoglobinuria	• Creatine kinase
	• Autoantibodies (e.g. ANCA for Wegener's granulomatosis, polyarteritis nodosa; or antiglomerular basement antibody for Goodpasture's syndrome
Radiological	
• Plain abdominal and chest X-ray	
• Renal ultrasound	**Other**
• Urography	• 12-lead ECG
• Isotope renography	• Renal biopsy
• CT scan	

A history should be taken and physical examination performed (see Table 8.8). For diagnosis and further management it is vital that the chronological sequence of events is ascertained. Coexisting diseases, which may have a causative or exaggerating effect, may be discovered. The patient may be taking medication which might affect the kidney or its vascular supply (e.g. angiotensin-converting enzyme inhibitors such as enalopril or captopril). The physical examination could reveal signs and symptoms of uraemia, anaemia, coagulopathy, and fluid overload all indicative of renal dysfunction.

Urinary investigations

The simple 'stick test' will reveal pH and specific gravity values, glucose, ketones, bilirubin, urobilinogen, protein, and blood. The presence of protein may indicate an underlying glomerulonephritis or interstitial nephritis. The presence of blood may indicate haemoglobin or myoglobin in the urine (i.e. intravascular haemolysis or rhabdomyolysis, respectively).

Table 8.8 History and physical examination

History	Physical examination
Taken from: patient, family members, case notes, the referring team *Including:*	*For:* (1) signs and symptoms of uraemia (e.g. drowsiness, coma, nausea, vomiting, pruritis);
(1) coexisting diseases (e.g. diabetes, heart failure, hypertension, vascular disease);	(2) bruising, possibly indicating platelet dysfunction;
(2) any potentially nephrotoxic medication (e.g. non-steroidal anti-inflammatory drugs, aminoglycosides);	(3) signs of metabolic acidosis (e.g. hyperventilation or 'air hunger');
(3) history of trauma	(4) pericarditis;
	(5) joint pain;
	(6) signs of fluid overload (e.g. raised jugular venous pressure, peripheral, and pulmonary oedema).

The urine can be examined directly for red and white blood cells or the urinary sediment after centrifugation for casts and crystals.

Acute nephritis	Acute tubular necrosis	Glomerulonephritis
White blood cells and white blood cell casts	Tubular epithelial cells and casts	Granular and red cell casts

Creatinine clearance using a 24-hour collection of urine and a plasma sample can be used to make an assessment of GFR. It is calculated as follows:

$$\frac{\text{Creatinine concentration (urine) } \mu mol/l \times \text{Urine volume ml/min}}{\text{Creatinine concentration (plasma) } \mu mol/l}$$

(Normal GFR = 120 ml/min)

Table 8.9 indicates urinary values for oliguria secondary to either renal or pre-renal causes. Caution must be exercised when interpreting such values if the patient has pre-existing renal disease and/or has received diuretics, as these can affect tubular concentrating ability and urinary electrolyte excretion.

Table 8.9   Diagnostic urinary indices for oliguria

Test	Pre-renal	Renal
Specific gravity	>1020	1010
Osmolality mOsmol/kg	>500	250–300
Sodium mmol/l	<15	>40
Urea mmol/l	>250	<160
Urine/Plasma osmolality ratio	>1.3:1	<1.1:1
Urine–plasma urea ratio	>10:1	<4:1
Urine–plasma creatinine ratio	>40:1	<20:1

In the clinical setting, the differentiation between the patient in pre-renal and established renal failure is not always as well defined as Table 8.9 would suggest. Many patients fall between the two categories, especially those with non-oliguric renal failure.

Blood investigations

The blood urea can be raised in the absence of a reduction in GFR, from:

(i) increased protein catabolism, as seen in burns, fever, and after surgery,

(ii) from increased protein intake (e.g. gastrointestinal bleeding with increased reabsorption of amino acids, and

(iii) dehydration.

Creatinine is produced by creatine breakdown and varies with muscle mass. Therefore, the plasma creatinine is reduced in the very young, the elderly, and in those with chronic wasting diseases.

Blood urea and creatinine levels have limitations in diagnosing renal dysfunction in that a 60% loss of renal function has to occur before a rise is detectable. It is important to remember that GFR declines with age and, if accompanied by a reduction in muscle mass, the serum creatinine can remain within normal values.

Table 8.10   Blood investigations in acute renal failure

Test	Normal value	Value in acute renal failure
Full blood count	Haemoglobin (Hb): 12–18 g/dl	Hb normal or low with anaemia or dilutional effect
	White blood cells (WBC): $4{-}11 \times 10^9/l$	WBC normal or raised if accompanying infection/ inflammation
Platelet count	$150{-}400 \times 10^9/l$	Normal (but function may be decreased) or low (e.g. systemic lupus erythematosis)
Sodium	132–144 mmol/l	Normal, high, or low
Potassium	3.3–4.7 mmol/l	Normal, high, or low
Urea	2.5–6.6 mmol/l	Raised
Creatinine	55–120 μmol/l	Raised
Phosphate	0.8–1.4 mmol/l	Usually raised
Glucose	Fasting <5.5 mmol/l	Normal
Osmolality	285–295 mOsm/l	Usually raised
Magnesium	0.75–1.0 mmol/l	Variable
Calcium	2.12–2.62 mmol/l	Normal or low

Blood gas analysis will often reveal a metabolic acidosis, with a reduced bicarbonate, a significant base deficit and a low pH value.

Approximately 95 per cent of the total body potassium is intracellular. Together with other cations (e.g. calcium and magnesium), potassium is responsible for maintaining osmotic pressure in the intracellular fluid compartment. In the extracellular fluid compartment, potassium is instrumental in neuromuscular and cardiac function. Hyperkalaemia is frequently seen in acute renal failure due to the accumulation of hydrogen ions within the cells, forcing potassium out of the cells to maintain ionic balance.

Calcium levels tend to fall as the phosphate level rises in acute renal failure. In health, the kidneys produce 1 α-hydroxylase which converts 25-hydroxycholecalciferol into 1,25-dihydroxycholecalciferol. This, in turn, promotes the reabsorption of calcium from bone and decreases urinary calcium excretion. (See Table 8.10 for blood investigations in acute renal failure.)

Radiological investigations

These include the following:

Renal ultrasound
Useful for estimating renal size, detecting an obstruction. Probably the most common and useful radiological investigation of acute renal failure in the ICU.

Urography
Renal size and presence of an obstruction, suspected trauma.

Isotope renography
Renal function, size, vasculature and outflow.

Computerized tomography (CT) scanning
If retroperitoneal disease suspected. Often used as an alternative to arteriography or venography.

Plain abdominal X-ray
Detection of renal calculi

Renal biopsy
If the acute renal failure is unexplained and a histological diagnosis is required. Renal biopsy is not advised if the patient only has one kidney. Any coagulation abnormalities must be corrected prior to biopsy and the patient monitored closely for 24 hours for signs of bleeding.

Priorities of care

As with any patient, the three main priorities are those of:

Airway, Breathing, and Circulation

Airway

The patient's conscious level may deteriorate in the presence of uraemia. Neurological observations should be performed when the patient is admitted to the ICU to provide a baseline and recorded frequently thereafter. The patient may lose the ability to maintain a patent airway. Although airway adjuncts, such as nasopharyngeal and oropharyngeal (Guedel) airways have their uses, the patient will probably require endotracheal intubation.

Breathing

The patient's respiratory status may be affected by pulmonary oedema from fluid overload, coexisting pulmonary insufficiency (e.g. adult respiratory distress syndrome; ARDS) or from neuronal effects of uraemia. If the patient is severely acidotic, 'Kussmaul' breathing (see Chapter 3) may be observed with the patient breathing rapidly and deeply. This may occur in the patient with or without a patent airway and may eventually necessitate intubation and ventilation if the acidosis cannot be corrected and the patient tires.

On admission, the patient's respiratory rate and pattern of breathing should be documented and recorded regularly thereafter. Continuous pulse oximetry is a simple and immediate form of assessing oxygenation in addition to arterial blood gas estimation and should also be monitored.

The patient's pulmonary secretions should be noted, in particular to detect pulmonary oedema, pulmonary haemorrhage (in the presence of coagulopathy), or 'pulmonary–renal syndromes', such as Wegener's or Goodpasture's syndrome.

Circulation

Continuous ECG and blood pressure monitoring should be standard. Non-invasive forms of blood pressure monitoring are useful prior to arterial cannulation. A method of measuring ventricular filling pressures is also essential to gauge volume load. At minimum, a central venous catheter should be inserted, though a pulmonary artery catheter is preferable as it can provide a wider range of information such as left heart filling pressure or cardiac output. The insertion of any intravascular lines should be performed under strict aseptic conditions to prevent infection.

The presence of uraemia (and potentially other system failures) could impair platelet function. Prior to intravascular catheter insertion, the bleeding and clotting times should be investigated and treated as appropriate. One dose of DDAVP (1-desamino-8-D-arginine vasopressin or desmopressin) can be given to improve platelet function transiently in the presence of uraemia if surgery is required.

An adequate circulating volume should be maintained at all times, together with an effective perfusion pressure.

Peaked T waves may be seen suggesting hyperkalae-mia, although this may be present without this sign. These and destabilizing arrhythmias should be treated swiftly. Hyperkalaemia can be treated with calcium resonium 30 g (orally or rectally); this non-absorbable ion exchange resin removes potassium from the circula-tion but it does not have a rapid effect (see also Table 8.11). For more immediate control of the effects of hyperkalaemia, 10 ml of 10% calcium chloride, can be given to stabilize the myocardial cell membrane. This is followed by 50 ml of 50 per cent glucose containing 10–12 units of soluble insulin infused over 30–60 min and repeated as necessary. Insulin promotes intracellular movement of potassium thereby lowering the blood levels. Untreated hyperkalaemia can lead to asystolic arrest. If the patient is not anuric/oliguric and fluid overloaded, sodium bicarbonate (50 ml aliquots of 8.4 per cent solution) may be useful as it will also lower the blood potassium level and provide symptomatic relief from the metabolic acidosis. However, ongoing treat-ment of the acid–base derangement is normally achieved with a form of renal replacement therapy.

Table 8.11 Agents used in the treatment of hyperkalaemia

Treatment of hyperkalaemia	Timing of effect
Glucose/insulin	Immediate effect
Renal replacement therapy	Immediate effect
Sodium bicarbonate	Immediate effect
Calcium resonium	Delayed effect

Principles of care

Monitoring urine output

A deteriorating urine output is usually the first indicator of a potential renal problem. In an adult, an hourly volume of 0.5 ml/kg/h is the minimum acceptable vol-ume. If the patient does not have a urinary catheter *in situ* then catheterization should be performed and a catheter left in place and connected to a drainage bag for further monitoring of urine volumes. The drainage bag tubing should be supported or fixed to the patient's leg to prevent drag on the urethra.

A fluid balance chart to record intake and output on an hourly basis should be maintained.

If a urinary catheter is already in place the possibility of catheter blockage should be excluded by bladder irrigation. If necessary, the catheter should be re-placed. If the patient is anuric, the presence of a urinary catheter may cause infection and it should be removed. Likewise, it is essential that in patients with nephrostomy tubes, ureteric stents or urostomies, the possibility of obstruction is ruled out.

If the patient has been admitted post-urological sur-gery or post-renal trauma, the possibility of blood and blood clots causing an obstruction must be strongly suspected. If the patient is oliguric, and circulating fluid volume has been optimized, the fluid intake should be restricted, to replace urine output plus insensible losses only. This is acceptable in the critically ill patient for only a short period of time as intense fluid restriction pre-cludes provision of adequate nutrition; renal replacement therapy is often implemented for this reason.

Care should be taken when administering hypertonic solutions, such as sodium bicarbonate, mannitol, or 10–50 per cent glucose, if the patient is oliguric. The hypertonicity will pull extravascular fluid into the circu-lation and the patient may become intravascularly fluid-overloaded.

Avoidance of pre-renal renal failure

If the urine output is less than 0.5 ml/kg/h per hour and the urinary catheter is patent, there may be a pre-renal cause of oliguria.

Avoidance of pre-renal renal failure

- Adequate circulating volume and organ perfusion pressure
- Adequate cardiac output
- Possible use of dopamine infusion at 1–3 µg/kg/min

It is essential that the patient has an adequate circulat-ing blood volume. The presence of tachycardia, hypo-tension, and cool peripheries may indicate that extra fluid is required. If so, the patient should be adminis-tered aliquotes of colloid fluid, 200–300 ml at a time (see Chapter 5 — 'Fluid challenge'). The patient's ventricular filling pressures (determined by either the central venous pressure and/or the pulmonary artery wedge pressure, as available) should be measured before and after each bolus of fluid.

If, 5–10 minutes following the bolus of fluid, the filling pressure rises $\geq$ 3 mmHg and remains at that level then the patient probably has an adequate circulation. How-ever, if there is no change or only a small increase then the optimal filling pressure may not have been achieved.

Further fluid should be administered as appropriate. When the patient has a pulmonary artery catheter, the stroke volume and cardiac output can be used to determine the optimal filling pressure (see Chapter 5).

The urine output should be reassessed in the light of an adequate circulating volume; if there is no improvement and the patient remains tachycardic, ± hypotension, and peripherally cool, attempts should be made to increase the cardiac output with a suitable inotropic or vasodilating agent (see Chapter 5). Cardiac output studies during this phase are useful to determine the effect of any inotropes administered. It is vital that attention be paid to the maintenance of an optimum cardiac output and circulating blood volume during all stages of the patient's illness.

Diuretic therapy

If the patient has a good circulating volume and an adequate cardiac output but remains oliguric, diuretics can be given in an attempt to promote a diuresis. The two classes of diuretics that can be given in this situation are:

(1) osmotic (e.g. mannitol), and

(2) loop (e.g. frusemide)

It has not been shown that either drug improves renal function but they can promote a diuresis. Mannitol may have a beneficial role in myoglobinuria, radiological contrast media-induced renal failure, and nephrotoxicity (Corwin and Bonventre 1988). However, the administration of mannitol can increase the extracellular fluid volume and may cause pulmonary oedema.

The administration of frusemide is also not without risk. If a diuresis is promoted, the fluid and solute loss can cause hypovolaemia and exacerbation of poor renal perfusion. Although frusemide may increase the urine output, there is no evidence that it increases survival (Corwin and Bonventre 1988). There is some evidence that these two agents may have a more effective role in the patient who is 'at risk', rather than in the patient who is in established renal failure (Lazarus 1990). (See Table 8.12 for the actions of mannitol and frusemide.)

Typical dosages of mannitol and frusemide in renal failure
Mannitol: 500 mg/kg (i.e. 5 ml/kg of 10% solution or 2.5 ml/kg of 20% solution)
Frusemide: 20–1000 mg bolus followed by an infusion of 2 mg/min up to a maximum of 500 mg

---

Table 8.12 Actions of mannitol and frusemide

Mannitol	*Frusemide*
May reduce cell swelling and decrease tubular cell injury	May increase intratubular flow, preventing obstruction
May increase extracellular volume and therefore cardiac output, may decrease blood viscosity and systemic oncotic pressure resulting in an increase in GFR	May cause vasodilatation of glomerular capillaries
May increase intratubular flow, preventing obstruction	May inhibit tubuloglomerular feedback, increasing GFR
May cause vasodilatation of glomerular capillaries, perhaps by increasing prostaglandin production	May decrease transport related oxygen consumption

Dopamine can be infused, at the so-called 'renal dose' of 1–3μg/kg/min. At this dose, dopamine will cause intrarenal vasodilatation as well as a diuresis, but again the overall effect on survival is not clear.

The administration of a diuretic may promote a diuresis and the development of established oliguric renal failure may be avoided. The patient may enter into a phase of non-oliguric acute renal failure, in which adequate volumes of urine are produced but renal function deteriorates as urine quality is poor. Investigations, as outlined in the acute renal failure section (p. 216) must be performed, a diagnosis made, and appropriate management stategies determined.

It is often at this point that patients are admitted to the ICU, when the renal failure is established and is no longer reversible.

Nutrition

The patient in acute renal failure is often extremely catabolic and the implementation of nutrition should be a priority as muscle mass is quickly broken down to provide an energy source.

Enteral nutrition is preferable with fewer complications (e.g. metabolic or feeding line-related sepsis); it also maintains gut integrity and may help to prevent translocation of bacteria and endotoxins.

If renal replacement therapy is in progress, there is no requirement to restrict protein (and hence restrict urea production), fluid volume, or potassium. Although the patient can be catabolic, there is no benefit in providing more than 2000–2500 kcal per day (Hartley 1992).

It can be useful to be able to calculate the patient's requirements with a metabolic computer (see Chapter 10). Protein requirements rarely exceed 14 g of nitrogen per day, except in the patient with burns. Extra protein losses occur with peritoneal dialysis and amino acid losses with haemofiltration, this should be allowed for in the feeding regime.

Electrolyte and trace elements should be titrated and supplied according to blood levels and not simply given as a routine. The B group vitamins are water-soluble and can be removed during dialysis and haemofiltration. They should therefore be supplemented regularly.

Skin integrity

The risk of tissue breakdown and the development of decubitus ulcers is high in this group of patients. The renal failure has often been caused by a state of hypoperfusion, where intense peripheral vasoconstriction occurs as a compensatory mechanism. In addition, these patients often require inotropic support which can further decrease blood supply to the skin and underlying tissue.

Lengthy periods of time spent inserting lines, investigating, and fluid resuscitating often require the patient to remain in one position which can aggravate the situation even further.

The patient should be examined and assessed for risk of developing pressure sores as soon as possible following admission. This should be documented, along with a preventative strategy or a treatment programme appropriate to the risk or the sore involved. It may be necessary to use a pressure-relieving mattress or bed if the patient is particularly vulnerable or is too cardiovascularly unstable to withstand frequent changes of position.

Care should also be taken with skin underlying ECG electrodes, lines, and endotracheal tapes as these can quickly break down in the presence of poor skin perfusion.

The patient may experience skin irritation arising from azotaemia (high blood levels of nitrogenous waste products). Care should be taken that the patient does not scratch him/herself causing disruption of skin integrity and supra-added infection.

Renal replacement therapy

The indications for commencing a form of renal replacement therapy (RRT) are as follows:

- Metabolic acidosis (pH < 7.3 and falling).

- Hyperkalaemia (> 6 mmol/l and rising).

- Fluid overload or to create space for nutrition.

- Severe uraemic symptoms (confusion, pericarditis, nausea, vomiting, etc.).

- Urea > 30 mmol/l and rising, creatinine > 300 μmmol/l and rising.

All the above indications are relative and individual cases may require earlier or later treatment.

The overall aims of any form of renal replacement therapy are:

- To relieve fluid overload, restore, and maintain fluid balance.

- To remove waste products (i.e. urea and creatinine).

- To correct and maintain metabolic and electrolyte balance.

Types of renal replacement therapy
- Haemofiltration (various types).

- Intermittent haemodialysis (IHD).

- Peritoneal dialysis (PD).

- A combination of IHD and haemofiltration.

Basic physiological principles common to all renal replacement therapies

Diffusion

The movement of solutes across a semi-permeable membrane from an area of high to low concentration. A concentration gradient is therefore always necessary for diffusion to occur.

Molecules with a smaller molecular weight will move across a semi-permeable membrane more readily than those with a larger molecular weight. A semi-permeable membrane has a defined pore size, any molecule exceeding this will not be able to pass through.

Diffusion will be affected by the resistance offered by the membrane, this is related to the thickness, size, and shape of the pores. Diffusion is utilized in peritoneal dialysis, haemodialysis, and haemodiafiltration (see Fig. 8.6).

Ultrafiltration

This a method of convective transport. It can be defined as the bulk movement of water together with permeable solutes through a semi-permeable membrane. Water molecules are small and can pass through all semi-permeable membranes.

Diffusion

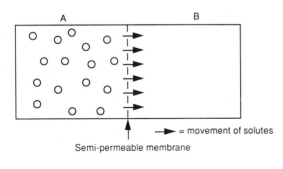

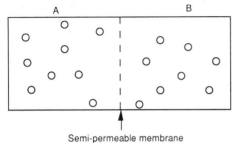

Fig. 8.6 The movement of solutes across a semipermeable membrane.

The driving force for ultrafiltration can be either an osmotic gradient or hydrostatic pressure (see Fig. 8.7).

Osmotic ultrafiltration
Water will be drawn across a semi-permeable membrane from a hypotonic solution into a hypertonic solution. The osmotic 'pull' is generated by the concentrated solute in the hypertonic solution.

Osmotic ultrafiltration is utilized in peritoneal dialysis.

Hydrostatic ultrafiltration
Water is forced across a semi-permeable membrane by a hydrostatic pressure exerted across the membrane. Hydrostatic ultrafiltration is utilized in haemofiltration and haemodialysis.

Ultrafiltration coefficient (KUF)
This indicates the permeability of the semi-permeable membrane. The KUF is defined as the number of millilitres of fluid per hour that will be transferred across the membrane per mmHg pressure gradient across the membrane.

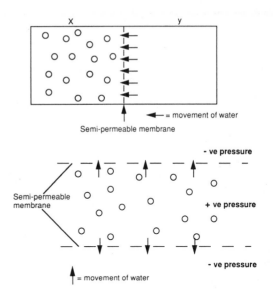

Fig. 8.7 Ultrafiltration: (a) osmotic; (b) hydrostatic.

Extracorporeal methods of renal replacement therapy

The majority of ICUs are now able to offer a vascular form of renal replacement therapy, including arteriovenous and venovenous methods. Haemodialysis and haemofiltration share some common principles and these will be discussed prior to addressing the techniques individually.

Buffers

To enable effective treatment of the metabolic acidosis which frequently accompanies acute renal failure, a buffer must be provided either in the dialysate fluid or in the replacement fluid (haemofiltration only).

Lactate is commonly used as the buffer for haemofiltration: it is metabolized by the liver into bicarbonate. Acetate, another buffer, is known to cause vasodilatation, a reduction in myocardial contractility, hypoventilation, hypoxaemia, and hypotension (Bihari and Beale 1991), rendering it inappropriate for most critically ill patients. Bicarbonate itself is also given as a buffer in haemodialysis. It can be used as the buffer for haemofiltration but this involves individual administration of other electrolytes, magnesium, and calcium.

Artificial membranes

There is a wide choice of artificial kidneys/filters available, all of which have differing membrane properties.

There are two main groups of membranes:

1. *Cellulose membrane*: cuprophane, cellulose hydrate, cellulose acetate.

2. *Synthetic membranes*: Polycarbonate, polysulfone, polyamide, polyacrylonitrile.

The cellulose membranes have traditionally been used for chronic haemodialysis (HD), having relatively low permeability with a cut-off at approximately 5000 daltons. The Cuprophane membrane in particular has been associated with complement activation, cytokine generation, white cell and platelet activation, all of which can lead to pulmonary and other organ dysfunction (Bihari and Beale 1991).

The synthetic membranes are, on the whole, not associated with such disturbances. Polyacrylonitrile, in particular, is a highly biocompatible and permeable membrane with a cut-off of approximately 35 000 daltons.

The artificial kidney itself can either be of a hollow fibre or a flat plate design.

Vascular access

Any of the 'spontaneous' extracorporeal methods of renal replacement therapy (i.e. without a blood pump in the circuit) require the vascular access to be arterial in origin so as to supply sufficient pressure to drive blood around the circuit and provide an adequate filtration pressure (Table 8.13.).

Once a blood pump has been incorporated, blood flow is not dependent upon arterial pressure and access may be gained from a vein.

For relatively short-term use in the ICU, a 'double lumen cannula' is commonly used. This is a Y-shaped cannula inserted into a large vein (e.g. femoral, internal jugular, or subclavian veins). One arm of the Y allows blood to be drawn away from the patient, while the other arm allows blood to be simultaneously pumped back into the patient further up the vein to prevent re-circulation (Fig. 8.8).

Anticoagulation

Most forms of extracorporeal circulation require anticoagulation to help prevent platelet and coagulation system activation as a response to contact with a foreign surface (i.e. the circuits and filter). There are methods

Table 8.13 Vascular access in renal replacement therapy

Access	Use	Comment
Separate artery and vein cannulation	Non-blood pump-driven methods.	Commonly femoral approaches used. Renders patient immobile, blood flow obstructed if legs bent.
Arteriovenous shunt (e.g. Schribner) Radial artery/cephalic vein or post-tibial artery/long saphenous vein	Pumped and non-pumped methods	Provides good blood flow. Cannot be changed, along with other patient lines if sepsis suspected.
Double lumen: Jugular vein access	Pumped methods.	Provides good blood flow. Position often uncomfortable for patient. Can be difficult to fix to the skin due to position.
Double lumen: Subclavian vein approach	Pumped methods.	Provides good blood flow. Allows greater patient mobility. Potential insertion complications: pneumothorax, brachial plexus injury. Longer-term complications: subclavian vein thrombosis/stenosis.
Double lumen: Femoral vein approach	Pumped methods.	Provides good blood flow — if legs kept straight. No proven increased risk of infection. Can be a difficult site to expose for observation.

during intermittent HD that allow for heparin-free dialysis. This is rarely successful for continuous techniques such as haemofiltration.

There are three main tests used to assess anticoagulation during renal replacement therapy.

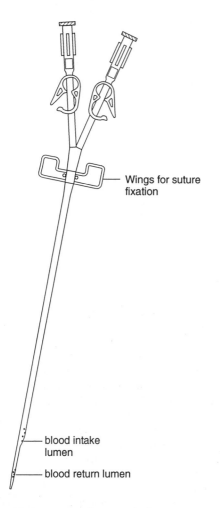

— Wings for suture fixation

— blood intake lumen

— blood return lumen

Fig. 8.8 Double-lumen vascular cannula for venovenous haemo(dia)filtration.

1. Activated clotting time (ACT)
Blood is added to a tube containing siliceous earth which accelerates the clotting process. A machine (e.g. Haemochron) is then used to automatically tilt/rotate the tube and to detect clot formation.

During HD, ACT is normally maintained at 200–250 seconds (baseline = 120–150 seconds).

During haemofiltration the ACT would normally be maintained at approximately 150–220 seconds (same baseline as above).

2. Whole blood partial thromboplastin time (WBPTT)
The clotting process is accelerated by the addition of 0.2 ml of actin FS reagent (Thrombofax) to 0.4 ml of blood. This is set in a heating block at 37 °C for 30 seconds and then tilted every 5 seconds until a clot forms. During HD, the WBPTT would be maintained at the baseline value + 40–80 per cent, approximately 120–140 seconds. During haemofiltration, a baseline value + 50 per cent would be maintained.

3. Lee White clotting time
In this method, 0.4 ml of blood is added to a glass tube which is inverted every 30 seconds at room temperature until a clot forms. A baseline would be 4–8 minutes with a desired value at 20–30 minutes. This is the least accurate or desirable method of assessing anti-coagulation status.

Heparin
This is the most frequently used anticoagulant. However, it is a difficult agent to titrate, particularly because its effects vary so dramatically between individuals. The half-life of heparin can range from 45 seconds to 4.5 hours without any predictable reason.

The most common type of heparin used is mixed molecular weight unfractionated heparin which is not cleared across artificial membranes fully due to its high negative charge and protein binding. There has been increased interest in low molecular weight heparin which, in theory, presents fewer haemorrhagic risks to the patient.

The dose of heparin required during haemofiltration is less than in HD. Commonly, doses of 5–10 iu/kg/h are infused proximal to the filter. If the patient has adverse reactions to heparin (e.g. thrombocytopenia) or is at risk from bleeding (e.g. post-surgery), prostacyclin or alprostadil (PGE$_1$) can be infused instead at 2.5–10 ng/kg/min. This allows the rate of heparin infusion to be decreased to $\leqslant$250 iu/h or stopped completely. If the patient develops heparin-induced thrombocytopenia syndrome (HITS) *all* heparin must be stopped, including that in flush lines. Low molecular weight heparin may be used as an alternative. Prostacyclin acts by inhibiting platelet aggregation (see Chapter 12). Heparin-bonded circuits are being developed but are currently very expensive.

Haemofiltration

Principles

Haemofiltration is a convective process in which there is mass movement of plasma water and solutes across a highly permeable membrane.

The blood on one side of the membrane exerts a hydrostatic pressure (from the presence of a pump or the patient's arterial pressure). This pressure allows plasma water and solutes to move across the membrane by hydrostatic ultrafiltration to become the 'filtrate'. The constant draining of the filtrate compartment ensures a negative pressure on the other side of the membrane, thus maintaining a pressure gradient. Much of the protein as well as cellular constituents of blood are prohibited from moving across the membrane due to their molecular size.

The process is not selective and the removal of waste products can only be achieved by the removal of an accompanying load of water and other solutes. The volume of filtrate removed can be over 2 litres per hour; to maintain cardiovascular stability, fluid must be replaced concurrently up to the desired fluid balance. The fluid used as replacement should be isotonic and should also aim to replace the solutes lost as filtrate that would otherwise be selectively reabsorbed by the normal kidney.

Typical constituents of haemofiltration replacement fluid

- Water
- Sodium 140 mmol/l
- Calcium 1.75 mmol/l
- Magnesium 0.75 mmol/l
- Chloride 100 mmol/l
- Lactate 45 mmol/l
- Variable potassium content
- Osmolality 287.4 mosmol

The amount of filtrate removed can, if wished, be controlled by using a volumetric pump distal to the artificial kidney.

Advantages

- Haemofiltration allows continuous control of uraemia and fluid balance which promotes cardiovascular stability.

- It does not require the utilization of specialist renal staff or equipment/water supplies.

- It can be performed in the ICU, negating the need to transfer critically ill patients to renal centres.

Disadvantages

- Haemofiltration restricts the patient's mobility and necessitates constant patient-centred activity which can disrupt rest and sleep patterns.

- Anticoagulation has to be continuous, albeit at a relatively lower dose.

- Removal and consequent administration of large volumes of fluid is nurse-intensive and open to potential error.

Types of haemofiltration

Haemofiltration can be spontaneous, where blood flow through the extracorporeal circuit depends on the patient's arterial pressure, or it can be assisted with the inclusion of a blood pump in the circuit.

Continuous arteriovenous haemofiltration

Continuous arteriovenous haemofiltration (CAVH) usually refers to a spontaneous method where arterial access and venous return is used. However, CAVH can also refer to a pumped method where for whatever reason, separate arterial and venous cannulation (or an arteriovenous shunt) is utilized (see Fig. 8.9(a).).

Continuous venovenous haemofiltration

Continuous venovenous haemofiltration (CVVH) refers to a pumped method which uses either a double lumen cannula sited in a large vein or two separate venous cannulae for blood access and return.

Once a blood pump has been included in the extracorporeal circuit, the alarm and monitoring devices common to dialysis machines must also be incorporated (see Fig. 8.9(b).).

CAVH is a relatively simple and inexpensive process but is totally dependent on the patient's systolic blood pressure to maintain an adequate blood flow and therefore filtration rate. In the highly catabolic patient, filtration may not be sufficient to achieve adequate control of uraemia (Wendon et al. 1989). In these patients, CVVH is preferred because far higher filtration rates can be maintained with the use of a blood pump. Whether CAVH or CVVH are used, the inadequacies, increased workload, and potential dangers of concurrent removal and replacement of fluid and solutes remain.

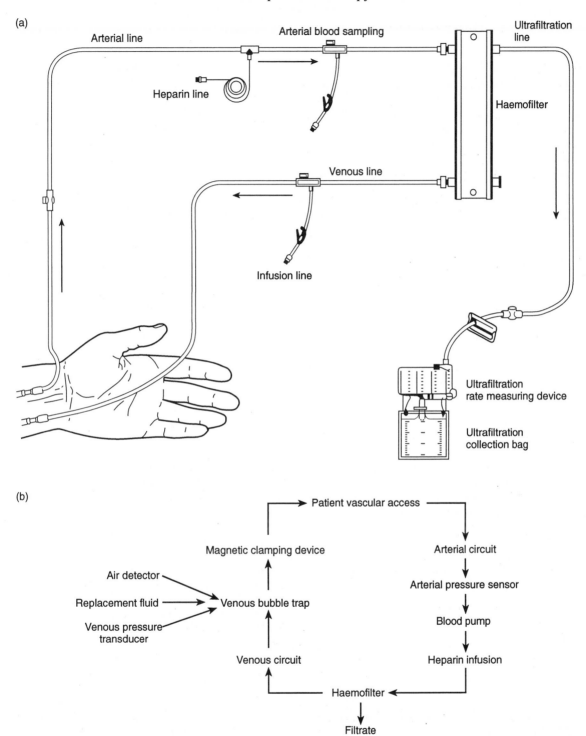

Fig. 8.9 (a) and (b) Continuous arteriovenous (a) and venovenous (b) haemofiltration (see text).

Continuous arteriovenous haemodiafiltration (CAVHD) and continuous venovenous haemodiafiltration (CVVHD)

Both CAVH and CVVH can be adapted by running a dialysate solution through the artificial kidney, in a counter-current direction to the blood and on the opposite side of the membrane. Filtration still occurs because a pressure gradient still exists (albeit to a lesser degree) but, in addition, diffusion can be utilized to facilitate the removal of solutes. This decreases the need to remove such vast volumes of fluid in order to achieve the same result.

The dialysate used is commonly the same as the replacement fluid or peritoneal dialysis fluid. The main disadvantage of using peritoneal dialysis fluid is that glucose can diffuse into the blood causing hyperglycaemia. The flow rate of the dialysate can be up to 2 litres per hour, depending on the clearance of solutes desired.

Assisted haemo(dia)filtration techniques

A number of machines are available for haemofiltration and their modes of operation differ. However, the principles of management are similar.

Fluid balance

Some haemofiltration machines operate on specific time cycles over a number of hours, others operate on an hourly basis. Whichever time unit is used, the patient's intake (nutrition, drugs, and infusions) must be balanced against any losses, including the filtrate. A target fluid balance (either positive or negative) is determined on the basis of clinical assessment of intravascular and total body fluid volume status. Most machines incorporate a pump for the infusion of replacement fluid. Spontaneous methods would utilize a separate volumetric pump.

Example 1

Intake		Output	
Enteral feed	120 ml	Wound drain	50 ml
Omnopon	5 ml	Filtrate	1500 ml
Insulin	2 ml		
	127 ml		1550 ml

The time cycles are hourly and the patient requires to be in a neutral balance at the end of each cycle. To achieve this, 1423 ml of replacement fluid should be given over the same time cycle (1550 − 127)

Example 2

Intake		Output	
Parenteral feed	100 ml	Nasogastric tube	50 ml
Adrenaline	5 ml	Filtrate	1800 ml
Fentanyl	5 ml		
Insulin	3 ml		
	113 ml		1850 ml

The time cycle is hourly and the patient requires to be in a balance of − 100 ml at the end of each cycle. The amount of replacement fluid to be given is:

1850 − 113 = 1737 ml (to achieve neutral balance)

1737 − 100 = **1637 ml** (to achieve a 100 ml/h negative balance)

Fluid balance recordings must be documented clearly to avoid confusion and checked carefully to avoid accidental hypo- or hypervolaemia.

If a form of haemodiafiltration is used, it must be remembered to subtract the volume of dialysate infused from the total filtrate volume to obtain the actual filtrate volume.

Haemodynamic monitoring

Continuous ECG and blood pressure monitoring are essential, primarily to detect signs of hypovolaemia (i.e. tachycardia and hypotension). If significant hypovolaemia occurs, an increase in core–peripheral temperature gap and decreased cardiac filling pressures (central venous pressure, pulmonary artery wedge pressure) would also be observed.

Relative hypovolaemia can be observed when instigating haemofiltration as the patient has to become accustomed to an additional circulation (the extracorporeal circuit). Prior to use, the haemofiltration circuits have to be primed (usually with heparinized saline) to remove air, to coat the circuit with heparin, and to flush the artificial kidney.

There are two options when commencing the technique. One is to attach the patient to both ends of the circuit which results in the patient receiving the prime solution remaining in the circuits (approximately 200 ml). This may not be desirable if the patient is severely overloaded. The second option is initially to attach the arterial end of the circuit only, allowing the patient's blood to move into the circuits and expelling any prime solution before attaching the venous circuit. This method can lead to relative hypovolaemia due to the patient losing blood into the circuit without receiving any back until the prime has been lost and the venous limb attached. If this method is used a colloid solution must be immediately available to be infused if hypovolaemia becomes apparent.

When the technique is established, hypovolaemia may occur if the patient's fluid requirements change. Critically ill patients experience fluid shifts and periods of vasoconstriction and vasodilatation, all serving to alter fluid status. The original fluid balance aims may not now be tolerated by the patient and should be reassessed. It should be borne in mind that any signs of hypo- or hypervolaemia could be caused by inaccurate fluid balance recordings and calculations should always be checked to guard against this.

Arrhythmias can also occur, as with haemodialysis due to hypo- or hyperkalaemia or hypovolaemia. Serum potassium values should be checked at least 4-hourly, especially with haemofiltration alone. If employing haemodiafiltration, electrolyte balance is less likely to present a problem as serum levels can equilibriate with the dialysate fluid. Therefore, if the dialysate fluid contains 4.5 mmol/l of potassium and the serum potassium falls below that value, potassium will diffuse across the artificial membranes into the patient until the serum potassium has reached 4.5 mmol/l. If the patient's potassium should rise above 4.5 mmol/l the reverse would happen. The same principle applies to all serum constituents which can diffuse across the artificial membranes. Notably, sodium losses during haemofiltration can exceed sodium intake and additional sodium may have to be infused. In haemodiafiltration, the sodium levels can be maintained by diffusion from the dialysate.

The patient's central temperature should be monitored and maintained at >36°C. The effect of circulating blood outside the body where it rapidly cools will reduce the patient's body temperature as can the infusion of large volumes of replacement fluid. Replacement fluid should be warmed (i.e. via a blood-warming device) prior to infusion. If required to maintain temperature, the dialysate fluid can also be warmed prior to use. Conversely, in the pyrexial patient, infusion of unwarmed replacement fluid can be used with therapeutic benefit. It is important to remain aware that an underlying pyrexia may be masked by the cooling effect of continuous haemofiltration and haemodiafiltration.

Nursing interventions

Rest and sleep
One significant disadvantage of continuous haemofiltration and haemodiafiltration is that the nurse's attention is focused around the patient continuously, night and day. This is unavoidable, but steps should be taken to allow the patient adequate periods of rest and sleep. If desired, the technique can be stopped during the night but this has to be weighed against the cost and nursing time implications of changing circuitry every 24 hours.

Psychological care
The sight of seemingly large volumes of blood in an extracorporeal circuit is often taken for granted by the ICU staff but can be frightening for both patient and relatives. This should be anticipated and necessary steps taken to reduce any anxiety. The possibility of haemofiltration as a treatment should be introduced to the patient and relatives prior to its commencement. If there has not been any previous discussion, the 'sudden' appearance of yet another piece of machinery can be viewed by the relatives as treatment which was not anticipated and as an 'emergency' (i.e. introduced as a result of a sudden deterioration in condition). It must be emphasized that giving the patient and relatives prior warning not only maintains their confidence in the ICU staff but also helps to minimize anxiety.

Changing the circuit
There are no specific guidelines regarding the frequency of changing circuits. Some authorities advise that circuits should be changed every 48 hours but there is little evidence to support this and many would not change until there is:

(i) a significant reduction in performance;

(ii) known or suspected bacteraemia;

(iii) evidence of a large clot in the filter or bubble trap which traps and consumes platelets and may provide a medium for bacterial growth.

Ideally, the decision to change the circuits should be made while it is still possible to return the 200 ml of blood in the circuit back to the patient. This is done by disconnecting the arterial circuit from the patient and attaching it to a bag of normal saline. The saline is then allowed to run through the circuit pushing the blood back into the patient via the venous circuit which remains attached. If the circuit has been changed because of clotting, the reason for clotting must be investigated prior to the connection of a new circuit.

If inadequate anticoagulation was the cause (as detected by coagulation tests), the rate of heparin infusion should be increased, perhaps accompanied by more frequent coagulation tests. Clotting in the venous bubble trap and artificial kidney may be detected by the

Table 8.14 Problems associated with haemofiltration

Problem	Cause	Action
Filtrate volumes in excess of ability to concurrently replace fluid.	Can be experienced with new circuits, usually settles down after 3–4 hours.	The filtrate outflow line can be partially clamped. The collecting vessel can be raised to a higher position (if using a spontaneous circuit). Blood flow rate can be reduced but should be maintained above 100 ml/min.
Filtrate volumes decreasing.	Inadequate blood flow (hypotension in spontaneous methods or slow blood pump speed). Clotting in the artificial kidney.	In spontaneous methods: (a) improve blood pressure, (b) lower level of filtrate collecting vessel or apply suction to filtrate collection vessel (increases − ve pressure in filter and therefore increases pressure gradient across semi-permeable membrane). In pumped methods: (a) check blood pump speed (> 100 ml/min). Clotting: see below.
Clotting of the circuit.	Low blood flow, intermittent blood flow (from poor access), cool blood, inadequate anticoagulation, inadequate priming technique, low blood antithrombin III level.	It is possible to continue with some clot present provided that: (a) sufficient volumes are produced for control of uraemia (b) clots are not encouraging further clinically significant platelet adherence (as detected by a continuing low serum platelet count and spontaneous bleeding from line sites etc.) (c) that the patient is not bacteraemic (clots in the kidney would provide a good medium for bacteria). If indicated, the circuit should be changed.

venous pressure monitor. Spontaneous methods can be severely hampered in hypotensive patients, even if the pressure gradient across the semi-permeable membranes in the artificial kidney has been enhanced by lowering the level of the filtrate collecting vessel or applying suction to the filtrate collection point. If this interrupted situation continues, a pumped method is preferable to gain a more constant blood flow and therefore an improved control of uraemia. In pumped methods, the blood flow must be maintained at greater than 100 ml/min to avoid clotting in the artificial kidney. While the speed of blood flowing through the circuit is important, so is the consistency of that speed. If, for example, the vascular access is a femoral vein cannula and the patient is bending his/her legs the flow of blood from the femoral vein will be intermittent and this can precipitate clotting in the artificial kidney. The arterial pressure monitor will detect significant decreases in blood flow from the vascular access. If the flow is severely obstructed, air can be seen being sucked into the arterial circuit by the blood pump. If the circuits are being changed frequently and vascular

access is thought to be the problem, it is sensible to review the site of access.

Often, when moving the patient, blood flow can be interrupted because of cannula movement. The effects of this can be reduced by slowing the blood pump speed for the duration of the move on the pretext that a constant blood flow, although at a slower speed, is preferable to no blood flow.

If clotting occurs soon after connecting the patient with no other obvious problem or alarm status, it is likely that the priming technique has been inadequate. One of the most important functions of priming is to flush the artificial kidney of any sterilizing and stabilizing materials and to open up the pores in the semi-permeable membranes. If this has not been achieved, at best there will be poor diffusive function of the membrane and, at worst, it will clot prematurely. Additionally, if clotting is a continual problem, it may be that the patient has a low plasma level of antithrombin III; this will disrupt the pathway through which heparin works. Options in this case include giving antithrombin III (which is expensive) or fresh frozen plasma which will replace a certain amount of antithrombin III. A less effective alternative is to use prostacyclin to anticoagulate. Failure to establish the cause of repeated clotting of the artificial kidney and circuits can be expensive, time consuming and, most importantly, allows only intermittent control of uraemia.

Safety

The importance of constant nursing attendance cannot be overemphasized. While the machines, cannulae, and circuits are now purpose-built, the consequences of disconnection somewhere in the extracorporeal circuit can be dire.

The spontaneous methods of haemofiltration, although simple, do not incorporate any alarm systems and extra vigilance is called for. Undetected disconnection can lead to exsanguination and/or air embolism. If air has been entrained, the patient should be placed in a head down position and, if possible, on the left side. The rationale for this positioning is that air will always move to the top of any fluid medium and the priority is to prevent air entering the pulmonary circulation.

The vascular access should be in easy view and inspected regularly. The circuits should be supported to avoid undue tension being placed on the cannula(e). Arteriovenous shunts should be kept warm and unkinked to guard against clotting of the shunt; periods of hypotension will also promote clotting in the shunt. The circuits and the haemofiltration machine (if being used) should be positioned to avoid being an obstacle to other necessary pieces of equipment, especially emergency items. The need to reach something quickly could result in the inadvertent removal of circuits and cannulae.

Infection

Critically ill patients who have acute renal failure are immunocompromised to a greater or lesser degree. Extra caution must be exercised when priming circuits and replacing bags of replacement fluid or dialysate fluid.

Strict asepsis must be adhered to when inserting and re-dressing lines. There is evidence to suggest that the skin is the most common source of microorganisms in line-associated bacteraemias. The vascular access must be sutured into position and, to avoid undue movement, be dressed with an adherent material. A suitable dressing should be transparent for ease of viewing.

If a local site infection is suspected, a swab for microbiology should be taken and the line removed and replaced at a different site, in an aseptic manner. If a septic focus is suspected blood cultures are sent with the line tip to the microbiology department.

Anticoagulation

Both haemodialysis and haemofiltration require anticoagulation. Ineffective anticoagulation will cause clotting in the artificial kidney. Although the effects of this are time-consuming, expensive, and provide inadequate therapy, it does not directly present a hazard to the patient. However, the infusion of too much anticoagulant can be extremely dangerous and the patient's coagulation status must be monitored frequently. Any signs of bleeding, from vascular access sites, the gastrointestinal tract, or mucosal membranes should be viewed with suspicion and investigated.

Drug removal

In addition to waste products and other solutes, therapeutic drugs can also be removed by the artificial kidney. There are a great deal of data referring to drug removal during haemodialysis but less so with haemofiltration. This is less of a problem in haemodialysis as, unless absolutely necessary, the giving of drugs can be avoided during the 3- or 4-hour dialysis session. In haemofiltration, unfortunately, this is not the case. It is known that protein-bound drugs are far less likely to be removed by the artificial kidney in view of the size of the drug–protein complex. It is important to remember this when titrating vasoactive drugs, sedatives, muscle relaxants, or analgesics when the patient's requirements may seem unusually high. Antibiotics, such as the aminoglycosides, and other drugs which can be monitored (e.g. digoxin and aminophylline) should be regularly measured to ensure therapeutic levels.

Intermittent haemodialysis (HD)

Principles

Blood is pumped into an extracorporeal circuit where it is anticoagulated prior to passage through an artificial kidney or dialyser. This contains multiple hollow fibres or sheets which form the semi-permeable membranes. Within the artificial kidney a dialysate fluid is pumped on the opposite side of the semi-permeable membrane to the blood and in a counter-current direction. Waste products move from the blood, across the membrane, into the dialysate by diffusion.

Blood flows of up to 600 ml/min can be achieved during haemodialysis. While the clearance of small molecules depends on the concentration gradient across the membrane, their clearance can also be improved by increasing the counter-current dialysate flow rate, which is commonly set at up to 500 ml/min.

Water is removed by ultrafiltration and this can be

achieved by the exertion of a pressure across the semi-permeable membrane, (the so-called 'transmembrane pressure' TMP). The TMP can be exerted in two ways: first, by the partial occlusion of the dialysate inflow line with the dialysate pump on the outflow line; and secondly, by generating a positive pressure in the blood compartment.

The dialysate is usually supplied in concentrated form and needs to be diluted with water. Proportionators mix the correct volume of water with the correct amount of dialysate concentrate and are either incorporated within each dialysis machine or are situated centrally in a unit and then pumped to individual machines.

Typical dialysate composition

- Sodium 140 mmol/l
- Potassium 1.5 mmol/l
- Calcium 1.5 mmol/l
- Magnesium 1.5 mmol/l
- Chloride 100 mmol/l
- Acetate 35 mmol/l
- Dextrose 12 mmol/l

Vast quantities of water, in the range of 120 litres per session, are required and it must be sterile. The water must also be specially treated, either by reverse osmosis or ion exchange resins. There are systems available which allow the spent dialysate to be recycled by passing it through a sorbent cartridge. This method utilizes 6 litres as opposed to 120 litres of water per session. It is, however, a relatively expensive option.

Advantages
- The most effective method of clearing waste products.

- Uses an intermittent technique, only requiring anti-coagulation during the procedure.

- The patient can be mobile between therapies.

- The intermittent nature incurs lower demands on nursing time.

- A closed-circuit ensures less risk to staff from hepatitis B or C, or HIV infection.

Disadvantages
- Nursing and medical staff need to be specifically trained in the technique.

- During a 2–4-hour period of HD, enough fluid has to be removed to allow nutrition and other infusions to be given throughout the following 24–72 hours between dialyses.

- The patient may require a negative fluid balance at the end of dialysis, necessitating rapid and significant fluid shifts leading to haemodynamic instability in the critically ill patient.

- Haemodialysis provides only episodic control of uraemia.

- Hypoxaemia, hypotension, and complement activation are associated with cheaper types of membrane and buffer solutions, all of which are undesirable in the critically ill patient.

- The equipment and water supply required can be expensive.

Nursing interventions

Many nursing interventions are focused on the detection and early treatment of complications. The dialysis machine incorporates numerous monitoring and alarm systems which must be observed, recorded, and acted on accordingly. (See Table 8.15.)

Complications

In addition to responding to the monitoring and alarms facilities provided by the dialysis machine, the patient must also be observed for the development of potential complications.

Hypotension
Hypotension in the patient receiving haemodialysis can be related to a variety of causes. It is commonly caused by hypovolaemia from the rapid and excessive removal of fluid. The use of acetate as the buffer is also known to precipitate vasodilatation and hypotension.

The critically ill patient receiving haemodialysis should have continuous blood pressure monitoring by either invasive or non-invasive methods to allow early detection of hypotension.

Cardiac arrhythmias
Arrhythmias, commonly due to hyper- or hypokalaemia or to hypovolaemia can occur during dialysis. Tachycardias may be seen as compensatory mechanisms in the event of hypovolaemia and hypotension. The patient should have continuous ECG monitoring.

Hypoxaemia
It is known that certain dialyser membranes can cause hypoxaemia, in particular the cuprophane membrane. The causes are thought to be cytokine activation, oxygen

Table 8.15 Haemodialysis monitors and alarms

Monitor/alarm	Function
Arterial pressure monitor	Situated proximal to the blood pump. Prevents excessive suction on the vascular access by the blood pump. Most common cause of alarm being insufficient blood flow due to malposition or malfunction of the access.
Venous pressure monitor	Situated distal to the dialyser. Prevents excessive resistance to blood returning to the vascular access. Clotting or obstruction of the venous blood line will activate the alarm.
Venous bubble trap and air detector	Situated distal to the venous pressure monitor. Prevents air being returned to the patient. Air entering the venous trap will lower the blood level and activate the air detector.
Dialysate conductivity	Monitors concentration of the dialysate. Prevents dialysing against a hyper- or hypo-osmolar solution. A common cause is a kink in the tubing directing water into the machine, leading to a concentrated dialysate.
Dialysate temperature	The dialysate is heated by the machine and this temperature is monitored to prevent patient hypo- or hyperthermia.
Bypass valve	Operates in the event of a conductivity or temperature alarm. The valve diverts the dialysate directly to the drain.
Blood leak detector	Situated on the dialysate outflow, detects blood in the dialysate which could occur if a leak develops in the dialyser membranes. 'False' blood leaks can be caused by air bubbles in the dialysate, bilirubin (in jaundiced patients) in the dialysate or a dirty sensor.
Dialysate outflow pressure	Can monitor the transmembrane pressure and therefore ultrafiltration rate.

removal and shunting. Continuous pulse oximetry, supported by arterial blood gas monitoring, if indicated, should be performed during dialysis.

Muscle cramps, nausea, and vomiting
The aetiology of cramps, nausea, and vomiting is largely unknown yet are experienced by many patients receiving haemodialysis. The critically ill patient, who may be sedated, could present with signs of restlessness, agitation, and tachycardia. The possibility of cramps or nausea should be considered. Common predisposing factors to cramps are hypotension, dehydration, and a low plasma sodium. Hypotension itself is a potent cause of nausea.

Disequilibrium syndrome
This is a rare yet serious potential complication of haemodialysis. It is thought to be caused by the rapid removal of urea and 'uraemic toxins' during dialysis which results in a much decreased concentration of

these substances in the plasma when compared to the cerebrospinal fluid (CSF). The osmotic gradient now existing between plasma and CSF allows water to move into the CSF and the brain tissue. The patient can present with headache, vomiting, restlessness, convulsions, and even coma. The severely uraemic patient should not experience a reduction in plasma urea of greater than 30% in the first instance to avoid this complication.

Acute haemolysis

This can be caused by overheated, hypotonic, or contaminated dialysate fluid. The patient may complain of back pain, tightness in the chest and dyspnoea. Blood in the venous circuit may take on a 'port wine' appearance in colour. If haemolysis is not detected early, hyperkalaemia can result from the release of potassium from the haemolysed red cells.

Plasma estimations of sodium, potassium, urea, and creatinine should be taken before and after dialysis, in addition to a coagulation screen. If possible, the patient should be weighed (perhaps on a 'weigh bed') before and after each session to estimate fluid status.

Peritoneal dialysis (PD)

Principles

Waste products from the body diffuse across the peritoneum (the semi-permeable membrane) into a dialysate fluid. Flow rates of 70–100 ml/min can be achieved across the peritoneum. Fluid is removed by osmotic ultrafiltration, the osmotic pull provided by varying concentrations of glucose in the dialysate. The higher the concentration of glucose, the stronger the osmotic pull and the more fluid is removed. Blood electrolytes can be manipulated by alteration of the electrolyte levels in the dialysate; diffusion again being the mode of transport.

A catheter, commonly a Tenckhoff catheter, is placed into the peritoneal cavity. This is a sterile procedure, performed using local anaesthetic. The catheter is positioned either in the midline, approximately 3 cm below the umbilicus, or to either side of the abdomen, usually lateral to the border of the rectus muscle. Prior to insertion, the bladder should be emptied and an examination performed to exclude any organ enlargement in order to prevent accidental perforation.

Dialysate fluid is infused via the catheter into the peritoneum. Diffusion of waste products and ultrafiltration of water occurs across the peritoneal membrane, into the dialysate which is then drained out via the catheter. The degree of diffusion and ultrafiltration can be con-

trolled by altering the time that the dialysate is allowed to remain in the peritoneal space, the so-called 'dwell time'. For the purposes of acute PD a typical pattern of treatment would be hourly cycles, 10 minutes for the dialysate to run in, 30 minutes dwell time, and 20 minutes for the dialysate to run out. The more rapidly these cycles are repeated the more diffusion is enhanced. The volume of fluid infused depends upon the size of the peritoneal cavity and how much can be tolerated by the patient. One litre is frequently used and tolerated. There are three concentrations of glucose generally available, 1.5% (standard), 2.5%, and 4.25% — the latter achieving the greatest osmotic pull and so the greatest water removal.

Typical pattern of peritoneal dialysis treatment

- 10 minutes for the dialysate to run in
- 30 minutes dwell time
- 20 minutes for the dialysate to run out

Concentrations of peritoneal dialysis fluid available

1.5% glucose (standard)

2.5% glucose

4.25% glucose

Automatic cycling machines are available which save considerable nursing time.

Advantages
- Relatively simple and inexpensive.
- Can be performed by relatively unskilled nurses.

Disadvantages
- Contraindicated in the presence of abdominal trauma, abdominal sepsis or post abdominal surgery.
- The presence of dialysate fluid in the peritoneum can cause abdominal distention and restrict diaphragmatic movement.
- Questionable control of uraemia, especially in the catabolic patient.
- Proteins can be lost across the peritoneum causing difficulties when attempting to maintain a positive nitrogen balance.
- Risk of peritonitis.

Nursing interventions

The peritoneal dialysate fluid must be warmed prior to infusion to prevent hypothermia. Blood glucose levels must be checked regularly as these can rise due to the diffusion of glucose from the dialysate into the body. If concentrated dialysate fluids are used the blood sugar levels must be checked more frequently.

Potassium (2–4 mmol/l) is often added to the dialysate to regulate body potassium.

One of the most common operational problems with PD is that of dialysate outflow failure. The dialysate fluid removed should at least equal, if not exceed the volume infused; failing this, steps should be taken to rectify the situation (Table 8.16)

Table 8.16 Outflow problems in peritoneal dialysis

Cause	Action
Kinking of the catheter	Re-establish good catheter position and secure in place
Decreased bowel motility	Use of laxatives, suppositories, enemas, and diet
Obstruction by fibrin plugs or strands	Add heparin to the dialysate 200–500 iu/l
Obstruction by fibrin, not responsive to heparin	Infuse streptokinase into the catheter(750 000 iu diluted in 30–100 ml normal saline) Clamp the catheter for 2 hours then reassess drainage
Peritonitis	Add appropriate antibiotics to dialysate

Strict asepsis must be adhered to when changing the dialysate bags or when disconnecting the circuit for any reason. Care must be taken to avoid infection of the catheter site. This can be achieved by preventing undue movement of the catheter by stabilization and by using aseptic technique when cleaning the site and changing the dressing. The patient should be observed for signs of abdominal pain which can indicate either peritonitis or over-distention from too great a dialysate volume per cycle.

If the patient is self-ventilating, care must be taken to position the patient such that the presence of dialysate fluid in the abdomen does not restrict diaphramatic movement. The respiratory rate should be checked at regular intervals.

Peritoneal dialysis, haemodialysis, haemofiltration, and haemodiafiltration are the most common forms of renal replacement therapy in the ICU today. There are some other techniques which are combinations of haemodialysis and haemofiltration (e.g. continuous ultrafiltration with periods of dialysis; CUPID). A purpose-built machine and circuits are used. Fluid removal is performed gently over the 24-hour period then, using the same set-up, dialysis can be performed periodically. The principles of management are as for dialysis and haemofiltration (Milne 1986).

Disorders associated with acute renal failure

Rhabdomyolysis

The association between acute renal failure and skeletal muscle damage was first described by Bywaters and Beal in 1941 (see Better 1990). It is a condition which combines pre-renal, nephrotoxic, and obstructive causes of acute renal failure.

The causes of rhabdomyolysis
Direct trauma, crush injury, burns
Muscle compression from prolonged immobility (surgery, coma)
Metabolic illness (diabetic metabolic decompensation)
Hypokalaemia, hypophosphataemia
Myxodema
Myositis
Temperature extremes
Toxins (alcohol, solvents, carbon monoxide, drug abuse (e.g. heroin or ecstasy)
Muscular dystrophies
Excessive muscle activity (e.g. prolonged seizures)

The damaged muscle can both release and absorb substances; this phenonemon has significant clinical consequences.

Substances released by muscle
Potassium	→	Hyperkalaemia
Hydrogen ions	→	Acidosis
Phosphate	→	Hyperphosphataemia
Creatine	→	High creatine kinase level
Myoglobin	→	Myoglobinuria

Substances absorbed by muscle
Calcium	→	Hypocalcaemia
Sodium	→	Hyponatraemia
Water	→	Dehydration

Management of rhabdomyolysis

The prime aims in management are:

 (i) the prevention of acute renal failure;

 (ii) the correction of electrolyte imbalances; and

 (iii) prevention of further muscle necrosis.

Myoglobin (an iron-containing pigment found in skeletal muscle) has nephrotoxic effects, especially in the presence of volume depletion and acidosis. Early and aggressive volume replacement combined with alkalinization of the urine (pH $\geqslant 7$) should be implemented as soon as possible.

Myoglobin can also obstruct the renal tubules and, in addition to the maintenance of a good circulating volume, mannitol and/or frusemide can be used to ensure a high urine throughput. Care should be taken to maintain patency of the urinary catheter, especially if the urine contains large amounts of myoglobin. The associated hyperkalaemia is often resistant to dextrose and insulin therapy; it may be the overriding initial indication for renal replacement therapy. These patients are also known to be highly catabolic and nutrition must be introduced at an early stage.

Special attention must be paid to any area of musculoskeletal damage. The patient may present with compartment syndrome in which a muscle compartment has been compressed resulting in a restricted neurovascular supply to the extremity distal to the injury and muscle necrosis. Urgent fasciotomy is indicated if compartment syndrome is present. Any extremities which may be affected should be observed frequently for the presence of pulses and impaired circulation as well as swelling and pain.

Hepatorenal syndrome

Hepatorenal syndrome (HRS) is a recognized syndrome in which renal failure accompanies liver failure, especially cirrhosis. The pathogenesis is not fully understood, however; the kidneys on examination appear normal and the resulting renal dysfunction appears to be in part due to a decreased blood flow because of vasoconstriction of the renal cortical vessels. Patients with acute liver failure as a result of hepatitis or paracetamol poisoning are also known to develop HRS.

HRS is characterized by the presence of a low urinary sodium (< 10 mmol/l) and increased urinary osmolality in the absence of proteinuria. Sodium and water conservation is intact, unlike acute renal failure with coexisting liver disease where urinary sodium is > 20 mmol/l.

The management of this condition includes renal replacement therapy, appropriate stategies for treatment of the liver failure and control of ascites (see Chapter 10).

Glomerulonephritis

The term 'glomerulonephritis' encompasses a large number of renal disorders. Patients can present with varying clinical features that can often be difficult to relate to histological findings. Circulating immune complexes that trigger inflammatory and complement reactions cause over 95 per cent of the cases of glomerulonephritis. In less than 5 per cent of cases an inflammatory response set up by circulating immunoglobulins is thought to cause the condition. Some forms of glomerulonephritis may be encountered in the critical care setting and these are described below.

Goodpasture's syndrome

This is an auto-immune disease seen more frequently in young men. It is often accompanied by haemoptysis, anaemia, proteinuria and renal failure. Bilateral lung opacities are seen on chest X-ray and the pulmonary involvement can necessitate intubation and ventilation. Steroids and plasmapheresis are the mainstays of treatment. It is diagnosed by a positive titre of antiglomerular basement membrane antibody in the blood.

Vasculitis

Vasculitis is often seen in polyarteritis, which often presents with asthma, fever, skin rashes, neuropathy, and abdominal pain. Renal failure can develop rapidly with haematuria, proteinuria, and nephrotic syndrome. Treatment is with steroids, cyclophosphamide, and plasmapheresis. Diagnosis is by histology or a raised P-ANCA test. (P-ANCA is the P form of antineutrophil cytoplasmic antibody).

Vasculitis can also accompany Wegener's granulomatosis which is a disease that can affect the respiratory tract and the kidney with vasculitic lesions. Again, steroids, cyclophosphamide, and plasmapheresis are used as treatments. Diagnosis is by histology or a positive titre to antineutrophil cytoplasmic antibody (C-ANCA) in the blood.

Systemic lupus erythematosus

Systemic lupus erythmatosus (SLE) is a systemic disease that can affect the kidneys and cause renal failure.

Females are affected more than males with presenting features of fever, rashes, and arthritis. Cerebral, hepatic, and myocardial involvement can be seen and may be the reason for admission into an ICU. Diagnosis is by positive titre to double-stranded DNA antibody in the blood, and treatment consists of steroids and immuno-suppressants.

References

Beaman, M. and Adu, A. (1992). Acute renal failure. In *Care of the critically ill patient*, (ed. J. Tinker and M. Zapol), 2nd edn, pp. 515–30. Springer, Berlin.

Better, O.S. (1990). Acute renal failure and crush injury. In *Acute renal failure in the intensive therapy unit*, (ed. D. Bihari and G. Neild), pp. 215–21. Springer, Berlin.

Bihari, D. and Beale, R. (1992). Renal support in the intensive care unit. *Current Science*, 272–78.

Cameron, J.S. (1986). Acute renal failure in the intensive care unit today. *Intensive Care Medicine* **12**, 64–70.

Corwin, H.L. and Bonventre J.V. (1988). Acute renal failure in the intensive care unit. Part 2. *Intensive Care Medicine* **14**, 86–96.

Hartley, G.H. (1992). Nutritional support in acute renal failure. *Care of the Critically Ill*. **8**, 18–20.

Lazarus, J.M. (1990). Prophylaxis of acute renal failure in the intensive care unit. In *Acute renal failure in the intensive therapy unit*, (ed. D. Bihari and G. Neild), pp. 280–309. Springer, Berlin.

Milne, A.D. (1986). Continuous ultrafiltration with periods of dialysis. *Care of the Critically Ill*, **1**, 168–76.

Neild, G.H. (1990). Endothelial and mesangial cell dysfunction in acute renal failure. In *Acute renal failure in the intensive therapy unit*, (ed. D. Bihari and G. Neild), pp. 77–89. Springer, Berlin.

Schieppati, A. and Remuzzi, G. (1990). Eicosanoids and acute renal failure. In *Acute renal failure in the intensive therapy unit*, (ed. D. Bihari and G. Neild), pp 115–29. Springer, Berlin.

Schrier, R.W., Abraham, W.T., and Hensen, J. (1990). Strategies in management of acute renal failure in the intensive therapy unit. In *Acute renal failure in the intensive therapy unit*, (ed. D.Bihari and G. Neild), pp. 193–214. Springer, Berlin.

Smithies, M. and Cameron, S. (1992). Renal failure following reconstructive arterial surgery. In *Surgical management of vascular disease*, (ed. P. Bell, C. Jamieson, and C. Ruckley), pp. 1027–48. W.B. Saunders, London.

Wendon, J., Smithies, M., Sheppard, M., Bullen, K., Tinker, J., and Bihari, D. (1989). Continuous high volume venous–venous haemofiltration in acute renal failure. *Intensive Care Medicine*, **15** 1–6.

9. Neurological problems

Introduction

Benner and Wrubel (1989) suggests that the holistic approach to neural organization views the brain as complex and dynamic. It is an organ capable of considerable growth, development, and change, both physiologically and in terms of its behavioural effects. Disruption of neurological function, therefore, has major implications for nursing intervention and often places overwhelming demands up patients and their family and friends.

Anatomy and physiology

Table 9.1 and Fig. 9.1 show the structure and function of the brain.

The prime function of the nervous system is the co-ordination and integration of all body functions and can be categorized on the basis of function and location.

Table 9.1 Structure and function of the brain.

Structure	Function
Cerebral hemispheres	
● Cortex	Higher mental functions (e.g. judgement, language, memory).
● Basal ganglia	Functions with other lower areas of the brain to provide co-ordination and smoothing of subconscious rhythmic movements and voluntary movements.
Diencephalon	
● Thalamus	Sensory and motor relay centre for impulses, gross awareness of sensation, contributory function to reticular activating system.
● Hypothalamus	Production of neurosecretory substances to stimulate or inhibit anterior pituitary secretion, contains centres to co-ordinate autonomic stimulation, and to regulate: (i)temperature, (ii) appetite, (iii) water balance by ADH, (iv) rhythmic activities such as sleep.
● Limbic system	Consists of hypothalamus, cingulate gyrus, amygdala, hippocampus, mamillary bodies, septum, and interconnecting fibre tracts (see Fig. 9.2). Functions to control emotional and behavioural activities and responses (e.g. excitement, rage, terror, pleasure). It also provides a connection between perception, higher brain function, and endocrine/autonomic responses.
Midbrain (mesencephalon)	Acts as a relay centre for motor signals to the cord and pons, forms part of the basal ganglia motor control system, controls eye movements particularly the reflex pupillary response to bright light. The periaqueductal gray nuclei are located here. These play a major role in the analysis and reaction to pain.
Pons	Contains the nuclei of several cranial nerves including vestibulocochlear (VIII) and abducens (VI) which transmit sensory signals from the ear and control eye movement. The pneumotaxic and apneustic centres (see Chapter 3) are located here with tracts connecting them to higher and lower centres.
Medulla	Contains autonomic centres controlling respiration and vasomotor response as well as vomit, gag, and cough reflexes. The vagus and glossopharyngeal nerve nuclei are located here.
Cerebellum	Receives signals from all ascending sensory input and all descending motor impulses. Matches intended motor stimuli against sensory data to co-ordinate smooth movement, maintain equilibrium, and smoothly control posture.

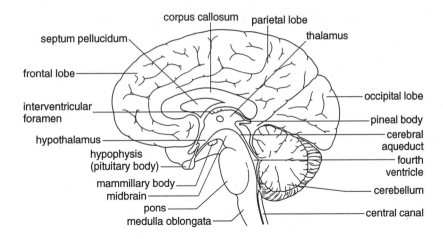

Fig. 9.1 The midline section of the brain. (Reproduced from Hudak *et al. Critical care nursing. A holistic approach.* 1990, with permission).

Function

1. Largely voluntary and automatic (somatic).

2. Largely involuntary (autonomic).

Location

1. Central nervous system (CNS).

2. Peripheral nervous system (PNS).

Cellular level

Nervous tissues comprise:

- motor neurones,

- sensory neurones,

- inter-(connecting) neurones.

Figure 9.3 is a diagram of a typical neurone.

Neural impulses are generated near the cell body and are conducted along the axon at variable speeds. The speed is dependent on:

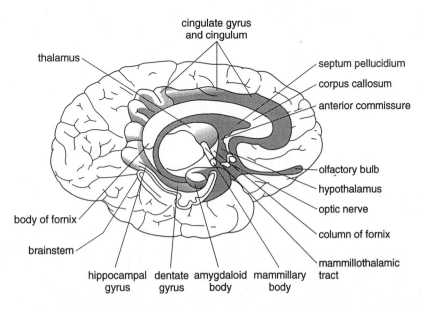

Fig. 9.2 The limbic system in the midportion of the cerebellum. (From Warwick and Williams, *Gray's anatomy*, (35th British edn), 1973; reprinted with permission.)

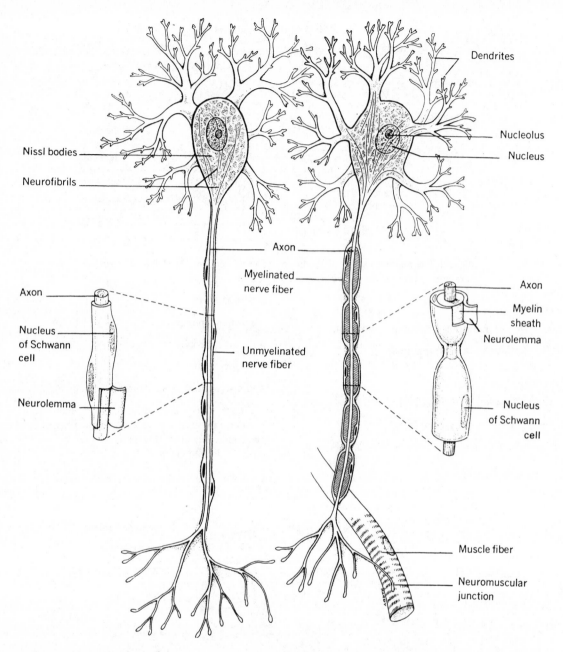

Fig. 9.3 Diagram showing the structure of typical efferent neurones. Reprinted from Chaffee and Lyttle *Basic anatomy and physiology* (1980) with kind permission.

1. The width of the axon.

2. The presence or absence of an outer myelin sheath.

   The presence of a myelin sheath will enhance the speed of neural conduction and provide a high degree of insulation of electrical impulses down the axon. Fifty per cent of all axons are myelinated (i.e. myelin-sheathed). Axons normally carry nervous impulses away from the cell body (efferent) in contrast to the dendrites which conduct the nerve impulses towards the cell body (afferent). Axons and dendrites may vary in size and length, ranging from microscopic areas on the cell body surface to cylindrical processes that can extend to over one metre in length.

Neurones are not structurally connected but the propagation of the nervous impulse is facilitated via a synapse which is dependent on a chemical neurotransmitter. Figure 9.4 is an example of a two neurone system with its specific neurochemical. The essence of the neural impulse is the action potential and its propagated conduction.

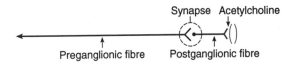

The pre- and postganglionic parasympathetic nerve fibres.

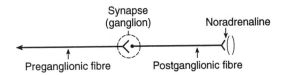

Fig. 9.4 The pre- and postganglionic sympathetic nerve fibres (From Green, *An introduction to human physiology*, (4th edn), Oxford University Press with permission).

The membrane of the neurone maintains a relative negative charge inside the cell using sodium pumps. The cytoplasm of the neurone contains large anions (negatively charged particles) that are too large to cross the membrane. These attract cations (positively charged ions), such as sodium and potassium, into the cell. The active transport enzyme system pumps out sodium ions almost as fast as they enter, retaining a relative negative charge. This is referred to as the resting polarity of the neurone and measures -85 mV. The sodium–potassium pumps are temporarily switched off by a stimulus which causes depolarization (loss of the electrical charge), and if this occurs in sufficient magnitude then depolarization will become self-propagating and spread throughout the entire neurone. This is a temporary event and the resting potential of the neurone will be restored by reactivation of the sodium pumps. This temporary alteration in electrical charge is known as an action potential. Neuronal electrical activity can be monitored at the surface of the brain producing waveforms which are recorded as an electroencephalogram (EEG).

The synapse

This is the junction between one neurone and the next across which an impulse is transmitted. Synaptic vesicles in the presynaptic terminal secrete either excitatory or inhibitory transmitter substances in response to an action potential. These substances cross the synaptic cleft (a microscopic space between the synaptic terminal and the receptor area of the effector cell). The transmitter substance changes the permeability of the receptor area postsynaptic membrane producing either excitation or inhibition of the receptor. While the transmitter substance is bound to the receptor site the neurone is either stimulated (depolarized or hypopolarized) or inhibited (hyperpolarized). The transmitter detaches from the receptor almost immediately after contact and is then either re-attached or inactivated (see Fig. 9.5).

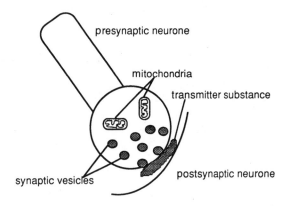

Fig. 9.5 Synaptic transmission.

Neurotransmitters

These are chemicals which transfer electrical impulses from a nerve cell to its target cell. The target cell can be another nerve cell, a muscle, or a gland cell (see Table 9.2). Most chemical transmitters are stimulators, and only γ-aminobutyric acid (GABA) is known to inhibit target cells.

Structural level

Figure 9.6 shows the protective coverings of the brain. The functions of these protective layers are complex and exert positive and negative influences on cerebral function.

Advantages
1. Protection of brain from externally applied forces (skull and cerebrospinal fluid).

2. Protection from infection.

3. Promotion of healing.

Table 9.2 Neurotransmitters and their secretion sites

Neurotransmitter	Site of secretion

Acetylcholine (ACh)
• Chief neurotransmitter of parasympathetic nervous system (NS)
	• Autonomic NS
	  – all preganglionic nerve endings
	  – parasympathetic postganglionic nerve endings
	• Sympathetic postganglionic nerve endings of sweat glands
	• Neuromuscular junctions (voluntary skeletal muscle)
	• Adrenal medulla

Noradrenaline • Chief neurotransmitter of the sympathetic NS	• Sympathetic postganglionic nerve endings (except sweat glands) • Systemic effect caused by release into bloodstream by adrenal medulla
Dopamine • Affects control of fine movement, sensory input integration, and emotional behaviour	• Extrapyramidal system of the basal ganglia • Sympathetic ganglia • Limbic system • Portions of retina • Median eminence and other parts of hypothalmus
Serotonin (5-hydroxytryptamine) • Control of heat regulation, sleep, hunger, behaviour, and some effect on consciousness	• Hypothalamus, limbic system, cerebellum, spinal cord
γ-Aminobutyric acid (GABA) • Inhibitory effect on brain, spinal cord, and retina • Present in large amounts in the grey matter of the brain • Regulates portions of available energy	• Cerebellum, cerebral cortex, neurones mediating presynaptic inhibitors, retina

Disadvantages

1. High vascularity — tendency to lacerating wounds and bleeding (scalp and meningeal vessels).

2. Restrictive structure leaving little room for expansion of contents (skull).

Meninges

These are three layers of tissue:

(i) pia mater, which lies confluent to the brain and spinal cord,

(ii) arachnoid layer, which supports a network of blood vessels,

(iii) dura mater, which is the thickest and most protective layer lying between the bones of the skull and spinal cord and the arachnoid layer.

Cerebrospinal fluid

Cerebrospinal fluid (CSF) has a similar composition to plasma, although with minimal large plasma proteins (0.1–0.4 g/l). It is secreted by the choroid plexus — a mass of capillaries embedded in the four ventricles of the brain. CSF occupies the thin subarachnoid space between the arachnoid and pia mater. Approximately 800 ml are formed each day producing a pressure in the CSF system of about 10 mmHg. CSF then flows through the third and fourth ventricles into the subarachnoid space. It circulates through the subarachnoid space of the brain via the foramina of Luschka and through the subarachnoid space of the spinal cord via the foramen of Magendie. Most of the CSF is reabsorbed into the arachnoid villi (projections from the subarachnoid space into the venous sinuses of the brain). The CSF then drains into the superior sagittal sinus. The major functions of the CSF are to act as:

(i) a protective shock absorber for the delicate brain tissue,

(ii) a nutrient supply to cellular compartments.

Specific neural physiology

The respiratory and cardiovascular systems transport glucose, the obligatory fuel for nervous tissue function.

$$O_2 + \text{Fuel (Glucose)} = \text{Energy} + CO_2 + H_2O.$$

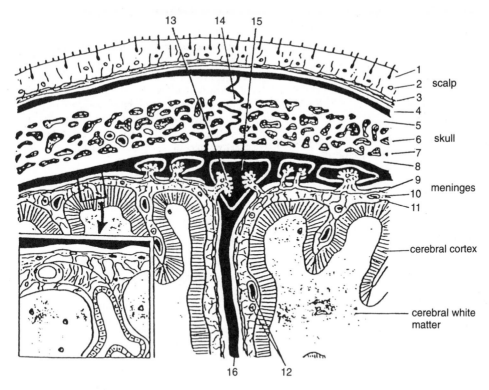

Fig. 9.6 Protective coverings and structures of the brain.

(1) skin	(7) inner table	(12) artery and vein
(2) subcutaneous tissue	(8) dura mater	(13) arachnoid granulation
(3) galea	(9) arachnoid	(14) sagittal suture
(4) periosteum	(10) subarachnoid space	(15) superior sagittal sinus
(5) outer table	(11) pia mater	(16) falx cerebri
(6) diploe		

(From Hinchcliffe and Montague 1989 *Physiology for nursing practice*, reprinted with permission).

Transport of nutrients and oxygen to the brain is dependent on adequate perfusion for optimum delivery. Adequate perfusion requires a level of pressure known as the cerebral perfusion pressure (CPP). CPP is derived by subtracting the intracranial pressure (ICP) from the mean arterial pressure (MAP):

$$CPP = MAP - ICP.$$

Changes in either MAP or ICP will inevitably affect CPP.

Intracranial pressure

Intracranial pressure is a reflection of the pressure exerted by the contents within a rigid structure (the skull). The contents comprise:

- Cerebrospinal fluid (CSF): 8–9%.

- Venous and arterial blood: 2–5%.

- Nervous tissue + water: 88–88.5%.

(Normal ICP: 0–12 mmHg.)

An increase in volume (and subsequent pressure) in any one of these three constituents without a compensatory reduction in one or both of the other constituents will result in an overall increase in ICP. The compensatory mechanisms are as follows.

Chief compensatory mechanisms:

1. Increased displacement of CSF into the subarachnoid space.

2. Decreased production of CSF.

3. Increased absorption of CSF into the venous system.

Minor compensatory mechanisms:

1. Reduction of blood volume: increased compression results in venous shunting into the venous sinuses and systemic circulation.

2. Displacement of brain tissue: may offer some compensation for slowly expanding space-occupying lesions. However, this is generally regarded as *decompensation*.

The extent of increase in ICP depends on a number of factors, the chief of which include:

1. The volume of the space-occupying lesions (haematoma, abcess, oedema).

2. The *rate* of expansion.

3. Total volume within the intracranial cavity.

4. Intracranial compliance.

Compliance relates to and is an indication of the volume — pressure relationship within the skull.

When compensatory mechanisms are operational then compliance is considered normal. However, when compensatory mechanisms fail, compliance is reduced and even very small increases in volume may produce significant increases in ICP.

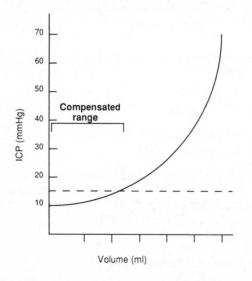

Fig. 9.7 Pressure–volume curve of intracranial pressure (ICP) and volume increase in cranial contents.

Autoregulation

The brain, in common with the kidney, has the ability to regulate its own blood flow. Fundamentally, the concept of autoregulation relates to the ability of the brain to regulate the diameter of the arterioles to maintain a mean consistent blood flow. Compensatory vasoconstriction or vasodilatation of the arterioles in response to increases or decreases in systemic MAP results in a concurrent reduction or increase in cerebral blood flow (CBF). However, in the presence of autoregulation, MAP appears to have little effect on CBF when the CPP is between 40 and 140 mmHg.

Autoregulation becomes impaired or non-functional when the ICP exceeds 40 mmHg. Equally, other factors can render autoregulation inactive:

1. Focal or diffuse cerebral injury.

2. Loss of blood–brain barrier.

3. MAP below 50 mmHg or above 180 mmHg.

Cerebral Vascular Resistance

The cerebral vascular bed is strongly influenced by the arterial partial pressures of oxygen (P_aO_2), and carbon dioxide (P_aCO_2). Metabolic stimuli will also override autoregulation.

The effects of hypoxaemia and hypercapnia on cerebral vasculature are critical and should always direct medical and nursing intervention. The consequences are an increased blood flow and volume and, subsequently a raised intracranial pressure (RICP). However, it is only when the P_aO_2 is less than 7 kPa (50 mmHg) or the P_aCO_2 greater than 5.5 kPa (40 mmHg) that marked increases in blood flow are observed.

Manipulation of P_aCO_2 was, until recently, one of the major therapeutic interventions in the management of potential or actual RICP, however the benefits of prolonged hyperventilation are now being questioned.

Assessment of the neurological patient

General assessment

This involves assessing the patient's behaviour, including:

1. Conscious level.

2. Mental state (e.g. alertness, agitation).

3. Speech patterns and thought processes.

It is important to avoid subjective, judgemental observation of the patient, for example, a recent excessive alcohol ingestion by the patient may cloud the issue and lead to misinterpretation of data.

Flexion (decorticate rigidity)

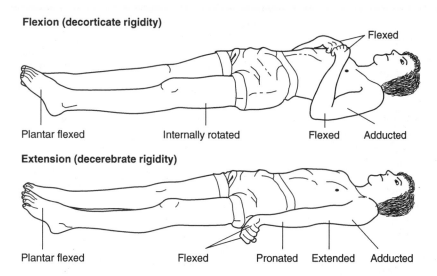

Plantar flexed   Internally rotated   Flexed   Adducted

Extension (decerebrate rigidity)

Plantar flexed   Flexed   Pronated   Extended   Adducted

Fig. 9.8 Abnormal Flexion, and extension.

There are a variety of scoring systems available which are designed to assess neurological status. The one most commonly used is the Glasgow Coma Scale (see Appendix 1). The scale is designed to assess the patient's level of consciousness in relation to responses to stimuli, plus best motor and verbal response.

Scoring systems are liable to subjectivity and should only be used as an aid to patient assessment. It is important that nurses are skilled in the interpretation and use of such scoring systems.

Assessing the patient's level of consciousness

Verbal response

This is designed to elicit the state of orientation or confusion present when the patient replies to a series of closed questions. This may range from no response, random, and disorganized replies to complete orientation.

It is important to establish the patient's acuity of hearing and understanding of language prior to assessing this response.

Responses to stimuli

This is designed to elicit eye opening or limb movement in response to a variety of commands and painful stimuli.

It is important to communicate the exact method employed to elicit the individual response when handing over care to a colleague, thus ensuring consistency.

Motor response (Fig. 9.8)

This is designed to establish the patient's ability not only to obey a command but to localize, withdraw, or assume abnormal body positions in response to the noxious stimuli or command.

It is important to distinguish between the following:

(a) Abnormal flexion of limbs — the patient assumes a decorticate posture.
(b) Abnormal extension of limbs — the patient assumes a decerebrate posture.
(c) Flaccid response — the patient does not respond at all.

Note. Any persisting effect of sedative or paralysing agents which may have been used in the immediate management of the patient, should be taken into account, particularly in the light of hepatic or renal impairment.

When assessing any changes related to the patient's intracranial pressure, early detection can be crucial to patient survival.

Pupil reaction

1. Pupillary dilatation represents direct involvement of the brain stem and compression of the 3rd cranial nerve. This may be present in the absence of raised ICP (e.g. with a direct 3rd nerve lesion).

2. Unequal pupillary action indicates a compensatory stage and is always ipsilateral (dilatation of the pupil

on the same side as the injury or space occupying lesion). This calls for immediate medical consultation and intervention.

3. Bilateral dilatation and fixation represents decompensation and is an indication of serious brainstem involvement.

Note. If a patient is fully orientated and alert there cannot be any possibility of an expanding lesion compressing the oculomotor nerve since pupillary change is a late sign of intracranial involvement. The influence of certain drug actions, such as atropine and neostigmine, on pupillary size and reaction should be considered as these are independent of intracranial pathology. The usefulness of assessing pupillary reaction in certain situations is debatable.

Haemodynamic changes

1. Narrowing of pulse pressure is regarded as compensatory and is important in that it may be a prelude to decompensation.

2. Hypertension is a late sign and signifies decompensation.

3. Changes in heart rate: slight irregularity and tachycardic episodes represent early stages of decompensation and are followed by profound bradycardia which calls for immediate intervention

Respiratory changes

Changes in respiratory depth and pattern are to be expected when pressure is exerted on the respiratory centre within the brainstem. Patterns of respiration and their characteristics help to localize specific involvements related to compensation and decompensation.

Patterns of breathing

Cheyne–Stokes
Rhythmic waxing and waning of rate and depth interspersed with briefer periods of apnoea may indicate deep, usually bilateral, lesions. May occur with upper brainstem involvement.

Neurogenic
Sustained, regular and rapid with forced inspiration, hyperventilation, and expiration. This may indicate low midbrain or upper pons involvement of the brainstem.

Apneustic
Prolonged inspiratory and expiratory phases with sig-

nificant pauses. This may indicate mid or low pons involvement of the brainstem.

Cluster breathing
Irregular clusters of respiration with longer periods of apnoea. This may indicate low pons or upper medullary involvement

Assessment of raised intracranial pressure

Clinical assessment for the presence of raised ICP is not always reliable or accurate, particularly in relation to cerebral oedema. There are several diagnostic tools which may help in determining the presence of a raised ICP:

- Skull radiography

- Computed tomography (CT scan)

- Magnetic resonance imaging (MRI)

- Direct ICP monitoring

- Electroencephalography (EEG)

- Cerebal function analysing monitor (CFAM).

Skull radiographs

These provide no useful information in screening for raised ICP in adults. However, in children up to the age of 8 or 9 years, they are valuable in determining both chronic and acute raised ICP. Splitting of the sagittal sutures and possible thinning of the skull vault would be evident in this age group as a result of raised ICP.

Computed tomography

Computed tomography is the single most useful investigation currently employed, given its safety and the speed at which it can be undertaken. Its value lies in determining brain shift with effacement of the subarachnoid spaces and compression of the ventricles. In addition, it is possible to diagnose discrete lesions (e.g. subdural haematoma). However, a normal CT scan does not exclude a raised ICP.

Magnetic resonance imaging

Magnetic resonance imaging (MRI) is another digitized diagnostic technique which has an increased sensitivity compared with computerized tomography, but its use is limited in head trauma on a purely practical level. The patient must be placed within a semi-circular magnet in

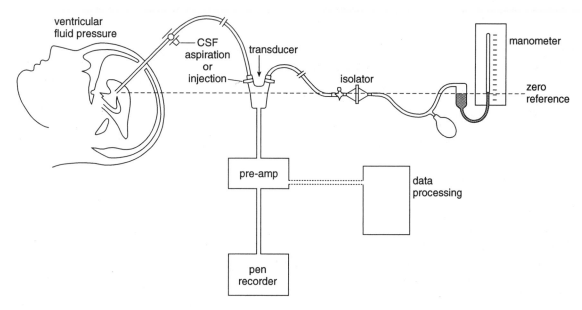

Fig. 9.9 Apparatus to measure intracranial pressure (ICP) using a disposable isolator (from North and Reilly 1990).

which a strong magnetic field is disturbed by radio-frequency signals. The transient realignment of tissue atomic protons results in release of energy spectra which can subsequently be analysed to create anatomical images. This may cause malfunctions in ventilator and IV pump systems. The procedure requires up to 45 minutes to complete, during which time, unless specially adapted monitoring facilities are available, close monitoring of clinical status is difficult. The patient must remain still during the procedure which can also be a problem.

One further disadvantage is that MRI does not detect the presence of blood during the first two hours following a cerebral event.

Direct ICP monitoring

As ICP varies from minute to minute particularly when it is raised, continuous monitoring is useful. The principles of monitoring *per se* have been previously discussed and a number of methods of monitoring ICP are available (see also Fig. 9.9).

Monitoring methods

1. *Intraventricular technique.* First reported in 1951, the technique requires placement of a catheter into the lateral ventricle via a burr hole. The catheter is connected via a fluid-filled system to a transducer. Pressure can then be displayed via any pressure monitoring system and CSF drainage and sampling can be carried out via the catheter.

Disposable fibre-optic systems (Camino catheter) allowing pressure measurement at the tip of the catheter have been developed eliminating the need for a fluid-filled transducer system.

2. *Subarachnoid (subdural) technique.* Measurement of ICP via a subarachnoid bolt or screw requires placement of the rigid bolt through a burr hole and connection to a fluid-filled system as for the ventricular catheter. Pressures obtained usually correlate reasonably well with intraventricular pressures. It is also possible to use the fibreoptic catheter system to measure subarachnoid/subdural pressure through the bolt. Subarachnoid/dural bolts are easier to insert than ventricular catheters but more prone to blocking and damping at higher pressures. CSF drainage and sampling is also possible via the bolt.

3. *Epidural technique.* An epidural device with either fibreoptic or transmitted information relay can be used for epidural placement and measurement of ICP via the CSF. However, there are problems of accuracy and stability and the technique is only used where coagulation problems make other forms of monitoring potentially hazardous (e.g. hepatic encephalopathy; Ward 1994).

4. *Parenchymal technique*. A fibre-optic catheter is inserted through a subarachnoid bolt, the dura and arachnoid mater are punctured and the catheter passed into the white matter of the brain. Brain tissue pressures are then monitored, these have been shown to correlate well with ICP.

The value of continuous ICP monitoring is controversial given the lack of concrete evidence in relation to patient outcome and the arguable weight of disadvantages over advantages.

Advantages:

- Excellent quality of recording.

- Rapid real time changes in pressure can be seen allowing prompt directed treatment.

- Ventricular access facilitates the withdrawal of CSF for temporary reduction of raised ICP in ventricular and subarachnoid monitoring.

Disadvantages:

- Risk of haemorrhage.

- Risk of infection.

- Lateral ventricle difficult to locate.

- Basal ganglia injury.

- Varying degrees of accuracy depending on method used.

Interpreting the ICP
Continuous monitoring of any physiological variable relies heavily upon the interpretation of data. Identification and interpretation of the waveform in relation to pressure changes must be carried out. Awareness of the causes of potential pressure changes both physiological and pathological is important and appropriate response is essential.

In interpreting the ICP waveforms both baseline level and any variations should be examined.

1. The normal upper limit of ICP would be expected to rise transiently during coughing and straining. The degree of rise and the length of time sustained is therefore important. It is also important to relate the ICP to the systemic blood pressure as current thinking suggests that the CPP should be maintained above 50–70 mmHg.

2. The appearance of the ICP waveform varies according to the type of monitoring and the patient's pathology.

Oscillations in the waveform associated with haemodynamic and respiratory pressure changes can be seen. Variations in the waveform associated with raised ICP have been categorized into A, B, and C waves.

A (or plateau) waves are associated with a baseline ICP of > 20 mmHg. They appear as large increases in ICP above 50–100 mmHg, lasting for 15–20 minutes. The presence of A waves indicates loss of intracranial spatial compensation and may be related to either an unstable CPP in the presence of relatively intact autoregulation or an increase in cerebral blood volume with a simultaneous decrease in cerebral blood flow. They may be produced by vasodilatation, or by non-specific stimuli such as pain, aroused mental activities, or changes in ventilation.

B waves are rhythmic oscillations associated with an ICP of up to 50 mmHg occurring at a frequency of 0.5–2.0/min. The waves correspond to changes in respiration and are often found in association with periodic breathing. They may disappear with mechanical ventilation.

C waves are low amplitude rhythmic oscillations of up to 20 mmHg occurring at a frequency of 4–8/min. They are related to blood pressure and reflect severe intracranial compression with limited remaining compensatory mechanisms.

Electroencephalopathy (EEG)

The EEG is a measure of spontaneous electrical activity recorded by electrodes placed on the scalp. Postsynaptic potentials and not action potentials in cortical grey matter are the sources of the EEG activity. Single neurone depolarization cannot be sensed from the surface of the brain but fluctuations in electrical current from large areas of cortical tissue can be detected.

The value of this non-invasive diagnostic aid is to interpret abnormal neural activity relating to pathology and loss of function. The central features in analysing the EEG concern the waveforms, their distribution, and the context in which they occur. It aids in seizure focus detection, localization of a source of irritation, such as a tumour or abscess, and in the diagnosis of metabolic disturbances and sleep disorders. It may also be used in determining whether the patient should be assessed for brainstem death tests.

Cerebral function analysing monitor (CFAM)

CFAM provides a method of continuous monitoring of the patient's cerebral function.

Biparietal electrodes monitor varying amplitudes of EEG signal and plot amplitude distribution with analysis of frequency of the waveform into beta (13–27 Hz), alpha (7.5–13 Hz), theta (3.5–7.5 Hz), and delta (1–3.5 Hz) wave bands. The recorder runs at 6–30 cm/h, which is much slower than the EEG, allowing analysis and prolonged monitoring. There are three areas of possible use in the ICU although none is frequently used:

(1) monitoring of seizure activity if the patient is on muscle relaxants which abolish any clinical evidence;

(2) monitoring of appropriate dose of cerebral metabolic depressant drugs in management of severe head injury;

(3) indication of impaired cerebral perfusion resulting from nursing procedures in haemodynamically unstable patients.

Use and interpretation of CFAM requires some skill but can provide a valuable addition to monitoring of cerebral function (Maynard and Jenkinson 1984)

Priorities of care for patients with actual or potential raised ICP

- Ensure optimum oxygenation.

- Avoidance of hypercapnia.

- Rationalization of essential nursing care.

- Recognition of ICP waveforms and signs of raised ICP.

- Respond appropriately to changing clinical events.

- Prevent infection.

- Support the family and relatives in coming to terms with the patient's condition.

Management of raised intracranial pressure

The management of a patient who manifests raised ICP is dependent on four key factors:

1. Ensuring optimum oxygenation ($P_aO_2 > 10$ kPa, $S_aO_2 > 90\%$).

2. Avoiding hypercapnia (maintaining $P_aCO_2 < 4.5$–5.0 kPa).

3. Modifying essential nursing care.

4. Optimizing sedation.

Optimizing oxygenation

Hypoxaemia increases intracranial pressure and therefore *must* be avoided at all costs. A fall in the P_aO_2 produces a rise in cerebral blood flow (CBF) due to vessel dilatation. The mechanisms responsible for changes in vessel diameter remain controversial but may involve the following (North and Riley 1990):

1. Tissue hydrogen iron concentration in the extracellular fluid (ECF).

2. Calcium, potassium, prostaglandins.

3. Adenosine.

The patient will generally be intubated and ventilated, sedated, and possibly paralysed. In the event of the patient not being mechanically ventilated or intubated then the nurse must ensure protection of the airway, administration of oxygen, and skilful neurological observation in order to identify and prevent further deterioration at an early stage.

Avoiding hypercapnia

Regional cerebral blood flow responds to the metabolic needs of the tissues and increases in P_aCO_2 act as a powerful vasodilating agent — the CBF doubles when the P_aCO_2 rises from 4.0 kPa and halves when P_aCO_2 falls below 3 kPa (North and Riley 1990).

In the past, this effect was used as the rationale for an established intervention of mechanical ventilation to hyperventilate the patient in order to control and limit P_aCO_2 levels. However, there are now a number of doubts about the effectiveness of this intervention (Kerr and Brucia 1993). These are:

(i) the effect may only be transient

(ii) the resulting decrease in blood flow associated with cerebral vasoconstriction may increase the risk of cerebral ischaemia

(iii) the cerebral vasculature may be unable to respond to alterations in P_aCO_2.

There remains a place for hyperventilation to control P_aCO_2 in the short term and as an acute response to raised ICP spikes, but the benefits of maintaining hypocapnia are debatable. When P_aCO_2 is allowed to increase, this should be done slowly to avoid sudden changes in cerebral blood flow.

Modifying essential nursing care

Studies have shown that certain nursing activities cause a significant rise in ICP and the triggering of A waves (see p. 246) during cerebral function monitoring (Walleck 1993; William and Coyne 1993). These include:

1. Suctioning and hyperinflation technique.

2. Indirect cuff blood pressure measurements.

3. Insertion of nasogastric tubes.

4. Positioning the patient.

5. Painful stimuli.

6. Pupillary light checks.

7. Mouth, eye, and pressure area care.

8. Discussion of the patient's condition at the bedside.

This list gives a guide for prioritizing care. However, it must be stressed that when the patient has significant lung pathology with potential for hypoxaemia, then aggressive physiotherapy and suctioning takes precedence, provided that the patient is well sedated. Rudy *et al.* (1991) found the mean ICP during suctioning increased with the number of suction passes. They recommended hyperoxygenation prior to suction and a maximum of two suction passes during each suction episode. Suctioning and hyperinflation may require the use of bolus supplements to sedation prior to intervention.

When positioning the patient the nurse must ensure that the patient's head is in alignment with his/her body during and after repositioning. This is to prevent obstruction of venous drainage. The patient's head should be elevated to 30 degrees for cerebral drainage unless otherwise instructed. The rationale for this is that about 75 per cent of the intracranial blood volume lies in the venous section of the vascular bed (capacitance vessels) and there is a direct connection between the cerebral veins, venous sinuses, and the large neck veins. Therefore, there is unimpeded transmission of any rise in venous pressure from the thorax and neck to the brain thus causing a rise in ICP. Although modifying essential nursing care is a priority when caring for a patient with raised ICP, it also important to remember that therapeutic care should *not* be forgotten or limited, such as expressive and therapeutic touch, music therapy, or other complementary therapies. All these therapies may contribute to reducing ICP (Johnson *et al.* 1989).

Optimizing sedation

In order to facilitate ventilation, thus optimizing oxygenation and avoiding hypercapnia, it is necessary to use a combination of sedatives $\pm$ neuromuscular blocking agents. The choice of drugs to optimize sedation has moved away from barbiturates, such as thiopentone, as studies have shown that they make no significant difference to patient outcome or long-term reduction of raised ICP.

Drugs in common use today are short acting, such as proprofol, midazolam, morphine, alfentanil, vecuronium, and atracurium, and should be prescribed on an individual basis. The most important point to remember is that the patient should be adequately sedated *before* being paralysed and that there should be continual assessment of the effectiveness of the drugs prescribed. At no time should patients 'fight' the ventilator since this will directly affect oxygenation and raise ICP. Those patients who are not mechanically ventilated should not generally be prescribed sedatives, or opiates. However, should an analgesic be required then judicious use of codeine phosphate is recommended. Pain relief is important as the ICP will rise if the patient is uncomfortable. Similarly, if sedation is required for an agitated patient, chlorpromazine may be used.

Additional therapies

Other therapies which may contribute to the management of a patient with raised ICP include:

1. Restricted fluid management: this should not be at the expense of cardiovascular or renal function.

2. Drug therapy.

3. Surgical intervention.

Restricted fluid management

This used to be the main method of management of raised ICP since the effects of osmotic diuresis were described early in the twentieth century. However, a restriction of fluids is now debatable as unnecessary hypovolaemia in patients, who may be already cardiovascularly compromised, will further reduce cerebral perfusion.

The nurse must therefore ensure that the patient achieves a neutral fluid balance unless otherwise instructed.

Drug therapy

These include:

(a) Osmotic diuretics.

(b) Renal diuretics.

(c) Corticosteroids.

(d) Anticonvulsants.

(e) Newer agents.

Osmotic and renal diuretics

The primary effect of osmotic diuretics (e.g. mannitol) lies in establishing osmotic gradients across the capillary wall thereby drawing fluid from the extracellular space. Because this action theoretically requires an intact blood–brain barrier it has been argued that osmotic diuretics remove water preferentially from normal brain tissue. However, recent studies suggest that the preference is for the removal of fluid from the oedematous brain. Further debate surrounds the action of osmotic diuretics on the specific gravity of the white matter brain water is reduced following head injury. The effect of osmotic diuretics is lost with successive doses, as the drug will cross the blood–brain barrier into the extracellular fluid, thus raising tissue osmolarity.

Additional effects of osmotic diuretics include the decrease in blood viscosity and subsequent reflex vasoconstriction and fall in ICP, reduction in CSF volume, and scavenging of oxygen-derived free radicals in brain tissue which has experienced an ischaemia–reperfusion injury.

It should be remembered that the infusion of osmotic diuretics may contribute to an increase in circulating volume. A renal diuretic (e.g. frusemide) can also be used which will augment the effects of the osmotic diuretics, in addition to reducing CSF formation directly.

Corticosteroids

There is no evidence that the use of corticosteroids improves the outcome of patients with head injury. However, they are effective in reducing swelling related to brain tumours and abscess.

Anticonvulsants

There is a risk of seizure following head injury and neurosurgery, the major consequences of which are cerebral hypoxaemia and its attendant complications.

Intravenous phenytoin (15–18 mg/kg at a rate no greater than 50 mg/min) is usually administered in the event of seizures or as prophylaxis following neurosurgery.

Newer agents

New agents currently being investigated especially in head-injured patients include calcium antagonists and a variety of oxygen radical scavengers.

Surgical intervention

There are a variety of methods available, these include:

(a) Craniotomy — surgical opening of the skull to allow access to the brain.

(b) Ventriculostomy — insertion of a drainage catheter into a cerebral ventricle to allow drainage of excess cerebrospinal fluid.

(c) Burr holes — a hole made in the cranium with a special drill for evacuation of an extracerebral clot.

The continuous and comprehensive monitoring of these patients is crucial if trends are to be identified and the effects of treatment evaluated. The aim of nursing care in these patients is observation and interpretation of the data with initiation of appropriate timely intervention.

In addition to the haemodynamic and neurological factors that have already been discussed, further consideration must be given to the following in relation to the maintenance of homeostasis:

1. Core temperature

2. Electrolyte and acid–base balance

3. Fluid balance.

Core temperature

An increase in core temperature will lead to an increase in cerebral oxygen demand. This increase in cerebral metabolism causes an increase in CO_2 production and subsequent vasodilatation. It has been shown that core temperatures in excess of 40 °C compound the hypoxaemic and hypercapnic insult.

The patient should be kept normothermic using various strategies such as tepid sponging, cool ambient temperature, and exposure. Specific drug therapy includes paracetamol and the use of paralysing agents to prevent shivering.

Electrolyte and acid–base balance

Derangements of plasma sodium would be expected to affect the osmotic gradient with implications for changes in total brain water.

Any alterations of acid–base balance, causing either an acidosis or an alkalosis, will have direct effects on cell membrane integrity and the propagation of nervous impulses. There will also be a reduction in oxygen availability with alkalosis potentiating the risk of cerebral hypoxia due to the shift to the left in the oxyhaemoglobin dissociation curve (see Chapter 3).

Hypoglycaemia can be rapid and can cloud the picture when assessing the patient. In addition, hypoglycaemia can cause further brain damage.

Fluid balance

Monitoring fluid balance can be complicated in the presence of diabetes insipidus which occurs with damage to the posterior pituitary gland. This can involve urinary losses well in excess of one litre an hour. During this process, urine becomes more dilute, specific gravity and urine osmolality decrease, while serum osmolality and serum sodium increase. Immediate treatment focuses on fluid replacement and, in moderate to severe cases, administration of antidiuretic hormone (ADH) replacement therapy.

Maintaining fluid balance requires vigilance.

Diabetes insipidus
Control of renal filtration is lost due to inadequate or absent secretion of antidiuretic hormone. This results in the excretion of up to 20 l/day of dilute urine

---

Antidiuretic hormone
Produced by the supraoptic and paraventricular nuclei of the hypothalamus and secreted by the posterior pituitary gland in response to increased blood osmolality. It acts on the distal renal tubules promoting reabsorption of water

---

Pain

The experience of pain is a complex phenomenon involving social, cultural, emotional, psychological, and physiological components.

Pain is aggravated in the intensive care unit (ICU) by:

(1) anxiety and fear;

(2) difficulty in communicating pain;

(3) life-saving priorities may displace the importance of pain relief (e.g. limiting opioid doses when blood pressure is low).

Pain contributes to the patient's stress and can increase confusion, paranoia, and delirium, as well as decreasing patient resistance to other stressors. Jones *et al.* (1979) reviewed patients' recollections of ICU and found that their greatest worries were pain and the inability to lie comfortably. Pain was also the leading cause of sleeplessness. This finding was reinforced by Simpson *et al.* (1989) who studied 59 patients following discharge from ICU. They found 36 per cent of the patient's negative recollections of ICU referred to pain or discomfort.

Puntillo (1990) suggests that pain is often inadequately assessed due to the patient's inability to communicate verbally and that nurses frequently underestimate the patient's analgesic requirements as a result.

Physiology of pain

The feeling of pain is caused by a noxious stimulus generated by release of products from tissue damage or nerve terminal damage. The products known to induce a noxious stimulus include bradykinin, histamine, prostaglandins, and hydrogen ions. They act by binding to nerve receptors and depolarizing the nerve membrane thus initiating an action potential and impulse generation in the nociceptive fibres. This impulse will produce both a spinal (reflex) and central response. (See Fig. 9.10 for pain pathways).

Pain is perceived at thalamic and forebrain levels and constitutes both sensory and reactive components. The thermal threshold is used as a determinant of sensory pain threshold and is remarkably constant between one person and another (44–45 °C). However, the individual's reaction to that sensation is greatly varied. The perception of pain by the individual may be altered according to other factors such as environment, experience, culture, mood, and pathology. Thus, the meaning any individual attaches to the pain they perceive will affect his or her response.

As a further factor in individual response to pain, the endogenous opioid (endorphin release) system will allow varying degrees of modulation of perceived pain. It is suggested that endorphin release occurs in response to pain, elevated blood pressure, fear, stress, restraint, and hypoglycaemia. Many of these factors are present in the critically ill and may allow for at least some reduction in perceived pain. Unfortunately, it is not possible to assess the level of endogenous opioid available or even to manipulate it and the patient's response to pain is the only method currently available to indicate requirements for analgesia.

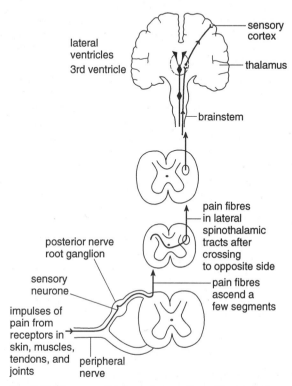

lateral
ventricles
3rd ventricle

sensory
cortex

thalamus

brainstem

posterior nerve
root ganglion

sensory
neurone

impulses of
pain from
receptors in
skin, muscles,
tendons, and
joints

peripheral
nerve

pain fibres
in lateral
spinothalamic
tracts after
crossing
to opposite side

pain fibres
ascend a
few segments

Fig. 9.10 Diagram of pain pathways (from Verran and Aisbitt *Neurological and neurosurgical nursing* 1988 reprinted with permission).

There are a number of theories of pain perception reflecting the complexity of the phenomenon. One of the most accepted and applicable of the current theories is Melzack and Wall's gate control theory (1965).

The pain perception transmitted by small diameter nerve fibres (these carry pain stimuli) can be inhibited by stimulation of large diameter nerve fibres (these carry innocuous information). The mechanism is postulated as follows:

(1) the small diameter fibres inhibit modulation by specialized tissue and excite cells which act as activators of central transmission of sensory and emotional aspects of pain. They therefore 'open the gate';

(2) the large diameter fibres inhibit the excitatory cell activity and 'close the gate' to pain;

(3) higher central nervous system processes can influence the gate control via inhibitory messages to the spinal cord.

The gate control theory explains the effects of many alternative pain therapies. Thus, rubbing, use of transcutaneous electrical nerve stimulation (TENS), and massage, preferentially stimulate large diameter fibres which inhibits, to a varying degree, central transmission of pain stimuli.

Assessment of the patient's pain

Nurses' assessment of the patient's pain has been shown to be influenced by a number of variables including ventilatory status, length of time after surgery (Gujol 1994), and the patient's ability to communicate (Puntillo 1990). Assessment within an ICU setting is extremely difficult, particularly in situations where the patient is unable to communicate verbally. Where non-verbal communication is impossible the nurse must rely on physiological variables, such as tachycardia, raised blood pressure, and physical responses (e.g. sweating, and lacrimation). Unfortunately, these responses are subject to an enormous range of contributory factors which limit their interpretation.

Even when patients are able to express pain verbally their response is frequently underestimated and analgesia withheld. Puntillo (1994) found that only 48% of a sample of 35 patients had analgesia administered in the hour prior to chest drain removal. The mean visual analogue score for the intensity of pain of the procedure was 6.6; and it was described by patients as 'tender', 'sharp', and 'heavy' pain.

Tittle and McMillan (1994) studied 44 patients in both an ICU and a surgical unit and found that patients continued to experience pain even following pain management interventions. An average of only 30% of the maximum possible prescription for opiate analgesia was administered to the ICU patients. Documentation was also minimal giving little idea of the patient's response to the dose administered or the intensity of the pain experienced. Use of a pain chart or of adequate recording in the patient's care plan is essential in order to allow evaluation of intervention and further pain relief when necessary.

Methods of pain relief

1. Analgesia

Opiates and synthetic opioids are the mainstay of pain relief for critical care patients. In the ventilated patient the added advantage of blunting of the respiratory drive is useful in managing modes of ventilation which are not physiological. Intravenous infusions produce a more consistent analgesia which can be titrated to patient response. Dose will depend on age, weight, haemodynamic status, and clinical effect. Use of IV boluses (small dose, delivered slowly) prior to any unpleasant procedure will provide increased analgesic effect over the short term.

2. Regional analgesia

Epidural analgesia is most advantageous following upper abdominal and chest surgery, when coughing, deep breathing, and mobility are facilitated. The epidural catheter is inserted between T7 and T10 for abdominal and thoracic pain or at L1–2 or L2–3 for lower abdominal and pelvic pain. Analgesia may be delivered either as a constant infusion or boluses.

3. Transcutaneous electrical nerve stimulation (TENS)

Large diameter afferent nerve fibres are stimulated by a low level electric current thus selectively inhibiting transmission of pain signals via small diameter nerve fibres. The effect on ICU patients seems to be limited and may only reduce pharmacological analgesic requirements, rather than providing complete pain relief.

4. Nitrous oxide

Inhalation of a gas consisting of 50 per cent nitrous oxide and 50 per cent oxygen (entonox) can provide good analgesic effect. It can only be used for short-term pain relief as bone marrow depression can occur after 36 hours. Its primary use at present is to provide pain relief to spontaneously ventilating patients who are able to use the demand valve system of delivery for analgesia during unpleasant procedures. It can also be delivered via a rigid oxygen mask but at a reduced percentage of nitrous oxide, due to entrainment.

It is possible to deliver the gas through a positive pressure ventilator but this requires special adaptation of the gas delivery system.

5. Localized warmth and/or cooling

Application of local warmth using warming pads or warmed bags of fluid can help relieve aching or muscular spasm pain. Alternatively, topical cooling using permeable gel dressing or cool (but not iced) dressings can relieve some of the pain associated with burns.

6. Relaxation techniques and massage therapy

Relaxation techniques may be useful in relieving anxiety-related distress in patients who are able to co-operate or who can be taught prior to admission about the techniques used. Miller and Perry (1990) studied the effectiveness of slow, deep-breathing relaxation in relieving post-operative pain after cardiac surgery. The study group of 15 patients showed significant decreases in blood pressure, respiratory rate, and descriptive report of pain, compared to the control group. However, there was no significant difference in analgesia requirement.

The effect of foot massage with and without aromatherapy on patient's anxiety following cardiac surgery has been evaluated (Stevensen 1994). Patients were significantly less anxious in the group treated with aromatherapy, although there was minimal difference in the reported level of pain.

7. The importance of communication

Attention to factors identified by the patient and his/her increasing anxiety (e.g. regarding pain, anxiety, and fear, need for information) is essential. Interventions such as these may assist in decreasing the 'distress' factor associated with pain perception and therefore increase the patient's ability to tolerate pain.

Pain associated with neuropathology

Much of the nervous tissue in the brain is completely insensitive to pain. However, certain structures are highly sensitive, these include:

- Cranial sensory nerves
- Meninges
- Large intracranial and extracranial arteries
- Venous sinuses.

Headache is a common phenomenon, sometimes in the absence of obvious organic cause. Occasionally, this type of headache may be intractable. Headache may persist following head injury.

Pain relief following neurosurgery and/or head injury

In a patient requiring hyperventilation to reduce raised ICP, necessitating sedation and/or paralysing agents, the nurse will only have changes in autonomic responses to rely on as an index of the patient's pain experience. These may well be complicated by haemodynamic changes of other origins, and using professional judgement is of paramount importance. In these circumstances, the use of opiates is entirely appropriate and would probably have been initiated already.

In the non-ventilated patient or those being weaned from mechanical ventilation then judicious use of small amounts of opiates or codeine phosphate intramuscularly should be employed.

Sedation in the critically ill

The goals of sedation in the critically ill patient are to:

(i) Allay anxiety

(ii) Relieve discomfort

(iii) Aid sleep.

The achievement of these goals will depend on appropriate pain relief (see above).

Indications for sedation have been described by Oh (1990):

(1) facilitation of mechanical ventilation;

(2) relief of anxiety;

(3) management of acute confusional states;

(4) implementation of treatment or diagnostic procedures;

(5) obtundation of the physiological response to stress to reduce tachycardia, hypertension, or raised intracranial pressure.

A sixth major indication is to prevent the patient being aware during paralysis. Opiate drugs are frequently given not only for their analgesic effect but also for anxiolytic and euphoric effects. They are often used in conjunction with sedative drugs to provide a combination of pain relief, drowsiness, and, when necessary, respiratory depression.

Assessment of the patient's level of sedation should be carried out at regular intervals using a sedation score (e.g. the Bloomsbury Sedation Score, see Table 9.3). The aim is to maintain a score of between 0 and 1, unless the patient is particularly unstable or requires a mode of ventilation which is difficult to tolerate.

Table 9.3 The Bloomsbury Sedation Score

3	Agitated and restless
2	Awake and uncomfortable
1	Aware but calm
0	Roused by voice, remains calm
−1	Roused by movement or suction
−2	Roused by painful stimuli
−3	Unrousable
A	Natural sleep

Types of sedative drugs

(1) Benzodiazepines

These are sedative–anxiolytics that promote amnesia. Used in combination with opiates, they can significantly reduce recall of unpleasant events and potentiate analgesic efficacy thus reducing analgesic requirements (Table 9.4). Other properties of benzodiazepines include:

(i) anticonvulsant,

(ii) muscle relaxant,

(iii) prophylaxis of alcohol withdrawal.

Reversal of benzodiazepine respiratory and central depressant effects can be accomplished in up to 80 per cent of patients using flumazenil, a competitive benzodiazepine receptor antagonist. Care must be taken to continue to observe the patient following administration due to the short half-life of flumazenil and the danger of re-sedation.

Propofol

Developed as an anaesthetic induction agent, propofol is now used as an infusion for short-term sedation in the critically ill (Table 9.5). It should be administered with caution in patients suspected of hypovolaemia or poor cardiovascular function as it has vasodilator and potent negative inotropic properties and can cause large falls in blood pressure.

It is not licensed for use in children and should not be administered to anyone under 12 years.

Chlormethiazole

Chlormethiazole has sedative, anticonvulsant, and antiemetic actions. It is useful for patients suffering from delirium tremens, acute agitation, confusional states, status epilepticus, and eclampsia (Table 9.6). Its cumulative effect may result in respiratory depression even when the dose remains unchanged.

Table 9.4   Sedative drugs: benzodiazepines

Drug	Bolus dose	Infusion rate	Cautions	Elimination half-life
Diazepam	0.15–0.2 mg/kg slowly	Not recommended	• Respiratory depression especially in the elderly • Hepatic and renal dysfunction prolongs action • Potentiates other CNS depressants • Potentiated by cimetidine • Active metabolites may prolong action • Paradoxical confusion/agitation with withdrawal symptoms in long-term use	20–90 h
Lorazepam	4 mg 4–6-hourly	Not recommended	• Respiratory depression especially in the elderly • Slower onset, longer duration of action	
Midazolam	50 μg/kg slowly	50–100 μg/kg/h titrated to response	• Respiratory depression especially in elderly • Hepatic and renal dysfunction prolongs action • Potentiated by cimetidine • 10% of patients are slow metabolizers • ↓ SVR, ↑ HR, and ↓ BP: increased in volume depletion, the elderly, and cardiac disease • Paradoxical confusion/agitation with withdrawal symptoms in long-term use	2–4 h extended after infusion due to accumulation in fat

Table 9.5   Sedative drugs: propofol

Drug	Bolus dose	Infusion rate	Cautions	Elimination half-life
Propofol	1.0–2.0 mg/kg slowly	1.0–3.0 mg/kg/h	• Negative inotropic effect • Large ↓ in BP especially with hypovolaemia or poor CVS function • Decreased clearance may occur in renal insufficiency and in the elderly • Seizures have been reported	3–6 h

Table 9.6   Sedative drugs: chlormethiazole

Drug	Bolus dose	Infusion rate	Cautions	Elimination half-life
Chlormethiazole	0.1–0.2 ml/kg/min	0.5–1.0 ml/min	• Metabolized in the liver • Increased bronchial secretions • Fluid overload possible • Causes haemolysis (? in higher concentrations) • Tachycardia • Respiratory and cardiac depression	8 h: may be extended after prolonged infusion

The relatively large fluid (electrolyte-free water) volume required for infusion can cause problems in the patient who is fluid-restricted. Hyponatraemia can also result. Infusion concentrations higher than 0.8 per cent have been associated with haemolysis.

Care should be taken if the infusion is administered for more than 2–3 days as there is a recognized degeneration, associated with chlormethiazole, of certain plastics used in the manufacture of venous cannulae.

Ketamine

This is an anaesthetic and sedative agent with potent analgesic properties. It directly stimulates the myocardium and sympathetic nervous system but has little effect on respiration although it reduces airway resistance by its action on β-receptors (Table 9.7). It can be used in unstable, critically ill patients, and particularly asthmatics, who will benefit from its bronchodilator effects.

Its use is associated with distressing and unpleasant nightmares which may be stimulated by external irritation such as noise, touch, etc. It should thus be used with benzodiazepines to provide an amnesic effect.

Types of muscle relaxants (paralysing agents, neuromuscular blockers)

There are four major indications for the use of muscle relaxants:

1. Facilitation of endotracheal intubation.

2. Assist the use of certain ventilatory modes (e.g. inverse ratio ventilation).

3. Prevention of activity associated with high levels of oxygen consumption (e.g. shivering) in patients with very poor respiratory function and high F_iO_2.

4. Reducing muscle spasm associated with tetany.

Muscle relaxants should only be given to patients who are either intubated or about to be intubated.

They should also only be used in conjunction with adequate sedation to avoid the terror of conscious paralysis. Levels of sedation should be assessed regularly by reducing or discontinuing the paralysing agent to allow assessment.

Atracurium and vecuronium are least likely to be associated with adverse cardiovascular effects and should be considered for haemodynamically unstable patients (Table 9.8).

Complications associated with muscle relaxants

Malignant hyperthermia
This is a rare genetic disorder which can be precipitated by the use of muscle relaxants (mostly suxamethonium) but usually in combination with an inhalational anaesthetic. The patient becomes rapidly pyrexial and develops severe muscle rigidity. There are gross metabolic derangements as a result of abnormal cellular calcium metabolism.

Treatment consists of stopping the muscle relaxant, aggressive cooling, and administering intravenous dantrolene.

The key to successful sedation of critically ill patients is constant assessment of their responsiveness and comfort. This should be carried out using a sedation score or structured format to allow comparison between different staff members. Adjustment of sedative doses should then be carried out according to agreed unit protocols.

Specific neurological disorders

The unconscious patient

Coma can be defined as an acute or chronic reduction in cerebral responsiveness from which a stimulus cannot elicit arousal. The common causes are wide-ranging (see box).

Coma should be distinguished from 'locked in' syn-

Table 9.7 Sedative drugs: ketamine

Drug	Bolus dose	Infusion rate	Cautions	Elimination half-life
Ketamine	1.0–2.0 mg/kg added doses of 0.5 mg/kg	3.0–10.0 μg/kg/min	• Tachycardia and ↑ catecholamine stimulation • Minimal depression of respiration unless really large doses • Nightmares and hallucinations	3–6

Table 9.8 Muscle relaxants

Drug	Bolus dose	Infusion rate	Cautions	Elimination half-life
Atracurium	0.6 mg/kg	0.1–1.0 µg/kg/h	• Anaphylaxis has been reported • Adequate sedation required • Accumulation of a metabolite may cause seizures after some days • Breakdown is delayed in hypothermia and acidosis	Short
Vecuronium	0.08–0.1 mg/kg	50–80 µg/kg/h (intermittent injection preferred)	• Anaphylaxis and prolonged effects reported • Renally excreted — use with caution in renal insufficiency	Short
Pancuronium			• Renally excreted • Metabolized in liver to active metabolites: should not be used in hepatic failure • May cause tachycardia and hypotension due to vagal blockade	Long

drome and psychogenic unresponsiveness such as catatonia. Psychogenic unresponsiveness may show voluntary eye closure, resistance to eye opening, corneal reflexes, nystagmus to cold caloric stimulus, and normally responsive EEG. Patients with 'locked in' syndrome are aware but cannot respond to stimuli except with vertical eye movements or blinking.

Causes of coma

- Cerebral hemisphere dysfunction: post-ictal stupor, CVA, closed head injury

- Damaged or depressed reticular activating system: compression by tumour or haemorrhage, tentorial herniation

- Metabolic encephalopathy

- Post-anoxic encephalopathy

- Ischaemic encephalopathy

- Meningoencephalitis

- Poisoning

- Hypo- and hyperthermia

- Septic encephalopathy

Assessment and investigations

A full physical examination should be carried out.

Laboratory investigations are listed in the box below. Other investigations include CT scan, chest X-ray, lumbar puncture, and EEG.

Laboratory investigations for cause of coma

- Arterial blood gases

- Blood glucose

- Urea, electrolytes, calcium, and liver function tests

- Full blood count

- Drug and poison screen

- Co-oximetry for carboxyhaemoglobin

Management

- Airway protection (position on side, oropharyngeal airway, possible intubation) and resuscitation are a priority.

- Investigation and assessment to identify cause and enable specific treatment to be carried out.

- Oxygenation should be monitored and supported. Intubation and ventilation should be instituted if necessary.

- Cardiovascular function should be optimized with electrolytes, fluid, and, where necessary, vasoactive therapy.

- Monitoring of neurological status should be carried out to allow early detection of deterioration.

- If raised ICP is suspected management and nursing care should follow the guidelines for raised ICP.

- Full supportive care as detailed in Chapter 2 should be carried out

Prognosis deteriorates with the length of coma, absent oculovestibular reflexes, and presence of decerebrate posturing and rigidity in non-trauma patients for greater than 24 hours.

The acutely confused patient

Many patients experience a phase of extreme agitation and disorientation following neurological injury or deficit. However, there are many other causes for this distressing condition (Table 9.9), and it is important to attempt to identify the underlying cause involved. Specific treatment is then based on this diagnosis.

Table 9.9 Causes of an acute confusional state

- *Infection*
  Chest, urinary, abdominal, neurological, cardiac (e.g. endocarditis, gynaecological, sinusitis, cellulitic)

- *Metabolic*
  Hyper-/hypoglycaemic, hyper-/hyponatraemic, hyper-/hypocalcaemic, hyper-/hypothermic.
  Uraemia, hepatic encephalopathy, dehydration

- *Neurological*
  Meningo-encephalitis, abscess, cerebral malaria, space-occupying lesion, concussion, post-ictal, vasculitis

- *Respiratory*
  Hypoxaemia, hypercapnia

- *Cardiac*
  Low output states, hypotension

- *Drug-related*
  Withdrawal from alcohol, opiates, benzodiazepines, drug abuse, use of sedatives, analgesics, anti-Parkinsonian drugs, diuretics in the elderly

Use of sedation at this stage is often difficult, due to the need to avoid clouding the assessment of neurological status or to concern over respiratory inadequacy. Management of this state is extremely demanding and can cause a considerable increase in the patient's requirements for nursing intervention. The very real danger that they may cause themselves harm during this period means that nurses must employ all possible strategies to limit this risk.

Management
- The patient should be assessed for any underlying causes of agitation (see Table 9.9). Specific intervention aimed at correcting the cause should be commenced.

- Correct hypoxaemia and, if possible, continually monitor oxygen saturation via pulse oximetry. The presence of an oxygen mask is often an extremely irritating stimulus and better patient compliance may be obtained with nasal cannulae. If a mask is essential, sedation may be required to facilitate tolerance.

- If sedation is absolutely necessary, chlorpromazine and haloperidol IV can be given as small boluses allowing 20 minutes, if possible, between each dose. Small subcutaneous doses of opiates may also be used. Occasionally, continuous infusions (e.g. chlormethiazole) are necessary to manage the patient.

Nursing interventions
- Provide a calm, peaceful environment, and, if possible, a single room. Music, distraction, and aromatherapy may all help to relieve the patient's agitation.

- Agitation is frequently associated with nightfall and the dark. If possible, the patient should be in a softly lit rather than dark environment.

- Familiar faces, such as members of the family, and familiar objects, will often have a calming effect.

- Continuous re-orientation of the patient to time, place, and events is required.

- Triggers of agitation should be avoided where possible.

- Use of tone of voice rather than physical restraint. Physical restraint frequently increases agitation and should be avoided until absolutely necessary

- Cot sides with pillows for padding should be in place. However, if they increase agitation, one side should be taken down providing a nurse can remain with the patient to prevent injury.

- Sedatives, such as chlorpromazine, diazepam, or haloperidol, can be given IV or IM if absolutely necessary. The patient's respiratory state must be continually observed following sedation. Use of pulse oximetry alone will not warn of hypercapnia.

● Physical restraint is an absolute last resort. It should only be used if the patient is in imminent danger of causing severe harm to themselves and where the use of pharmacological restraint is not possible. Bandaging the hands will prevent removal of ET tubes, central venous cannulae, urinary catheters, etc. The bandages should be removed frequently to allow movement of the fingers and prevent stiffness. Limb restraints should ideally be purpose-made but if these are not available, foam or gauze protection of the skin under the ties is essential.

The family are an important part of managing the patient but are likely to be distressed by the patient's condition. Where possible, they should be given a full explanation of the cause and the importance of their help in caring for the patient should be stressed. They may then be able to respond positively.

Most patients respond well to continuous psychological support and calming interventions. However, they are extremely demanding patients to nurse and the nurse in charge should remain aware of the need for high levels of support for the nurses at the bedside.

Neuromuscular disorders

Acute infective polyneuritis (Guillain–Barré syndrome)

The aetiology of this autoimmune disorder remains unclear but, essentially, it is a reversible disease characterized by weakness and/or paralysis of the voluntary muscles. Sensation may also be involved. The involvement of muscles can develop in an ascending or descending manner but the classic picture is one of rapid weakness of peripheral nerves progressing to involvement of those muscles above the diaphragm. The need for respiratory monitoring, mechanical ventilation, or plasma exchange are all indications for ICU admission. In the early stage there may also be autonomic involvement characterized by labile blood pressure and a tachycardia–bradycardia syndrome which will require specific intervention.

The pathological changes are:

1. Loss of Schwann cells.

2. Widening of the nodes of Ranvier.

3. Loss of conduction.

Nursing and medical intervention

The key to the management and care of these patients lies in the multi-disciplinary approach and high standards of meticulous nursing care. There is no specific treatment although plasmapheresis has been shown to accelerate recovery of muscle fatigue and paralysis in some patients if carried out promptly following onset of symptoms. It is thought this is related to the reduction of circulating antibodies.

Successful patient outcome depends on prevention of the complications of long-term bedrest, mechanical ventilation when necessary, invasive monitoring techniques, and provision of nutrition. Comprehensive physiotherapy plays an important role, particularly in the prevention of contractures. It is vital that the patient who is not yet ventilated has continuous respiratory monitoring because deterioration can be acute. The vital capacity should be measured frequently by spirometry and if it drops below 10–15 ml/kg mechanical ventilation should be considered.

Pain relief in patients with neuromuscular disorders

While many of these patients have both sensory and motor deficits, muscle spasm is still a frequent cause of distress and often difficult to deal with from both a nursing and patient perspective.

A variety of agents are employed and depend on local prescribing and resources:

● diazepam;

● antispasmodics (e.g. baclofen);

● transcutaneous electrical nerve stimulation (TENS);

● complementary therapies, such as massage.

Obviously, each patient is an individual who will respond uniquely to any intervention and establishing a successful regime is often a matter of trial and error.

Organization of the delivery of nursing care

Organization of essential nursing care is paramount. Team or primary nursing would seem to be an obvious choice given the debilitating and prolonged nature of this disorder. The patient may feel that progress often seems minimal and the feelings of loss of control are often overwhelming.

A dynamic nurse–patient relationship, which involves a number of innovative approaches to care, can significantly change the patient's experience in the ICU; nurses can derive enormous satisfaction from such creativity. Several models exist which nurses can adapt in designing an eclectic framework which mirrors the corporate philosophy of the unit (Fig. 9.11).

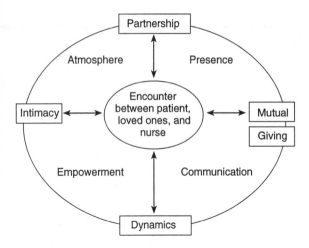

Fig. 9.11 A conceptual framework for therapeutic nursing intervention.

Rehabilitation is a challenge for health care professionals, family, and friends and the reader is advised to refer to specific texts.

Myasthenia gravis

This autoimmune disorder is characterized by a muscle weakness directly proportional to the use of the muscle and due to an abnormality of neurochemical transmission. It would appear that these patients have high levels of circulating antibodies to acetylcholine receptors on the cell membrane, thereby reducing the number available and resulting in a proportional loss of action potential and rapid degradation of the existing acetylcholine by cholinesterase. Treatment is aimed at reducing muscle work and preventing the rapid degradation of acetylcholine by blocking the action of cholinesterase.

It should be remembered that this is a progressive disease and the priority when patients are admitted to ICU is the early recognition of acute ventilatory failure. Care and treatment is therefore directed at optimizing alveolar ventilation.

Achieving alveolar ventilation in these patients requires careful selection of a range of options. Some patients will require tracheostomy, thereby reducing anatomical dead space and the work of breathing.

Mechanical ventilation

The mode of mechanical ventilation needs careful consideration in this group of patients and may include the following:

1. Synchronized intermittent mandatory ventilation (SIMV).

2. SIMV with pressure support.

3. Pressure support.

4. Patient trigger with titration of sensitivity.

Assessment

- Confirmation of impairment of neuromuscular transmission is achieved by a positive edrophonium (Tensilon) test. This should be done with full emergency facilities and an anaesthetist available as it may precipitate profound weakness.

Edrophonium test

- Atropine 0.6 mg (IV) is given to prevent muscarinic side-effects

- Edrophonium chloride 1 mg (IV) is given followed by a further 5 mg (IV) if there is no response

- Any unequivocal improvement in weakness is considered positive

---

- The single most useful index of ventilatory function is the measurement of the patient's vital capacity which should be recorded on a separate progress grid in order to identify trends and which should direct care and intervention. A vital capacity of < 10–15 ml/kg is an indication for ventilation.

- Identifying the patient's best motor response is also a useful tool in assessing the patient's progress.

Management

- Medical management includes:

  (i) anticholinesterase drugs such as pyridostigmine

  (ii) steroids, and

  (iii) azathioprine.

Thymectomy is advocated early in the progress of the disease and plasmapheresis should be considered for severe exacerbations.

- Chest physiotherapy to:

  (i) improve airway clearance (bronchial secretions are increased by anticholinesterase drugs),

  (ii) prevent infection,

(iii) maintain alveolar access and gas exchange.

- Intervention to limit patient's muscular workload either by assisting or taking over activities.

- Provide psychological support.

Myasthenic crisis

A life-threatening episode of acute deterioration in patients with myasthenia gravis. Requires increased doses of anticholinergic drugs, steroids, and in some cases, plasmapheresis.

Cholinergic crisis

A condition induced by overadministration of anti-cholinergic drugs. Deterioration following edro-phonium in a known myasthenic is an indication of cholinergic crisis.

Requires atropine 1 mg (IV) repeated every 30 mins to a maximum of 8 mg.

This group of patients often present a major challenge to nursing staff as with any patient with a neuromuscular disorder. Of greater significance, however, is that it is progressive in nature and sudden onset of ventilatory failure is extremely frightening for patients.

The relationship between the patient and nurse is again of vital importance in order to support therapeutic nursing intervention. Mutual goal-setting is the pivot to the successful management and care of these patients.

Miscellaneous neuromuscular entities

There are a wide variety of syndromes and disorders affecting individuals resulting in the need for short- or long-term intensive care nursing and medical management. Many of these syndromes are particularly rare and further information on these should be obtained elsewhere.

Acute cerebrovascular accident

Acute cerebrovascular accident (CVA) manifests as a neurological deficit which develops over a brief period of time (typically between minutes and hours) and remains over 24 hours. If the patient is young or active surgical treatment is indicated and transfer to the ICU may be appropriate.

Causes include:

(i) Vascular obstruction: (a) thrombotic or (b) embolic (usually cardiac in origin), 85 per cent of cases.

(ii) Haemorrhage usually secondary to hypertension, 10–12 per cent of cases.

Management

- Maintenance of the airway is a priority as in any unconscious patient.

- Oxygenation should be supported with oxygen therapy.

- Blood glucose levels should be ascertained to rule out hypoglycaemia

- Frequent neurological observations for early identification of deterioration.

- Intervention to control blood pressure should be limited to severe hypertension (MAP > 140 mmHg / diastolic > 120 mmHg). MAP should not be lowered to < 130 mmHg and diastolic not less than 110 mmHg, in the first 48 hours.

- Cardiac output should be supported, if necessary, by treating arrhythmias, optimizing fluid load, and haemoglobin levels.

- Full supportive care should be instigated (see Chapter 2) including physiotherapy, pressure area care, hygiene, psychological support, prevention of infection, nutrition, pain relief, rehabilitation.

- If an embolic cause is likely, thrombolysis and/or anticoagulation therapy should be considered.

Subarachnoid haemorrhage

Subarachnoid haemorrhage (SAH) refers to bleeding occurring within the subarachnoid space. This is most frequently due to rupture of cerebral aneurysms. Other causes include rupture of vascular malformation and rupture of weakened vessels secondary to systemic hypertension.

Clinical presentation

Patients may complain of sudden onset of severe headache, followed by loss of consciousness, and meningism (neck stiffness, photophobia, vomiting, and Kernig's sign). Transient neurological deficits may be seen or early gross deficits related to cerebral ischaemia or intracerebral haematoma.

The World Federation of Neurological Surgeons (WFNS) have proposed a universal grading scale for SAH based on the Glasgow Coma Score (GCS) to allow classification of risk and poor prognosis (see Table 9.10).

Management

Management of the patient is aimed at:

(i) prevention of further bleeding,

(ii) prevention of cerebral vasospasm,

(iii) limitation of further neurological dysfunction.

1. Maintenance of blood pressure within normal limits

Hypertension should be controlled unless there is evidence of cerebral vasospasm. Primary interventions are relief of agitation, anxiety, and pain in conjunction with antihypertensive agents (beta blockers, methyldopa, and hydralazine). Calcium-channel blockers, specifically nimodipine, may provide a dual role in reducing hypertension and preventing cerebral vasospasm. Nimodipine has been shown to improve outcome in SAH (Pickard *et al.* 1989).

2. Maintenance of oxygenation

Optimal oxygenation is essential to limit any effects of ischaemia. Inspired oxygen levels should be titrated to maintain P_aO_2 at normal levels.

3. Prevention or treatment of vasospasm

Cerebral vasospasm can be diagnosed by excluding other causes of neurological deficit, analysing time of onset, and rate of development of neurological deficit. Other investigations, such as angiography, which is the most effective, transcranial Doppler, and cerebral blood flow studies can indicate vasospasm.

The most consistently effective treatment for vasospasm is hypervolaemia and induced arterial hypertension (Thompson 1990) although some favourable results have been obtained using nimodipine (a calcium-channel blocker). If hypervolaemia is undertaken, early surgery is necessary to prevent inducement of further bleeding.

4. Management of cerebral oedema

Cerebral oedema is managed in the same way as raised intracranial pressure (see p. 247).

5. Surgery

The most frequent form of surgery is clipping of the aneurysm, although alternative methods, such as reinforcement with mesh, are in use. Timing of surgery is a contentious issue with some preference for allowing stabilization before intervention (usually at 7–10 days) as opposed to early intervention within 3 days. However, there may be an increased risk of rebleeding if surgery is delayed. At present, there is little supporting evidence that early intervention is more effective than late.

Table 9.10 Classification of subarachnoid haemorrhage

Clinical neurological classification		Proposed WFNS scale		
Grade	Signs	WFNS grade	GCS	Motor deficit
I	Conscious patient +/− meningism	I	15	Absent
II	Drowsy patient with no significant neurological deficit	II	14–13	Absent
III	Drowsy patient with neurological deficit: probably intracerebral clot	III	14–13	Present
IV	Deteriorating patient with major neurological deficit (because of large intracerebral clot)	IV	12–7	Present or absent
V	Moribund patient with extensor rigidity and failing vital centres	V	6–3	Present or absent

(6) Prevention of rebleeding

The risk of rebleeding depends on:

   (i) site of aneurysm,

   (ii) presence of clot,

   (iii) degree of vasospasm,

   (iv) age and sex of patient.

Rebleeding is most likely to occur between days 4–9 following the primary event and there is a 40% mortality associated with the second haemorrhage. Antifibrinolytic therapy has been shown to reduce rebleed rates by 30–50 per cent but has had little effect on mortality, due to other problems associated with its use (cerebral ischaemia, hydrocephalus, thrombosis).

Nursing care of the patient

• Frequent neurological assessment should be carried out for early identification of deterioration.

• A quiet environment should be provided with sedation to minimize anxiety or agitation.

• If the patient is unconscious then maintenance of the airway is essential and full essential nursing care, as detailed in Chapter 2, is required.

Seizures

The pathology is of a sudden discharge of a group of neurones either focally (partial seizure) or bilaterally (generalized seizure) within the brain. In the normal brain, a balance between excitatory and inhibitory synaptic influences on the postsynaptic neurones ensures that areas of excessive depolarization do not occur. During seizures, the neurones are subjected to a random discharge of electrical activity. These are known as paroxysmal depolarization shifts (PDS). Hypotheses surrounding the aetiology of PDS include:

1. Derangement of the sodium pump mechanism.

2. Acetylcholine–cholinesterase imbalance.

3. Abnormal conversion of glutamic acid to GABA (γ-aminobutyric acid).

It is thought that cessation of seizures is facilitated by neural fatigue (depletion of glucose and oxygen) and/or active inhibition by specific structures within the brain itself.

Types of generalized seizures

Absence seizure (petit mal) — transient loss of consciousness or contact with the environment

Tonic–clonic seizure (grand mal) — bilateral tonic extension of extremities followed by synchronous bilateral jerking movements

Myoclonic seizure — synchronous, asymmetrical rapid jerking of one or more extremity, the trunk or a specific muscle group

Atonic seizure — brief episode of loss of consciousness involving transient loss of muscle tone

---

Management

This centres around identification of the underlying cause and its treatment. It is vital, however, that regardless of the cause, prompt action be taken to abolish the seizure to prevent further brain damage from depletion of glucose and oxygen.

   Seizures are the most common sequelae of head injury and/or surgery and pharmacological intervention includes administration of anticonvulsants such as phenytoin. This may be continued, possibly in conjunction with other drugs, (e.g. sodium valproate, phenobarbitone), during rehabilitation and following discharge.

Status epilepticus

This medical emergency exists when there is incomplete recovery between seizures of 30 minutes or more duration (Mitchell 1989), and which may not respond to anticonvulsant therapy.

Causes of status epilepticus

• In the established epileptic:

(1) non-compliance with therapy;

(2) change in anti-epileptic drug dosage or type;

(3) febrile illness;

(4) interaction with anti-convulsant therapy from other drug or disorder.

• In the patient without a history of epilepsy:

(1) cerebral tumour;

(2) metabolic disorders: hypoglycaemia/ hyponatraemia/ hypocalcaemia/ hypomagnesaemia/ hepatic encephalopathy/ uraemia;

(3) head injury;

(4) subarachnoid haemorrhage;

(5) intracerebral haemorrhage;

(6) encephalitis, meningitis;

(7) acute alcohol or drug withdrawal;

(8) drug overdose (e.g. amphetamines, tricyclic anti-depressants);

(9) hypoxic encephalopathy;

(10) hyperthyroidism;

(11) eclampsia.

Management

• As with any emergency the priorities are airway, breathing, and circulation.

• The patient should initially be placed in the recovery position and receive high-flow oxygen via a facemask.

• An urgent blood glucose measurement should be performed.

• It is likely that the patient requiring ICU intervention will also require intubation and mechanical ventilation. Oxygen saturations of < 90 per cent and evidence of poor airway protection are indications for intubation and ventilation.

• Central venous access should be established to allow effective delivery of drug therapy and fluid management.

• An arterial line will facilitate the monitoring of arterial blood gases and blood pressure.

• A full range of investigations (serum electrolytes, calcium, and magnesium; full blood count; and tests specific to the patients condition) should be carried out to establish the cause of status epilepticus

• Mechanical ventilation is usually instituted.

Alternative anticonvulsant drugs

• Diazepam/midazolam — for status epilepticus rather than prophylaxis. Usually given in 2.5–5 mg boluses or, in the intubated, ventilated patient, as an infusion.

• Chlormethiazole — for status epilepticus rather than prophylaxis. Given at first as an infusion at between 40–100 ml over 10 min followed by between 40–100 ml/hr.

• Carbamazepine

• Sodium valproate

• Barbiturates (thiopentone) — if the above do not control seizures a thiopentone infusion may be used starting at 2 mg/kg/h and titrated upwards until seizures are controlled.

• Magnesium

• Clonazepam (primarily used for myoclonic seizures).

Rhabdomyolysis is a serious complication of muscle damage associated with prolonged seizures (see Chapter 11). Following status epilepticus there is usually a profound lactic acidosis due to the intense muscular activity with or without hypoxaemia. It generally reverses quickly on cessation of seizures.

It is important that nursing and medical staff are aware that convulsive status epilepticus may include tonic–clonic muscle activity or muscle twitching. Status epilepticus may be evident on an EEG in the absence of clinical evidence. CFAM monitoring may be used to determine seizure activity when clinical evidence is obscured by use of paralysing agents.

Status epilepticus should also be considered when a patient does not wake up as expected following craniotomy.

Spinal cord compression

There are two main categories of non-traumatic causes of spinal cord compression:

1. Disease of the vertebral column
   (secondary carcinoma; cervical spondylosis; primary neoplasms, such as myeloma; osteitis).

2. Other causes: extradural abscess; arachnoiditis; infiltration of the meninges; extramedullary, and intramedullary tumours.

Secondary carcinoma is the commonest cause and produces collapse by erosion of the spongy portions of the vertebra leading to cord compression. Protrusion of intervertebral discs are another cause of cord compression produced by tumours or abscesses.

Clinical manifestations depend on the lesion and the level of vertebra involved. Patients with acute collapse complain of severe pain and paresthesiae with tenderness of the spine on pressure or percussion. Autonomic symptoms can occur producing excessive sweating, as well as poor regulation of body temperature and blood pressure.

An urgent CT and/or MRI scan or myelography is

required to determine the level of cord compression and the intervention required.

For further management and nursing care refer to Chapter 11.

Spinal abscess

This is an emergency situation, which if untreated, will cause irreversible paraplegia. The abscess is usually due to either staphylococcal infection which is blood-borne, vertebral osteomyelitis or tuberculosis.

Symptoms for abscess are back pain, fever, leucocytosis, and spinal tenderness. Management requires surgical exploration and decompression with appropriate antibiotic treatment for the abscess.

Meningitis

A wide variety of bacteria, viruses, parasites, and fungi may cause this distressing and serious illness (see Table 9.11). Modes of transmission vary (Fig. 9.12).

Table 9.11 Causes of meningitis

Bacterial	Fungal
Meningococcus (*Neisseria meningitidis*)	*Crytococcus neoformans*
Pneumococcus (*Streptococcus pneumoniae*)	**Viral**
Haemophilus influenzae	Enteroviruses (poliovirus, echovirus, coxsackievirus)
Listeria monocytogenes	Herpes simplex type 2, varicella zoster
Staphylococcus aureus	Mumps
Mycobacterium tuberculosis	HIV
Escherichia coli	

Clinical manifestations

The onset is generally rapid and is characterized by severe frontal or diffuse headache peaking in a few hours. There is nausea, vomiting, fever, and photophobia. The patient's conscious level may be impaired or they may be confused, agitated, or fitting. Meningism may not necessarily be present.

> **Meningism**
> Neck stiffness and a positive Kernig's sign with normal CSF pressure
> (Kernig's sign — extension of one knee with hip fully flexed produces pain and spasm of the hamstrings)

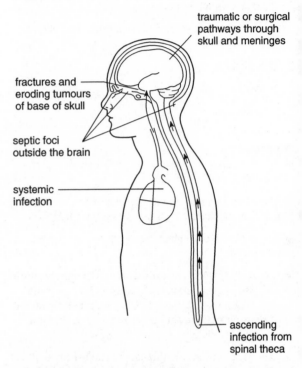

traumatic or surgical pathways through skull and meninges

fractures and eroding tumours of base of skull

septic foci outside the brain

systemic infection

ascending infection from spinal theca

Fig. 9.12 Meningitis: routes for infection of the brain (from Verran and Aisbitt 1988). Reprinted with permission.

As involvement of the meninges progresses, pain in the neck (nape) descends to the back and legs and irritability may be profound, especially on attempted neck movement. A high-pitched scream is characteristic in children and overt crying may be seen in adults, — such is the severity of pain.

Further deterioration is rapid and irritability may progress to drowsiness, stupor, and coma in a few hours. Opisthotonus may be seen frequently in children (see Fig. 9.13).

Management of meningitis

The onset of coma may necessitate admission to the ICU. Investigations should include CT scan, blood cultures, and, on exclusion of raised ICP, lumbar puncture should be performed. The CSF pressure should be measured and

CSF should be sent for culture and sensitivity. CSF should also be sent for glucose and protein levels (see Table 9.12). A blood glucose should be sent at the same time. Appropriate antibiotics should be commenced as soon as possible, based either on clinical assessment or on organism and sensitivities, if known.

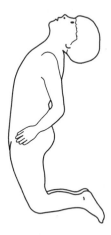

Fig. 9.13 Meningitis: opisthotonous is seen frequently in children (from Verran and Aisbitt 1988). Reprinted with permission.

Table 9.12 Typical cerebrospinal fluid values in meningitis

	Pyogenic	Viral	TB
Appearance	Turbid	Clear	Fibrin web
Predominant cell type	Polymorphs	Lymphocytes	Lymphocytes
Cell count/mm^3	>1000	<500	50–1500
Protein (g/l)	>1	0.5–1	1–5
Blood glucose	<0.6	>0.6%	<0.6%

(i) Meningococcal

This is primarily seen in children and young adults. There may be a distinctive petechial or sometimes purpuric rash. Benzylpenicillin or Cefotaximé are the antibiotics of choice, or chloramphenicol if the patient is allergic to penicillin.

(ii) Pneumococcal

This is primarily seen in older adults. There is no rash. Treatment is as for meningococcal meningitis.

(iii) Viral

If no organisms are isolated and there is a high lymphocyte count in the CSF, viral meningitis or a partially treated bacterial meningitis may be suspected. The treatment is acyclovir.

Steroids (dexamethasone) have been shown to reduce the incidence of complications and improve the outcome in bacterial meningitis in children. There is no data as yet in adults.

Nursing management

The patient should be nursed in quiet surroundings in a single room with barrier nursing precautions. Careful neurological assessment is required to follow trends and to allow for early detection of complications.

Temperature is labile and cooling measures including anti-pyretics and traditional nursing interventions should be employed.

The key to the outcome for these patients is meticulous essential nursing care.

Repositioning should be accomplished with the utmost gentleness without unnecessary jerking or bumping movements, even if the patient is sedated.

Complications of pyogenic meningitis

1. Adhesions between the pia and arachnoid meninges causing obstruction of CSF flow

2. Development of intracranial abscess causing raised ICP.

3. Cranial nerve palsies.

4. Corticothrombophlebitis causing seizures and hemiparesis.

These patients may be left with considerable neurological deficit in sensory, motor, and cognitive function.

Close contacts of patients with meningococcal or haemophilus meningitis should be given oral rifampicin for 2–4 days to clear carriers of the organism.

Brainstem death, organ donation, and care of the relatives

Brainstem death

This is the irreversible loss of neural function above the foramen magnum evidenced by apnoeic coma with absent brainstem reflexes (Pallis 1983).

There is little doubt both ethically and physiologically that the irreversible cessation of all central neurological function constitutes death. In most ordinary deaths, brain death occurs following cessation of respiration and heart beat, however, where brain death occurs as the primary event this sequence is reversed. The ability to support respiration and cardiac function has led to the situation where patients who are brain dead could be maintained on ventilators in intensive care for a number of days before finally succumbing. Patients diagnosed as brain dead eventually develop asystole at some point following brainstem death (Jørgensen 1973; Jennet et al. 1981).

The need to develop rigid diagnostic criteria which allowed establishment of braindeath without doubt, and the possibility of utilizing cadaveric organs for transplantation, produced the code of practice for cadaveric organs for transplantation (*Working party on cadaveric organs for transplantation — A code of practice* 1983). Following these criteria, patients can be diagnosed brain dead and mechanical ventilation withdrawn, or organs offered for transplantation, with confidence that there is no chance of error in diagnosis.

Death of the brainstem can occur as a result of:

(1) severe head injury;

(2) spontaneous intracerebral haemorrhage;

(3) cerebral hypoxia due to cardiac arrest, respiratory arrest, smoke inhalation or carbon monoxide poisoning, cerebral hypoperfusion,

(4) Brainstem infarct,

(5) Cerebral tumour,

(6) Drug overdose,

(7) Air or fat embolus,

(8) Intracranial infection.

Note. Spinal reflexes may remain producing limb movements in response to irritant stimuli — these are not an indication of higher function and the family should be made aware of this if they occur.

It has been recommended that testing is performed twice to ensure that there has been no observer error. Tests should be carried out by two senior doctors, one of whom should be a consultant. Where a consultant is not available another senior doctor who has been registered for more than five years and who has adequate experience in these cases can carry out the tests.

On completion of the second set of brainstem tests the patient is legally dead and this is the time of death recorded on the death certificate. The family should be informed of the outcome of the tests and the appropriate moment for removal of ventilatory support be decided with them. Relatives should not be asked to agree to turning off the ventilator as this may lead to further psychological stress and possible feelings of guilt.

If the patient has been identified as a potential organ donor and the family have agreed, the patient remains ventilated until the organ(s) have been removed.

Brainstem death is only diagnosed following a strict set of criteria (see Appendix 2). These are divided into two main sections:

1. The preconditions

Patients should only be considered for the diagnosis of brainstem death in the following circumstances:

(a) The patient is deeply comatose.
Metabolic or endocrine causes of coma must be excluded; there should be no suspicion of drug-induced coma and the patient should not be hypothermic (body temperature $> 35\,^{\circ}$C).

(b) The patient is being maintained on a ventilator because spontaneous respiration has ceased altogether.
Muscle relaxants and other drugs must be excluded as a cause of respiratory failure.

(c) There is no doubt that the patient's condition is due to irremediable structural brain damage.

If the preconditions are not fulfilled, for whatever reason, the testing stage cannot be implemented.

2. Tests for the absence of brainstem function

Brainstem death tests (Table 9.13) are designed to test the brainstem reflexes and ensure that these are definitely absent.

Organ donation

Patients can be considered for organ donation if they fit the criteria for brain stem death and there are no absolute contraindications (see Table 9.14).

Other factors, such as diabetes or poor renal function, are not necessarily a contraindication but should be discussed with the transplant co-ordinator. At this point, the question of brain death should be raised with the relatives and where appropriate, the possibility of

Table 9.13   Tests for brainstem death

Diagnostic tests	Cranial nerve	Area of brainstem tested
Fixed diameter pupil, unresponsive to sharp changes in light intensity	Cranial nerve III	Midbrain
Absent corneal reflex: no blink occurs when cornea is brushed with gauze	Cranial nerve III — oculomotor and IV — trochlear	Midbrain
Absent vestibulo-occular reflex: no eye movement occurs during or following slow injection of 20 ml ice-cold water into each external auditory meatus (ensure the tympanic membrane is visible, i.e. no blockage or perforation)	Cranial nerve VIII — vestibulocochlear	Pons
No motor response within the cranial nerve distribution in response to stimuli	Cranial nerve VII — facial or XI — accessory	Pons/Medulla
No gag reflex or cough reflex in response to suction catheter passed down the trachea, no slowing of heart rate	Cranial nerve IX — glossopharyngeal, or X — vagus	Medulla
No respiratory movements occur when disconnection from the mechanical ventilator allows P_aCO_2 to rise above 6.65 kPa: sufficiently high to stimulate respiration (oxygen levels are maintained by insufflation of oxygen through a suction catheter placed in the trachea)		Respiratory centre in the medulla

Note. Spinal reflexes may remain producing limb movements in response to irritant stimuli — these are not an indication of higher function and the family should be made aware of this if they occur.

organ donation. This should be done by a senior member of the medical staff accompanied by a nurse who is familiar with the patient's relatives. The condition and the nature of the tests should be explained. It is likely that this will need repeating on several occasions and written information, such as that provided by transplant co-ordinators, should be made available to the relatives.

Table 9.14   Absolute contraindications to organ donation

1. Patients from high-risk groups (as defined by the Department of Health)

2. History of malignancy — except primary brain tumour

3. HIV positive patients

Management/preparation of the potential organ donor

When organ donation is a possibility there are a number of factors which may limit the suitability of

the patient. These should be discussed with the transplant co-ordinator as soon as possible in order to ensure that the patient is a suitable donor.

Factors affecting the ability to donate organs:

(1) Malignancy (except primary brain tumours)

(2) Long-standing diabetes mellitus

(3) Chronic hypertension

(4) Hepatitis or positive hepatitis B status

(5) Tuberculosis

(6) AIDS or HIV

(7) Sepsis

(8) Sustained hypotension leading to oliguria or anuria which is unresponsive to intervention.

Principles of care of the potential donor

1. Maintenance of haemodynamic stability
In order to maintain the organs in optimal condition, perfusion should be supported with either fluid or

Table 9.15 Preconditions and contraindications for specific organs

Organ	Age (yrs)	Preconditions and contraindications
Kidneys	2–75	No relevant medical history, very few contraindications
Heart	0–55	No relevant medical history, no prolonged asystole or high inotropic support
Heart and lungs	0–55	No relevant medical history, recent clear chest X-ray with good gas exchange
Lungs	0–55	No relevant medical history, each lung assessed and can be used individually
Liver	0–65	No relevant medical history, such as drug or alcohol abuse
Liver and small bowel	0–30	No relevant medical history
Small bowel	0–30	No relevant medical history
Pancreas	12–55	No relevant medical history (e.g. diabetes or pancreatitis)
Cornea	0–100	No history of neurological disease of unknown aetiology (e.g. Alzheimer's), no history of untreated viral infection
Heart valves	0–65	No history of valve disease
Bone	18–60	No relevant medical history
Skin	0–70	
Research		Only with specific consent from family

inotropes as required. Hypotension can be a frequent problem due to hypovolaemia, derangement of vasomotor control mechanisms, endocrine abnormalities, and left ventricular dysfunction. Support of renal perfusion should be monitored using urine output as a guide and low-dose dopamine infusion may be used to maintain perfusion.

2. Maintenance of adequate oxygenation
Oxygenation should be optimal to maintain donor organs. Ventilation and inspired oxygen levels should be adjusted according to blood gases and supportive physiotherapy carried out. If the lungs are being considered for donation, prophylactic antibiotics may be required.

3. Prevention or treatment of arrhythmias
Electrolytes should be monitored and maintained and arrhythmias treated as necessary. There are many contributory factors including myocardial ischaemia, raised ICP, and inotropic infusions. Bradycardia in the brainstem dead patient is usually resistant to atropine.

4. Anaemia
Transfusion may be required to maintain the haemoglobin at $\geqslant 10$ g/dl

5. Diabetes insipidus
Urine volume and electrolyte losses should be replaced using a hypotonic solution, such as 0.45 per cent saline or dextrose 5 per cent, to avoid hypernatraemia. If urine output continues to be excessive, DDAVP (desmopressin) should be given.

6. Prevention of infection
Infection control measures and strict adherence to aseptic protocols should be followed to prevent any infection likely to harm the recipient.

7. Temperature fluctuation
Control of body temperature is lost with brainstem death and patients may cool to near ambient temperature unless this is controlled for them. Warming blankets and constant monitoring of temperature is important to prevent hypothermia.

Care of the relatives

The offer of organ donation to a potential donor family allows the nurse to experience with them a positive end to a tragic beginning. For this to happen it is imperative that the donor family is cared for within a therapeutic nursing framework. Nurses, therefore, need to assess accurately and respond to the individual, and be knowledgeable as to the process of organ donation if they are to care in a therapeutic manner.

When a patient has been diagnosed as brainstem dead, the main aim of care is directed at the preservation of the organs so that they are in optimum function for the recipient. There also should be a subtle shift of focus of care from the patient to the relatives so that the whole family now becomes the pivot for the nurse's therapeutic intervention. This can only be achieved if the nurse is aware of the ethical, legal, moral, cultural, spiritual, and mythical issues surrounding organ donation and has developed values and beliefs in relation to the essence of caring for both patients and their loved ones. The provision of psychological and physiological comfort should be developed as the primary intervention for the family of the brainstem dead patient to make this unique and individual experience as positive as possible. Fig. 9.14 highlights the specific needs of the relatives of the organ-donating patient.

> RESPECT to be shown for the donating patient
>
> To UNDERSTAND the necessity for essential nursing care to continue
>
> KNOWLEDGE that their decision is not irrevocable
>
> DIGNITY of the patient to be maintained once the organs have been retrieved
>
> OPPORTUNITY to say goodbye again after organ removal
>
> INFORMATION as to how the organs have been used

Fig. 9.14 The specific needs of relatives of the organ-donating patient.

References

Bastnagel Mason, P. (1992) Neurodiagnostic testing in critically injured adults. *Critical Care Nurse*, **12**, 64–75.

Bates, B. (1983). *Guide to Physical examination*, (3rd edn), J.B. Lippincott, Philadelphia.

Benner, P. and Wrubel, J. (1989). *The primacy of caring*, p. 322. Addison-Wesley, Menlo Pk.

Chaffee, E.E. and Lytte, I.M. (1980). Basic *Physiology and anatomy*. J.B. Lippincott, Philadelphia.

Frisby, J.R. (1990). Status epilepsy. In *Intensive care manual*, (3rd edn) (ed. T.E. Oh). Butterworth, Sydney.

Gujol, M.C. (1994). A survey of pain assessment and manage-ment practices among critical Care nurses. *American Journal of Critical Care*, **3**, 123–8.

Health Departments of Great Britain and Northern Ireland working party. (1983). *Cadaveric organs for transplantation: A code of practice including the diagnosis of brain death*. HMSO, London.

Hudak, C.M., Gallo, B.M., and Benz, J.J. (1990). *Critical care nursing: A holistic approach*, (5th edn). J.B. Lippincott, Philadelphia.

Green, J.H. (1992). An introduction to Human physiology, (4th edn). Oxford University Press, Oxford.

Hinchcliffe, S. and Montague, S. (1989). *Physiology for nursing practice*. Ballière Tindall, London.

Jennett, B., Gleave, J., and Wilson, P. (1981). Brain death in three neurosurgical units. *British Medical Journal*, **282**, 533–9.

Jones, J., Hoggart, B., Witney, J., Donaghue, K., and Ellis, B.W. (1979). What the patients say: a study of reactions to an intensive care unit. *Intensive Care Medicine*, 89–92.

Johnson, S.M., Omery, A., and Nikos, D. (1989). Effects of conversation on intracranial pressure in comatose patients. *Heart and Lung*, **18**, 56–63.

Jørgensen, E.O. (1973). Spinal man after brain death. *Acta Neurochirugica*, **28**, 259–73.

Kerr, M.E. and Brucia, J. (1993). Hyperventilation in the head-injured patient: An effective treatment modality? *Heart and Lung*, **22**, 516–21.

Melzack, R. and Wall, P.D. (1965). Pain mechanisms: a new theory. Science, **150**, 971–8.

Maynard, D.E. and Jenkinson, J.L. (1984). The cerebral func-tion analysing monitor. *Anaesthesia*, **39**, 678–90.

Miller, K.M. and Perry, P.A. (1990). Relaxation technique and post-operative pain in patients undergoing cardiac surgery. *Heart and Lung*, **19**, 136–46.

North, B. and Reilly, P. (1990). *Raised intracranial pressure: a clinical guide*. Heinemann, Oxford.

Oh, T.E. (ed.) (1990). *Intensive care manual*. Butterworth, Sydney.

Pallis, C. (1983). An ABC of brain stem death. *British Medical Journal*, **286**, 123–4.

Pickard, J.D., Murray G.D., Illingworth, R., Shaw, M.D., Teasdale, G.M., Foy, P.M., *et al.* (1989). Effect of oral nimodipine on cerebral infarction and outcome after subar-ochnoid haemorrhage: British aneurysm nimodipine trial. *British Medical Journal*, **298**, 636–42.

Puntillo, K.A. (1990). Pain experiences of intensive care unit patients. *Heart and Lung*, **19**, 526–33.

Puntillo, K.A. (1988). The phenomenon of pain and critical care nursing. *Heart and Lung*, **17**, 262–73.

Puntillo, K.A. (1994). Dimensions of procedural pain and its analgesic management in critically ill surgical patients. *American Journal of Critical Care*, **3**, 116–22.

Rudy, E., Turner, B., Baun, B., Stone, K., and Brucia, J. (1991). Endotracheal suctioning in adults with head injury. *Heart and Lung*, **20**, 667–74.

Simpson, T.F., Armstrong, S., and Mitchell, P. (1989). Patients' recollections of critical care. *Heart and Lung*, **18**, 325–32.

Stevensen, C.J. (1994). The psychophysiological effects of aromatherapy massage following cardiac surgery. *Complementary Therapies in Medicine*, **2**, 27–35.

Thompson, W.R. (1990). Acute cerebrovascular complications. In *Intensive care manual*, (ed. T.E. Oh), pp. 270–80. Butterworth, Sydney.

Tittle, M. and McMillan, S.C. (1994). Pain and pain-related side effects in an ICU and on a surgical unit: Nurses' management. *American Journal of Critical Care*, **3**, 25–30.

Verran, B., and Aisbitt, P. (1988). *Neurological and neurosurgical nursing*. Edward Arnold, London.

Walleck, C. (1993). Patients with head injury and brain dysfunction. In *Critical care nursing*, (ed. J. Clochesy and E.B. Rudy). Saunders, Philadelphia.

Ward, J.D. (1994). Intracranial pressure: Its measurement and treatment. In *Yearbook of intensive care and emergency medicine*, (ed. J.-L. Vincent) pp. 631–7. Springer, Berlin.

Williams, A. and Coyne, S.M. (1993). Effects of neck position on intracranial pressure. *American Journal of Critical Care*, **2**, 68–71.

Appendix 1

The Glasgow Coma Scale

Response	Score
Best eye-opening response	
Spontaneously	4
To speech	3
To pain	2
No response	1
Best verbal response	
Orientated	5
Confused conversation	4
Inappropriate words	3
Garbled sounds	2
No response	1
Best motor response	
Obeys commands	6
Localizes stimuli	5
Withdrawal from stimulus	4
Abnormal flexion (decorticate)	3
Abnormal extension (decerebrate)	2
No response	1

Appendix 2

CHECKLIST OF CRITERIA FOR DIAGNOSIS OF BRAIN DEATH

Diagnosis to be made by two independent doctors one a consultant and the other a consultant or senior registrar. Diagnosis should not normally be considered until at least 6 hours after the onset of coma or, if cardiac arrest was the cause of the coma, until 24 hours after the circulation has been restored.

Name ....   Unit No ....

PRE-CONDITIONS

Are you satisfied that the patient suffers from   Time of onset
a condition that has led to irremediable brain   of unresponsive
damage? Specify the condition: coma:

Dr A ....

Dr B ....

Are you satisfied that potentially reversible causes for the patient's condition have been adequately excluded, in particular:

	Dr A	Dr B
Depressant drugs		
Neuromuscular blocking (relaxant) drugs		
Hypothermia		
Metabolic or endocrine disturbances		

TESTS FOR ABSENCE OF BRAIN-STEM FUNCTION

	Dr A		Dr B	
	1st testing	2nd testing	1st testing	2nd testing
Do the pupils react to light?				
Are there corneal reflexes?				
Is there eye movement on caloric testing?				
Are there motor responses in the cranial nerve distribution, in response to stimulation of face, limbs or trunk?				
Is there a gag reflex? (If the test is practicable)				
Is there a cough reflex?				
Have the recommendations concerning testing for apnoea been followed?*				
Were any respiratory movements seen?				

	Dr A	Dr B
Date and time of first testing		
Date and time of second testing		

(As stated in paragraph 30 of the Code of Practice the two doctors may carry out the tests separately or together.)

Dr A Signature ....   Dr B Signature ....

Status ....   Status ....

*Diagnosis of Brain Death. Brit Med J 1976, ii, 1187-8.
See note (b) on page 35 of the Code of Practice

10. Gastrointestinal problems; and nutrition

Introduction

The gastrointestinal (GI) tract has been not always been considered an area of vital importance in the care of the critically ill. However, its effectiveness as a defence system and an essential resource for other organs is increasingly recognized and support of these functions is now considered an essential part of global treatment of the critically ill.

Anatomy and physiology

The anatomy and physiology of the GI tract will be described briefly, with particular reference to those aspects which have relevance to the critically ill. The GI tract acts as both a point of access and a protective barrier to the external environment. Its functions include breakdown of complex nutrients, absorption of predigested molecules, movement of foodstuffs through the digestive tract, elimination of waste matter, recycling of materials used in digestion, and protection of vulnerable internal organs from ingested organisms.

The GI tract is mostly under the control of the autonomic nervous system. The oropharyngeal cavity, upper oesophagus, and external anal sphincter are under voluntary control via somatic motor fibres. Most of the GI tract is supplied by both sympathetic and parasympathetic nerves.

Sympathetic stimulation will decrease gut motility, increase sphincter tone, and decrease exocrine secretions (i.e. discharged via a duct). Parasympathetic stimulation will increase motility, decrease sphincter tone, and increase exocrine secretions. Sympathetic and parasympathetic response can be altered by psycho-emotional stimuli mediated by higher neuronal centres. Thus, fear may increase the viscosity of saliva and decrease the amount secreted producing the characteristic dry mouth, while any strong emotion may increase gut motility.

Gut function

(1) Oropharyngeal cavity:
- mechanical breakdown of food,
- swallowing of food bolus (voluntary),

- saliva production (saliva = mucus + salivary amylase, a starch-digesting enzyme). The mucus lubricates and binds food and the amylase breaks down carbohydrate to simple sugars. The saliva is increased by parasympathetic stimulation and decreased by sympathetic stimulation

(2) Oesophagus
- secretion of mucus (lubrication and protection),
- propulsion of food (peristalsis).

(3) Lower oesophageal sphincter (last centimetre of oesophagus)
- prevention of reflux of gastric contents by continuous smooth muscle contraction (the muscle relaxes in response to peristalsis to allow food to pass through).

(4) Stomach

The stomach has a primary digestive function but its highly acidic environment also acts as an effective barrier to foreign organisms

- breakdown of food by pepsin and gastric acid (hydrochloric acid; HCl),
- production of intrinsic factor (facilitates absorption of vitamin B_{12} by the small intestine),
- production of gastrin (promotes growth and repair of gastric mucosa and stimulates secretion of pepsinogen and HCl)

Gastric acid secretion is stimulated by:

(i) histamine via the H_2-histamine receptors in the gastric mucosa,

(ii) alcohol and caffeine via the gastric chemoreceptors and intramural nerve plexuses in the stomach wall,

(iii) hypoglycaemia via the brainstem and vagal fibres.

Protection of the gastric epithelium from gastric acid is vital as the gastric luminal pH is maintained at a potentially damaging value of 2–3.

This protection is achieved by:

(i) The luminal surface membranes of gastric mucosal cells fit tightly together forming a barrier against HCl damage. The barrier is impermeable to hydrogen ions maintaining a concentration gradient between epithelium and lumen. This barrier can be disrupted by, among others, bile salts, alcohol, aspirin, and steroids. Mucosal blood flow and thus oxygenation is an important factor in maintaining mucosal integrity (see later).

(ii) Secretion of mucus/bicarbonate gel by mucosal cells to cover mucosal epithelium. The gel is capable of maintaining a pH gradient from approximately 2 on the gastric lumen side to approximately 7.3 on the epithelial side.

Endogenous prostaglandins play a role in maintaining gastric mucosal integrity by influencing mucosal blood flow, stabilizing the mucosal barrier, and stimulating mucus/bicarbonate secretion. The prostaglandin inhibition by non-steroidal anti-inflammatory drugs may result in gastric erosions or deeper ulceration.

Enteral nutrition or the presence of any food in the stomach may also be important in maintaining mucosal integrity (see later).

(5) Pancreas

The pancreas secretes both exocrine and endocrine substances.

Exocrine function:

- secretion of water to dilute chyme (a mixture of semi-digested food and gastric enzymes) and increase nutrient absorption,

- secretion of bicarbonate to neutralize post-gastric chyme,

- secretion of inactive forms of enzymes including:

  (i) protein-digesting trypsin, chymotrypsin, elastase, and carboxypeptidase,

  (ii) fat-digesting lipase and esterase,

  (iii) starch-digesting amylase,

  (iv) nucleic acid–digesting nuclease.

In the duodenum, trypsin is activated by the intestinal mucosal enzyme, enterokinase, and trypsin then activates other pancreatic enzymes.

Endocrine secretions, such as insulin and glucagon, are discussed fully in Chapter 13.

(6) Gallbladder

- holds and concentrates bile.

  (i) Bile emulsifies fat into small droplets for degradation by lipase and esterase into micelles (particles with a fatty core and water-soluble coat). Micelles are then transported across the intestinal lumen leaving the bile behind.

  (ii) Bile ionizes fat-soluble vitamins into absorbable forms.

  (iii) Bile acts to suspend cholesterol, triglycerides, and medium-density lipoproteins in the blood, preventing precipitation and deposition.

(7) Duodenum and jejunum

- secretion of water to further dilute chyme,

- secretion of bicarbonate to neutralize postgastric acidic chyme,
  (water and bicarbonate are secreted by Brunner's glands in the mucosa),

- mucus secretion to protect the duodenal lumen,

- secretion of enterokinase to convert trypsinogen (inactive form) to trypsin (active form),

- secretion of secretin and cholecystokinin (CCK) in response to acidity and proteins. These act to stimulate pancreatic secretion and gallbladder release of contents,

- secretion of maltase, lactase, and sucrase to convert carbohydrates to simple sugars,

- mixing of chyme to allow exposure of all molecules to the absorptive surface,

- peristalsis to propel chyme along the small intestine,

- absorption of carbohydrates by active and passive transport across the intestinal lumen into the bloodstream,

- absorption of protein as amino acids and protein fragments by active (assisted movement across a concentration gradient) and passive (movement from high to low concentration) diffusion,

- absorption of fats in the form of fatty acids and monoglycerides by passive transport in the duodenum and the first half of the jejunum.

Effect of tonicity of gastrointestinal contents
Tonicity is defined as the effective osmotic pressure of a fluid in relation to plasma. Further details about osmosis and osmotic pressure can be found in Chapter 8.

The gastrointestinal tract is highly permeable in both directions to water. Water is absorbed passively throughout the stomach and small and large intestines and also secreted into chyme. If the gastrointestinal contents are hypertonic, then osmosis (the movement of water from an area of low solute concentration to an area of high solute concentration across a semi-permeable membrane) into the lumen will occur. If the contents are hypotonic then there will be movement of water from the gastrointestinal contents into the bloodstream. This can obviously affect the fluid balance of the body but it will also affect the amount of fluid in the gut contents. Thus, a hypertonic enteral feed may well produce diarrhoea due to the movement of water into the gut lumen via osmosis.

(8) Colon
- secretion of mucus to lubricate faecal material and protect mucosa,
- mixing of contents to allow exposure to absorptive surface and peristalsis to propel contents,
- mass movement to propel faecal matter rapidly into the rectum from the sigmoid and descending colon,
- absorption of water, potassium and chloride,
- absorption of folic acid,
- absorption of ammonia.

(9) Rectum
- defecation.

The immune function of the gut

The dual functions of: (i) connection with, and (ii) protection from, the external environment requires both accessibility (for absorption of required substances) and protection from external harmful organisms.

Protection is achieved by the following mechanisms:

1. The gut mucosa acts as a physical barrier against systemic invasion by bacteria which colonize the gut.

2. The gut epithelial cells prevent migration of organisms.

3. The intestinal walls contain high levels of lymphocytes and macrophages.

4. The mesentery is filled with regional lymph nodes.

5. Secretory (immunoglobulin A) (IgA) is produced intraluminally by specialized cells (Peyer's patches). This prevents adherence of bacteria to mucosal cells and is the principal component of the gut mucosal defence system.

6. Kupffer cells (fixed organ-specific macrophages) in the liver and macrophages in the spleen, trap and phagocytose bacteria and toxic products if penetration does occur.

In the healthy person this protection is highly organized and effective but when the patient becomes critically ill a number of factors may compromise the system and allow migration of invading organisms into the circulation (bacterial translocation). These factors are:

(1) Altered permeability or loss of integrity of the intestinal mucosa as a result of hypovolaemic ischaemia, sepsis or endotoxaemia (the presence in the blood of endotoxin — part of the outer membrane of Gram-negative bacteria, — see Chapter 14).

(2) Decreased host defence mechanisms such as immuno suppression.

(3) Increased bacterial numbers within the intestine caused either by overgrowth or intestinal stasis. The normal gut maintains a balance of commensal bacteria which restricts the numbers of any one type. This balance can be disturbed by antibiotics preventing the growth of one organism and thus allowing overgrowth of another.

All of these factors are found frequently in the critically ill patient who is therefore highly vulnerable to overwhelming bacterial invasion.

Protein malnutrition may also affect the integrity of gut mucosa or the immunocompetence of the gut and contribute to an increased risk of bacterial translocation although this has not been definitely established (Pingleton 1991). Early enteral feeding may protect against loss of mucosal integrity (Moore *et al.* 1989).

Absorption and storage of digested food

(1) Carbohydrate

Digestion reduces carbohydrate polymers to monosaccharides (mainly glucose). The intestinal epithelial cells contain enzymes which split polysaccharides into monosaccharides. Monosaccharides are absorbed in the intestine by combining with a carrier substance which also binds with sodium. Sodium is then moved through the cell by its own active transport mechanism and the monosaccharide is pulled with it. This active transport allows absorption to occur against a concentration gradient.

Glucose is carried in the bloodstream to the individual cells where it is transported through the cell membrane by a process known as facilitated diffusion (see Fig. 10.1).

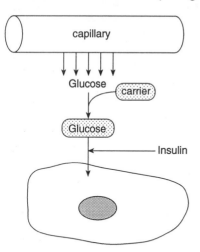

Fig. 10.1 Diagram showing the mechanism of facilitated diffusion of glucose through the cell membrane.

Glucose is stored as glycogen either in the liver or in muscle cells. This is usually sufficient to maintain blood glucose levels for about 24 hours under normal fasting conditions.

(2) Fat

Digestion of fat is by hydrolysis catalysed by the enzyme lipase. The end-products are fatty acids, glycerol, and glycerides. These molecules are highly soluble in the brush border of the epithelial cells and diffuse readily from the intestinal lumen. The molecules are re-synthesized and expelled into the lymph system via the central lacteals of the villi as small globules of fat called chylomicrons. Lymph is milked from the central lacteals into the abdominal lymphatics by rhythmic contraction of the villi. The chylomicrons are then transported via the thoracic lymph duct to empty into the bloodstream at the junction of the left internal jugular and subclavian vein.

Fat is stored in modified connective tissue cells as triglycerides (see Fig. 10.2). Triglycerides are broken down and re-synthesized continuously under the influence of the enzyme lipase. Net breakdown or synthesis is controlled by blood levels of glucose, insulin, catecholamines, and glucagon. High levels of glucose and insulin will increase synthesis and high levels of catecholamines or glucagon will increase breakdown.

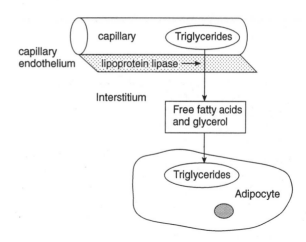

Fig. 10.2 Diagram showing the mechanism of triglycerides (fat) storage in adipocytes.

(3) Protein

Protein is digested in the stomach by pepsin to form small protein molecules (proteoses, polypeptides, peptones). These are further split by trypsin and other enzymes into amino acids and dipeptides and absorbed by active transport into the bloodstream using the sodium co-transport system utilized by monosaccharides.

The liver and many other cells of the body have the ability to store amino acids and to release them into the bloodstream when levels fall. As a result amino acids are in a state of continual flux from one part of the body to another (Fig. 10.3).

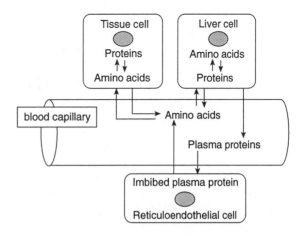

Fig. 10.3 Diagram showing the mechanism of the storage and breakdown of amino acids (proteins) (from Guyton *Anatomy and physiology* 1985 reprinted with permission).

The liver

The liver is one of the most important organs of the body and a wide variety of metabolic functions are performed by the hepatocytes (liver cells). As one of the most essential organs in the body the liver has the ability to regenerate itself. It has both an arterial and venous blood supply with approximately three–quarters of the blood flowing through the liver coming from the portal vein which supplies venous blood. The arterial blood is supplied via the hepatic artery.

The portal vein drains blood from the alimentary canal, spleen, pancreas, and gallbladder containing:

(a) nutrients for storage and synthesis,

(b) debris, including bacteria, for filtration and phago-cytosis.

Function of hepatocytes
1. Carbohydrate metabolism:

   (i) glycogen storage

   (ii) gluconeogenesis

   (iii) release of glucose into plasma.

When exogenous carbohydrate is not available the blood glucose concentration is maintained by endogenous glucose production, 90% of which is derived from the liver by glycogenolysis or gluconeogenesis. This response is affected by levels of circulating insulin, cortisol, glucagon, adrenaline, and thyroxine.

Gluconeogenesis
Formation of glucose from proteins through a series of chemical reactions in the liver cells

Glycogenolysis
The breakdown of glycogen stored in the muscle and liver cells to glucose by enzymes in the liver cells

---

2. Degradation of many drugs (including alcohol, benzodiazepines, tranquillizers, phenobarbitone, phenytoin, warfarin). Most drugs metabolized are fat-soluble and their conversion by the liver into water-soluble substances facilitates excretion in bile or urine.

Drugs are principally metabolized by hepatic enzymes in a specialized part of the hepatic cell. Two main kinds of chemical change occur:

(a) non-synthetic — the molecule is changed by oxidation, reduction, hydrolysis,

(b) synthetic — the molecule is conjugated with other substances such as glucuronic acid, acetic acid, and sulphate.

The pharmacological consequences of drug metabolism vary according to the drug and the reaction it undergoes. Conjugation almost always causes loss of activity (salicylates, paracetamol, and morphine). Acetylation of sulphonamides makes drugs less soluble and therefore potentially more harmful. When two drugs are metabolized by the same microsomal enzymes there may be prolongation of drug action.

Drug metabolism may be impaired in liver disease. The extent to which individual drugs are metabolized in an altered manner is highly variable and care must be taken to avoid overdosage, particularly with sedative drugs.

3. Elimination of bilirubin: 80% of bilirubin is derived from haem following the breakdown of haemoglobin in the liver, spleen, and bone marrow. It is not water-soluble and is carried in the plasma bound to albumin. In the liver it is transported into the hepatocytes, conjugated with glucuronic acid, and excreted by active transport into the bile. In the terminal ileum and colon bacteria reduce bilirubin to stercobilinogen which is excreted in the stool. A small amount is reabsorbed and excreted in the urine as urobilinogen.

4. Fat metabolism:

   (i) lipoprotein synthesis from cholesterol, phospholipid, and triglyceride combined with apoproteins,

   (ii) cholesterol and other lipid molecules synthesis,

   (iii) conversion of protein and carbohydrate to fat.

5. Mineral (up to 60% of excess iron) and vitamin storage including vitamin A, D, K, B_{12}, and folate

6. Production of bile: the primary bile acids (cholic and chenodeoxycholic acid) are produced from cholesterol. They are secreted into bile and then reabsorbed into the portal blood at specific sites in the terminal ileum.

7. Protein metabolism:

   (i) synthesis of plasma proteins including albumin, globulins (other than gamma-globulins), transferrin, and components of the complement system,

   (ii) deamination (breakdown) of proteins and conversion of ammonia to urea,

(iii) transamination (movement of amino acids from one molecule to another).

8. Steroid catabolism (hormones, including cortisol, oestrogens, and contraceptive drugs).

9. Synthesis of coagulation factors (I, fibrinogen; II, prothrombin; V, proaccelerin; VII, proconvertin; IX, plasma thromboplastin component; X, Stuart factor.)

10. Reticuloendothelial function

Kupffer cells:

● phagocytosis of bacteria, debris, and other foreign matter in the hepatic sinus blood,

● back-up defence mechanism against bacterial translocation into the portal vein.

Assessment of the patient

This should be performed with two goals in mind. The first is to assess the patient's nutritional status and the second is to assess potential gastrointestinal (GI) dysfunction.

History

Useful information can be obtained from the patient (or relatives) about nutritional status immediately prior to admission. In particular, recent weight loss, change in eating habits, and appetite. Other areas including bowel function, dental hygiene, and previous GI problems should also be covered.

Physical examination

The patient's general appearance can give a limited evaluation of nutritional state. Obvious signs of obesity and emaciation are easily discernible but muscle wasting (suggesting protein deficiency) may be obscured in the obese patient. Generalized oedema may also mask recognition of muscle wasting and it may only be in the resolution stage of the illness that the degree of loss is apparent. Features of individual vitamin and trace element deficiency, such as dryness, reddening, and haemorrhage of the skin in vitamin C, K, or A deficiencies, may be attributed to other causes such as coagulation disorders.

Jaundice and the almost green tinge associated with bile duct obstruction may be indicators of hepatic dysfunction although there may be few overt signs until hepatic dysfunction is quite severe.

Examination of the oral cavity

This should be done as part of a general assessment of the patient and includes assessing the condition of the mucosa, teeth (or dentures), and the lips. Signs of inflammation, fungal infection, such as *Candida albicans*, apthous ulcers, and herpetic lesions should be noted and swabs taken for culture if necessary. Medical staff should be informed.

Teeth need to be examined for blackening, dental caries, wobbling, or loose sockets, and plaque or debris. The gums can be assessed at the same time for signs of inflammation, recession, bleeding and overgrowth. Bleeding may be related to poor dental hygiene or to coagulation disorders and should be considered in context with the patient's underlying condition. Medical staff should be informed of loose teeth, bleeding gums, and very severe tooth decay, as a dental referral may be necessary.

The patient's breath should also be assessed and any unusual odour such as hepatic foetor (a sweet, musty odour) or ketones (a sweet smell of acetone) should be noted and reported.

Abdominal assessment

The abdomen should be examined for symmetry, size, evidence of distension (taut, swollen skin often with an everted umbilicus), and signs of pulsation (usually visible epigastrically). Dilated veins may be visible and any rashes, scars, or lumps should be noted.

Auscultation of the abdomen to assess bowel sounds should be carried out with the diaphragm of the stethoscope. The absence of bowel sounds cannot be confirmed unless auscultation continues for at least 3 minutes.

Palpation can be carried out to assess tenderness, muscle resistance, masses, and a fluid thrill (present in ascites). (For details of abdominal palpation see Hudak *et al.* 1990, p. 652.)

Rectal examination may be necessary if the patient complains of constipation or has diarrhoea that may constitute faecal overflow.

Specific problems associated with the gastrointestinal tract

Acute gastrointestinal bleeding

This may be manifested either by:

(1) haematemesis — this is usually related to a bleeding point above the duodenojejunal junction, or

(2) melaena — altered blood appearing black and tarry from passage through the upper GI tract. If bleeding is copious and current, the patient may pass virtually unaltered blood per rectum.

Assessment

Initial assessment of the patient should include the following areas:

● Physical
Skin — colour, evidence of perspiration, temperature.
Mucosa — evidence of anaemia.
Degree of weakness or obtundation.
Level of anxiety, mental state.

● Haemodynamic
Heart rate, blood pressure, temperature.

● Fluid status
If there is a central venous catheter assess CVP, if there is a urinary catheter, assess urine output. If there is a pulmonary artery catheter assess PA pressures, cardiac output, stroke volume.

● Respiratory state
Respiratory rate, oxygen saturation, arterial blood gases — degree of metabolic acidosis, evidence of respiratory compensation.

See Table 10.1 for causes of GI bleeding.

If the patient is able to give a history, details should be determined of the frequency and volume of haematemesis or melaena.

Priorities of management

(1) Resuscitation. This refers primarily to replacing and stabilizing blood loss but may also necessitate intubation and ventilation if the patient is unable to sustain adequate blood gases or protect the airway. Supplemental oxygen should always be given.

It includes placing large-bore IV access, preferably so that CVP or pulmonary artery occlusion pressure can be monitored, although large peripheral vein access can be used. Fluid is replaced as rapidly as necessary to maintain an adequate circulation.

Table 10.1 Causes of gastrointestinal bleeding

Problem	Area affected by problem			
	Upper GI bleeding		Lower GI bleeding	
	Oesophagus	Stomach	Small intestine	Large bowel and rectum
Varices	✓	✓ (less common)	✓ (less common)	
Inflammation	✓	✓ (gastritis)		✓ (ulcerative colitis)
Ulcers	✓	✓	✓	
Tumours	✓	✓		✓
Mallory–Weiss tear	✓			
Angiodysplasia		✓ (less common)	✓	✓ (less common)
Crohn's disease			✓	✓
Diverticula			✓ (Meckel's)	✓
Haemorrhoids				✓
Rectal fissures				✓

In the first instance, colloid is given urgently while blood is being cross-matched. If the haemoglobin is very low (<5–7 g/dl) and the patient is compromised then group-specific or at the extreme O-negative blood is necessitated.

(2) Monitoring and assessment of the patient's vital signs should be carried out and bloods taken to allow evaluation of arterial blood gases, haemoglobin, clotting, platelets, calcium, and urea and electrolytes.

(3) If the patient is aware he/she will require frequent and repeated reassurance and explanation as to what is going on.

Further management

(1) If the patient remains hypotensive, in spite of continued fluid resuscitation, investigation of uncontrolled bleeding should be instigated as soon as possible. Otherwise this may be left until the patient's condition has stabilized. Investigation of bleeding may require endoscopy for upper GI bleeding, sigmoidoscopy/colonoscopy for lower GI bleeding, angiography, or even laparotomy.

(2) Even if oesophageal varices are suspected, a large-bore nasogastric tube should be inserted to allow drainage and assessment of upper GI bleeding, prevent gastric dilatation, and allow administration of medication. The patient should remain nil by mouth initially in case surgery is required.

(3) Treatment can be either surgical, conservative, or using endoscopic or angiographic methods of haemostasis.

Conservative treatment

H$_2$-receptor antagonists (e.g. ranitidine) or proton pump inhibitors (e.g. omeprazole) are administered to reduce gastric acidity and the accompanying irritation of ulcers. Therapeutic results are best achieved if the gastric pH is kept above 4 and this should be checked 4-hourly. Antacids may have to be administered as well in order to achieve this.

Endoscopic treatment

Sclerosis (fibrosis) of the bleeding point(s) can be performed via the endoscope using either sclerosing agents (adrenaline or alcohol) or, where this is available, electrocoagulation or laser therapy. Preparation of the patient may require iced water lavage to minimize and clear any active bleeding so that points may be clearly identified and treated.

Oesophageal varices

Aetiology

Oesophageal varices occur when obstruction to the portal vein produces portal hypertension. This may be due to destruction of the hepatic vasculature as in cirrhosis or to obstruction of the portal vein itself. The back pressure produced is transmitted throughout the portal system and has the effect of producing dilatation of the surface blood vessels in the lower oesophagus and, occasionally, the fundus of the stomach and the duodenum (Fig. 10.4). The protruding veins can then become eroded and bleed. Varices should be suspected in patients with acute GI bleeding particularly with a history/physical examination suggestive of chronic liver damage.

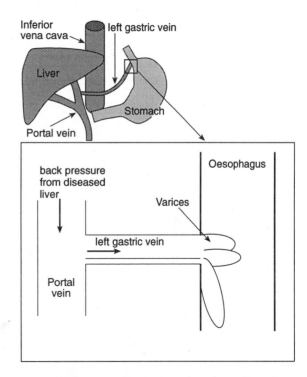

Fig. 10.4 Diagrammatic representation of oesophageal varices.

Priorities of management

(1) As before, resuscitation of the patient with colloid and blood is of paramount importance.

(2) An infusion of vasopressin (antidiuretic hormone) temporarily controls variceal bleeding in 60% of cases. It works by constricting the splanchnic arterioles and increasing their resistance to flow which reduces the

amount of blood entering the portal venous system. Its side-effects are systemic hypertension and intestinal colic and it may cause severe ischaemia in the intestine, skin, and heart. Simultaneous infusion of glyceryl trinitrate reduces the coronary and splanchnic vasoconstriction side effects.

Somatostatin or octreotide (a somatostatin analogue) is also commonly used as a first-line splanchnic vaso-constrictor. It is much more expensive although probably no more effective than vasopressin.

(3) If bleeding is severe a Sengstaken–Blakemore or modified Sengstaken (4-lumen Minnesota) tube should be inserted (Fig. 10.5). This tube is inserted through the nose or mouth and fed into the stomach. It has two balloons which when positioned correctly can apply local pressure to the cardia and the oesophagus. The Seng-staken tube has a lumen for gastric aspiration and the Minnesota tube has an extra lumen in the oesophagus for oesophageal aspiration.

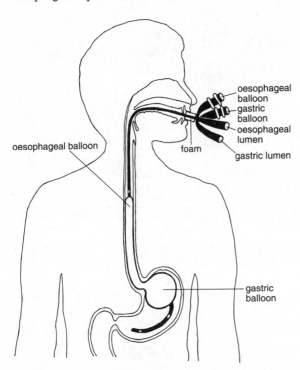

Fig. 10.5 The Sengstaken (modified) tube.

Insertion and care of the Sengstaken tube

This is a difficult manoeuvre which is usually complicated by the agitation of the patient and persistent haematemesis. Particular care should be taken to prevent contamination by blood splashes and all staff involved in the procedure should wear full-face visors, gloves, and plastic aprons.

Sengstaken (modified) tube: equipment required for insertion

- Sengstaken or equivalent tube (red rubber or latex tubes should be firmed by placing in a freezing compartment for at least 15 min prior to the procedure)
- Laryngoscope
- Tongue depressor
- Magill's forceps
- Anaesthetic spray
- Lubricating jelly
- Tape to fix the tube
- Piece of sponge, weight, or splint to apply traction
- 50 ml syringe

- The patient requires explanation and preparation for the procedure (see below). They are likely to be considerably distressed and may also be experiencing a degree of hepatic encephalopathy with alterations of perception and behaviour.

Sengstaken (modified) tube: points to explain to the patient prior to insertion
(1) Where the tube is going
(2) How it is going to work
(3) The sensations that the patient will experience (e.g. fullness in the stomach, a tube in the mouth and back of the throat, not being able to swallow saliva)
(4) Likelihood of success: 90% if the tube is used properly

- Prior to insertion the balloons should be checked for leaks and patency.

- The tube is inserted with the patient sitting at an angle of about 30° or alternatively in the left lateral position. The choice of position will depend on the patient's conscious level and ability to co-operate.

- When the tube is in position the gastric balloon is inflated with 150–200 ml of air and drawn back until it sits firmly against the cardia of the stomach.

- The tube should be secured with tape and splints or foam applied at the exit point from the nose or mouth in order to maintain traction Alternatively, firm traction can be maintained using a weight.

- The oesophageal balloon is not usually inflated unless bleeding continues in spite of the gastric tamponade. If it has to be inflated a manometer should be used to ensure that pressures are not greater than 30–40 mmHg (4.5–5.4 kPa). It should not be left inflated for longer than 24 hours as the risk of oesophageal wall ischaemia is high.

- If the tube has an oesophageal aspiration lumen this should be aspirated frequently or placed on continuous suction in order to prevent build-up of secretions and the danger of aspiration.

- The patient is unable to swallow and saliva will require removal by suction if the patient is unable to spit. Mouth care is essential although difficult to achieve if the tube is placed orally.

Once bleeding is controlled the patient will usually be referred for sclerotherapy, variceal banding, or surgery.

Removal of the Sengstaken tube
- The procedure should be explained to the patient.

- The patient should be sitting upright. If there is any concern over the patient's ability to protect his/her airway the medical staff should be consulted to ensure adequate back-up is present to prevent aspiration of any gastric contents.

- If the oesophageal balloon has been inflated this should always be deflated first. Frequently, a period of time is allowed between deflating the oesophageal balloon and removing the tube to ensure that bleeding does not recur.

- Immediately prior to removing the tube the gastric (and oesophageal if this is present) lumens should be aspirated to clear any gastric contents.

- The gastric balloon is then deflated and the tube removed by smooth firm traction.

Stress ulceration

The incidence of histological stress ulceration in ICU patients is high although the clinical significance of these lesions is much lower. The number that actually cause life-threatening GI bleeding has declined over the last decade.

Risk factors associated with stress ulceration
- Hypoperfusion
- Sepsis
- Head injury
- Renal failure
- Multiple trauma
- Respiratory failure
- Severe burn injuries
- Major surgical procedures
- Fulminant hepatic failure or severe hepatic dysfunction
- Drugs (e.g. non-steroidal anti-inflammatories)

Pathogenesis

A number of factors have been implicated in the development of stress ulcers.

(1) Decreased mucosal blood flow
Mucosal blood flow is vital in the maintenance of the gastric mucosal barrier but even a short period of ischaemia may be enough to disrupt the protective function of the mucosa. The mechanism is thought to be a decrease in intramural pH associated with a decreased blood flow limiting removal of hydrogen (H^+)ions, ischaemia, and development of anaerobic metabolism leading to intramural acidosis.

(2) Mucosal barrier breakdown
Disruption of the mucus-producing cells and reduction in mucus and bicarbonate production, and secretion allows back-diffusion of H^+ ions into the mucosa.
Factors affecting mucosal breakdown:

- Bile salts and urea damage the epithelial cells.

- Salicylates and local prostaglandin production inhibit active ion transport and bicarbonate secretion thus reducing the pH gradient between mucosa and gastric lumen.

- Ethanol decreases the thickness of mucus and stimulates histamine release which increases acid secretion.

- Corticosteroids alter the composition and decrease the production of mucus and cause an increase in acid secretion

(3) Increased intraluminal acid levels

The level of intraluminal pH is not necessarily a causative factor in itself. Stress ulceration seems to be related to other factors such as the integrity of the mucosal defence mechanisms.

(4) Decreased epithelial regeneration

Decreased cellular proliferation and deoxyribonucleic acid synthesis in the gastric mucosa have been shown to occur during stress. Thus, regeneration of the mucosal barrier for protection against intraluminal acid is compromised and may lead to ulceration.

(5) Lowered intramural pH

It is suggested that the intramural (intramucosal) pH which reflects local ischaemia is a better indicator of the development of stress ulceration than intraluminal pH (Fiddian-Green 1988). The decrease in intramucosal pH can be related to a number of mechanisms which result from poor mucosal blood flow and ischaemia:

(i) As luminal ions accumulate, they leak back into the mucosa causing a decrease in pH.

(ii) Decreased blood flow causes anaerobic metabolism with a further reduction in pH.

(iii) Vascular permeability is affected by the decrease in mucosal pH causing oedema. This is accentuated by release of histamine and serotonin which cause permeability changes and increased acid secretion.

(iv) Pepsinogen is activated by increased back-diffusion of H^+ ions leading to autodigestion of the mucosa.

While the pathogenesis of stress ulceration remains complex and, as yet incompletely explained, prevention of bleeding from stress ulcers has concentrated on two particular factors. The first is the presence of an acidic intraluminal environment and the second is the protective mucosal barrier.

Neutralizing the acidic intraluminal environment
● Antacids

These act as a base (a substance able to combine with H^+ ions) to neutralize gastric acid. They are effective in reducing the incidence of bleeding providing the pH is kept above 4. Side-effects include diarrhoea, hypermagnesaemia, increased plasma aluminium levels, and alkalosis. An increased incidence of aspiration pneumonia has been associated with their use, possibly as a result of bacterial overgrowth (Tryba 1991). The requirement of 1

to 4-hourly monitoring of gastric pH and administration of antacid is time-consuming (Konopad and Noseworthy 1988) and there may be difficulty aspirating a representative sample of gastric contents if a fine-bore feeding tube is used.

● Histamine (H_2)-receptor antagonists

Histamine release is thought to be the method by which increased gastric acid secretion is stimulated. The acid-secreting cells within the stomach respond to the presence of histamine via the H_2-receptor and acid is produced. Ranitidine and cimetidine are the most commonly used H_2-antagonists and have been shown to decrease the incidence of bleeding in selected groups of patients. However, there is no evidence that their use improves the overall survival of ICU patients.

Side-effects include drug interactions, suppression of ADH release, and reports of mental confusion. In addition, cimetidine has caused dysrhythmias, hypotension, and bradycardia, reversible bone marrow depression, and inhibition of cytochrome P450 in the liver, resulting in altered drug metabolism of diazepam, phenytoin, and propanolol.

The increase in intraluminal pH associated with H_2-receptor antagonist use may also result in bacterial overgrowth and an increased incidence of aspiration pneumonia.

Improving the protective mucosal barrier
Sucralfate

Sucralfate (the basic aluminium salt of sucrose octasulphate) forms a protective barrier over the gastric mucosa and facilitates healing of ulcers while gastric pH is maintained. It has been shown to be effective in the treatment of duodenal ulcers and in the prevention of gastric ulcers (Tryba 1991), however, evidence is conflicting with regard to stress ulceration. There may be less risk of nosocomial pneumonia associated with sucralfate probably due to the maintenance of gastric pH. It has few side-effects as it is not absorbed from the GI tract.

Enteral feeding has also been suggested as a method of protection from stress ulceration. However, until further studies comparing this with accepted methods have been carried out it is probably advisable to add an alternative form of stress ulcer prophylaxis for high-risk patients such as those with coagulopathies and previous history of gastric or duodenal ulcers.

The incidence of acute GI bleeding from ulcers in the critically ill patient has been dramatically reduced. However, it is likely that this is due as much to general improvements in support of the intensive care patient as to the use of any specific pharmacological agent.

The liver

Hepatic failure

(1) Fulminant hepatic failure

This is defined as severe impairment of hepatocellular function with concomitant hepatic encephalopathy (see below) in an individual with no evidence of previous liver disease (Levy *et al.* 1991). It can be further subdivided into acute and subacute depending on the length of time from onset to full symptoms. Common causes include viral hepatitis (A, B, C) and paracetamol overdose. Other causes include idiosyncratic drug reactions, acute fatty liver of pregnancy, inhalation of carbon tetrachloride or halothane, and Wilson's disease. Prognosis is poor and mortality can be as high as 80%.

(2) Acute on chronic hepatic failure

This is defined as an acute exacerbation of existing liver disease precipitated by a specific cause. Causes include: infection, gastrointestinal haemorrhage (varices, peptic ulcer), administration of sedatives, surgery, high protein load, or any other cause of decompensation of the liver. Short-term survival is better than in fulminant hepatic failure.

Problems associated with acute hepatic failure

Disturbance in conscious level
(see box for grades of encephalopathy)
Encephalopathy is associated with hepatic failure. It is uncertain exactly what causes it but many factors have been implicated. Free fatty acids, mercaptans, phenols, bilirubin, and bile acids have been shown to be toxic. Gamma-aminobutyric acid (GABA), 'middle molecular weight' compounds, and aromatic amino acids have also been associated with encephalopathy. In grades III–IV, cerebral oedema is common (>80% of patients with grade IV coma have cerebral oedema) and is the major cause of death (Hawker 1990). Prognosis is worse as the grade of encephalopathy increases.

Grades of encephalopathy
  0 Normal awareness
  I Mood change, confusion
 II Drowsiness, inappropriate behaviour
III Stuporose but rousable
 IV Unrousable to minimal stimuli or no response
     to noxious stimuli; decerebrate or decorticate
     posturing

Coagulopathy
This can cause bleeding at any site including the brain, lungs, and GI tract, as well as retroperitoneal haematoma. Liver synthesis of fibrinogen and factors V, VII, IX, and X is impaired. This is evidenced by prolongation of the prothrombin time which is used as a prognostic index (the greater the prolongation the worse the likely outcome).

Alterations in platelet count and function have also been associated with fulminant hepatic failure.

Renal failure
This occurs in approximately 50% of patients and up to 75% of those with grade IV coma. Hepato–renal syndrome refers to a functional renal failure probably due in the majority of cases to generalized intense renal vasoconstriction, the exact mechanism of which is unknown. The blood urea is often low and does not reflect renal function. This is because urea is produced by the liver and production is affected by hepatic failure.

Hypoglycaemia
This is probably related to failure of hepatic gluconeogenesis and can develop rapidly in the early stages.

Acid–base and electrolyte imbalance
Hypokalaemia due to inadequate potassium intake, vomiting, and secondary hyperaldosteronism occurs in the early stages of failure. It may later be replaced by hyperkalaemia if renal failure occurs. Hypomagnesaemia, hypophosphataemia, and hypocalcaemia can all develop and may exacerbate neurological complications.

Metabolic alkalosis may occur as a response to hypokalaemia and gastric acid loss through vomiting or aspiration. It can also be due to an inability to deal with amino acids in the urea cycle: i.e. removal of the amino radical ($-NH_2$) by conversion into ammonia which combines with carbon dioxide to form urea which is excreted renally.

Lactic acidosis is also possible.

Respiratory problems
The patient's airway may be compromised due to a decreased conscious level and the ventilatory response to hypoxia is decreased. Patients can develop pulmonary oedema which is thought to be related to alterations in membrane permeability and is associated with cerebral oedema (Levy *et al.* 1991). Furthermore, they develop intrapulmonary shunting leading to ventilation/perfusion mismatch and hypoxaemia. This is due to diffuse dilatation of the pulmonary vascular bed.

Cardiovascular problems

Hypotension due to vasodilatation and hypovolaemia can occur and arrhythmias related to electrolyte disturbances are common.

Sepsis

The patient is immunocompromised and bacteraemia and fungaemia are common. This is related to reduced reticuloendothelial clearance, impaired leucocyte function, and deficient complement activity.

Management

Due to the high-risk nature of some of the causes of fulminant hepatic failure, source isolation barrier nursing precautions should be followed when caring for these patients.

(1) Encephalopathy

- The absorption of nitrogen should be minimized by low protein intake. A high carbohydrate diet to prevent endogenous protein breakdown may also help.

- Magnesium sulphate enemas and oral lactulose should be given regularly to empty the bowel and therefore reduce reabsorption of protein.

- Sedation should be avoided unless absolutely essential (if necessary use chlormethiazole, diazepam, barbiturates, or short-acting anaesthetic agents).

- Reduce ICP (aim < 20 mmHg) and maintain cerebral perfusion pressure (aim > 50 mmHg) using hyperventilation and mannitol. If these measures prove ineffective, thiopentone may be administered (see Chapter 9). Hypotension, hypoxaemia, and hypercapnia should be avoided as these all cause cerebral vasodilatation and thereby increase ICP.

- Continuous assessment of the patient's mental state is important so that alterations in conscious level are quickly detected. Patients in the early stages of encephalopathy may be confused and difficult to manage. Considerable nursing time and expertise may be needed to avoid using sedation unless absolutely necessary and to prevent the patient coming to harm.

- Reduce sensory load by ensuring a quiet environment with minimal handling and providing reassuring and calming speech and touch (see Chapter 9).

(2) Coagulopathy

- Avoid procedures likely to cause bleeding (e.g. pro-

longed or excessive suction, vigorous mouth care, IM injections).

- Administer H_2-antagonists, with or without antacids, to maintain gastric pH > 4.

- Administer FFP, whole blood and platelets as prescribed. The aim is to keep the haemoglobin 8–12 g/dl and to treat bleeding problems.

- Vitamin K (IV) is usually prescribed on a daily basis for 2–3 days.

(3) Renal failure

Prevention is the most important aspect by:

(i) correction of precipitating causes (especially hypovolaemia),

(ii) use of mannitol to promote diuresis,

(iii) avoidance of nephrotoxic drugs and high-dose frusemide, and

(iv) use of dopamine to promote renal perfusion.

(4) Hypoglycaemia and nutrition

- Monitor blood glucose levels hourly. If blood glucose is < 3.5 mmol/l, 10–20% glucose should be infused, to maintain normoglycaemic blood levels.

- Nutrition should consist of low-protein, high carbohydrate feed.

- Some authorities suggest higher than normal levels of vitamins.

- Enteral feeding is possible providing the patient has not recently bled and the GI tract is functioning.

- There is little evidence at present that use of high-branched chain, low aromatic amino acid feed formulae improves the level of encephalopathy.

(5) Acid–base and electrolyte management

- Monitor potassium levels frequently and correct as necessary.

- Consider correction of metabolic alkalosis by correction of potassium deficiency.

- Respiratory alkalosis associated with hyperventilation and metabolic acidosis does not usually require treatment

(6) Respiratory problems

- The patient may need to be intubated in order to

protect the airway. If severe hypoxaemia, hypoventilation, or fitting occurs the patient should be ventilated. Airway pressures should be kept as low as possible and use of PEEP minimized, IPPV may be used to hyperventilate to reduce ICP in severe cerebral oedema.

(7) Cardiovascular problems

- Optimal intravascular volumes should be maintained using either CVP or PA pressure measurements

- Treat any causes of hypotension, such as hypovolaemia, arrhythmias and, if necessary, maintain the circulation with inotropes and/or vasopressors.

(8) Risk of infection

- Scrupulous attention should be paid to infection control measures. Infective complications occur in 20–36% of patients probably due to impaired neutrophil function, low serum complement concentrations, and decreased humoral response (Vargo and Rudy 1988).

- Regular cultures should be taken and appropriate antibiotics prescribed if organisms are found.
Note. There is a high incidence of fungal infections which need to be recognized and treated early.

Chronic hepatic failure

Chronic hepatic failure is characterized by jaundice, ascites, and encephalopathy. The two main causes of chronic failure are persistent hepatitis and cirrhosis. It is most likely that patients admitted with chronic hepatic failure to the ICU will either have suffered an acute decompensation most commonly due to GI bleeding or infected ascites. There may be an alternative cause for admission and the chronic liver failure is a secondary pathology.

Causes of cirrhosis of the liver

- Alcohol

- Infection

- Metabolic disorders (fibrocystic disease, Wilson's disease, glycogen storage disease)

- Drugs (methotrexate, methyldopa)

- Cholestasis

- Immunological factors

- Congestion (hepatic venous outflow obstruction)

Problems associated with chronic hepatic failure

Encephalopathy
The mechanism for development of encephalopathy is presumed to be similar to that of acute hepatic failure but development is slower and cerebral oedema is rare. It is usually known as portal-systemic encephalopathy in chronic failure due to the development of a portal-systemic collateral circulation (caused by portal hypertension). This allows bypassing of the liver by the blood supply of the GI tract and direct entry of toxins to the systemic circulation. The problem is often precipitated by an increased protein load in the gut, particularly following GI haemorrhage.

Ascites
This is not solely due to portal hypertension in cirrhosis. Sodium and water retention are increased by a decreased renal blood flow, and increased release of renin leading to secondary aldosteronism. The secondary aldosteronism is intensified by failure of the liver to metabolize aldosterone and vasopressin. Hypoalbuminaemia due to liver failure will lower colloid osmotic pressure and encourage the formation of oedema.

Oesophageal varices
The pathogenesis of oesophageal varices and their management are discussed on p. 279.

Management

Treatment of the precipitating factor is the most important aspect of management. Blood cultures and diagnostic paracentesis should be taken to rule out infected ascites and active measures should be carried out to prevent further GI bleeding.

(1) Encephalopathy
Management is as for acute hepatic failure (p. 284) except that cerebral oedema is less likely to be a problem.

(2) Ascites

- Sodium restriction of < 40 mmol/24h.

- Fluid restriction of 1500 ml/24h.

- Diuretic therapy.

- Paracentesis (drainage of ascites via an indwelling catheter) with or without infusion of salt-poor albumin.

(3) Oesophageal varices

Management is described in the section on acute GI bleeding (p. 279).

Jaundice

This word 'Jaundice' refers to the yellow appearance of the skin and mucous membranes seen with an increased bilirubin concentration in the body fluids. It is detectable when the serum bilirubin concentration exceeds 50 μmol/l.

Causes of jaundice are either haemolysis, obstruction, or hepatocellular.

(1) Haemolytic jaundice

An increased rate of destruction of red blood cells produces increased amounts of bilirubin which is excreted by the liver until its capacity is overwhelmed. The jaundice is usually mild, as the healthy liver can excrete up to six times the normal bilirubin load. Causes of haemolytic jaundice include drugs, erythrocyte abnormalities (e.g. sickle-cell disease) and malaria.

(2) Obstructive jaundice

Jaundice occurs due to obstruction of the excretion of bilirubin anywhere between the biliary canaliculi and the ampulla of Vater. Causes of large duct obstruction include gallstones in the common bile duct, biliary duct strictures, sclerosing cholangitis, carcinoma of the head of the pancreas, and other tumours. Causes of small duct obstruction include drugs and alcohol, which damage liver cells and bile ducts, primary diseases of the hepatocytes, such as viral hepatitis, severe bacterial infections, Hodgkin's disease, primary biliary cirrhosis, and pericholangitis associated with ulcerative colitis.

Jaundice can be prolonged and severe and the patient will pass pale or clay-coloured stools due to the lack of bilirubin entering the gut. Urine will be dark due to renal excretion of conjugated bilirubin.

(3) Hepatocellular jaundice

Jaundice results from the inability of the liver to transport bilirubin into the bile as a result of liver cell damage. Common causes are alcohol, drugs, and hepatitis B. Drugs, such as salicylates, oral contraceptives, and rifampicin, can interfere with bilirubin metabolism. The mechanisms are:

(i) displacement of bilirubin from protein binding in the blood (e.g. salicylates),

(ii) impairment of bilirubin uptake and transport (e.g. rifampicin),

(iii) blockage of excretion into the canaliculi (e.g. oral contraceptives).

Liver dysfunction

Critically ill patients may develop liver dysfunction as part of multiple organ failure. This can be either as a result of circulatory disturbance or as a reaction to one or more of the drugs used in treatment. Factors involved are numerous and may produce both hepatocellular damage and intrahepatic cholestasis. Decreased hepatic perfusion and hypoxia are a likely cause although cholestasis due to extrahepatic bile duct obstruction may also occur.

Management depends on the precipitating cause but is usually dependent on treating the underlying disease. If drugs are suspected as a cause then they are discontinued and an alternative used.

Liver transplantation

This procedure is necessary in patients who have severe acute liver failure, or chronic, irreversible and progressive liver disease which does not respond to alternative medical and surgical interventions.

Conditions in which liver transplant may be appropriate

- Biliary atresia
- Inborn errors of metabolism
- Chronic active cirrhosis
- Primary biliary cirrhosis
- Sclerosing cholangitis
- Primary hepatic malignancy
- Acute liver failure
- Subacute hepatic necrosis

Major contraindications are extrahepatic malignancy, severe sepsis, and active alcoholism.

Relative contraindications are portal vein thrombosis, severe cardiopulmonary or renal disease, age over 55 years, past multiple abdominal operations, psychological instability, and positive hepatitis B e-antigen.

Donors

The same criteria for approach to donation are required as for any other organ (see Chapter 9 and Hawker 1990).

Clinical criteria for cadaveric liver donors (from Hawker 1990)

- Age less than 55 years
- No hepatobiliary disease or severe liver trauma
- Acceptable liver function tests and coagulation profile
- Size and ABO compatibility with available recipient
- No extracerebral malignancy
- No active systemic or hepatic infection
- Negative HIV and hepatitis B serology
- Negative cytomegalovirus (CMV) serology

Transplantation

Orthotopic (replacement of the recipient's liver with that of the donor) transplantation is the usual method. Donor livers can be maintained for between 8 and 20 hours using a perfusion solution.

Blood loss can be high and transfusion requirements may range from 10–100 units. Fresh frozen plasma (FFP) and platelets are also required in large quantities.

Post-operative management

(1) Haemodynamic problems

- Monitoring and management of intravascular volume is vital and patients have pulmonary artery catheters *in situ* to allow assessment of fluid status as well as cardiac output. Sub-optimal circulating volumes are corrected using blood, colloid, and crystalloid as appropriate.

- Hypotension not related to low intravascular volume is corrected using inotropes. The specific inotrope will depend on peripheral vascular resistance and cardiac output (see Chapter 5).

- Hypertension occasionally occurs and must be controlled to protect the integrity of the vascular anastomoses. Treatment is usually related to the underlying cause, such as inadequate sedation or continuing cerebral oedema, in patients with previous acute hepatic failure. Occasionally, antihypertensive agents are required.

- Hypothermia is common due to the length of operation and the use of bypass. Gradual warming is instituted using foil blankets.

(2) Respiratory problems

The majority of patients are ventilated post-operatively to allow optimal respiratory support. PEEP at moderate levels is used to minimize basal atelectasis. Active chest physiotherapy is then required to prevent further problems. Pleural effusions are common and the majority resolve spontaneously or with diuretic therapy. Development of ARDS is associated with intra-abdominal sepsis, allograft rejection, and hepatic artery thrombosis.

(3) Metabolic disturbances

- Hypokalaemia can be severe due to absorption of potassium into the reperfused hepatocytes. Potassium supplements are given routinely unless serum levels are high.

- Hyperglycaemia may require insulin to maintain normal blood glucose levels.

- Metabolic alkalosis is probably related to the large amounts of citrate in transfused blood as well as hypokalaemia.

(4) Bleeding and coagulopathy

Continuous bleeding is usually surgical in origin and may necessitate a return to theatre. Coagulopathy can usually be controlled using FFP and platelet infusions.

(5) Immunosuppression

The exact programme and timing of immunosuppression varies but the primary agents used are prednisolone, azathioprine, and cyclosporin. Newer agents, such as polyclonal and monoclonal antilymphocyte globulin preparations, are used in some centres as initial immunosuppression which is then followed by cyclosporin long term. Cyclosporin is a highly effective immunosuppressant but its use carries the risk of a number of side-effects (e.g. nephrotoxicity), some of which can be severe.

(6) Infection

The patient will be susceptible to infection due to his/her

chronic ill health state or acute liver failure pre-operatively. This will then be compounded by the introduction of immunosuppressive drugs.

Bacterial infections occur frequently post-operatively and are treated with the appropriate antibiotics. Fungal infections (*Candida albicans* and *Aspergillus* most commonly) are treated with amphotericin B. Viral infections can also occur and require acyclovir.

Patients should be nursed in side-rooms with protective isolation. Scrupulous care is required for all clean and aseptic procedures.

(7) Renal dysfunction

This occurs in up to two-thirds of transplant patients post-operatively. It may result from continued bleeding and poor renal perfusion, sepsis, and poor allograft function. The drugs used for immunosuppression and to treat infection can be highly nephrotoxic. Management consists of maintaining intravascular volume and infusing dopamine at 2–5 µg/kg/min to support renal perfusion. The aim is to produce 0.5 ml/kg/h urine.

(8) Neurological dysfunction

Patients who have undergone transplant for acute liver failure will require continual ICP monitoring throughout the post-operative period. Neurological assessment is regularly carried out to monitor status in all liver transplant patients. Complications, such as fitting, can occur which are usually associated with cyclosporin neurotoxicity or hypomagnesaemia. Other neurological problems may occur as a result of intracerebral haemorrhage, hepatic or metabolic encephalopathy, and opportunistic infection.

(9) Pain

An opiate, such as morphine, is usually given as an infusion or intravenous bolus. Some centres also use a sedative, such as diazepam, to reduce patient awareness of discomfort and facilitate ventilation.

(10) Psychological problems

There are numerous psychological problems associated with adjusting to transplantation. The nearness of death will have caused fear and anxiety and a necessity to confront their own mortality. The adjustment to accepting the presence of another person's organ within their own body may also take considerable support and rationalization. Patients require trained counselling and support which must be an important part of any transplant programme.

(11) Nutritional deficit

Patients are often severely malnourished pre-operatively due to prolonged liver disease. Energy expenditure is significantly raised by the stresses associated with transplantation and patients are hypercatabolic in the post-operative phase. Nutrition is therefore urgently required and can be given either enterally or parenterally.

(12) Liver dysfunction

Liver function usually returns to normal soon after transplantation but up to two-thirds of patients suffer some degree of liver dysfunction. In the extreme situation the graft fails to function immediately due to ischaemic injury and there is total hepatic failure. Re-transplantation is the only possible course although prognosis is poor. There may be some lesser degree of failure related to technical complications, such as bleeding, and these may be repaired on return to theatre. Rejection is the commonest cause of graft dysfunction and occurs to some extent in most patients usually 2–3 weeks later. Rejection can occur slowly and progressively or acutely. Treatment consists of increasing levels of steroids and use of antilymphocyte globulin or monoclonal antilymphocyte antibody (OKT3). Survival following liver transplant is now around 80% at 1 year and 60% at 5 years. It is an accepted form of treatment both in end-stage liver disease and acute liver failure.

Acute pancreatitis

This condition occurs in about one in ten thousand people and is largely associated with alcohol abuse or gallbladder disease (75% of cases).

The exact aetiology of the disease is unknown but its pathogenesis involves the activation of pancreatic enzymes within the pancreas rather than in the duodenum (see p. 273). This leads to autodigestion and an acute inflammatory response. It is thought that in the case of alcohol this is caused by irritation and protein precipitation which obstructs the acinar ductules and traps enzymes within the pancreas. The irritant factor in gallbladder disease is thought to be bile which due to biliary tract abnormalities may reflux back and irritate the pancreas. Blockage of the pancreatic duct by gallstones may also precipitate pancreatitis. Many of the multi-system problems associated with pancreatitis (respiratory complications, cardiac abnormalities, impaired renal function, disseminated intravascular coagulation, etc.) are related to the transfer of enzymes and products of pancreatic tissue destruction to the circulation. This is thought to happen via the lymphatic drainage of the pancreas.

Signs and symptoms of acute pancreatitis

- Acute epigastric and peri-umbilical pain

- Nausea and vomiting

- Abdominal distension associated with a small bowel ileus or pseudocyst in severe disease

- Low grade pyrexia, occasionally hypothermia

- Shock: ↑ pulse, ↓ BP, etc.

- Retroperitoneal haemorrhage showing as either:
  - Grey-Turner sign — grey discoloration (bruising) over the flanks, or
  - Cullen's sign — bruising in and round the umbilicus

Diagnosis of pancreatitis is difficult and is usually based on a number of differential diagnoses as well as the interpretation of laboratory data.

Laboratory data associated with acute pancreatitis

- Serum amylase is high (usually > 1000 iu/l)

- Serum lipase is high in 75% of cases

- Total calcium levels are decreased (this may be due to hypoalbuminaemia or extravascular precipitation)

- Ionized calcium levels may also decrease due to intraperitoneal combination with free fatty acids

- Hyperglycaemia is common (this is related to either hyperglucagonaemia or, more commonly, insulin deficiency)

- Hyperbilirubinaemia

- Raised transaminase and alkaline phosphatase levels

- Hypoalbuminaemia

Strategies for management

(1) Correction of hypovolaemia and fluid volume imbalances

The release of vasoactive substances following auto-digestion of pancreatic tissue causes alterations in permeability of the capillary membrane. This leads to large losses of fluid into the extravascular space and particularly into the peritoneal space. Fluid losses lead to a low circulating blood volume with reactive constriction of the splanchnic (abdominal organ) blood vessels resulting in poor perfusion of the pancreas, further damage to pancreatic tissue and a continuing downward spiral in the patient's condition.

Further fluid losses related to nasogastric aspiration and vomiting must also be taken into account.

- Adequate volume loading is essential in the management of these patients and should be given under CVP or PA pressure monitoring. The fluid of choice will depend on the clinical situation and can be crystalloid or colloid, although blood may be used in haemorrhagic pancreatitis if the haemoglobin is low.

- Crystalloid fluid replacement should continue at a rate suitable for the patient's normal fluid requirements. The aim is to preserve organ perfusion and maintain renal function with a urine output > 0.5 ml/kg/h.

(2) Correction of electrolyte imbalances

Imbalance in calcium, magnesium, phosphate, and potassium are also related to alterations in capillary permeability, nasogastric losses, vomiting, and diarrhoea. Calcium levels are reduced as a result of intraperitoneal saponification (combination to form a soap-like compound) with free fatty acids released during fat necrosis. Alcohol abusers may also suffer from diet-related decreases in these levels.

- Levels should be monitored and corrected as required.

- The patient should also be observed for signs of hypocalcaemia. (Chvostek's sign: twitching of the lip and cheek in response to tapping of the side of the face over the facial nerve in the parotid gland or Trouseau's sign: carpopedal spasm with wrist and metacarpophalangeal joints flexed and interphalangeal joints extended when a blood pressure cuff placed on the same arm is inflated to just above systolic pressure. (The response should occur within 2 minutes).

- Continuous ECG monitoring is useful for signs of, and arrhythmias associated with, hypokalaemia and hypomagnesaemia. Regular measurements of electrolytes from arterial blood samples should be taken to monitor potassium levels.

(3) Haemodynamic disturbances

These are related to the acute inflammatory process as

well as hypovolaemia, hypocalcaemia, hypokalaemia, and possible myocardial depressant factors.

- There is a need for continuous monitoring of blood pressure, ECG, CVP or PA, and cardiac output if myocardial depression is suspected.

- Ideally, the patient should be catheterized in order to monitor urine output.

- Intravascular volume should be optimized and electrolyte levels corrected. If cardiac output remains low, inotropes will be required or vasopressors if in high output shock.

(4) Compromised respiratory function

Hyperventilation may occur as a response to the acute pain associated with pancreatitis.

- Pain relief is important in limiting this response.

Respiratory complications occur in 30–50% of patients and up to 70% are hypoxaemic. There are a number of possible contributory factors:

(i) Increased likelihood of developing ARDS (see Chapter 3). Non-cardiogenic pulmonary oedema occurs in 10–30% of patients.

(ii) Pleural effusions may form from the passage of pancreatic exudate via lymph channels into the chest, or extravasation of exudate through the diaphragm.

(iii) Pseudocysts or abscesses may form a fistula into the chest cavity.

(iv) Atelectasis may occur as a result of hypoventilation due to pain-related splinting of the abdominal wall.

- Management consists of supporting respiratory function with appropriate oxygen therapy and ventilation when necessary.

- Monitoring should include pulse oximetry and frequent arterial blood gases.

(5) Pain

The epigastric and peri-umbilical pain in acute pancreatitis is caused by extravasation of inflammatory exudate and enzymes into the retroperitoneum. This may lead to digestion of the fat in the pancreatic bed and surrounding tissue. Another cause may be distension of pancreatic ducts and obstruction of the ampulla of Vater or swelling of the head of the pancreas producing duodenal obstruction.

- Analgesia is essential; usually by opiate infusions. Pethidine is the opiate of choice and morphine should be avoided due to its increased ability to cause spasm of the sphincter of Oddi.

- Localized analgesia, such as nerve blocks or ganglion blocks, may be useful although epidurals should be used with caution.

- Other methods of pain relief, such as warmth, positioning, and relaxation, may have a minimizing effect but are unlikely to take the pain away completely.

- Continuous nasogastric aspiration and nil by mouth should be instituted in order to limit pancreatic stimulus to release enzymes.

(6) Hyperglycaemia

This can occur secondary to hyperglucagonaemia and insulin deficiency.

- Insulin infusion titrated to blood glucose levels should be used.

(7) Nutrition

Oro- or naso-gastric nutrition is contraindicated in acute pancreatitis because of the stimulant effect food may have on the pancreas. However, the duodenal route can be used for feeding without pancreatic stimulation and some centres have infused elemental feed intragastrically without apparent harm (Schlichtig and Ayres 1988). The feed should be high in carbohydrate and low in fat to minimize pancreatic secretion. Patients with small bowel obstruction should not receive enteral feed.

- In general, patients with acute pancreatitis requiring intensive care are likely to need parenteral nutrition. This should be started as soon as possible particularly in view of the potentially poor nutritional state of alcohol abusers.

(8) Surgery or drainage of abcesses/necrosis

Surgical debridement or radiologically-guided drainage is occasionally indicated, particularly if the general state of the patient deteriorates.

Endoscopy

Oesophagogastroduodenoscopy is the examination of the upper GI tract using a flexible fibreoptic instrument which is passed into the mouth and down the oesophagus to allow direct visualization of the mucosal surface. It is also possible to carry out procedures, such as sclerosis of varices, and to take biopsies of lesions, such as ulcers, via an instrument channel within the scope.

The critically ill patient is most likely to require endoscopy for investigation of GI haemorrhage, epigastric pain, and possibly to carry out haemostasis of bleeding varices or ulcers.

Indications for endoscopy

- Acute gastrointestinal haemorrhage (identification of site and haemostasis)
- Biopsy of lesions such as tumours and ulcers
- Placement of duodenal and jejunal feeding tubes
- Sclerosis of oesophageal varices
- Removal of ingested foreign objects
- Studies of biliary and pancreatic ducts

Preparation of the patient for endoscopy

The patient should be adequately resuscitated from any bleeding prior to endoscopy. In addition, an explanation of the procedure, reasons for it, and likely sensations should be given. Routine gastric lavage prior to the procedure is unnecessary. Increased levels of sedation may be required during the procedure. Endoscopy can cause hypoxaemia in any patient with cardiorespiratory compromise and monitoring of ECG, arterial blood pressure and oxygen saturation should continue throughout the procedure. If necessary, the inspired oxygen concentration may have to be increased.

Following the procedure, the patient should be observed for signs of further bleeding and/or perforation. (See Table 10.2 for haemostasis.)

Delivery of nutritional support

Most ICU patients are unable to meet their own nutritional requirements in the normal way. They must therefore be assessed and the most appropriate type of support decided on the basis of that assessment.

Assessment of the patient's nutritional status and requirements

This is difficult in the critically ill patient; problems are caused not only by the alteration in metabolic function associated particularly with sepsis and trauma, but also

Table 10.2 Haemostasis of bleeding points

1. *Chemical methods*	2. *Thermal methods*
Injection of sclerosants, such as adrenaline and alcohol, directly into the base of an ulcer	Electrocoagulation: monopolar and bipolar diathermy
	Heater probe
Use and efficacy	Laser photocoagulation
Can control arterial bleeding in over 90% of cases	*Use and efficacy*
	Haemostasis of most vessels apart from brisk arterial bleeding.
	Can control arterial bleeding from peptic ulcers
	Effective in 80–90% of ulcer bleeds. Can reduce the incidence of arterial rebleeding from ulcers

with other stressors (for details see Chapter 2). Most of the methods for assessing nutritional status and requirement were produced for a relatively well population and may not apply to the critically ill. Suggested methods are described below with details of their application in intensive care.

(1) Anthropometry

Daily weight is not a reliable measure of nutritional status in the critically ill. The fluid balance fluctuations associated with the illness or therapy may produce considerable changes in weight which are unrelated to nutrition. Weight loss itself also gives little indication of the composition of that loss. Thus, a 2 kg weight loss in starvation may have a ratio of fat to protein of 2:1, but in the hypercatabolic patient the ratio may be 1:4 (Berger and Adams 1989) with much graver consequences.

Measurement of skinfold thickness and midarm muscle circumference have also been used to gauge muscle mass (for details of the technique see Goodinson 1987) but this too has problems in the critically ill patient. Oedema may seriously alter the measurement, changes develop slowly, and there is considerable inter-operator variation.

Measurements of hand-grip muscle strength by dynamometry and respiratory muscle strength using maximal inspiratory force have been used but are affected by other variables such as patient co-operation, and respiratory muscle fatigue.

(2) Assessment of nitrogen balance

Nitrogen balance, as the end-product of amino acid break-down can provide an insight into whether protein (and therefore lean body mass) is being gained or lost. Intake of nitrogen (usually in the form of protein) is compared to nitrogen losses as urinary urea in a 24-hour urine collection. The difference between the two is termed the nitrogen balance and may be neutral or negative but is rarely positive in the critically ill (Schlichtig and Ayres 1988).

(ii) movement of proteins into extravascular spaces through leaky capillary membranes,

(iii) dilution by infusion of artificial colloids,

(iv) decreased liver production due to liver dysfunction associated with the disease state.

Thus, despite the absence of significant malnutrition, low albumin levels may be found.

Calculation of nitrogen balance

Nitrogen balance ($=$ intake $-$ loss/24 h)

$$\text{Intake (g/24 h)} = \frac{\text{Protein}}{6.25} \text{ (g/24 h)}$$

Loss (g/24 h) = Urinary urea (mmol/l) $\times$ Urinary volume/24 h (l) $\times$ 0.028

Estimation of faecal losses of 4 g/day of nitrogen has been suggested. However, in the parenterally fed patient with minimal or absent stools this will overestimate the losses and vice versa in the patient with diarrhoea. It must therefore be added to the nitrogen balance calculation with caution.

The usefulness of nitrogen balance in assessing the patient's nutritional state is debatable. Assumptions are made that a steady state exists within the body pool of nitrogen but this may not be the case. For instance, a rising blood urea in acute renal failure will affect the amount of urinary urea lost giving a falsely low level of nitrogen loss. Correct interpretation of nitrogen balance is therefore important and assessment of the patient's overall nutritional status must be made in order to evaluate the results correctly.

(3) Levels of serum proteins as nutritional indicators

Most investigators have concluded that levels of serum proteins do not accurately assess whole body nutritional status in individual patients (Schlichtig and Ayres 1988). There are a number of other factors involved in the critically ill patient which alter the levels of these proteins without affecting nutritional status. The most commonly used indicator has been albumin, however albumin levels are frequently low in the critically ill due to:

(i) fluid shifts producing comparative dilution,

Plasma proteins used to assess nutritional state

Serum albumin
May fall precipitately in the critically ill without significant nutritional deficit. It rises slowly in repletion.

Serum transferrin
Can also be raised in iron deficiency. It frequently underestimates nutritional status in the critically ill. It rises earlier than albumin in repletion.

---

(4) Indirect calorimetry

This may be the only clinical method currently available that can provide a reasonably accurate assessment of the individual patient's energy requirements. It is a technique whereby the patient's energy expenditure is calculated from the inspired and expired gases (i.e. the amount of oxygen consumed and the amount of carbon dioxide produced by the patient). These gases are consumed and produced during the oxidation of food substances and the amount of oxygen and carbon dioxide can be directly related to the amount of food oxidized to produce energy.

$C_6H_{12}O_6 + 6O_2 = 6H_2O + 6CO_2 + Energy(kcal)$
(carbohydrate)

It requires a metabolic monitor, such as the Datex Deltatrac, or a ventilator that incorporates metabolic monitoring such as the Engström Erica or Elvira ventilators. It is also possible to use the technique of mass spectrometry (different constituents of a gas are detected by passing them through an electron beam which ionizes them, and then a magnetic field which separates the ionized molecules by their mass and electric charge), however, this is a very expensive alternative and is rarely available clinically.

The advantages of indirect calorimetry for assessment of energy expenditure are that:

(i) it is accurate for the individual patient (as opposed to formulae and tables which are accurate for a population of patients),

(ii) if continuous measurements are performed, changes in metabolic rate (for instance, as a result of activity or drugs) are measured (Weissman et al. 1989),

(iii) it gives an immediate answer to the patient's energy requirements rather than waiting for laboratory analysis, etc.

Other information may be gained from the use of indirect calorimetry such as an indirect measure of the work of breathing. If the patient is being weaned from the ventilator and support is decreased, providing no other changes in the patient's condition are occurring, then the increase in oxygen consumption will reflect the increased work required from the patient to compensate for the decrease in ventilatory support.

The disadvantages of indirect calorimetry for assessment of energy expenditure are that:

(i) its accuracy decreases with increasing inspired oxygen concentrations; an error $> 5\%$ exists with $F_iO_2 > 0.6$. It is therefore more inaccurate in the critically ill patients who are least able to tolerate either the effects of over- or underfeeding,

(ii) the assumption that steady state conditions exist may not always apply. In particular, body carbon dioxide pools are likely to increase and decrease if there are pH imbalances and this may produce an inaccurate reading,

(iii) if the patient is on haemofiltration, there may be carbon dioxide loss across the filter membrane in solution in the ultrafiltrate and as bicarbonate. This results in underestimation of carbon dioxide production by the indirect calorimeter and therefore underestimation of energy expenditure,

(iv) hypoventilation and hyperventilation will also affect the measurement of expired gases as carbon dioxide accumulates or is blown off. This results in over- or underestimation of energy expenditure,

(v) a major disadvantage of this method is the cost of the equipment which may make its routine use prohibitive.

If used correctly, indirect calorimetry is the most accurate way of assessing the individual critically ill patient's energy needs (Weissman et al. 1986; Van Lanschot et al. 1986; Carlsson et al. 1984).

Markers of gut function

A number of factors are used in assessing the function of the gut but some are more useful than others and all should be assessed before a decision is made.

(1) Presence or absence of bowel sounds

These are frequently used as an absolute indicator of gut function but their presence or absence should be interpreted with caution. Bowel sounds are produced by the disruption of the gas–fluid interface of the intestinal and gastric lumen by peristaltic waves. The largest areas of gas-fluid interface are in the stomach and the colon — the two areas of the bowel most sensitive to loss of function. In some circumstances, gastric and colonic function may be affected but small bowel function may continue or return more quickly following an insult. Bowel sounds may thus be absent although only parts of the gut are non-functioning. As the small bowel is the major site for absorption of nutrients it may still be possible to feed the patient enterally using a nasoduodenal tube or jejunostomy tube placed directly into the small bowel. Bowel sounds should therefore be interpreted in context with other indicators of bowel function such as pain, distension, vomiting, gastric aspirate, and diarrhoea.

Indications for parenteral nutrition
1. GI tract obstruction (adhesions, hernia, carcinoma of the oesophagus or colon, intussusception, volvulus, and diverticular disease)
2. Prolonged paralytic ileus (post-surgery, peritonitis, post-spinal injury)
3. Enterocutaneous fistulae
4. Malabsorption and short-bowel syndromes
5. Inflammatory intestinal disease (some patients with Crohn's disease, or ulcerative colitis)
6. Pancreatitis and cholecystitis

Table 10.3 Factors involved in deciding the mode of nutritional support

Gut function	Oral/oesophageal route	Mastication and swallowing	Patient ability
Gut is fully functioning	Oral/oesophageal route is patent	Patient is able to masticate and swallow	Patient can eat a normal diet
Gut is functioning although tolerance of certain foods may be affected	Oral/oesophageal route is patent	Patient may have difficulty with mastication but can swallow	Patient can eat a modified diet
Gut is functioning although tolerance of certain foods may be affected	Oral/oesophageal route may have some degree of restriction or damage so that whole foods are not tolerated	Patient may have difficulty with mastication but can swallow	Patient can take nourishing fluids only
Gut is functioning although tolerance of certain foods may be affected or parts of the gut, such as the stomach, may not function	Oral/oesophageal route may be restricted or damaged or gastric function may be absent	Patient has difficulty masticating or swallowing	Patient requires enteral feed via a nasogastric/duodenal tube or gastrostomy/jejunostomy tube
Gut is *not* functioning or requires rest from stimulation			Patient requires parenteral nutrition

(2) High volumes of nasogastric aspirate

There is no definitive level at which the amount of aspirate clearly indicates loss of gut function. Volumes used as a cut-off point reflect the amount of feed being given and the likely amount of gastric secretions. Gastric secretions are approximately 2 litres per day in the healthy person but can be increased by stimulation, such as the presence of a nasogastric tube (Guyton 1985, p.678). The amount of aspirate used in some ICUs as a cut-off point for continuing or commencing enteral feed is less than 200 ml after a 4-hour period without aspiration (McClave *et al.* 1992). (Again, this must be considered in context with other factors.)

(3) Vomiting/regurgitation of feed

This is a dangerous situation if the patient is unable to protect his/her airway as the risk of aspiration is considerable. Endotracheal intubation should not be considered totally protective as aspiration of feed is not uncommon in intubated patients despite fully inflated cuffs. Enteral feeding should always be stopped and the patient assessed for other signs of intolerance such as abdominal distension, pain, and diarrhoea. If there is no evidence of an abdominal disorder then drugs that increase gastric motility and emptying, such as metoclopramide, may be given to improve gastric emptying, and feed re-started cautiously at a low rate.

Assessment of nasogastric aspirate or vomit.
The colour, amount, pH, and consistency of nasogastric aspirate or vomit can provide useful information. It should be observed and recorded. Gastric or duodenal bleeding will either appear as a normal red colour if it has spent little time in the stomach itself or will be altered to the so-called 'coffee grounds' (brownish-black particles) if it remains in the stomach for any length of time. Normal biliary and gastric secretions appear green. Bile that has had little time in the stomach, and is therefore unaltered, is yellow.

(4) Diarrhoea

Between 25% and 40% of critically ill patients develop diarrhoea (Dobb, 1986; Belknap Mickschl *et al.* 1990). Many of the causes are not simply related to intolerance of enteral feed although this may aggravate the situation. The patient should be investigated and treated for likely causes prior to discontinuing enteral feeding for diarrhoea. For further details see care of the enterally fed patient (p. 304).

Assessment of bowel movements
There is a considerable variation in the normal frequency of bowel movements between individuals and the patient's history should be referred to before deciding whether there is a problem with constipation or diarrhoea. Information can be obtained from a thorough assessment of the patient's stools and a record of frequency, consistency, and texture should be recorded in the nursing record (see Table 10.4).

Factors that have been implicated in diarrhoea include

- Lactose intolerance (Berger and Adams 1989)

- Antibiotic therapy (Schlichtig and Ayres 1989)

- Other drug therapy such as digoxin (Koruda *et al.* 1987)

- Zinc deficiency (Schlichtig and Ayres 1989)

- Feed osmolality (Keohane *et al.* 1984)

- Low serum albumin levels (Brinson and Pitts *et al.* 1989)

- Bacterial contamination of feeds

- Infection such as *Clostridium difficile*

- Fat malabsorption

Table 10.4   Types of diarrhoea

Frequency	Colour	Texture	Cause
Occasional	Black	Tarry	Old bleeding: melaena
Frequent, depending on the rate of bleeding	Dark red	Viscous but liquid	Fresh bleeding: melaena
Constant	Bright red	Liquid	Rectal bleeding, haemorrhoids
Frequent	Green/ khaki	Soft stool or liquid	Infective: *Clostridium difficile*, Salmonella
Frequent	Pale brown/ clay coloured	Loose, bulky, may float or be frothy	Malabsorption, obstruction of the biliary duct
Frequent	Bloody	Loose with obvious blood	Ischaemic or infarcted bowel
Frequent	Flecks of blood and mucus	Loose with mucus	Ulcerative colitis, Crohn's disease

(5) Pain

Acute abdominal pain is frequently associated with gut dysfunction and should always be treated seriously. It is an important sign in ileus, peritonitis, obstruction etc and if accompanied by other signs such as abdominal distension, and vomiting, feed should be stopped immediately and medical staff informed.

Conditions producing abdominal pain/tenderness
(Perforated) peptic ulcer
Dissecting or ruptured aneurysm
Pancreatitis
Ruptured ectopic pregnancy
Cholecystitis
Acute renal infections
Crohn's disease
Pelvic inflammatory disease
Ulcerative colitis
Hepatitis
Diverticulitis
Occlusion of mesenteric artery
Appendicitis
Ileus
Bowel obstruction
Peritonitis

Rare but recognized extra-abdominal causes
Myocardial disease
Respiratory disease
Diabetic or thyroid crisis
Spinal cord lesion
Acute intermittent porphyria
Pneumonia
Lead poisoning
Endometriosis
Sickle-cell disease
Trauma to spleen and kidney

(6) Distension

The abdomen may be distended for a number of reasons and care should be taken in assessing this. However, when associated with pain, vomiting, or diarrhoea it should be taken as a sign of gut dysfunction, any enteral feeding should be discontinued and senior medical staff informed.

Priorities of care

There are two major categories in priorities of care:

1. Prevention of gastrointestinal problems associated with critical illness

2. Maintenance of nutritional intake

Causes of abdominal distension

- Intestinal obstruction

- Malabsorption

- Peritonitis

- Abdominal haemorrhage (see Chapter 11)

- Ascites

- Gas

- Paralytic ileus

- Gut wall oedema

Prevention of gastrointestinal problems

(1) Aspiration of stomach contents

The incidence of aspiration in critically ill patients has been quoted as high as 38% (Winterbauer et al. 1981). It is a potentially lethal complication leading to pneumonia or ARDS, and it is important to avoid any potentiating circumstances.

Increased risk of aspiration is associated with:

- ↓ level of consciousness

- Diminished or absent cough or gag reflexes

- Incompetent oesophageal sphincters

- Delayed gastric emptying (such as that associated with diabetes or malnutrition)

- Paralytic ileus

- Displacement of enteral feeding tube either into the oesophagus or into the pharynx itself (can be associated with vigorous coughing or retching)

It is should always be borne in mind that even intubated patients or those with tracheostomies can aspirate gastric contents in spite of an inflated cuff.

Strategies to avoid aspiration include:

- Use of a small-bore feeding tube. Aspiration is still possible but the oesophageal sphincter is less compromised by the smaller diameter and reflux is less likely (Elpern et al. 1987).

- Monitor gastric residual volumes (the amount of gastric aspirate in the stomach) 4-hourly when feeding

is being established and 8-hourly once it is established (note: some individual ICU feeding protocols may differ).

- Check gastric residual volumes prior to any vigorous head-down procedures such as postural drainage.

- Nurse the patient in a 30–40 degree upright position to reduce the risk of reflux, providing cardiovascular status allows.

- Monitor the tube position externally by marking the entry site with tape or ink on the tube and checking that this has not migrated outwards.

- Monitor the tube position internally by performing gastric aspiration and confirming a satisfactory position on chest X-ray.

Use of duodenal/jejunal feeding tubes may reduce the risk of aspiration but must still be monitored closely to ensure they are correctly placed.

(2) Nosocomial pneumonia

Bacterial transfer from the stomach to the oropharynx and trachea is recognized as a major factor in the development of nosocomial pneumonia in ventilated patients. Increased growth of organisms in the stomach is associated with an increase in gastric pH (Pingleton 1991). A rise in gastric pH can be due to the use of H_2-receptor antagonists, antacids, and enteral feeding. In a small study, Lee et al. (1990) found an incidence of 54% of nosocomial pneumonia in ventilated patients who were continuously enterally fed.

The use of selective decontamination of the digestive tract (SDD) has been successful in reducing the incidence of nosocomial pneumonia in certain ICU populations (Meijer et al. 1990). In particular, the multiple trauma patient, patients with > 5 day stays in ICU and surgical ICU patients (Van Dalen 1991). However, it has not made any difference to length of stay in ICU nor to mortality in all but a small subgroup of patients (multiple trauma patients).

Strategies to reduce the incidence of nosocomial pneumonia include:

- Elimination/reduction of the factors contributing to the incidence of aspiration (see above).

- Avoidance of exogenous bacterial contamination (see Chapter 2).

- Avoidance of use of antacids or H_2-antagonists if possible (see p. 282).

- In certain groups of patients (see above), use of SDD may be appropriate.

- It may be appropriate to discontinue enteral feeding for a period (up to 8 hours) in each 24 hours to allow gastric pH to return to its bactericidal normal level.

(3) Stress ulceration and acute bleeds

This is discussed in the section on acute GI bleeding (p. 281).

Maintenance of nutritional intake

Nutritional support does not constitute part of first-line life-saving interventions but has an essential role in the treatment and recovery of the critically ill patient. Progressive weight loss adds to debility, and patient mortality and morbidity correlate closely with loss of body weight. Loss of greater than 30% of body weight is usually fatal (Apelgren and Wilmore 1983).

The goal of nutritional therapy in the acute phase of critical illness is to provide sufficient calories and protein to maintain body weight and reduce nitrogen loss. It is not usually possible to replenish body stores until the recovery phase of critical illness due to the levels of catabolic hormones associated with the stressed state.

Nutritional support is indicated in the first instance in:
Hypercatabolic patients: burns, multiple trauma, sepsis, and major operations
Patients with greater than 10% body weight loss

Nutritional support may be unnecessary in the first instance in:
Acute but quick resolving illness, e.g.
 – cardiac surgery on relatively healthy patients
 – some major surgery requiring short-term ICU intervention
 – some drug overdoses, etc.

Modes of nutrition

Provision of complete nutritional support can be accomplished in two ways: parenterally or enterally. Considerable debate exists as to the advantages and disadvantages of each method, but neither can be used exclusively in the ICU. The decision as to which method is best for the individual patient must be made on the basis of GI function, metabolic problems, and the knowledge of the potential risks and advantages of each route. One method may have to be substituted for the other as the patient's condition changes. Nevertheless, there are a number of good reasons for attempting to use enteral nutrition where possible.

- Advantages of enteral nutrition

(1) more physiological, using the normal route for absorption and subject to the checks and balances associated with the uptake of oral nutrition,

(2) cheaper (an important aspect in view of limited resources),

(3) does not require central venous access with the associated risks of insertion, infection, etc.,

(4) preservation of gut mucosal integrity,

(5) possible role in modifying the immune response to stress if administered in the early stages following trauma (Moore et al. 1989)

- Disadvantages of enteral nutrition

(1) an association with diarrhoea (41%, Dobb 1986). This can cause dehydration, electrolyte imbalance, skin excoriation, and discomfort as well as increasing nursing workload considerably.

(2) in many cases, patients who are enterally fed do not always receive the amount of feed prescribed; in some cases they may not receive even basic metabolic requirements (Petrosino et al. 1989; Keohane et al. 1984; Rapp et al. 1983). This appears to be related to functional problems (Adam 1990) associated with the technique including:

  (i) stopping feeds for an hour each time absorption is checked,

  (ii) keeping patients nil by mouth for excessive periods prior to procedures,

  (iii) poor systems for checking that the amount prescribed is actually delivered.

(3) possibly an increased risk of nosocomial pneumonia associated with continuous enteral feeding. The mechanism is thought to be related to the increase in gastric pH which allows bacterial colonization of the stomach and retrograde migration of the organisms via the oesophagus to the respiratory tract,

(4) not all patients will be capable of absorbing enteral feed.

It is possible to feed a high percentage of critically ill patients enterally but this requires a commitment to the method and a willingness to tackle associated problems.

Differences in metabolism between parenteral and enteral feeding

The assimilation of digested enteral feed occurs via the portal system and the liver. Parenteral feed passes directly into the circulation.

Amino acids, with the exception of branched chain amino acids, are extracted by the liver from the enteral route. Branched chain amino acids pass directly into the systemic circulation and are taken up primarily by muscle. However, in parenteral administration, all amino acids enter the systemic circulation although the same pattern of uptake is then followed.

Carbohydrate normally passes directly from the intestine to the liver but in parenteral feeding, it first passes into the circulation, which may have an effect on the levels of insulin-mediated uptake by the liver.

The metabolism of fat may also be affected by parenteral administration as hepatic steatosis (fatty liver) is a complication which is not seen in enterally fed patients. The mechanism is not known but is related to high levels of glucose feeding previously more common prior to the introduction of lipid solutions.

Complications associated with enteral feeding

(1) *Mechanical* due to:

- knotting of the tube,
- clogging or blockage of the tube due to;
  - (i) fragments of inadequately crushed tablets;
  - (ii) adherence of feed residue,
  - (iii) incompatibilities between feed and medication given (e.g. phenytoin),
- incorrect placement (usually in the bronchial tree),
- nasopharyngeal erosions and discomfort,
- sinusitis and otitis,
- oesophageal reflux and oesophagitis,
- tracheo-oesophageal fistula,
- ruptured oesophageal varices,
- pyloric or intestinal obstruction by gastrostomy or jejunostomy tubes

(2) *Nausea and vomiting*, due to:

- high infusion rates,
- large gastric volumes,
- fat or lactose intolerance,

- hyperosmolality,
- delayed gastric emptying.

(3) *Aspiration* (see priorities of care, p. 296)

(4) *Diarrhoea* (see markers of gut function, p. 294)
Diarrhoea has been particularly associated with enteral feeding in the critically ill. It does not necessarily indicate that the gut is unable to function and the patient should be assessed for precipitating factors which can be dealt with before feed is discontinued.

(5) *Abdominal distension/delayed gastric emptying*, due to:

- formula (associated with high density, high lipid content),
- medication (opiates),
- ileus,
- gastric atony,
- medical conditions such as pancreatitis, diabetes, malnutrition, or post-vagotomy

(6) *Cramping*, due to:

- lactose intolerance,
- high fat content formulae,
- malnutrition-related malabsorption

(7) *Constipation*: rarely occurs but can be related to:

- previous laxative abuse,
- long-term feeding regimens (particularly low-fibre formulae)

(8) *Hyperglycaemia*: this is associated with age, renal insufficiency, diabetes, steroid therapy, high caloric density formulae, sepsis

High rates of infusion, or inadequate endogenous insulin production and inadequate exogenous insulin supplementation can also induce hyperglycaemia. Prolonged hyperglycaemia may develop into hyperosmolar, hyperglycaemic non-ketotic dehydration, and coma (HHNK), although this is unlikely to develop in the ICU.

(9) *Hypercapnia*

High levels of carbohydrate in feeds can produce large amounts of CO_2 that require increased minute volumes and respiratory rate in order to be excreted. This may precipitate ventilatory failure in the patient with compromised respiratory function or in the weaning patient

(10) *Electrolyte and trace element abnormality*

- hypernatraemia: due to high sodium intake and dehydration

- hyponatraemia: due to overhydration and GI water loss (diarrhoea, drains, etc.) as well as insufficient sodium intake,

- hyperkalaemia: usually associated with renal insufficiency and metabolic acidosis,

- hypokalaemia: usually associated with diarrhoea, high-dose insulin, or diuretics, but can also be due to insufficient intake or replacement,

- hyperphosphataemia: usually caused by renal dysfunction in tube-fed patients,

- hypophosphataemia: occurs in the same way as hypokalaemia but may also be seen in malnourished patients along with low serum levels of zinc, copper, and magnesium.

Complications associated with parenteral feeding

(1) *Insertion of central venous catheter*

- pneumothorax

This is a recognized complication, the frequency of which is usually associated with the expertise of the operator. It is most likely to occur on the left as the left pleural dome is higher. There is an increased risk with mechanical ventilation, CPAP, obesity, and chest deformities.

- arterial puncture

Accidental puncture of the carotid artery often only requires digital pressure. However, significant bleeding can occur if the subclavian artery is punctured especially in patients with coagulation abnormalities, including platelet dysfunction. Accidental injury to the thoracic duct may produce chylothorax and, although rare, can occur with a left-sided approach.

- catheter misplacement

This is usually misdirection up into the neck from the subclavian approach and is more common with right-sided approaches because of the abrupt descent of the vena cava from the junction point of the right subclavian vein. Occasionally, the catheter may pass down the subclavian vein from a jugular approach. It is also possible to perforate a vessel and place the catheter into the neck tissue, mediastinum, or pericardium. This may result in a large haematoma, upper airway obstruction, hydro- or haemopneumothorax or pericardial tamponade.

(2) *The presence of a central venous catheter*

- infection

Bacterial and fungal infections occur in between 3% and 7% of patients. The infecting organism is commonly *Staphylococcus aureus* (a skin commensal). Most infections are thought to be due to poor insertion technique or failure to observe infection control protocols (see Chapter 2).

(3) *Metabolic*

- hyperglycaemia

Causes include persistent gluconeogenesis, blunted insulin response, decreased sensitivity to insulin, impaired peripheral utilization of glucose or phosphate, and chromium deficiency. Late development in a stable patient may signal a new infection or complication.

- hypoglycaemia

A sudden discontinuation of feed may induce hypoglycaemia, particularly if the patient is receiving insulin concurrently. The insulin should usually be discontinued or reduced prior to stopping the feed and, if this is not possible 10–20% glucose may be commenced. Blood glucose should be frequently monitored.

- hyperlipidaemia

Lipid clearance may be impaired in liver disease. Rapid infusion of lipid may also result in transient hyperlipidaemia.

- hepatic dysfunction

Abnormal liver function tests (LFTs) and fatty infiltration of the liver can develop in carbohydrate-based parenteral nutrition. It is treated by reducing the amount of calories or increasing the proportion of fat.

- acid–base disturbances

Hyperchloraemia can develop from amino acid metabolism but the resulting acidosis is usually mild and most amino acid preparations contain acetate as a buffer. Metabolic alkalosis can be seen with diuretic use, continuous nasogastric drainage, or corticosteroid therapy if concomitant replacement of sodium, potassium, and/or chloride ions is inadequate.

• electrolyte imbalance

Generally, sodium, potassium, chloride, and bicarbonate are monitored and corrected before problems occur. However, significant body deficiencies may not be reflected by plasma levels due to the effect of pH and serum albumin levels or hormonal influences, such as aldosterone or ADH, which are often altered in the critically ill. Occasionally, magnesium, calcium, and phosphate may become imbalanced. Hypophosphataemia is often seen when parenteral nutrition is first started following a period of semi-starvation due to poor prior intake, increased glucose phosphorylation, and augmented intracellular transport of phosphates. Plasma phosphate levels below 0.3–0.5 mmol/l can cause haemolysis, rhabdomyolysis, respiratory failure, and hamper weaning attempts. This may persist for several days after adequate replacement. Other effects include arrhythmias, decreased myocardial contractility, 2,3-DPG deficiency, seizures, diminished tissue sensitivity to insulin, abnormal calcium and magnesium metabolism, decreased sensitivity to vasoactive drugs, generalized tissue hypoxia, and ATP deficiency.

Other complications associated with parenteral feeding

(1) Precipitation of ventilatory failure and failure of weaning due to excessive carbohydrate administration (see p. 298).

(2) Hyperosmolar states with an excessive osmotic diuresis.

(3) Abnormal platelet function and hypercoagulability states.

(4) Anaemia after prolonged use of IV lipids.

Many of the potentially serious complications associated with parenteral feeding can be avoided or controlled by rigorous monitoring and observation of the patient. A high index of suspicion for complications should also be maintained.

Nutritional requirements (Tables 10.5–10.9)

It is only possible to give an approximate guide to the amount of nutrients required by the individual patient.

Table 10.5 Monitoring nutritional support

Variable	Enteral nutrition	Parenteral nutrition
Electrolytes	Daily	Daily
Serum magnesium, calcium, phosphate	Twice weekly	Twice weekly
Acid – base status	Daily	Daily
Gastric residuals (aspirate)	4-hourly when starting feeding; 8-hourly when established	As required by pathology
Abdominal function (distension, vomiting, nausea, diarrhoea, constipation)	Continuously	As required
Flow rate and volume infused	Hourly	Hourly
Blood glucose	8-hourly	1–2-hourly at first; when stable 4–6-hourly
Urinalysis for glucose and ketones	Daily	Daily
Urea and creatinine (plasma)	Daily	Daily
Urea and creatinine clearance (urinary)	24-h urine collection weekly	24-h urine collection weekly
Weight (if mobile or on a weigh bed)	For fluid status: daily For nutritional status: weekly	For fluid status: daily For nutritional status: weekly
Haematological and coagulation screens	Every 1–2 days	Every 1–2 days
Serum albumin, proteins, LFTs, trace elements. (e.g. copper, zinc, etc.)	Weekly	Weekly

Table 10.6   Daily nutritional requirement during enteral and parental nutrition

Nutrient	Amount per day	Influencing factors
Protein (nitrogen)	0.7–1.0 g/kg/day (0.15–0.3 g/kg/day)	Hypermetabolism can increase protein requirements to 1.5–2.0 g/kg/day.
Carbohydrate	Need will depend on the patient's energy requirements two-thirds of which are usually provided by carbohydrate, and one-third by fat	Patients with respiratory insufficiency or those who are weaning after long-term ventilation may not cope with the high carbon dioxide levels associated with high intakes of carbohydrate. Energy requirement can then be supplied as one-half fat and one-half carbohydrate
Fat	The minimum amount of fat necessary to prevent fatty acid deficiency is 1 litre of 10% fat emulsion (e.g. intralipid) weekly. However, usually the amount of fat providing calories is adjusted to between one-third and one-half of total calories required	

Note. This table represents only a rough guide, and each patient should be assessed individually.

Table 10.7   Electrolyte requirements during enteral or parenteral nutrition

Electrolyte	Typical daily requirement	Additional factors
Sodium	70–100 mmol/day	More may be needed with loop diuretic therapy or increased losses such as diarrhoea, fistulae, etc. Less may be required in oedema and hypernatraemia
Potassium	70–100 mmol/day	More may be needed during early repletion, post-obstructive diuresis, with loop diuretic therapy and increased GI tract losses. Less may be required in renal failure
Magnesium	7.5–10 mmol/day	As above
Calcium	5–10 mmol/day	
Phosphate	20–30 mmol/day	More may be needed during early repletion when there may be dramatic falls in serum phosphate (see p. 300). Less may be required in renal failure

Factors, such as age, weight, sex, severity of illness, use of catecholamines, body temperature, and injury, will all affect nutrient and energy needs. Electrolyte and fluid balance are also important factors in deciding the composition of feeds.

The exact requirements for trace elements in the critically ill have not been determined but deficiency can have significant effects on a number of metabolic processes. Most enteral feeds contain stated amounts of most essential trace elements. Multiple additives for parenteral feeding may be supplemented as necessary.

Insertion of nasogastric and duodenal feeding tubes

Enteral feeding tubes are normally inserted blind by appropriately experienced nursing staff. However, the presence of an endotracheal tube cuff increases the difficulty of entry to the oesophagus by pressing on its soft walls and decreasing its size. It may therefore be necessary to insert the tube under direct visualization of the pharynx. This is usually carried out by senior medical staff.

Table 10.8　Trace element requirements during enteral and parenteral nutrition

Trace element	Recommended daily dietary allowance (mg)	Effects of deficiency
Zinc	15	Impaired cellular immunity, poor wound healing, diarrhoea
Chromium	50–200	Insulin-resistant glucose intolerance, elevated serum lipids
Copper	2–3	Hypochromic microcytic anaemia, neutropenia
Iron	10 (men) 18 (women)	Anaemia
Iodine	150	
Selenium	50–200	Cardiomyopathy
Molybdenum	150–500	
Manganese	2.5–5	CNS dysfunction
Fluoride	1.5–4	

Table 10.9　Vitamin requirements during enteral or parenteral nutrition

Vitamin	Recommended daily dietary allowance
A (retinol)	5000 iu
B_1 (thiamine)	1.5 mg
B_2 (riboflavin)	1.7 mg
B_6 (pyridoxine)	2.2 mg
B_{12} (cyanocobalamine)	3 mg
C (ascorbic acid)	60 mg
D (cholecalciferol)	400 iu
E (δ and α tocopherol)	30 iu
Folic acid	400 mg
K (phytomenadione)	70–140 mg
Pantothenic acid	4–10 mg
Biotin	100–200 g

Note. The ET tube cuff does not provide complete protection against inadvertent tracheal intubation with the nasogastric tube.

The technique for insertion will differ slightly according to the type of tube but the principles are the same.

Principles of insertion.

- Explanation to the patient is required whether they are sedated or awake. This should include: the need for the tube, where the tube will be placed, likely sensations that the patient may feel and how long the tube is likely to be in place.

- Insertion is treated as a clean rather than aseptic technique with hand-washing prior to commencement and non-sterile gloves worn for protection of the operator.

- Measurement of the length of tube required to ensure placement within the stomach or duodenum. This can be fairly accurately measured using the formula shown in Fig. 10.6 (91% of tubes placed within the stomach, Hanson 1979).

- Placement in the duodenum requires insertion of at least 85 cm of feeding tube to allow direct passage or to allow a coil in the stomach which may then be passed into the duodenum. (Whatley *et al.* 1984)

- Lubrication is necessary to promote atraumatic insertion. Some tubes are pre-lubricated and require placing in water to activate the lubricant, others require lubricating jelly.

- The tube is inserted along the floor of the nose; this avoids the sensitive conchae and will provide a guide through the nasal cavity to the nasopharynx. If the patient is conscious they may assist insertion by swallowing once the tube is felt at the back of the nasopharynx.

- Once the tube has been inserted, the position should be checked. The following methods are suggested, although the only certain method of checking placement for fine-bore tubes is by X-ray.

  - Auscultation over the epigastric region during insufflation of 20 ml of air into the tube. Bubbling air should be clearly heard. *Note.* It is still possible to hear bubbling air if the tube is in the lung (Metheny *et al.* 1990)

  - Aspiration of gastric contents and testing of the pH of fluid withdrawn. Care must be taken with critically ill patients and those receiving H_2-antagonists or antacids, as the gastric pH may be as high as 5–6. It is also possible to withdraw tracheobronchial secretions in certain conditions with a low pH, e.g. pH 7.0–7.29 (malignancy) pH 6 (oesophageal rupture) and pH 5.5 (empyema).

- If the tube has a guidewire it should be removed once the tube is in the correct position. If there is difficulty withdrawing the guidewire, 1–2 ml water inserted into the tube may assist in lubricating its passage.

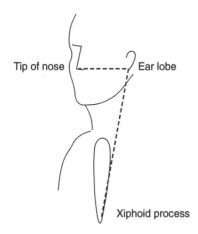

distance from Nose to Earlobe to Xiphoid = NEX
Formula for length of NG tube
$$= \frac{NEX - 50 \text{ cm}}{2} + 50$$

Fig. 10.6 Calculation of the length of the nasogastric tube.

Care of the enterally fed patient with a nasogastric tube

(1) Checking gastric residual volumes (aspirate)

- Residual volumes should be checked 4-hourly when feeding is first commenced and then 8-hourly once the feed has been running without large amounts of residual volumes. This may differ according to unit protocols.

- It is unnecessary to stop feeds for an hour in order to check residual volumes. The minimal time necessary to demonstrate reduced absorption has not yet been determined but it is probably less than 30 minutes even with reduced gastric motility.

- If all is well following a check for residual volumes, the rate of feed delivery should be increased to cover delivery of the feed missed prior to the check.

- It is possible to aspirate fine-bore nasogastric tubes of 1.5–2.0 mm internal diameter. A 50-ml syringe should be used which exerts less pressure and is therefore less likely to cause the tube to collapse.

- Gastric residual volumes of less than 200 ml have been found to be an acceptable cut-off limit in practice. There is little published research in this area and recommendations range from 'more than 1.5 times the previous hour's input of feed' (Koruda *et al.* 1987) to '< 200 ml.' (Armstrong *et al.* 1991, McClave *et al.* 1992).

- If residual volumes of 200 ml or more are obtained, the feed is either held at the current level if feeding is just building up, or reduced to a lower rate if the feed has been in progress for some time. Volumes are then checked again 4 hours later and the manoeuvre repeated. If this occurs three times in succession, or is accompanied by abdominal pain or distension, the medical staff should be informed and the feed stopped.

- Stimulants of intestinal motility may be used including metaclopramide and cisapride if the patient has no acute signs of feed intolerance but continues to have high volumes of gastric residuals.

- Feeding into the duodenum may still be possible and should be tried if there is no evidence of general gut dysfunction (pain, distension, vomiting). Care should be taken when duodenal feeding to assess gastric contents regularly by aspiration, either using a double lumen tube with a gastric port or by inserting a nasogastric tube.

(2) Prevention of tube obstruction

- Avoid giving crushed tablets down the enteral tube. Any drugs given in the nasogastric tube should be either soluble or in the form of linctus. A 20–30 ml flush of water should be given following administration of drugs; more may be required if crushed tablets are given.

- Some authorities recommend flushing the tube with at least 30 ml of water every 4 hours during continuous feeding (Kohn and Keithley 1989).

- Water is the most appropriate fluid for flushing tubes. (Metheny et al. 1988)

- Use a continuous delivery method of feeding (drying and encrustation between feeds may obstruct the tube).

- Use a polyurethane or PVC material tube as these have a larger internal diameter and better flow rates than silastic tubes (Metheny et al. 1988).

(3) Prevention of tube displacement

- Use a firm but easily removable tape to attach the tube to the nose or face.

- The point of entry into the nose should be marked on the tube with fine tape once correct placement has been established. This can then be checked to ensure it is in the same place. *Note.* This does not guarantee the tube has remained in the stomach. It is possible for it to be brought up by vigorous coughing or retching and sit coiled in the mouth or oropharynx.

- Check tube placement after any vigorous coughing or retching using the methods described above.

(4) Diarrhoea

Causes are frequently multi-factorial in the critically ill patient so the whole patient should be reviewed to identify all relevant factors as follows.

(i) Drugs

- Drugs that have been particularly associated with diarrhoea are: antibiotics, magnesium-containing antacids, electrolyte elixirs, large amounts of hypertonic sugary elixirs, digoxin, methyldopa, and laxatives.

- The patient's drugs should be reviewed and alternatives sought where possible, to those which may be implicated in diarrhoea. Hypertonic elixirs can be diluted prior to administration.

- Addition of a *Lactobacillus acidophilus* preparation, such as live yoghurt, may help restore normal gut flora.

- It may be appropriate to give antidiarrhoeal drugs, such as loperamide, diphenoxylate, and codeine phosphate for drug-related diarrhoea, with the exception of antibiotic-related diarrhoea. Cholestyramine has been suggested for diarrhoea caused by *Clostridium difficile* toxin (Koruda et al. 1987).

(ii) Bacterial contamination

- Potential sources of bacterial contamination should be investigated and a stool specimen sent for culture, sensitivity, and *Clostridium difficile* toxin.

- Feed should not be hung at room temperature for more than 12 hours and feed bags should not be 'topped up'. Feed-giving sets should be changed every 24 hours.

Ready-made feed should be used wherever possible. If feed has to be re-constituted on the unit, care should be taken to maintain sterility.

(iii) Feed constituents

- High osmolality, high fat content, and high lactose content feeds have all been associated with diarrhoea. In fact, most formulae no longer contain lactose and research has shown conflicting evidence of the link between high osmolality and diarrhoea (Keohane et al. 1984). Problems with fat tolerance are more likely with special feeds such as Pulmocare (50% of non-protein calorie content from fat, 50% from carbohydrate). If appropriate, an alternative feed with less fat or a lower osmolality may be tried instead.

- In some cases, a bulking agent, such as methylcellulose or psyllium hydrophilic mucilloid, has been used to good effect (Heather et al. 1991).

(iv) Albumin levels

- Hypoalbuminaemia may cause osmotic diarrhoea if it is associated with a lowering of capillary oncotic pressure (COP). However, artificial colloids may maintain an adequate COP despite a low albumin level. If the COP is reduced, feed within the intestinal lumen creates an osmotic gradient with fluid moving into, rather than out of, the intestine, resulting in a loose watery stool.

(v) Intestinal effects of malnutrition and parenteral nutrition

- Malnutrition is associated with a loss in the number and height of intestinal villi and decreased levels of brush border enzymes. The effect of this is a reduction in the absorptive capability of the intestine. Similar effects can be seen following long periods of parenteral feeding (Koruda *et al.* 1987). There is also some evidence to show that intestinal epithelial cells may benefit from direct uptake of glutamine from feed given via the intestinal tract as a source of energy, for maintenance of the intestinal barrier and the gut's immune function.

- Commencement of enteral feeding in a malnourished patient may require very slow increase in delivery rates and use of a peptide-based formula which is more easily absorbed.

- In some cases, it may be appropriate to co-feed enterally and parenterally to encourage return of gut function and to maintain a suitably high level of nutritional intake.

Many critically ill patients with diarrhoea associated with enteral feed can be managed simply by altering the feed formula, reviewing implicated factors, and adjusting treatment accordingly. Frequently, enteral feeding can be continued at a reduced level until the appropriate treatment has been started. Diarrhoea should not prevent enteral feeding unless it is associated with severe absorptive disorders or infection such as *Clostridium difficile*.

(5) Evaluating delivery of feed

There is good evidence to suggest that patients do not always get the amount of feed that is prescribed and some may get only a small proportion of what is prescribed (Koruda *et al.* 1987; Petrosino *et al.* 1989; Keohane *et al.* 1984). Evaluation of the feed delivery should include a method of comparing feed delivered to feed prescribed on a daily basis. If no mechanism exists for this and no review is carried out the patient may become malnourished before the deficit is detected.

- Feed should be prescribed in *calories* per 24 hours rather than *millilitres* per hour.

- The total calorie intake over 24 hours should be calculated by the nurse; any large deficit or excess and the reasons for it, should be reported to the dietitian or medical staff.

- Nursing evaluation should include details of the patient's ability to absorb and tolerate enteral feed.

The most important aspects of feeding are that the patient receives what he/she requires in the form best suited to his/her ability to absorb and utilize it.

Care of the parenterally fed patient

(1) Insertion of the central venous catheter

Details for insertion of a central venous catheter are given in Chapter 4. In some units, a dedicated port of a triple lumen line is considered adequate for short-term parenteral feeding. However, long-term feeding should be either via a tunnelled feeding line or a Hickman catheter. Debate continues as to whether the risk of inserting a tunnelled feeding line into a critically ill patient outweighs the (slightly increased) incidence of infection in triple lumen lines.

(2) Infection of central venous catheters: mechanisms and management.

(i) Migration of organisms down the dermal tunnel, preceded by colonization of the skin surrounding the site of insertion. Colonization may occur from insertion or during redressing.

Strategy

- Scrupulous aseptic technique (surgical gowns, sterile gloves, povidone-iodine skin preparation, removal of any blood from insertion site prior to dressing) when inserting or dressing the catheter.

- Use of an occlusive dressing which should be redressed according to unit policy.

(ii) Bacterial colonization of the tip. This is generally as a result of bacteraemia from another source. The problem is then compounded by the formation of a fibrin sheath within 3 days of insertion which acts as a shield to bacteria against systemic antibiotics.

Strategy

- Maintenance of a high index of suspicion for catheter infection.

- Removal of the catheter if patient shows evidence of infection and send tip for culture — appropriate systemic antibiotics can then be prescribed if indicated.

● Change non-tunnelled lines if there is evidence of infection at the site or systemically.

(iii) Colonization of the hub or intraluminal segment of the catheter. This is generally due to contamination during tubing changes or by the infusion of contaminated solutions.

Strategy

● Scrupulous aseptic technique (sterile field, surgical gloves, spray hub, and connections with isopropyl alcohol) during changes of administration set or infusions.

● Change the administration set every 24 hours unless using pre-mixed 48-hour infusion bags when the administration set should be changed with the infusion bag.

(iv) Infected infusate. This is less likely than in many other IV infusions due to the amino acid content of the feed which decreases the pH. However, if lipid emulsion is present in the bag, bacterial and fungal growth will be supported. Lipid emulsion alone is almost as good a growth medium as that normally used to culture organisms.

Strategy

● Pre-mixed bags prepared in sterile conditions should be used wherever possible. If not, scrupulous aseptic precautions should be taken in setting up individual bottles and bags for concurrent infusion.

● Infection rates have been shown to be reduced to between 1% and 2% by employment of specially trained personnel. This is probably due to both an understanding of the risks as well as a high level of competence in manipulating lines. The same standards should be expected of the ICU nurse in order to limit the likelihood of infection in the highly vulnerable patient.

(3) Prevention of intolerance of glucose load

Hyperglycaemia associated with stress (see Chapter 2) is often exacerbated by infusing exogenous glucose. Insulin levels may rise in response to the glucose but are either insufficient to maintain normoglycaemia or appear not to function adequately to allow sufficient glucose uptake in the liver and tissues. This may be compounded by the failure of glucose infusions to suppress hepatic gluconeogenesis in the critically ill. The response to a glucose infusion may reflect the patient's degree of illness and reduction in insulin requirements may be an early sign of recovery. Conversely, increasing insulin requirements may indicate a new wave of sepsis. This should be interpreted with caution in patients with accompanying liver disease as gluconeogenetic mechanisms are impaired.

Strategy

● Regular monitoring of blood glucose is essential with hourly or more frequent measurements when parenteral nutrition is first commenced and following any sharp rise or fall.

● Intravenous insulin infusions should be titrated to maintain blood glucose < 10 mmol/l.

● Large changes in insulin infusion rates are not recommended because of the dangers of hypo- and hyperglycaemia. Insulin infusions should not be stopped abruptly even when the blood glucose is very low; it is better to infuse more glucose in order to maintain blood levels and reduce insulin as necessary.

● Infusion rates of glucose should be kept within the limits of metabolic requirements and if tolerance limits the amount below acceptable levels for nutrition, further calories should be given as lipid infusion.

● Infusion should be continuous and via an infusion pump to deliver a constant rate of feed.

● Consideration should be given to discontinuation of insulin infusions at least one hour prior to stopping parenteral nutrition in order to avoid hypoglycaemia.

(4) Prevention of problems from volumes of fluid infused

Due to its hypertonicity, most parenteral feed requires a considerable amount of fluid volume to deliver the nutritional requirements of the patient. This may cause fluid overload in the patient in renal failure or critically ill patients who have problems with oedema. Parenteral nutrition may have to be discontinued until either renal replacement therapy is commenced or the patient passes sufficient volumes of urine, and fluid overload is less of a problem.

Strategy

● Accurate calculation of fluid balance and hourly monitoring of intake and output are essential.

(5) Psychological aspects

Many of the psychosocial problems associated with parenteral nutrition (see box) do not apply to the critically ill as they may have little awareness of the need for food or lack of it. It is also unlikely that parenteral feeding will continue in the long term.

During the convalescent phase the patient may become more aware and the route for feeding, reason, and length of time it will continue should be carefully explained.

Psychosocial effects of parenteral nutrition

- Dependence on catheter and infusion pump

- Loss of potential comfort source

- Loss of taste and pleasure associated with eating

- Anxiety about whether it will ever be possible to eat again

- Anxiety about effects of the feed itself and its ability to provide adequate nutrition

- Loss of social aspects of eating (togetherness, communication, family relationships)

References and bibliography

Adam, S.K. (1990). An investigation into nutritional delivery, prescription and need in the ventilated, enterally fed ITU patient. M.Sc. thesis. King's College, University of London.

Apelgren, K.N. and Wilmore, D.W. (1983). Nutritional care of the critically ill patient. *Surgical Clinics of North America*, **63**, 497–507.

Armstrong, R.F., Bullen, C., Cohen, S.L., Singer, M. and Webb, A.R. (1991). *Critical care algorithms*. Oxford University Press.

Belknap Mickschl, D., Davidson, L.J., Flournoy, D.J. and Parker, D.E. (1990). Contamination of enteral feedings and diarrhea in patients in intensive care units. *Heart and Lung*, **19**, 362–70.

Berger, R. and Adams, L. (1989). Nutritional support in the critical care setting (part 1). *Chest*, **96**, 139–50.

Berger, R. and Adams, L. (1989). Nutritional support in the critical care setting (part 2). *Chest*, **96**, 372–80.

Brinson, R.R. and Pitts, W.M. (1989). Enteral nutrition in the critically ill patient: role of hypoalbuminemia. *Critical Care Medicine*, **17**, 367–70.

Brown, A. (1991). Acute pancreatitis: Pathophysiology, nursing diagnosis, and collaborative problems. *Focus on Critical Care*, **18**, 121–30.

Carlsson, M., Nordenstrom, J. and Hedenstierna, G. (1984). Clinical implications of continuous measurement of energy expenditure in mechanically ventilated patients. *Clinical Nutrition*, **3**, 103–10.

Dobb, J. (1986). Diarrhoea in the critically ill. *Intensive Care Medicine*, **12**, 112–15.

Elpern, E.H., Jacobs, E.R. and Bone, R.C. (1987). Incidence of aspiration in tracheally intubated adults. *Heart and Lung*, **16**, 527–31.

Fiddian-Green, R.G. (1988). Splanchnic ischaemia and multiple organ failure in the critically ill. *Annals of the Royal College of Surgeons of England*, **70**, 128–34.

Fromant, P. and Farman, J. (1987). Looking after the liver patient. *Care of the Critically Ill*, **3**, 34–7.

Goodinson, S.M. (1987). Anthropometric assessment of nutritional status. *Professional Nurse*, **2**, 388–93.

Guyton, A.C. (1985). *Anatomy and physiology*. Holt-Saunders, Philadelphia.

Hanson, R.L. (1979). Criteria for length of masogastric tube insertion for tube feeding. *Journal of parenteral and enteral nutrition*, **3**, 160–3.

Hawker, F. (1990). Liver transplantation. In *Intensive care manual*, (ed. T.E. Oh), (3rd edn), pp.240–5. Butterworth, Sydney.

Heather, D.J., Howell, L., Montana, M., Howell, M., Hill, R. (1991). Effect of a bulk-forming cathartic on diarrhoea in tube-fed patients. *Heart and Lung*, **20**, 409–13.

Hudak, C.M., Gallo, B.M. and Benz, J.J. (1990). *Critical care nursing: A holistic approach*, (5th edn). Lippincott, Philadelphia.

Keohane, P.P., Attrill, H., Love, M., Frost, P. and Silk, D.B.A. (1984). Relation between osmolality of diet and gastrointestinal side effects in enteral nutrition. *British Medical Journal*, **288**, 678–80.

Kohn, C.L. and Keithley J.K. (1989). Enteral nutrition: potential complications and patient monitoring. *Nursing Clinics of North America*, **24**, 339–51.

Konopad, E. and Noseworthy, T. (1988). Stress ulceration: A serious complication in critically ill patients. *Heart and Lung*, **17**, 339–48.

Koruda, M.J., Guenter, P. and Rombeau, J.L. (1987). Enteral nutrition in the critically ill. *Critical Care Clinics*, **3**, 133–53.

Laurence, B.H. (1990). Acute gastrointestinal bleeding. In *Intensive Care Manual*, (ed. T.E. Oh), (3rd edn), pp.219–24. Butterworth, Sydney.

Lee, B. Chang, R.W.S. and Jacobs, S. (1990). Intermittent nasogastric feeding: a simple and effective method to reduce pneumonia among ventilated ICU patients. *Clinical Intensive Care*, **1**, 100–2.

Levy, G.A., Chung, S.W. and Sheiner, P.A. (1991). Approach to the patient with severe liver failure. In *Update in intensive care and emergency medicine*, Vol. 14, (ed. J.L. Vincent), pp. 590–7. Springer, Berlin.

McClave, S.A., Snider, H.L., Lowen, C.C., McLaughlin, A.J., Greene, L.M., McCombs, R.J., *et al.* (1992). Use of residual volume as a marker for enteral feeding intolerance: prospective blinded comparison with physical examination and radiographic findings. Journal of parenteral and enteral nutrition, **16**, 99–105.

Meijer, K., Van Saene, H.K.F. and Hill, J.C. (1990). Infection control in patients undergoing mechanical ventilation: traditional approach versus a new development — selective decontamination of the digestive tract. *Heart and Lung*, **19**, 11–20.

Metheny, N., Dettenmeier, P., Hampton, K., Wiersma, L. and Williams, P. (1990). Detection of inadvertent respiratory placement of small-bore feeding tubes: a report of 10 cases. *Heart and Lung*, **19**, 631–8.

Metheny, N., Eisenberg, P. and McSweeney, M. (1988). Effect of feeding tube properties and three irrigants on clogging rates. *Nursing Research*, **37**, 165–9.

Miller, T.A. (1987). Mechanisms of stress-related mucosal damage. *American Journal of Medicine*, **83** (6A), 8–14.

Moore, F.A., Moore, E.E., Jones, T.N., McCroskey, B.L. and Peterson, V.M. (1989). TEN versus TPN following major abdominal trauma — reduced septic morbidity. *Journal of Trauma*, **29**, 916–23.

O'Grady, J.G. and Williams, R. (1989). Aspects of intensive care following liver transplantation. *Care of the Critically Ill*, **5**, 67–9.

Petrosino, B.M., Christian, B.J., Wolf, J. and Becker, H. (1989). Implications of selected problems with nasoenteral feedings. *Critical Care Nursing Quarterly*, **12**, 1–18.

Pingleton, S.K. (1991). Enteral nutrition and infection: Benefits and risks. In Vincent, J.L. (Editor) *Update in intensive care and emergency medicine*, Vol. 14, (ed. J.L. Vincent), p.581–9. Springer, Berlin.

Rapp, R.P., Young, B., Twyman, D., Bivins, B.A., Haack, D., Tibbs, P.A., *et al.* (1983). The favourable effect of early parenteral feeding on survival in head-injured patients. *Journal of Neurosurgery*, **58**, 906–12.

Schlichtig, R. and Ayres, S.M. (1988). *Nutritional support in the critically ill*. Year Book Medical Publishers, Chicago.

Sheiner, P.A., Greig, P.D. and Levy, G.A. (1990). Perioperative management of the liver transplant patient. In *Update in intensive care and emergency medicine*, Vol. 10, (ed. J.L. Vincent), pp.706–19. Springer, Berlin.

Tryba, M. (1991). Sucralfate versus antacids or H_2-antagonists for stress ulcer prophylaxis: A meta-analysis on efficacy and pneumonia rate. *Critical Care Medicine*, **19**, 942–49.

Van Dalen, R. (1991). Selective decontamination in ICU patients: benefits and doubts. In *Update in intensive care and emergency medicine*, Vol. 14, (ed. J.L. Vincent), pp.379–86. Springer, Berlin.

Van Lanschot, J.J.B., Feenstra, B.W.A., Vermeij, C.G. and Bruining, H.A. (1986). Calculation versus measurement of total energy expenditure. *Critical Care Medicine*, **14**, 981–5.

Vargo, R.L. and Rudy, E.B. (1988). Infection as a complication of liver transplant. *Critical Care Nurse*, **9**, 52–62.

Weissman, C., Kemper, M., Damask, M.C., Askanazi, J., Hyman, A.I. and Kinney, J.M. (1984). Effect of routine intensive care interactions on metabolic rate. *Chest*, **86**, 815–18.

Weissman, C., Kemper, M., Askanazi, J., Hyman, A.I. and Kinney, J.M. (1986). Resting metabolic rate of the critically ill patient: measured versus predicted. *Journal of Anaesthesiology*, **64**, 673–9.

Weissman, C., Kemper, M., Elwyn, D.H., Askanazi, J., Hyman, A.I., Kinney, J.M. (1989). The energy expenditure of the mechanically ventilated critically ill patient: an analysis. *Chest*, **89**, 254–9.

Whatley, K., Turner, W.W., Dey, M., Leonard, J. and Guthrie, M. (1984). When does metaclopromide factilitate transpyloric intubation? *Journal of Parenteral and Enteral Nutrition*, **8**, 679–81.

Winterbauer, R.H., Durning, R.B., Barron, E. and McFadden, M.C. (1981). Aspirated masogastric feeding solution directed by glucose strips. *Annals of Internal Medicine*, **95**, 67–8.

11. Trauma

Introduction

The management of the trauma patient demands considerable skill from the many disciplines involved in the patient's care. Injuries may range from simple, single organ damage to severe multiple injuries, and initial management is centred on the immediate identification of life-threatening injuries and the maintenance of the airway, breathing, and circulation. Continuous reassessment of the patient's clinical state and adequate monitoring of vital signs are essential from the moment the patient arrives in the emergency department.

> The aim of continuous reassessment and intensive monitoring is the early detection of deterioration and the prevention of secondary complications

The initial management of the trauma patient can be considered as four distinct phases (ACS 1984). These strategies begin at the scene of the trauma and continue until the patient is stabilized prior to transfer to the ICU.

Initial management

There are four stages in the initial management of the trauma patient:

1. Primary survey.

2. Resuscitation phase.

3. Secondary survey.

4. Definitive care phase.

Primary survey

This takes place at the scene of the trauma by pre-hospital staff and continues on arrival in the casualty department. The primary survey is concerned with the identification and management of life-threatening injuries and the following areas must be *simultaneously* assessed:

- Airway maintenance and cervical spine control.

- Breathing and ventilation.

- Circulation and haemorrhage control.

- Dysfunction of the central nervous system — the neurological status.

- Exposure — the patient is completely undressed for rapid assessment of injuries.

The patient's vital functions must be assessed quickly and treatment priorities established.

Airway

A patent airway must be established by chin-lift or jaw-thrust manoeuvres and debris and loose-fitting false teeth should be removed from the mouth. High concentration oxygen therapy ($F_iO_2 \geqslant 0.60$) should be immediately instituted by facemask. There is no place for low concentration oxygen administration in the trauma patient as urgent correction of hypoxaemia is imperative. Endotracheal intubation, cricothyroidotomy, or tracheostomy may be required to maintain a patent airway. The possibility of cervical spine injuries should always be suspected, particularly in patients with multiple trauma or blunt trauma above the clavicle (including whiplash injuries). The patient's head should not, therefore, be hyper-extended to maintain the airway.

Breathing

The chest must be exposed to assess respiratory movements as ventilation may be impaired even though the patient has a patent airway.

The following are the most common traumatic conditions that compromise ventilation and must be considered if ventilation is inadequate:

- Tension pneumothorax.

- Open pneumothorax.

- Flail chest with pulmonary contusions.

- Severe head injuries.

Circulation

A rapid assessment of the patient's haemodynamic status is essential. Initial observations include heart rate, blood pressure, skin colour, and capillary return. Hypotension following trauma is presumed to be due to hypovolaemia until proven otherwise. External haemorrhage should be controlled by direct pressure on the wound or by the use of pneumatic splints. Pneumatic antishock garments (e.g. military antishock trouser (MAST) suit) may be useful in controlling haemorrhage from injuries to the abdomen and lower extremities.

Haemorrhage into the thoracic and abdominal cavities, and around fracture sites, may account for major blood loss.

Dysfunction of central nervous system

A rapid neurological assessment must be made in order to evaluate the patient's level of consciousness and pupillary size and reaction. A more detailed neurological examination is made in the secondary survey (see later).

Exposure and examination

The patient should be undressed and a rapid assessment of injuries is made.

Resuscitation phase

The management of shock must be initiated, patient oxygenation reassessed, and haemorrhage control re-evaluated. Hypovolaemic shock is corrected by replacement of lost intravascular volume by blood or colloids and, if not contraindicated, a urinary catheter may be inserted to monitor output. Life-threatening conditions identified in the primary survey should be constantly reassessed as management continues.

Secondary survey

This begins after the life-threatening conditions have been identified and treated and shock therapy has begun. The secondary survey involves a head-to-toe thorough examination and assessment of the patient where each region of the body is examined in detail. In this phase, laboratory studies, X-rays, scans, and special investigations such as peritoneal lavage are carried out.

Definitive care phase

In this phase, all of the patient's injuries are managed comprehensively: fractures are stabilized, the patient is transferred to the operating theatre if immediate operative measures are necessary, or the patient is stabilized in preparation for transfer to the ICU or specialist area.

Arrival at the intensive care unit

The ICU staff should be informed in advance of the impending arrival of the patient. The time prior to receiving the patient must be spent preparing the bed area and assembling the necessary equipment. The nurse must anticipate all eventualities.

- If the patient is to remain spontaneously breathing, prepare equipment for administering humidified oxygen.

- If mechanical ventilation is required, ensure the ventilator is functioning correctly and is set appropriately for delivery of oxygen, minute or tidal volume, and respiratory rate. The patient may then be connected on arrival. If possible prepare appropriate infusions of sedation and/or analgesia.

- Suction equipment must be tested and ready for use. A manual rebreathing bag should be connected to the oxygen supply.

- Other basic supplies and apparatus should be available as per ICU protocol.

Depending on the patient's injuries, an appropriate bed or pressure-relieving mattress may be required (e.g. Stryker frame for spinal injuries).

If required, prepare traction in advance and ensure this can be affixed to the particular bed used.

Prepare a range of volumetric pumps for the immediate administration of drugs and fluids. Pressure bags for rapid volume transfusions may be needed. If continuous pressure monitoring is required, these too should be prepared in advance.

Continuous ECG monitoring will be essential. Ensure the monitor is working correctly, set the alarm limits, and have skin electrodes ready to attach on the patient arrival.

If the patient is haemodynamically stable in the casualty department, manual blood pressure recordings may be sufficient. Ensure that a sphygmomanometer and stethoscope, or a semi-automatic sphygmomanometer are at the bedside. Pulse oximetry is extremely useful as an immediate guide to patient oxygenation, especially prior to the insertion of an intra-arterial cannula for blood gas analysis. A variety of temperature probes may be required. An oral thermometer may be adequate but consider the need for recording core temperature if the patient is hypothermic. Skin probes may be required if there is vascular injury to the limbs.

Anticipate the need for central vein cannulation, prepare a trolley with the necessary catheters (e.g. triple lumen central venous, pulmonary artery).

Checklist for equipment preparation

- Humidified oxygen/ventilator

- Suction

- Rebreathing bag

- Special bed or pressure-relieving mattress

- Traction

- Volumetric pumps

- Pressure bags

- Skin electrodes for ECG monitoring

- Sphygmomanometer, stethoscope

- Pulse oximeter

- Temperature probes (skin/rectal), thermometer

- Transducers for invasive monitoring

- Trolley for central venous/arterial cannulation

When the patient arrives on the ICU, the clinical state may vary from conscious, alert, breathing spontaneously, and haemodynamically stable to unconscious, endotracheally intubated, mechanically ventilated, hypoxaemic, and shocked. The subsequent nursing and medical management will therefore depend entirely on the extent of the patient's injuries and alterations in clinical state. Constant reassessment of the patient's condition is essential. Continual monitoring of vital signs is important for the early detection of deterioration and the institution of appropriate treatment quickly and effectively.

The extent of the use of invasive and non-invasive monitoring devices will depend on the degree of the patient's injuries and the facilities available on the ICU. For a full description of patient monitoring refer to Chapters 4 and 5.

> When the patient arrives the immediate nursing priorities are to the **A**irway, **B**reathing, and **C**irculation, all of which should have been stabilized prior to transfer but may have deteriorated during transport

---

If the patient is breathing spontaneously and requires oxygen therapy, attach to the prepared humidified oxygen system, via facemask or T-piece if intubated, at the prescribed concentration and flow. If the patient requires mechanical ventilation, confirm that the ventilatory settings are correct then attach to the ventilator. Ensure that the alarm limits are set and chest expansion is adequate and symmetrical.

Connect the patient to the ECG monitor and note the heart rate and rhythm. If a central venous catheter is *in situ*, attach to the prepared transducer or manometer. Ensure that infusions in progress are running correctly and that any wound or chest drains, or urinary catheter, are correctly positioned. Check that chest drains are not clamped and ascertain if suction is required. If available, attach a pulse oximeter probe.

Record immediate baseline observations of:

- Heart rate and rhythm

- Blood pressure

- Central venous pressure

- Respirations or ventilator recordings

- Temperature

- Neurological status

The correct positioning of the patient must be considered and will depend on the injuries sustained. For instance, a spontaneously breathing patient with a flail chest should sit erect if his/her cardiovascular status and other injuries allow. Patients with actual or suspected fractures of the neck or spine will need extreme care in positioning and must remain flat with the appropriate area immobilized. Fractured limbs must be carefully positioned and supported. Any traction must be correctly fitted and the end of the bed elevated if appropriate and not contraindicated (e.g. spinal injury).

If the patient is stable at this point and no immediate treatment is necessary, a full nursing assessment should now be carried out. If the patient is haemodynamically unstable, ventilatory support inadequate, or the patient is in pain, then these aspects must be corrected first.

General nursing assessment

This involves a thorough head-to-toe examination of the patient by the nurse and will provide the starting point from which any change can be determined. The nurse must continually observe and reassess, document, and report changes, and be aware of the significance of deviations from the baseline measures.

Respiratory injuries

For a full description of respiratory assessment refer to Chapter 3.

The following are essential observations in the trauma patient.

Respiratory rate and depth

Record the respiratory rate if the patient is breathing spontaneously. Note the depth of respirations. Is the patient using accessory muscles to aid breathing? Is there stridor? (a sign of upper airway obstruction). A respiratory rate greater than 20 breaths per minute should alert the nurse to the possibility of respiratory compromise. Pulse oximetry and blood gas analysis should be used as an adjunct to observation and examination.

Chest movements and air entry

Is the chest moving symmetrically with each respiration? Is there air entry in all regions? If chest movement is unilateral, or air entry poor in any region, consider an obstruction in the right or left main bronchus, malposition of the endotracheal tube (if intubated), pneumothorax, haemothorax, rupture of a bronchus, or pulmonary contusions. Bear in mind that the patient may have underlying respiratory disease such as asthma, chronic obstructive airways disease.

If the patient has multiple rib fractures and/or a flail segment this may impair chest wall movement. If the patient is breathing spontaneously, paradoxical chest wall movement may be evident over the flail segment (see the section on chest injuries p. 325).

Respiratory pattern

Note the pattern of respiration. Is it regular? Particular patterns of respiration are characteristic of particular head injuries (e.g. Cheyne–Stokes respirations: periodic rapid and slow breathing) in bilateral cerebral hemi-sphere damage, hyperventilation in midbrain injuries, apneustic (prolonged inspiration) in pontine injuries, and ataxic (random) in medullary injuries. For further details see Chapter 9.

Skin

Examine the skin of the chest for bruising, lacerations, and abrasions which may indicate underlying injuries (e.g. seat-belt marks). Feel for subcutaneous emphysema which is due to air leaking into the subcutaneous tissues either from external (e.g. stab wound) or from internal (e.g. fractured ribs lacerating underlying lung) injuries.

Pain

Does the patient complain of pain or tenderness over any particular area of the chest? Does he/she have pain on inspiration that limits chest movement? If chest drains are *in situ*, note the contents (e.g. blood, haemoserous), and the presence of bubbling and swinging of the fluid level with respirations.

Summary of respiratory assessment

- Respiratory rate and depth

- Chest movements and air entry

- Respiratory pattern

- Skin (bruising, lacerations, emphysema)

- Pain

Cardiovascular injuries

A 12-lead ECG should be performed. Continuous ECG monitoring should be in progress in order to detect immediately any change in rate or rhythm. Feel the pulse from time to time. Is it rapid, thready, irregular, or full and bounding? Are all central pulses present? Bear in mind that the patient may have underlying cardiovascular disease that is being treated (e.g. beta blockers, a permanent pacemaker).

The frequency of blood pressure recordings will depend on the extent of the patient's injuries. Continuous monitoring by means of a transduced intra-arterial cannula allows changes in blood pressure to be detected immediately. This is essential in multiply-injured or shocked patients if rapid treatment is to be effected. However, manual recordings are sufficient if the patient is haemodynamically stable and the blood pressure can be taken with ease. Changes in blood pressure should not be taken in isolation but always related to changes in other variables, such as heart rate, central venous pressure, pulmonary artery pressures, and stroke volume. Consider the effects of drug therapy as a cause of the change in blood pressure (e.g. analgesia or sedation; a fall may be accentuated in a hypovolaemic patient).

Note if there is bleeding over wound sites and drains and measure these losses frequently.

Summary of cardiovascular assessment

- Heart rate and rhythm

- Blood pressure

- Central venous pressure, pulmonary artery pressure

- 12-lead ECG

- Central and peripheral pulses

- Bleeding (drains, wounds, etc.)

Neurological injuries

A full neurological assessment must be undertaken as soon as possible. This will indicate the severity of the injury and provide the baseline for sequential appraisal and the detection of deterioration. The Glasgow Coma Scale provides a quantitative measure of the level of consciousness and is the sum of the scores of three areas of assessment: (1) eye opening, (2) best motor response, and (3) best verbal response, each being graded separately. For a full description refer to Chapter 9.

Pupil size and their response to light must also be evaluated. A difference in pupil diameter of more than 1 mm is abnormal. A sluggish or lack of response to light may indicate intracranial injury, however, the effect of medications (e.g. atropine, opiates) must be considered.

The nurse should observe any spontaneous limb movements for equality though limb fractures or injuries may inhibit movement. The muscle tone should be assessed for flaccidity and asymmetry. Spasticity (e.g. following spinal cord transection) is a late sign. If spontaneous movements are minimal the response to painful stimuli must be determined. A decrease in the amount of movement or the need for more stimulus on one side is significant and may suggest an intracranial, spinal or nerve injury.

The frequency of recording of neurological observations will depend on the patient's neurological status and the presence of actual or potential head injury. The nurse should also examine the scalp for lacerations, bruising,

and obvious deformity. Bruising behind the ears may indicate bleeding into the mastoid spaces — a late sign of a basal skull fracture. The presence of otorrhoea or rhinorrhoea is also suggestive of a basal skull fracture. Leakage of cerebrospinal fluid can be confirmed by measurement of the glucose level which is at least half that of the blood glucose level.

Summary of neurological assessment

- Conscious level: Glasgow Coma Scale

- Pupillary response

- Limb movement and response to stimuli

- Examine scalp (lacerations, cerebrospinal fluid leakage, bruising)

Renal injuries

Unless the patient is fully conscious and haemodynamically stable, urine output will usually be monitored hourly by means of a urinary catheter and collecting system. However, certain conditions contraindicate the use of a urethral catheter; these include trauma, or suspected trauma, to the urethra. Observe for urethral bleeding. In this case, a suprapubic catheter is usually inserted.

Routine urinalysis should be carried out on all patients and the urine observed for frank haematuria, clots, debris and colour change. Haematuria is an important sign of potential genitourinary trauma. Note the urine colour — a black urine suggests myoglobinuria which follows muscle damage and breakdown (rhabdomyolysis). Examine genitalia and note any bruising, lacerations, or oedema which may indicate underlying injury. Urine output should be maintained at a minimum of 0.5 ml/kg/h in adult patients.

Summary of renal assessment

- Urine output

- Urinalysis

- Urine colour (haematuria, myoglobinuria)

- Examine genitalia

Gastrointestinal injuries

All mechanically ventilated patients should have a nasogastric tube inserted unless this is contraindicated (e.g.

nasal or basal skull fractures), in which case, an orogastric tube should be inserted. Gastric dilatation is common after major trauma as well as in ventilated patients. The gastric aspirate should be left to drain freely and should be aspirated regularly. Observe aspirate and test for blood.

Examine the abdomen for bruising, grazes and lacerations, particularly in the regions of the liver, spleen, and kidneys, which may indicate underlying organ damage. Is the abdomen painful in any particular region? Does the abdomen look distended? Is it rigid on palpation? Is there any evidence of bleeding per rectum (or per vagina)?

Assess the nutritional state and consider the need for early feeding (see Chapter 10).

Summary of gastrointestinal assessment

- Oro- or nasogastric tube (if not contraindicated)

- Measure gastric aspirate and test for blood

- Examine abdomen (bruising, pain, rigidity)

- Note bleeding per rectum (or per vagina)

Skin and limbs injuries

Note any bruising or lacerations. Feel the skin temperature and note the colour. The hypovolaemic patient may appear ashen-faced with cool, pale extremities. Look for cyanosis — peripherally in the nail beds and centrally in the lips and tongue. The efficiency of capillary refill in each limb can be tested by pressing the tip of a digit on the skin to blanch it and observing the return of colour. This is immediate in the well-perfused patient. Note if any limb is particularly cool. Check that distal pulses are present, and that pressure dressings, splints, plaster casts, or traction on limbs are not impeding the circulation. Ensure that pressure is not exerted on healthy skin by plaster casts or traction devices (observe for tissue swelling and breaks in the skin).

Summary of skin and limb assessment

- note bruising and lacerations

- skin temperature and colour

- peripheral perfusion and pulses

- check plaster casts, splints, traction

The patient and relatives

A concise medical and social history will need to be taken from the patient or relatives to aid the planning of your nursing care. Do not ask relatives to repeat information if this is already contained within the medical notes, although it is vital that correct addresses and telephone numbers of next-of-kin are confirmed.

Establish a short-term plan of action from the medical staff and relay this information to the patient and relatives. Encourage them to ask questions, explain the use of any equipment attached to the patient, and ensure that they are regularly informed of progress and developments. Document what information the patient or family have been told by medical staff concerning the injuries and outcome. A greater understanding of the patient's injuries and a good rapport with nursing and medical staff will help relatives cope with the frightening environment of the ICU.

Trauma is always sudden and unexpected and, unlike the routine post-operative patient who has a planned admission to the ICU, there can be no preparation time to allow the patient or relatives to adjust mentally. The patient's injuries may have a profound effect on normal daily living and family life. Financial and work problems may ensue. Emotional and perhaps professional support will be needed to help the family cope with these. Social workers, ministers of religion, and external organizations (such as those for head- and spine-injured patients) can offer great comfort, support and advice. Never forget that amidst the abundance of wires and tubes is a person who will need your constant care and reassurance and who is probably frightened about his/her injuries and worried about their effects on his/her future.

Head injuries

Head injuries are a common consequence when trauma results from vehicular or sports accidents, or falls in the home or work place.

Many patients with head injuries are, however, managed in general ICUs which have no facilities for monitoring intracranial or cerebral perfusion pressure. Severe head injuries still have a high morbidity and mortality and the management of such patients must be directed at preventing secondary brain damage and providing the best conditions for recovery from any brain damage already sustained. (See Table 11.1 for types of head injury.)

Table 11.1 Types of head injury

Scalp • Abrasions • Contusions • Lacerations • Avulsions	The rich blood supply to the scalp may cause wounds to bleed profusely. Always suspect underlying fractures and potential intracranial damage. Is there any foreign body (e.g. glass) remaining?
Fractures • Simple, linear	Impact causes a simple crack in the bone with no break in the skin.
• Simple, depressed	A portion of bone is pushed inwards.
• Compound, depressed	A violent blow causes pieces of bone fragment to be driven into the intracranial cavity.
• Open	A direct pathway or opening through the scalp laceration into the cerebral substance. The dura is torn; CSF may leak from the wound or the brain tissue may be visible. This type of fracture is an important source of intracranial infection.
• Basal	Characterized by CSF leakage from the ear (otorrhoea) or nose (rhinorrhoea) which may be mixed with blood. Ecchymosis (bruising) in the mastoid area behind the ear ('Battle sign') is a late sign appearing several hours after the injury. Periorbital ecchymosis ('raccoon eyes') is a sign of cribriform plate fracture.
Diffuse • Concussion	Caused by stretching of axonal shafts in white matter with reversible loss of function. Results in temporary confusion or loss of consciousness.
• Diffuse axonal	Microscopic damage throughout brain caused by tearing or stretching of axonal tracts. Not amenable to surgery. Characterized by prolonged, deep coma, often decerebrate/decorticate posturing, commonly autonomic dysfunction causing high fever, sweating, hypertension. Overall mortality 33%.
Focal • Contusion	Macroscopic damage occurring in a relatively local area, often beneath an area of impact (coup contusions) or areas remote from impact (contrecoup contusion). Often prolonged periods of coma, mental confusion, or obtundation. May cause herniation and brainstem compression if large or associated with pericontusional oedema. Alcoholic patients are prone to delayed bleeding into contusions.
• Intracranial haemorrhages (i) acute epidural	Bleeding from a tear in a dural artery or in the dural sinus. Rare but may be rapidly fatal. Causes loss of consciousness followed by lucid period, then a secondary depression of conscious level. A hemiparesis develops and a fixed dilated pupil on the side opposite the haematoma.
(ii) acute subdural haematoma	Bleeding commonly from rupturing of bridging veins between cerebral cortex and dura. Also seen with lacerations of the brain or cortical arteries. Often seen as underlying brain injury. Causes decreased level of consciousness and possible epileptic fits if the clot irritates the cerebral cortex.
Lacerations • Impalements and bullet wounds	Impaled objects must be removed at operation. Outcome depends on location, size of injury, and the patient's condition. Patients in coma following bullet wounds have a high mortality. The larger the calibre and the higher the velocity of the bullet the more likely death will occur. A bullet that does not penetrate the skull may still result in an intracranial injury.

Pathophysiology

See Chapter 9 for the detailed anatomy and physiology of the brain.

The brain, cerebrospinal fluid, blood, and extracellular fluid are contained within the rigid structure of the skull. The brain is poorly anchored within the skull and its soft consistency renders it liable to move in response to acceleration or deceleration. Bruising (contusions) can occur when there is contact between the interior skull and the surface of the brain; internal shearing forces can cause axonal tracts within the white matter to stretch and tear. Mild stretch injury, with reversible loss of function, is responsible for the transient disturbance of consciousness known as 'concussion'.

Skull fractures alone do not cause neurological disability and severe brain injuries can occur without skull fractures. A patient with a skull fracture is, however, at risk of having, or developing, intracranial damage. Close observation is necessary in order to detect early signs of neurological deterioration.

The contents of the skull are incompressible and, since the volume within the cranial vault is constant, increasing the volume (by oedema, haemorrhage, or haematoma), directly increases the intracranial pressure (ICP). Increases in ICP are initially compensated for by movement of cerebral venous blood into the systemic circulation. As the pressure rises further, there is compression of brain tissue and decreased cerebral arterial blood flow. If this continues, the ICP rises at the expense of cerebral blood flow and results in brain ischaemia. Brain tissue dies when its blood supply is interrupted for only a few minutes. The brain also has no metabolic reserves and is thus wholly dependent on arterial blood flow to meet its metabolic needs. The cerebral perfusion pressure (CPP) is measured by subtracting ICP from mean arterial pressure. CPP is thus decreased by a raised ICP and it may fall below the perfusion pressure necessary to maintain cerebral blood flow. Ischaemic injury resulting from a decreased CPP may involve all cerebral tissue or any focal areas. When compartmental pressure gradients develop from local areas of injury, brain shifts can occur within the cranial cavity, the most important being uncal or tentorial herniation (coning) which causes brainstem compression and catastrophic neurological injury.

Changes in vital signs in patients with raised intracranial pressure

As ICP increases, the heart rate and respiratory rate decrease and blood pressure and temperature rise. There may be irregular patterns of respiration with Cheyne–

> **Consequences of raised intracranial pressure**
>
> - Alterations in the level of consciousness
> - Headaches, photophobia, nausea, vomiting
> - Bradycardia and hypertension
> - Coma
> - Brain death

Stokes or Kussmaul breathing (see Chapter 3). If brain compression causes the circulation to fail, the pulse and respiration become rapid and temperature usually rises but does not follow a consistent pattern. The pulse pressure (the difference between systemic systolic and diastolic pressure) widens. Immediately preceding this, there may be a period of rapid fluctuations in pulse varying from a slow rate to a rapid one. Death will now ensue unless interventions are achieved. These changes in vital signs must, however, be assessed in relation to the patient's responsiveness (for more details of recognition and management of raised intracranial pressure see Chapter 9).

> **Cardiovascular signs of raised intracranial pressure**
>
> - Decreased heart rate
> - Decreased respiratory rate
> - Raised blood pressure
> - Raised temperature
> - Widened pulse pressure

Secondary brain damage

The brain requires continuous perfusion with well-oxygenated blood. A reduction in mean arterial blood pressure to below 60–80 mmHg, particularly when the intracranial pressure is raised, may cause ischaemic neuronal damage if sustained for more than a few minutes. The brain is normally able to regulate its own blood supply to maintain a constant perfusion pressure despite wide variations in systemic blood pressure. However, when injured, the brain loses this capacity. The brain is thus particularly vulnerable to ischaemic damage in the presence of hypotension, hypoxaemia, or hypovolaemia. Secondary brain damage can often be caused by extracranial or intracranial insults and may be prevented by rapid treatment (see Table 11.2).

Table 11.2 Causes of secondary brain damage

Cause	Secondary to
Extracranial	
• Hypoxia	• Brainstem damage causing decreased respiratory drive
	• Haemo/pneumothorax
	• Pulmonary contusions
	• Rib fractures
	• Aspiration pneumonitis/infection
	• Fat emboli/pulmonary emboli
	• ARDS
• Hypotension	• Hypovolaemic shock
Intracranial	
• Compression from haematomas	• Subdural
	• Extradural
	• Intradural (intracerebral/ subarachnoid)
• Venous engorgement leading to cerebral oedema	
• Secondary infection	• Meningitis
	• Brain abscess

Treatment

Basic requirements

The first priority in dealing with any patient with a head injury is to stabilize the airway, breathing, and circulation and thus prevent further secondary cerebral damage resulting from hypotension and hypoxia. Management thereafter will depend on the patient's condition and the presence of other injuries. Cervical spine injuries should always be suspected in all patients. Particular care must be taken to stabilize the cervical spine until neck injury has been excluded by X-rays and a specialist opinion.

Not all unconscious patients will require intubation; a Guedel or nasopharyngeal airway may be adequate to maintain a patent airway as long as a gag reflex is present. However, adequate blood gas tensions must be maintained and so the patient should be intubated, and mechanically ventilated if necessary, to prevent the patient becoming hypoxaemic. Obviously, other causes, such as a pneumothorax, should first be excluded.

Hyperventilation

This may be required if a patient's condition is deteriorating because of raised ICP. The question of hyperven-

tilation in head injury is a subject of some controversy. The objective is to induce hypocapnia since the arterial P_aCO_2 level profoundly affects cerebral blood flow. When the P_aCO_2 is abnormally elevated, cerebral vasodilatation occurs, increasing intracranial blood volume and thus ICP. A reduction in P_aCO_2 hence reduces intracranial blood volume and ICP. Hyperventilation to produce a P_aCO_2 of 3.4–3.7 kPa is generally recommended. This usually requires endotracheal intubation, mechanical ventilation and, often, neuromuscular blockade. Hyperventilation should be performed early in the comatose patient. Excessive hypocapnia can, however, reduce cerebral circulation to the point where cerebral ischaemia occurs. Blood gases must therefore be carefully monitored. Spikes in ICP can be treated with aggressive short-term hyperventilation.

Some authorities maintain that all cases of head injury with a raised ICP should be hyperventilated although some studies suggest that therapeutic hyperventilation does not improve outcome. The cerebral vasoconstrictor response to hypocapnia does not last for more than 24–48 hours and therefore prolonged hyperventilation must be reviewed regularly. The cerebral vascular resistance appears to normalize within 4–6 hours of hyperventilation. The P_aCO_2 should therefore be elevated slowly when discontinuing hyperventilation in order to prevent rebound cerebral vasodilatation and increased ICP.

Nursing procedures

See Chapter 9 for details of ICP monitoring.

The patient with a raised ICP should not be stimulated unnecessarily and should be nursed in a quiet environment. The ICP is raised by agitation, coughing, and pain and nursing procedures should therefore be aimed at minimizing these. In the intubated patient with a raised ICP, endotracheal suction should be carried out only as often as is necessary for clearance of secretions. If secretions are minimal the frequency of suctioning should be reduced. Chest percussion and physiotherapy will also increase ICP. Blocking the ICP response to these procedures can be achieved by careful positioning of the patient with head-up tilt at 30 degrees and with the neck in a neutral position. Tapes securing the endotracheal tube should not be tied too tightly as venous return may be impeded thus increasing ICP. Ventilate with 100% oxygen immediately prior to, and after, suctioning. In the unconscious patient, passive limb movements and regular turning must be instituted and a pressure-relieving mattress may be required. Bladder catheterization will also be necessary.

Always anticipate complications arising from the head

injury. Nursing management should be directed towards identification and prevention of these potential problems. Should complications develop, immediate medical or surgical intervention may be necessary.

Assessment

Frequent neurological assessment of the head-injured patient is vital to detect changes early and to effect rapid treatment. These may initially be performed at 15–30 minute intervals (see Chapter 9 for assessment procedures). Any deterioration must be reported and documented immediately.

Sedation and analgesia

Narcotics and non-depolarizing muscle relaxants do not alter cerebrovascular resistance and will not raise ICP provided blood gas tensions remain unaltered. Ideally, short-acting agents should be used which can be stopped to allow a fairly rapid assessment of underlying neurological function. Antagonist agents, such as flumazenil and naloxone, should be used with caution after head injury as they may induce epileptic fits and increase cerebral metabolism. Sedation and analgesia is often a problem as both opiates and benzodiazepines may cause respiratory depression in spontaneously breathing patients and thus enhance the possibility of secondary brain damage. Paracetamol, dihydrocodeine, or codeine phosphate are usually safe and effective. In the mechanically ventilated patient, analgesia should not be withheld, especially if other injuries such as limb fractures have been sustained. Heavy sedation may be employed instead. Propofol infusions are being used more often as the drug has a short half-life and does not alter pupillary response. Although propofol is potentially epileptogenic, this does not appear to be of major clinical concern. In the case of a raised ICP which does not respond to hyperventilation and dehydration therapy (see later) the use of intravenous barbiturates, such as thiopentone, should be considered as these reduce cerebral metabolism and oxygen consumption.

Dehydration therapy

The ICP can also be controlled by dehydration therapy using the osmotic diuretic mannitol ± frusemide. Following an infusion of 100 ml 20% mannitol (or 200 ml of 10% solution), a reduction in ICP is seen within 10–20 minutes as brain water follows the osmotic gradient into the vasculature with a consequent diuresis. The duration of reduction in ICP following mannitol may last from 2 to 6 hours and repeated boluses may be required to maintain the ICP below 20 mmHg. Mannitol does cross the blood–brain barrier and will therefore lose some of its efficacy with repeated use. Furthermore, a serum osmolality of 310–320 mOsm/kg should not be exceeded. Maintenance fluids are reduced to approximately half the daily requirement. Careful monitoring of heart rate, blood pressure, CVP, and blood electrolytes is essential during such therapy in order to avoid excessive hypovolaemia and electrolyte disturbances. This is especially important if the patient has sustained other injuries causing haemodynamic instability.

PEEP

Positive end expiratory pressure (PEEP) may be necessary in the hypoxaemic mechanically ventilated patient. However, PEEP will raise intrathoracic pressure which may impede cerebral venous return and thus elevate ICP. Without ICP monitoring it is difficult to assess the magnitude of this effect though PEEP levels of up to 10 cmH$_2$O are usually well tolerated.

Seizures

Epileptic fits may occur with any head injury either from direct irritation of the cortex or from secondary causes such as hypoxia, hypotension, and hypoglycaemia. Prolonged or repetitive fitting may be associated with intracranial haemorrhage. Fits are usually treated aggressively since they may cause cerebral hypoxia, brain swelling, and raised ICP. Respiratory function, length of time, and a description of the fits must be carefully documented on a 'fit chart'. Appropriate medication should be instituted (usually intravenous phenytoin). Ensure the safety of the patient at all times; side-rails should be used on the bed and padded with pillows to prevent injury.

Metabolic

Stress-induced diabetes mellitus may be a complication of head injury. Blood and urine should be regularly tested for glucose and insulin therapy prescribed as necessary. If impaired glucose tolerance persists, a diabetic diet should be instituted.

Diabetes insipidus is caused by damage to the hypothalamus or posterior pituitary gland. It occurs quite commonly in severe head injuries, and particularly brain death, but may follow fairly minor trauma. This results in failure of appropriate antidiuretic hormone (ADH) secretion resulting in the passage of large volumes of dilute urine. Intravenous fluid replacement will usually be necessary to prevent hypovolaemia and vasopressin therapy is usually required (see Chapter 8). Vital signs and blood electrolytes should be carefully monitored and the urine specific gravity should be regularly ascertained. Fluid balance must be carefully documented. Conversely, inappropriate ADH secretion may occur with head injury resulting in oliguria and fluid retention.

Infection

Infection may be a complication of head injury, either directly from an open head wound or skull fracture, especially if CSF leakage is present, or from cannulae and drain sites. These may give rise to meningitis or brain abscesses. Careful monitoring of temperature and bacteriological culture of potential sites of infection is necessary. Prophylactic antibiotic therapy, such as benzyl penicillin, is now considered only for those with basal skull fractures or compound vault fractures. Tetanus prophylaxis should not be overlooked when lacerations or penetrating injuries occur.

Miscellaneous

Gastric dilatation is common after any trauma and the risk of aspiration cannot be overemphasized. Vomiting and retching will increase the ICP and should be avoided by the use of antiemetics (e.g. metoclopramide). All semiconscious or unconscious patients should have gastric aspiration performed regularly by placement of a oro- or nasogastric tube. A nasogastric tube is never inserted in patients with frontal basal skull fractures because of the risk of passage of the tube into the cranium. Feeding should be commenced as early as possible; this should ideally be by the enteral route unless otherwise contraindicated (see Chapter 10). Glucose is a vital metabolic requirement of the brain and although the injured brain has a lowered cerebral metabolism it is more susceptible to lack of this substrate. Prolonged deprivation may cause secondary brain damage. Regular blood glucose measurements are therefore essential and supplemental intravenous glucose may be required. Early institution of feeding will also prevent the development of stress ulceration. Prophylactic ulcer medication is not generally indicated unless there is a coagulopathy or a relevant past history (e.g. known peptic ulceration, indigestion, alcohol abuse).

Myocardial ischaemia and injury are common in head-injured patients, either due to associated chest trauma and cardiac contusions, or to an association with elevated plasma catecholamines causing tachycardia, hypertension, and increased cardiac output, thus imposing excess work on the heart. A 12-lead ECG must be taken and continuous ECG monitoring should be in progress.

Hyperthermia is harmful to the head-injured patient since elevations in body temperature increase the metabolic rate of the brain and will elevate carbon dioxide levels. The higher the temperature, the greater the risk to the patient. Methods of cooling should be instituted immediately (e.g. antipyretics, fanning, tepid sponging, cooling mattress).

Agitation and restlessness may be a sign that the unconscious patient is getting better or, more ominously, that the patient is deteriorating. Restless patients must not be sedated without excluding hypoxia, hypotension, metabolic derangement, a full bladder, or pain from other injuries. The patient must be assessed for the development of any focal change (e.g. unequal pupils, non-use of one or more limbs). The patient should be prevented from harming himself (e.g. by using padded side-rails) or from dislodging cannulae and tubes.

Maxillofacial and upper airway trauma

Maxillofacial and upper airway injuries are common and the majority result from vehicular accidents, physical violence, or sporting injuries. Many patients with severe maxillofacial injuries will have other associated injuries; cervical spine trauma must always be suspected. Consequently, extreme care must be taken to stabilize the neck when the airway is being secured. Sharp trauma, such as knife and gunshot wounds, cause lacerations and penetrating injuries which may damage the air passages, blood vessels, nerves and oesophagus. Blunt trauma may cause bone fractures and damage to the larynx and trachea leading to severe airway problems.

Injuries to the face and neck can be life-threatening because they may severely compromise the airway and cause major haemorrhage. The management priorities are to therefore secure and maintain a patent airway and to prevent hypovolaemic shock due to massive bleeding from the facial skeleton and soft tissues. Airway management poses particular problems in these patients because the very nature of the trauma means that access may be obstructed. Once the airway has been secured and haemorrhage controlled, further definitive management should be deferred until other potential life-threatening injuries have been dealt with.

Airway management

Initial management will include assessment of the injury,

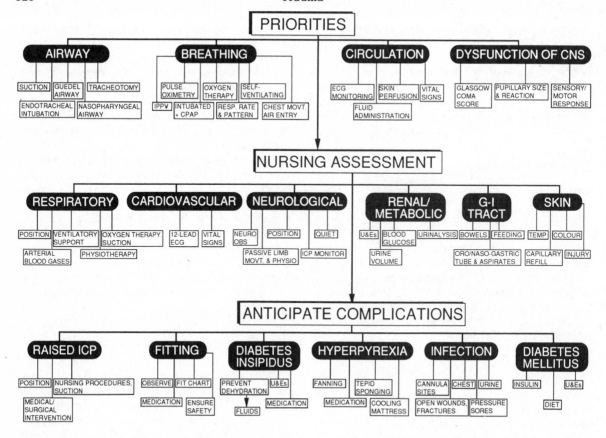

Fig. 11.1 Schema of head injury management.

the patient's conscious level, colour and ability to maintain a patent airway. Suction can be applied but, depending on the site and extent of the trauma, particular problems may be encountered.

Oral intubation or emergency tracheotomy may be required if a patent airway cannot be maintained. This may be particularly necessary in the following circumstances in order to maintain effective gas exchange:

- Bilateral anterior mandibular fracture or symphyseal fracture may cause the tongue to lose its anterior insertion. In the supine patient the tongue may then drop back and occlude the oropharynx. To open the airway a suture is placed through the tongue and secured with tape to the side of the face.

- The oral cavity or airway may be blocked by teeth, dentures, vomitus, bone fragments, blood, or foreign bodies. These can also block the larynx, trachea, or main bronchi. Attempts should be made to scoop out debris with a gloved finger and suction applied with a large-bore Yankauèr suction catheter.

- A maxillary fracture may be displaced and block the nasal airway. To open the airway the maxilla must be disimpacted by pulling it forwards.

- Haemorrhage may obstruct the airway and results from bleeding vessels in open wounds or from the nose if the maxillary artery or ethmoidal vessels are damaged. Direct pressure to wounds and suction are required to open the airway.

- Soft tissue swelling and oedema may obstruct the airway. Although not usually an immediate phenomenon, early intubation may prevent airway obstruction.

Trauma to the larynx or trachea may cause obstruction of the airway by swelling or displacement of structures (e.g. vocal cords or epiglottis). If the airway is threatened and anatomical disruption makes intubation difficult or impossible, an emergency cricothyroidotomy or a tracheostomy must be performed. Nasal intubation is never attempted when mid-facial injuries are present or a basal skull fracture is suspected.

Specific maxillofacial fractures

Mandible

This is easily fractured because of its prominent position. May cause airway obstruction if fractured bilaterally at the angle or body of the mandible. Often causes haematoma and swelling of the neck and floor of mouth. Definitive treatment consists of internal wiring or plating.

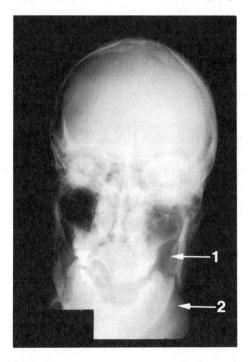

Fig. 11.2 X-ray showing fracture to mandible.

Maxilla

This injury is often accompanied by airway obstruction and fracture of nasal bones, orbit, zygoma, soft tissue injury, and ocular damage. Le Fort classified these fractures into three types, but there may be a combination:

Le Fort I: The least severe. A dento-alveolar fracture which separates the palate from the remainder of the facial skeleton.
Le Fort II: The fracture extends from the lower nasal bridge through the medial wall of the orbit and crosses the zygomatic-maxillary process.
Le Fort III: The most severe. The fracture completely separates the midfacial skeleton from the base of the upper nasal bridge, most of the orbit, and across the zygomatic arch. The fracture involves the ethmoid bone and may affect the cribriform plate at the base of the skull.

Le Fort II and III fractures are often associated with basal skull fractures and may lead to CSF leakage, meningitis, and pneumocranium. Nasal intubation (nasotracheal or nasogastric) must never be carried out due to the risk of passing the tube through the cribriform plate into the cranial cavity. Definitive surgery involves internal fixation with wiring and plating and intermaxillary fixation. External fixation is often required.

Zygoma and orbit

Fracture and displacement of the zygoma can disrupt the lateral wall and floor of the orbit. Subconjunctival ecchymosis and periorbital swelling may be present. Unstable fractures require internal or external fixation, stable fractures can be reduced by operation and no other active management is usually required. Fractures of the orbital walls may tear or compress the optic nerve and blindness is usually immediate and permanent.

Nasal

This injury is very common. Haemorrhage may be severe and nasal packing may be required. Closed reduction and external splinting may be required.

Larynx

Fractures of the larynx are usually caused by blunt trauma. These may severely compromise the airway and necessitate immediate tracheostomy. Surgical exploration and repair is then necessary.

Specific nursing management

Airway and breathing

Constant and careful observation of the airway is essential in any patient with faciomaxillary injuries. Soft tissue swelling and oedema rarely presents as an immediate problem but swelling can increase insidiously. Always remember that a patient who does not have an endotracheal tube or tracheostomy *in situ* is at risk of developing airway problems at a later stage.

Depending on the patient's injuries, the airway may be maintained by the patient him/herself, by a Guedel or nasopharyngeal airway, an endotracheal tube, or a tracheostomy. Humidified oxygen therapy will usually be required, but the patient may not necessarily require mechanical ventilation unless his/her injuries are severe or there are other injuries that necessitate this.

Ensure that oxygen masks are not tight-fitting if there are facial fractures or wounds. Nasal prongs may be more comfortable in some patients but oxygen cannot be humidified by this method. Never use nasal prongs if there is evidence of rhinorrhoea.

Specific respiratory assessment will include observation for any difficulty in breathing and evidence of stridor or increasing oedema of the neck, face, and mouth. If available, pulse oximetry is a useful guide to patient oxygenation but an intra-arterial cannula may be required for monitoring blood gases.

A patient who is tachypnoeic, tachycardic, and in respiratory distress may have a foreign body lodged in a main bronchus. A chest X-ray and bronchoscopy will be required if no other cause is apparent.

In general, patients are best nursed in an upright position if other injuries and the haemodynamic status allows. This encourages drainage of blood, saliva, and CSF away from the airway, reduces venous pressure and encourages fluid reabsorption.

Circulation

Significant haemorrhage can occur in patients with closed injuries to the bony structures of the middle third of the face (maxilla, nose, and ethmoids). Steady bleeding from the nose and oral cavity into the soft tissues of the face can cause profound swelling of the cheeks and a tense skin. Careful monitoring of blood pressure and pulse are essential. Even a small puncture wound that is continually trickling arterial blood can cause significant blood loss and may be overlooked. It is important to be aware of the potential for raised intracranial pressure if there are associated head injuries.

Wounds

Clear guidelines must be obtained from the medical staff regarding specific wound management. Check the scalp for lacerations, bruising, and foreign bodies, such as glass fragments. All wounds should be observed for signs of haemorrhage, haematoma formation, and infection. Monitor temperature regularly and swab and culture any suspected sites of infection. If external fixation has been used to stabilize fractures ensure that pin sites are kept clean and dry.

Mouth

The mouth must be kept clean, moist, and free of infection. This may be difficult in the patient who has his/her jaws wired together or is unable to take oral fluids. Patients who have had major oral surgery and have sutures or skin grafts within the oral cavity may require very frequent mouth care (hourly) and this must be carried out with great care in the immediate post-operative period.

If the jaws are wired together a pair of wire cutters must be available at the bedside and the nurse must be aware as to which wires should be cut if the airway is compromised. Anti-emetics should be given regularly if the patient is nauseated as vomiting must be prevented. A Yankauer suction catheter should be at hand.

Eyes

Observe for peri-orbital swelling (associated with fractures of the zygoma or maxilla) and subconjunctival ecchymosis (haemorrhage) which may be due to direct trauma to the globe or a fracture of the zygoma. A 'blow out' fracture is caused by a direct blow on the eyeball which causes such a rise in intra-orbital pressure that the orbital contents are forced through the orbital floor and herniate into the antrum. As well as bruising and endophthalmus, this causes a tethering of the eyeball where the muscles become trapped in the hernia limiting elevation of the eye and causing diplopia.

Pooling of tears in the eye may indicate damage to the lacrimal apparatus. If present, proptosis or exopthalmus suggests haemorrhage within the orbital walls. Ask the patient if he/she can see clearly. Does he/she have diplopia? Ascertain the normal visual acuity (does he/she wear spectacles normally?). Is there a contact lens or foreign body in the eye? Small particles that have sufficient force to penetrate the tough wall of the eyeball are generally metallic. Retained iron particles in the eye will gradually dissolve and the brown pigment is then dispersed through the ocular tissues but the sight is destroyed. Glass may remain inert for years. Pyrogenic infection of the eyeball often follows penetrating injuries.

Nose

Observe for bleeding or rhinorrhoea. If present, rhinorrhoea suggests a cribriform plate fracture. Never pass a nasogastric or nasotracheal tube in such a patient as the cranial cavity may be intubated. Ask the patient if he has any difficulty breathing through his/her nose. Does the nose look deformed in any way?

Ears

Observe for bleeding or otorrhoea. Look behind the ears for bruising over the mastoid process (Battle sign) which may indicate a basal skull fracture.

Spinal injuries

The most common causes of spinal injuries are vehicular accidents (including motorcycles), diving accidents, and falls. Less commonly they occur as a result of gunshot wounds and sporting activities.

They are often associated with other injuries, particularly to the head and chest. Any unconscious multiply-injured patient must be assumed to have spinal damage until this is excluded by an expert opinion. The first aid management is extremely important as considerable damage to the spinal cord can be caused by inexpert care at the scene of the trauma and in the transfer of the patient to hospital. This section will not discuss the first aid management of spinal injuries but will be concerned with the acute management of the patient on the ICU.

The spinal cord is most often damaged in the cervical region but the thoracolumbar region is also at risk. In this region the spinal canal is narrower relative to the width of the spinal cord and any vertebral displacement is more likely to cause damage to the cord. Injury to the cord leads to bruising or mechanical destruction of the nerves, haemorrhage, and oedema. Some of the cord damage may be reversible but up to four weeks will be required to assess the degree of final damage.

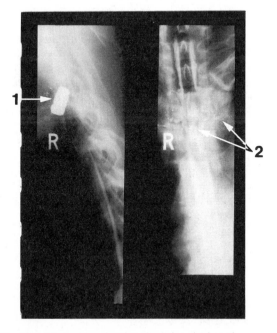

Fig. 11.3 Myelogram showing thoracic spinal cord disruption by a bullet injury. The track of the bullet is visible by the debris (*arrowed*).

The management of the airway, breathing, and circulation must take priority. However, spinal injury must be considered when establishing these priorities and precautions should be taken to prevent exacerbation of any neurological damage.

Nursing priorities

Airway with cervical spine control

In high cervical spine injuries intubation may be required in order to protect the airway or to provide a means of ventilatory support. Vertebral fractures above C5 lead to loss of diaphragmatic function and those above C8 to loss of intercostal function. There may also be other injuries to the head or chest that necessitate intubation in order to maintain effective oxygenation or to secure the airway. The intubation procedure must be carried out by an experienced anaesthetist with an assistant responsible for controlling the head and neck, and minimizing spinal movement. A difficult intubation should be anticipated and the necessary accessories such as a fibreoptic laryngoscope or bronchoscope should be at hand. In patients with acute cervical cord injury, pharyngeal stimulation by a Guedel airway, endotracheal tube or suction may provoke a vagal reflex causing severe bradycardia or asystole. This should be anticipated and can be prevented by the administration of atropine prior to the procedure. In patients with actual or suspected cervical spine injuries the neck must be stabilized at all times using a rigid collar of an appropriate size that grips the chin. However, collars alone are inadequate and lateral support must be given by the use of a sandbag each side of the head (with the head in a neutral position) or by manual stabilization during movement of the patient or during specific procedures. In the ICU, stabilization of the neck and spine must be continued throughout any procedures (e.g. X-rays, insertion of CVP lines). If X-rays confirm spinal damage, more definitive stabilization may be considered such as the use of skull tongs, halopelvic traction, or spinal fusion.

Breathing

The patient with a cervical spine injury who is breathing spontaneously requires very careful observation of his/her respiratory function. Ascending oedema of the traumatized cervical cord may result in deterioration of respiratory status shortly after admission and equipment for manual ventilation must be at the bedside.

Blood gas analysis and/or pulse oximetry should be used to identify hypoxaemia as early as possible.

Hypoxaemia can lead to neurological deterioration and must be avoided

It may be necessary to monitor vital capacity if there is any doubt that respiratory function is inadequate or could possibly deteriorate. This is particularly so in patients with fractures above C8. A forced vital capacity of less than 10–15 ml/kg body weight may indicate the need for ventilatory support.

Patients with spinal injuries should be nursed on a specific type of bed capable of lateral tilting and longitudinal elevation whilst keeping the spine straight (e.g. Stoke Mandeville, Parragon, or Stryker frame). This will ensure that the spine is always in a neutral position and the patient can be tilted head up and feet down to an angle of approximately 45 degrees. This will increase functional residual capacity and is particularly important in patients who have other chest trauma but are breathing spontaneously. Atelectasis is common and the ability to expectorate may be impaired. Regular physiotherapy is therefore essential and the use of narcotic drugs which further suppress respirations should be avoided.

Circulation

All patients with an acute spinal injury should have continuous ECG monitoring. Patients with injury to the cervical or high thoracic cord may have reduced sympathetic outflow between the T1 and L2 segments. This will cause hypotension and bradycardia and is known as neurogenic or 'spinal' shock. Atropine may be needed if the heart rate falls below 50 bpm with associated hypotension (systolic BP < 80 mmHg). This type of shock is purely neurogenic in origin and must be distinguished from hypovolaemic shock which may also be present in the multiply injured patient (characterized by hypotension and tachycardia). Aggressive fluid replacement is detrimental in patients with purely neurogenic hypotension as it precipitates pulmonary oedema. Patients with bradycardia and hypotension may be subjected to a fluid challenge with close monitoring of central venous (and/or pulmonary artery wedge) pressure. The response should be observed and measurements made before more fluid replacement is given. Hypotensive patients unresponsive to fluid replacement may need vasopressor support.

Hypotension and inadequate tissue perfusion may lead to irreversible neurological damage — careful monitoring of vital signs is therefore essential

Abdominal or other occult trauma may not be easily recognized in the tetraplegic patient since the abdominal wall is anaesthetized and flaccid. The classical signs of a rigid, painful abdomen following visceral perforation or haemorrhage may not therefore be apparent. Close monitoring of vital signs and an awareness of potential injury is important. Peritoneal lavage, ultrasound, and X-ray procedures may be performed if there is a suspicion of abdominal trauma. Some patients may feel shoulder tip pain if abdominal injury is present.

Specific nursing management

Paralytic ileus and gastric dilatation are common after spinal cord trauma. A nasogastric tube should be passed (unless contraindicated) and aspirated regularly. Enteral feeding may take time to become established because of this.

Acute urinary retention will develop in tetraplegic and paraplegic patients unless the sacral segments have been spared. A urethral catheter should be inserted (unless contraindicated) and urine output monitored closely. Infection of the urinary tract can become a major problem and catheterization should be carried out under strict aseptic conditions. Regular urinalysis, testing for the presence of white cells, and microbiological culture should be performed. Body temperature should be monitored.

The prevention of pressure sores is vital and meticulous attention must be paid to regular changes of position. Proper positioning is important to prevent pressure on heels and bony prominences, with padding (such as a pillow) placed between the inner surfaces of the knees and between the medial malleoli of the ankles. The skin should be kept clean and dry and hypoalbuminaemia avoided by an adequate nutrition.

The patient will develop atrophy of the extremities owing to disuse and, if their condition allows, passive exercises should be carried out with a range of movements that preserve joint motion and stimulate circulation. The positioning of joints and limbs is important in order to prevent deformities such as footdrop. The patient must be maintained in proper alignment at all times, however, there may be limitations to positioning and limb movements in the multiply-injured patient.

Chest injuries

The majority of chest injuries are caused by blunt trauma. Such injuries may result from a high velocity impact (e.g. a rapid deceleration as seen in road traffic accidents), a low velocity impact (e.g. a direct blow to the chest), or from crushing trauma to the chest. Less commonly, penetrating injuries, such as knife and gunshot wounds, are also seen. Many patients with severe intrathoracic injuries, such as laceration of the heart, aorta, or major airways, do not survive to reach hospital. Patients with chest trauma also often have other injuries such as head, spinal, abdominal, and faciomaxillary damage. Some will be multiply-injured. The priorities of management are, as always, maintenance of airway, breathing, and circulation, with identification and correction of life-threatening injuries.

Nursing priorities

Airway and breathing

A patent airway must be secured; intubation or tracheostomy may be required, depending on the patient's injuries. Chest injury often leads to tissue hypoxia. This may be caused by diminished blood volume, failure to ventilate the lungs adequately, ventilation/perfusion mismatch, or changes in intrapleural pressures, which lead to lung collapse with displacement of mediastinal structures. Hypoxia must be corrected and interventions are aimed at ensuring that adequate amounts of oxygen are delivered to the parts of the lung that are capable of normal ventilation and perfusion. If intubation is necessary to secure the airway, mechanical ventilation will normally be required. IPPV will be necessary in patients who are unconcious, have severe respiratory distress, or associated head injuries, where hypoxia must be avoided. A chest X-ray will have been taken as a matter of priority in the casualty department of any patient with suspected chest injuries. Many serious injuries including fractures, haemo- or pneumothorax, cardiac tamponade, ruptured diaphragm, dissecting aorta, and major airway disruptions can be diagnosed. Pneumothoraces should ideally be identified and drained before mechanical ventilation is instituted, although this may not always be possible. Close monitoring of arterial blood gases is essential and appropriate levels of oxygen must be administered to correct hypoxaemia.

In the self-ventilating patient careful and continuous monitoring of respiratory function must be made. Signs of respiratory distress may indicate the need for further interventions (see Chapter 3). Note that central cyanosis may be a late or absent sign of hypoxaemia in patients with a decreased haemoglobin as a result of haemorrhage.

Circulation

Patients with major cardiac or vascular lacerations may have had haemorrhage arrested by a tamponade effect. Rapid transfusion and the subsequent increase in arterial and intracardiac pressures may result in uncontrollable and fatal bleeding. Such injuries must be identified before resuscitation elevates the systolic blood pressure > 100 mmHg.

Continuous ECG and monitoring of vital signs is essential. Myocardial contusions are common in chest injuries and may give rise to tachyarrhythmias and conduction abnormalities. Large blood losses may result from haemothoraces and tearing of thoracic vessels. Observe for signs of hypovolaemia (see Chapter 5). Is the patient peripherally cool and poorly perfused? Look at the patient's colour. Is he/she pale? Are there signs of obvious bleeding (e.g. from chest or wound drains)?

Specific chest injuries

Pulmonary contusions

These occur when shearing or crushing forces are applied to the thoracic cage and cause disruption of the microcirculation. Extravasation of red cells and plasma occurs and these fluids fill the alveoli. This results in interstitial haemorrhage and alveolar collapse in the contused area. Gas exchange is impaired as perfusion is maintained in the unventilated lung segments causing intrapulmonary shunting and subsequent hypoxaemia. The infiltrates are usually absorbed after 3–5 days but may progress in complicated cases. A chest X-ray will reveal localized areas of contusion and haemorrhage.

Management is aimed at ensuring adequate ventilation and treating hypoxaemia. If severe, intubation and mechanical ventilation may be required. Pain control is important. Intercostal nerve blocks or epidural analgesia are extremely useful. A patient with adequate pain relief will breathe more deeply, be co-operative with physiotherapy, and clear secretions more effectively. Supplemental oxygen therapy should be given and blood gases monitored. If the patient is mechanically ventilated, manoeuvres to improve oxygenation are aimed at reducing the shunt (e.g. postural changes), increasing the F_iO_2, increasing the functional residual capacity by the use of PEEP, and improving tracheobronchial toilet by effective suctioning and physiotherapy.

Rib fractures

Blood loss and disruption of the underlying lung tissue are associated with rib fractures. The sharp edges of the fractured rib may lacerate the underlying lung causing haemorrhage. Any number of ribs may be fractured and if several ribs are fractured in more than one place or the broken ribs are combined with fracture dislocations of the costochondrial junctions or sternum, this is known as a flail segment and moves independently of the rib cage. The negative intrapleural pressures generated on inspiration will pull this segment inwards creating a paradoxical movement and thus compromise ventilation by reducing tidal volume. A flail segment itself is not an indication for mechanical ventilation but the functional consequences must determine the necessity for ventilatory support. Recent studies have shown a decreased mortality in patients with extensive rib fractures using a conservative approach to pain relief as opposed to routine mechanical ventilation, provided that the P_aO_2 remains above 6.6 kPa on an F_iO_2 of 0.5, vital capacity remains above 10 ml/kg and respiratory rate below 40 breaths/min.

Adequate analgesia is absolutely essential in patients with rib fractures. Pain will inhibit inspiration and lead to atelectasis in the basal segments, prevent adequate coughing, and clearance of secretions, and limit effective physiotherapy. If there are few unilateral rib fractures, oral analgesia, intercostal nerve blocks, or thoracic epidural analgesia may be sufficient, but in multiple fractures intravenous analgesia may be needed in addition. A mini-tracheotomy may prevent intubation if there is difficulty in clearing secretions. Chest strapping is no longer recommended as this will only serve to inhibit effective ventilation.

Close monitoring of blood gases will be required and pulse oximetry will be useful. Careful observation of respiratory function is vital. Assist with physiotherapy, encourage the patient to breathe deeply and cough to clear secretions. Position the patient in an upright and comfortable position if his/her condition allows. Assess the effect of any analgesia given and review this if pain persists.

Pneumothorax (simple, open, tension) and haemothorax

Chest injuries are often accompanied by either the collection of blood in the chest cavity (haemothorax) from torn intercostal vessels or haemorrhage from lacerated lung tissue, or the escape of air from injured lung into the pleural cavity (pneumothorax). Often both blood and air are found in the pleural cavity (haemopneumothorax). The lung on that side of the chest is compressed and ventilation is impaired. A small pneumothorax can be allowed to resolve spontaneously provided it is not compromising ventilation and is not

enlarging. A chest drain will however usually need to be inserted, particularly if the patient requires mechanical ventilation.

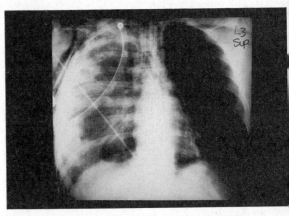

(a)

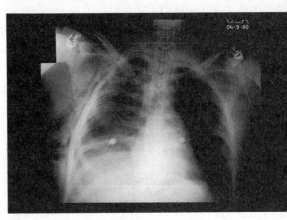

(b)

Fig. 11.4 X-ray showing fractured ribs, pulmonary contusions and pneumothorax. Before (A) and after (B) insertion of chest drain on left side.

A tension pneumothorax is a medical emergency and requires immediate decompression. In this situation, air is drawn into the pleural space from a lacerated lung or through a hole in the chest wall. Air that enters with each inspiration is trapped and cannot be expelled, therefore tension builds up. The lung is compressed and collapses, pushing the mediastinal structures (heart, trachea, and great vessels) towards the unaffected side of the chest (mediastinal shift), impairing ventilation in the other lung. Thus, tension pneumothorax results in impairment of cardiovascular as well as respiratory function. Collapse and electromechanical dissociation may rapidly result. The diagnosis of tension pneumothorax is made clinically; there is no time to take a chest X-ray before treatment is instituted. The patient will become hypoxaemic and may be tachycardiac and hypotensive. Air entry will be absent over the affected area and chest movement reduced. The trachea may be deviated, the neck veins distended, and the patient will become progressively cyanosed. Immediate decompression is obtained by inserting a needle into the second intercostal space in the mid-clavicular line of the affected hemithorax. The ability to aspirate air into the syringe attached to the needle will confirm the diagnosis and converts the injury to a simple pneumothorax. A chest drain should now be inserted. If there is failure to aspirate air from the needle, the needle and syringe should be withdrawn but the possibility of a pneumothorax now exists as a result of the needle insertion.

Massive blood loss may result from haemothoraces and these are usually caused by penetrating injuries lacerating systemic or pulmonary vessels. Such injuries are accompanied by hypovolaemic shock and insertion of a chest drain may reveal a considerable amount of blood in the chest cavity. Concurrent drainage of the haemothorax and volume resuscitation is required. Some patients will require surgical intervention and this is usually dependent on the continuing rate of blood loss. Very careful measurement of blood in the chest drain is required (every 15–30 minutes) and continuous monitoring of vital signs as fluid replacement is given.

An open pneumothorax is caused by a penetrating injury to the chest which leaves an open hole between the atmosphere and the chest cavity. Equilibrium between intrathoracic pressure and atmospheric pressure is immediate and if the opening in the chest wall is more than two-thirds the diameter of the trachea air will pass preferentially into the chest through the hole (causing a 'sucking' chest wound). Ventilation is impaired and the patient will become hypoxaemic. The hole must be sealed immediately with an occlusive dressing and taped securely on three sides only. Leaving one side of the dressing open will allow air to escape as the patient exhales, but as the patient breathes in the dressing is occlusively sucked over the wound preventing air from entering. If the hole is sealed completely, air will accumulate in the thoracic cavity resulting in a tension pneumothorax. This is a temporary measure; a chest drain should be inserted remote from the open wound. Surgical closure of the wound is often required.

Low pressure suction (up to 10 kPa) may be applied to chest drains in order to aid evacuation of air and blood from the pleural cavity. Pressure levels must be checked regularly and chest drain tubing may need to be 'milked'

frequently to prevent blood clots blocking the tubing and impairing drainage (for comprehensive care of chest drains refer to Chapter 3). If the patient is making any inspiratory effort, two chest drain clamps must always be available at the bedside in case of accidental disconnection of the tubing. A tension pneumothorax or a pneumothorax drain that is bubbling excessively must not be clamped or air will build up in the chest cavity.

Cardiac tamponade

This results from penetrating or blunt trauma which cause the pericardium to fill with blood from the heart or great vessels. The pericardium is a fibrous structure and even relatively small amounts of fluid in the pericardial sac will restrict cardiac filling. Cardiac tamponade is characterized by an increase in heart rate and central venous pressure, and a decrease in blood pressure and cardiac output. Peripheral perfusion will be poor and the neck veins may become distended due to the increase in central venous pressure. Pulsus paradoxus (disappearance or weakening of the radial pulse on inspiration) may be palpated. Large, cyclical, beat-to-beat variations may also be seen in the monitored systemic blood pressure trace that is related to the phases of the respiratory cycle.

Treatment is by pericardiocentesis where blood is aspirated by needle and syringe from the pericardium. If the blood in the pericardium is clotted, however, aspiration will be impossible. If the patient is moribund open thoracotomy may be required. Cardiac tamponade caused by penetrating trauma will need surgical exploration and repair.

Myocardial contusion

This is caused by blunt trauma to the chest or deceleration trauma, and is comparable in diagnosis and treatment to a myocardial infarction. ECG changes will be apparent: usually non-specific ST segment and T wave changes. Dysrhythmias are common and may be fatal. Tachyarrhythmias, multiple premature ventricular ectopics, and conduction disturbances (heart block and bundle branch block) often occur. Serial cardiac enzymes will be elevated. Continuous ECG monitoring is essential as the onset of dysrhythmias may be sudden. Cardiogenic shock rarely results from myocardial contusions, but if it does, inotropic support and intra-aortic balloon counterpulsation may be required to maintain systemic arterial pressure.

Diaphragmatic rupture

This usually follows penetrating or blunt trauma to the abdomen and may result in the abdominal contents being forced into the chest through a laceration in the diaphragm. The liver usually prevents herniation through the right hemidiaphragm and it is therefore most commonly seen on the left side. Herniation of the stomach into the chest may become evident when a nasogastric tube is seen in the chest cavity on X-ray. Early IPPV may mask the signs of respiratory distress that would be evident in the self-ventilating patient. Penetrating injuries into the abdomen may lacerate the diaphragm and cause a haemothorax. Most patients with a diaphragmatic rupture will require surgical exploration and repair.

Major airway injuries

Blunt or penetrating trauma may cause rupture of the trachea or bronchus, or tears and punctures of the lung tissue. The presence of surgical emphysema is a sign of airway injury and in transection of the trachea or bronchus this may be extensive in the mediastinum and subcutaneous tissues. Pneumothorax and haemothorax are commonly associated and usually require drainage. Rupture of a large bronchus may cause haemoptysis and atelectasis of the affected lung. Patients with complete transection of the trachea often die rapidly of asphyxia but an adequate airway may exist and treatment is usually by surgical repair. Patients with tracheal rupture may have stridor, aphonia, and respiratory distress. Considerable problems may be encountered in endotracheal intubation. Blind intubation may prove fatal and fibreoptic intubation may be required.

Penetrating injuries are often accompanied by injuries to the oesophagus, carotid artery, and jugular vein; missile injuries may cause extensive tissue destruction.

Aortic rupture

This usually occurs as a result of deceleration trauma but occasionally from penetrating trauma. Tears of the aorta and pulmonary arteries are frequently fatal: 90% of patients will die at the scene of the injury. Most survivors will have had the blood loss contained by a haematoma, and an intact adventitia (outer wall) may prevent immediate death. Initial severe hypotension will occur with the loss of up to 1000 ml of blood and the patient will usually respond to rapid fluid resuscitation. However, hypotension may be recurrent or persistent and blood transfusion will be necessary to maintain oxygen carrying capacity and arterial pressure. A chest X-ray may show a widened mediastinum, tracheal shift to the right, and blurring of the aortic outline. Early angiography would be indicated if the patient's condition permits but urgent surgical repair may be required.

Abdominal and pelvic injuries

Penetrating injuries, particularly stab and gunshot wounds, are common causes of abdominal trauma in young men. Blunt trauma most often results from road traffic accidents and falls; many of these patients will have associated injuries to the head, spine, chest, and genitourinary system. These injuries will complicate management, and it must be remembered that patients with abdominal injuries have the potential for severe haemorrhage and an increased risk of post-traumatic sepsis. Injuries resulting from blunt trauma to the abdomen are the most difficult to diagnose and, in the multiply-injured patient, the signs of intra-abdominal injury (pain, guarding) may be difficult to assess or masked by other injuries.

The immediate management is aimed at identifying the presence of abdominal injury rather than making an accurate diagnosis of a specific injury. The liver, spleen, and kidneys are the major organs involved in blunt trauma. Visceral disruption can occur as a result of rapid deceleration, a direct blow or shearing forces. The compulsory use of seat belts in vehicles has reduced mortality from head and faciomaxillary injuries but has significantly increased the incidence of damage to the thoracic cage, liver, spleen, and mesentery.

Diagnosis can be aided by various procedures such as peritoneal lavage, computerized tomography, ultrasonography, X-rays, and selective angiography. Peritoneal lavage is performed by installation of a litre of normal saline into the peritoneal cavity through a percutaneous catheter; this fluid is then drained out through the same catheter and examined for blood. The technique is accurate in 95% of cases in detecting intra-abdominal haemorrhage (including bleeding from pelvic fractures) and is helpful in evaluating the need for laparotomy.

Injuries sustained from penetrating trauma will depend upon the type of weapon or object, its path or trajectory, and in the case of gunshot wounds, the velocity and calibre of bullet. Stab wounds will penetrate adjacent structures but bullets may have a circuitous or tumbling action causing extensive tissue damage involving multiple organs.

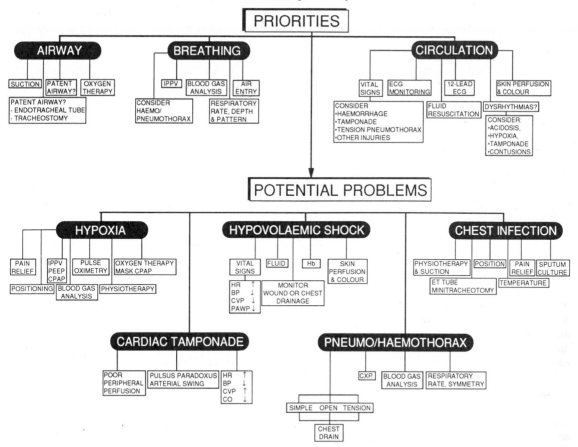

Fig. 11.5 Schema of chest injury management.

Abdominal injuries

Initial resuscitation priorities of the patient with abdominal trauma are maintenance of airway, breathing, and circulation. Specific treatment of abdominal injuries should not delay correction of hypoxaemia and tissue perfusion. Urgent laparotomy may be indicated if hypovolaemia persists after adequate fluid replacement and the cause cannot be attributed to other injuries. In the ICU the patient must be carefully observed for increasing abdominal pain, rigidity or tenderness. Continuous monitoring of vital signs is essential. It is important to be alert for haemodynamic changes that indicate haemorrhage (tachycardia, hypotension, low CVP, poor peripheral perfusion, pale colour) or the need for excessive fluid replacement that does not improve the cardiovascular status. The abdominal cavity is a potential reservoir for major occult blood loss and injury must always be suspected if there is bruising or superficial

lacerations (e.g. from seat belts) which may indicate damage to underlying organs.

Unless contraindicated, a urethral catheter should be inserted in patients with severe abdominal trauma in order to monitor urine output. The presence of haematuria is an important sign of potential genitourinary damage although such damage can occur without any subsequent haematuria. Similarly, a naso- or orogastric tube should be inserted (unless contraindicated) in order to decompress the stomach, reduce the risk of pneumonic aspiration of stomach contents, and detect the presence of upper gastrointestinal injury (if blood is aspirated). Remember that patients whose prime insult is not to the abdomen may still have the potential for abdominal injury. Trauma to the lower chest (e.g. rib fractures or stab wounds) may damage the underlying abdominal viscera. This is because at full expiration the diaphragm rises to the level of the 4th intercostal space. Up to 60% of gunshot wounds and 25% of stab wounds in this region of the chest will cause abdominal injury.

Pelvic fractures

Pelvic fractures may cause massive and sometimes un-controllable haemorrhage (up to 4 litres of blood may be lost). However, 75% of patients will become haemo-dynamically stable after initial fluid resuscitation. The associated muscles are also very vascular and major veins and arteries in the pelvis can easily be disrupted by trauma. The mortality of patients with open pelvic fractures exceeds 50% and associated rectal and geni-tourinary injuries are common. Approximately 30% of patients with pelvic fractures also have a ruptured bladder and torn urethra.

Severe haemorrhage may be difficult to control and pneumatic antishock garments (e.g. MAST suit) may be useful in initial resuscitation. Immobilization and inter-nal/external fixation may help control bleeding but surgical repair of torn vessels or angiography and em-bolization may be required.

Signs of haemorrhagic shock

- Tachycardia

- Hypotension

- Low CVP

- Low PAWP

- Poor peripheral perfusion

Genitourinary injuries

Upper genitourinary injuries (kidneys, upper ureters, and renal vessels)

Injuries to the kidneys are most often caused by blunt trauma (sporting injuries, falls, vehicular accidents, and assaults): 40% of patients will have associated or multiple injuries that may obscure the signs and symptoms of renal trauma. Penetrating trauma directly to the kidney from stab or gunshot wounds are easy to diagnose but may cause injury to other organs, such as the spleen, liver, pancreas, bowel, and duodenum, or perforate the dia-phragm. Damage from penetrating trauma can be severe and extensive, particularly from gunshot wounds causing laceration of the renal vessels, kidney, and ureters.

Direct blows to the back resulting in bruising and abrasions may indicate underlying renal damage and in any patient sustaining deceleration trauma there is potential for genitourinary injury. Rapid deceleration (as in falls) may cause tearing of the renal vessels, intimal tearing, or rupture of the ureters at the pelviureteric junction. Direct blows to the abdomen can crush the kidney between the anterior end of the 12th rib and the lumbar spine. Fractures to the lower ribs or spinal processes should therefore raise suspicion of renal in-jury. Vehicular accidents may cause renal injury if a seat belt, steering wheel, or other external mechanical forces crush the kidney anteriorly between the abdominal wall and the paravertebral muscles.

Renal trauma can be categorized into minor, major, or critical injuries. Minor injuries are limited to minor parenchymal damage, contusions, and superficial lacera-tions to the kidney. These are the most common and constitute 85% of renal trauma. Major injuries are considered to be deep lacerations involving the pelvi-calyceal system and/or tears of the capsule. They result in major parenchymal damage and constitute 10% of renal injuries. Critical injuries include renal fragmentation and pedicle injuries (renal artery thrombosis, pelviureteric rupture, or avulsion of renal vessels) and occur in 5% of renal trauma. Major blood loss can occur in these patients with consequent hypovolaemic shock.

The patient sustaining a direct blow to the flank may elicit signs of bruising or swelling over the lower thoracic, loin, or upper abdominal areas. The patient will often complain of loin pain, and the anterior abdominal wall may be rigid on the affected side. Haematuria may be present and painful ureteric colic may occur if blood clots are passed through the ureter.

The initial management of the patient will depend on his/her clinical state. The airway, breathing, and circula-tion must be stabilized before attention is directed to a specific diagnosis of renal injury or lengthy X-ray in-vestigations are carried out. Renal trauma alone rarely causes severe hypovolaemic shock or threatens life. If hypovolaemia is present other injuries must be consid-ered beforehand as the prime cause. Once the patient's oxygen requirements and circulation are stabilized, diag-nostic X-ray procedures can be undertaken. Intravenous urography is usually carried out in all patients with haematuria and a systolic blood pressure less than 90 mmHg. Renal ultrasonography is used on patients who are clinically stable but require evaluation of renal damage. Occasionally, a retrograde ureterogram may be required in patients with suspected disruption of the pelviureteric junction and selective renal arteriogra-phy may be performed in patients with persistent hae-maturia (longer than one week) or those with vascular pedicle injuries.

Patients with critical renal injuries or penetrating trauma will require surgical exploration. Lacerations to the renal vessels may then be repaired and partial or total nephrectomy will be required for patients with fragmented kidneys. Patients with a renal artery thrombosis that has been identified within 10 hours of the trauma may be considered for thrombectomy.

All patients with renal injuries, however minor, must be observed closely.

Vital signs should be recorded frequently, urine output monitored and observed for haematuria. Pain must be assessed and adequate analgesia administered. Any loin swelling should be observed for change in size and prophylactic antibiotics are usually given. Strict bedrest is enforced until the vital signs are stable, haematuria has ceased, and any perirenal swelling has clinically resolved.

Lower genitourinary injuries (bladder, urethra, genitalia)

Injuries to the bladder, urethra, and genitalia can be caused by penetrating trauma (particularly gunshot) but more commonly from blunt trauma. In patients with suspected lower genitourinary trauma injuries, the urethral meatus must be inspected for blood, the abdomen examined for signs of peritonism, and the perineum for signs of bruising. A urethral catheter must not be inserted in patients with suspected trauma or major pelvic fractures until advised by a urologist. If blood is present in the meatus, intravenous urography (antegrade or retrograde) will be required to detect a perforated or displaced bladder before suprapubic catheterization. Pelvic fractures are a common cause of injury to the bladder and urethra due to perforation from a bony segment. Signs of urethral injury are blood in the urethral meatus, inability to void, and perineal bruising. If these are present a urethral catheter must not be passed as the urethra is often traumatized and devascularized when torn and may be eroded by the catheter, disintegrate around it, or the catheter may be passed through the tear. The catheter would also prevent haematoma drainage and may introduce infection. A suprapubic catheter must therefore be inserted.

In patients with pelvic fractures but no evidence of blood in the meatus, a urethral catheter may be passed and a cystogram used to exclude bladder rupture. Patients who are shocked, have peritonism (a rigid, painful abdomen), and in whom cystography shows bladder rupture will require laparotomy. In women, the urethra is rarely damaged from pelvic fractures and a urethral catheter can usually be passed, following which cystography may be performed to exclude bladder injuries.

Bulbar injuries are usually caused by direct trauma (e.g. a straddle impact) and such patients will have blood in the urethral meatus and perineal bruising. A urethral catheter must never be passed as this will introduce infection and aggravate the injury. The patient should be allowed to pass urine naturally, but if retention occurs a suprapubic catheter should be inserted. Prophylactic antibiotics should be given. Injuries to the scrotum and penis can also occur. Scrotal tears heal very well and do not normally require suturing but direct blows to the scrotum can cause large scrotal haematomas and damage to the testes which may require surgical repair.

Specific nursing management

The nursing management of the patient with abdominal trauma (including pelvic fractures) will depend on the patient's specific injuries. Those patients with severe abdominal injuries will probably undergo explorative laparotomy and definitive surgery before they are admitted to the ICU. Care will then be directed towards anticipating potential problems relating to the specific surgery.

All patients will require careful monitoring of vital signs, urine output, wound drainage, and blood gas analysis. It is essential to always be aware of potential haemorrhage even after surgery as coagulation defects are common after major trauma and large blood transfusions. Anticipate complications arising from the hypoperfusion of major organs if large blood losses have occurred. Management must always be directed to restabilizing vital functions and optimizing oxygenation and tissue perfusion. Blood glucose levels must be monitored, particularly after surgery to the pancreas or liver, and the need for parenteral nutrition considered if the enteral route cannot be used for some time.

Patients with pelvic fractures may pose particular problems in the care of pressure areas. Clear instructions must be obtained from the surgeons as to the degree of mobility that the patient is allowed. Nursing is made considerably easier if the fracture is stable or externally/internally fixed. However, some type of pressure-relieving mattress will be required as movement will still be considerably limited.

Patients with abdominal and pelvic injuries are more susceptible to infection, particularly if the injury results from penetrating trauma. Contamination may occur from foreign material (such as clothing in missile injuries) and if the gastrointestinal tract is disrupted the bowel contents may be distributed into the peritoneal cavity. Such patients are at risk from local infection (abscess formation), septicaemia, and multi-organ failure. Patients who have undergone total splenectomy are at risk from overwhelming bacterial sepsis due to diminished humoral immunity and operative measures now attempt to preserve some splenic tissue. Prophylactic antibiotics should be administered to patients with

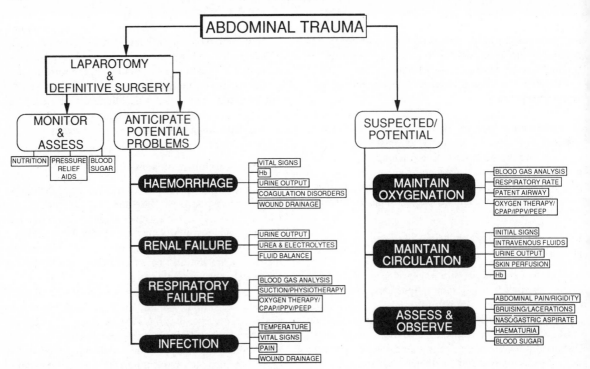

Fig. 11.6 Schema of abdominal trauma management.

penetrating trauma and the patient must be monitored for potential infection (e.g. temperature, signs of peritonism, presence of purulent discharge from wounds or drains).

The measurement of abdominal girth as an indication of intra-abdominal haemorrhage remains controversial. The abdominal cavity is capable of containing a significant amount of blood without distension and large blood losses can occur retroperitoneally. An increase in girth may, therefore, be a late sign of haemorrhage or be due to the presence of air and/or fluid in the bowel. Girth is often inaccurately measured, particularly post-operatively if wounds are re-padded or dressings changed. Today, when accurate and continuous haemodynamic monitoring can be made, where changes in vital signs can be detected almost immediately, and where haemoglobin and haematocrit measurements can be carried out rapidly, there is no place for girth measurement in the detection of intra-abdominal bleeding — rather, it should be used as an adjunct to changes in haemodynamic parameters that suggest haemorrhage.

Musculoskeletal injuries

Musculoskeletal injuries themselves are rarely life-threatening but their associated injuries can be. Up to 70% of multiply-injured patients will have injured limbs, fractures, or dislocations. The management of limb trauma is always secondary to resuscitation and control of the airway, breathing, and circulation. Only when the multiply-injured patient is stable is attention directed to the definitive care of the limb injury. At this point a thorough head-to-toe examination is carried out and limb X-rays are taken. Certain musculoskeletal conditions are considered life-threatening. These include traumatic amputations (particularly of a whole limb), major haemorrhage from vascular injuries or open fractures, severe crush injuries to the pelvis and abdomen, and multiple long bone fractures.

Blood loss from open wounds may seem obvious but large amounts of blood can be lost in closed fractures. Major haemorrhage can occur in closed fractures of the humerus and tibia (up to 1.5 litres each) and femur (up to 2.5 litres). Rapid resuscitation is vital to replace lost circulatory volume, however, the cause of haemorrhagic shock must never presumed to originate solely from skeletal injury — other potential injuries must be considered. Open wounds or fractures may have bled extensively from the time of the injury and blood loss may be difficult to assess. Generally, for open fractures the blood loss is 2–3 times greater than that of closed fractures. Direct pressure should be applied to any bleeding, open wounds by compression bandage or hand pressure, until definitive treatment can be carried out.

A fracture also produces damage to the muscles surrounding the injured bone and to the blood vessels and nerves in its vicinity. Penetrating trauma and local contusions may disrupt blood flow; furthermore, peripheral circulation may be poor in the hypovolaemic patient. Vascular impairment and neurovascular bundle injury may therefore compromise the survival of a limb and must be identified without delay. Bleeding or thrombosis in a blood vessel can impair the distal circulation and cause limb ischaemia. Vascular injury should be identified promptly by close and regular observation before ischaemia develops. Peripheral limb pulses must therefore be evaluated regularly to assess circulation and an absent or diminished pulse reported without delay. Skin perfusion should be assessed by the capillary return, temperature and colour of the limb distal to the injury. A low skin temperature indicates inadequate perfusion. Check that plaster casts, traction, and compression bandages are not impairing circulation.

If nerve damage has occurred sensation will be impaired. This sensation is lost early if ischaemia is present. Nerve injury may be caused by direct severing of nerve fibres by penetrating trauma or by stretching or compression of the nerve fibres causing variable degrees of paralysis.

Dislocations may produce neurovascular injury by stretching nerves and compressing blood vessels causing muscle injury. They should be reduced promptly, particularly at the knee, elbow, and ankle. Angiography may be required if vascular injury is suspected. Obvious and complete arterial occlusion will however, require prompt surgical exploration.

Musculoskeletal injuries

Check limbs for:

- Colour

- Temperature

- Pulses

- Sensation/pain

- Local compression (plaster-of-Paris, splints, bandages)

Compartment syndrome and rhabdomyolysis are specific complications following musculoskeletal injuries and are discussed fully on pp. 233 and 336.

Specific management

Open fractures

In this type of fracture a wound in the skin communicates directly with the broken bone. The most important factor in management is to prevent infection thus open fractures should be definitively treated within 8 hours of the injury. The fracture should be aligned and splinted and the wound covered with a sterile dry dressing. Antibiotic therapy should be instituted and tetanus prophylaxis administered. Surgery will include the thorough cleaning of the wound and debridement of non-viable tissue. Wounds are often left open for 5–7 days to prevent a rise in tissue pressure which contributes to wound hypoxia and infection. Open fractures are often unstable; rigid stabilization will promote tissue healing and a variety of methods can be used.

Closed fractures

In this type of fracture there is no open wound. In the multiply-injured patient early fixation of fractures (within 24 hours) can reduce mortality and morbidity from ARDS, fat embolism, and systemic sepsis. Nursing of the patient is made considerably easier and analgesia requirements can be reduced.

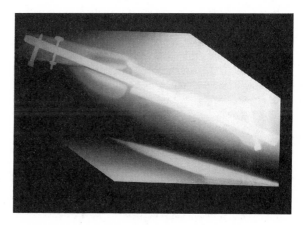

Fig. 11.7 Repair of compound femoral structure (intramedullary nail).

Dislocations

Dislocations must be reduced promptly to prevent potentially irreversible damage to neurovascular bundles and plexus injuries.

All dislocations are extremely painful. Adequate analgesia must be given, although occasionally with caution in the presence of other injuries. The limb should be supported on a pillow or immobilized with traction whilst awaiting definitive treatment.

Table 11.3 Types of dislocations and associated complications

Dislocation	Associated complication
Knee	Popliteal artery/nerve injuries
Ankle	Skin pressure and necrosis
Elbow	Ulnar and median nerve damage
Shoulder	Brachial plexus injury
Hip	Aseptic necrosis of femoral head

Specific nursing management of musculoskeletal injuries

Specific nursing care will be dictated by the extent of the patient's injuries and his/her degree of immobility. Several methods can be used to maintain reduction of fractures depending on the nature of the fracture; for example, plaster casts, splints, continuous traction, pin and plaster techniques, and internal fixation devices (nails, plates, wires, screws, and rods). Continuous traction can be by means of skin traction or skeletal traction using wires, pins, or tongs placed through the bone with a system of ropes, pulleys, and weights. Space does not permit a comprehensive explanation of the nursing management of orthopaedic injuries. However, the patient in the ICU frequently has multiple injuries or has some other serious injury as well as a fracture that necessitates his/her stay on the unit.

The following are basic points to remember:

1. The patient in traction
- Check the skin around the traction device for evidence of circulatory impairment.

- Frequent and meticulous attention to pressure areas. Use a pressure-relieving mattress if available.

- Inspect pin sites daily and keep clean and dry.

- Passive/active exercises to non-immobilized joints.

- The knots on the traction rope should be secure and the supporting apparatus free of the pulleys.

- Check that the ropes are in the wheel groove and the weights hang free.

- The weights should not be removed when the patient is moved. One nurse must support the weights without relieving the traction if a patient is moved up the bed.

2. The patient with a plaster cast

Constriction due to swelling may cause circulatory impairment, pain, and pressure on healthy tissue. Therefore, check skin temperature, colour, pulses, and sensation in the affected limb. Check skin integrity around the edge of the cast. Pressure points may need extra padding.

Pain under the cast may be due to pressure on a bony prominence, nerve, or blood vessel. Supracondylar fractures of the elbow are often accompanied by considerable swelling which may impair circulation in the forearm and hand. The radial pulse must be checked frequently in the first 24 hours. Elevating the limb on a pillow may alleviate swelling but if severe the plaster may need to be split.

3. Anticipate complications
- *Haemorrhage* — monitor vital signs, observe wounds and drains for bleeding, monitor haemoglobin.

- *Compartment syndrome* — observe limb frequently for tense swelling, pain, and diminished sensation.

- *Infection* — monitor temperature, inspect wounds, cannulae, and pin sites. Swab and culture if necessary.

- *Deep vein thrombosis* — inspect calves for pain and swelling. Consider antiembolic stockings and prophylactic anticoagulation. Passive/active limb movements may help prevent thrombosis.

- *Rhabdomyolysis* — monitor urine output, daily urinalysis, observe urine for myoglobinuria, measure plasma creatine kinase (CPK). Keep patient well hydrated and maintain a good diuresis. Monitor urea and electrolytes, including magnesium, calcium and phosphate.

Complications following trauma

Complications secondary to trauma can result from:

1. Shock causing hypoperfusion of vital organs (e.g. renal and circulatory failure). The origin of the shock may be:

- hypovolaemic (e.g. haemorrhage),

- septic,

- neurogenic (e.g. spinal injury),

- obstructive (e.g. pulmonary embolus),

- cardiogenic (e.g. direct myocardial contusion).

2. Specific types of trauma causing rhabdomyolysis, compartment syndrome, air embolism, and fat embolism syndrome (e.g. long bone fractures, chest injuries, crush injuries).

3. Transfusion of large amounts of blood causing anaphylactic reactions, ARDS, multi-organ failure, coagulopathies, and hypocalcaemia.

4. Infection causing septicaemia and multi-organ failure.

5. Immobility causing pressure sores, deep vein thrombosis (DVT), and pulmonary embolism.

6. Hypoxaemia from chest, head, and neck injuries causing respiratory failure and multi-organ failure.

Shock

Although shock is generally described as hypotension and tachycardia, a more accurate definition is inadequate tissue oxygen delivery due to hypoperfusion. Hypotension need not necessarily be present to indicate organ hypoperfusion. At a cellular level, inadequately perfused cells compensate initially for the lack of oxygen supply by shifting to anaerobic metabolism. This results in lactic acid formation and thus development of a metabolic acidosis. If shock is prolonged, cellular swelling occurs, leading to cellular damage and death. Management is directed at reversing this phenomenon with adequate oxygenation, appropriate fluid resuscitation, and vasoactive drug support as necessary.

Hypovolaemic shock

All types of shock may be present in the trauma patient but the vast majority of injured patients in shock are hypovolaemic — usually haemorrhagic.

Early haemodynamic responses to blood loss are compensatory (i.e. progressive vasoconstriction of cutaneous, visceral, and muscle regional circulations in order to preserve blood flow to the kidneys, heart, and brain). A young person can lose over 30% of his/her circulating blood volume before showing any significant change in heart rate and blood pressure, especially if supine. Only when intravascular depletion is so great as to exhaust these compensatory mechanisms does hypotension ensue. The body also compensates for intravascular volume loss by redistributing fluid from the extravascular compartments into the blood stream.

The direct effect of haemorrhage depends on the percentage of acute blood volume lost and can be considered in four classes:

Class 1. Loss of up to 15% of blood
Clinical signs are lacking. Minimal tachycardia, no measurable changes in blood pressure, pulse pressure, respiratory rate, or capillary refill test. Replacement of the primary fluid losses will correct the circulatory state.

Class 2. 15–30% blood loss
This would represent 800–1500 ml of blood loss in a 70 kg adult.

Clinical symptoms may include tachycardia, tachypnoea, a decrease in pulse pressure (the difference between the systolic and diastolic pressures), and a minimal change in systolic pressure. Other changes include subtle central nervous system changes, such as anxiety, fright, or hostility. Normally urine output is only mildly affected — usually 20–30 ml/h in the 70 kg adult.

Class 3. 30–40% blood loss
This would represent about 2000 ml loss in an adult and its clinical effects can be devastating. Patients present with classical signs of inadequate perfusion — marked tachycardia, tachypnoea, significant changes in mental state, and a considerable fall in blood pressure.

Class 4. More than 40% blood loss
This degree of blood loss is immediately life-threatening. Symptoms include a marked tachycardia, significant fall in blood pressure, a very narrow pulse pressure, or an unobtainable diastolic pressure. Urinary output is negligible and mental status markedly depressed. The skin is cold and pale. Such patients require rapid transfusion and immediate surgical intervention. Blood loss of over 50% of the patient's blood volume results in loss of consciousness, pulse, and blood pressure.

Management of hypovolaemic shock

Hypovolaemia must be promptly diagnosed and treated. Vascular access must be obtained immediately using large-bore cannulae. In severe cases, the peripheral veins may be collapsed and cannulation may prove impossible. Either an intravenous cut-down on to a peripheral vein, or cannulation of a central vein can be performed. Difficulty can sometimes be experienced with a jugular or subclavian approach with an increased risk of complication (e.g. pneumothorax). In these cases, the femoral vein is usually readily accessible and safer.

Baseline observations of vital signs and sequential monitoring are crucial. It should be noted that the central venous pressure may purely reflect the body's continuing ability to vasoconstrict rather than an adequate circulating blood volume. The central venous pressure will be elevated while fluids are being rapidly infused; a 5–10 minute period of cessation will allow equilibration between intra- and extravascular compartments and give a better idea of total body fluid balance.

Normalization of blood pressure, heart, and respiratory rate, cerebration, peripheral circulation, and core-toe temperature gradient indicate that organ perfusion is improving. A good urine output and disappearance of metabolic acidosis are sensitive markers of the adequacy of resuscitation.

It is important to treat the cause rather than the effects of hypoperfusion. Thus bicarbonate should not be given to treat the metabolic acidosis nor frusemide to increase the urine output. Likewise, inotropes should be withheld until adequate fluid has been administered. The patient may respond to either pain or a metabolic acidosis by hyperventilating; attention should therefore be directed towards adequate analgesia and proper fluid management.

Fluid administered for resuscitation should be a combination of both colloid and blood. Colloid (e.g. gelofusin, haemaccel, hespan, human albumin solution) is a better intravascular volume expander, while the blood provides the necessary haemoglobin replacement to carry oxygen to the tissues.

Ideally, blood should be fully cross-matched and this can be achieved within 30 minutes. In dire situations either O-negative (universal donor) or, preferably, group-specific (antibody-untested) blood can be given while awaiting a more formal cross-match. The blood should be transfused if possible through a warming device if large amounts are required. Calcium gluconate 10% 5–10 ml may be given for every 6 units of blood transfused. This is because the citrate used as an anticoagulant in stored blood may induce hypocalcaemia with resulting tetany and decreased muscle contractility. Stored blood contains few platelets or clotting factors; consideration should be given to separate administration of fresh frozen plasma and platelets if large volumes are needed. Although the blood potassium may rise following infusion of stored blood, this will rarely cause a significant hyperkalaemia.

Compartment syndrome

This is due to swelling, bleeding, or ischaemia within the fascial compartments of the arm and/or leg. As these compartments are unable to expand to any significant degree, interstitial tissue pressure will rise. When this pressure exceeds that of the capillary bed, local ischaemia of nerve and muscle occurs. Rhabdomyolysis, permanent paralysis, or gangrene may result. This typically occurs after crush injuries, closed or open fractures, or sustained compression of a limb in an immobile patient.

If able, the patient will complain of increasing pain in the affected limb, despite immobilization of fractures. Pain on passive stretching of muscles within the affected region may also be evident. There will be tense swelling of the involved fascial compartment(s) and possibly reduced sensation over the dermatomes supplied by the affected nerves. The absence of distal pulses does not identify a compartment syndrome as these may be intact until late in the progression of the syndrome after irreversible damage has been done. Restricting dressings should be released. Development of a compartment syndrome may not be an immediate complication and careful observation of limbs for swelling, abnormal perfusion, or pain should be performed.

If recovery is not rapid, urgent fasciotomy should be considered to relieve the pressure. Compartmental pressures can be monitored with needle manometry and pressures greater than 30 mmHg are considered abnormal. Fasciotomies should be performed when the intra-compartmental pressure exceeds 40 mmHg (or the diastolic blood pressure minus 30 mmHg) and remains at that level for more than 8 hours. Considerable blood loss may occur following fasciotomy.

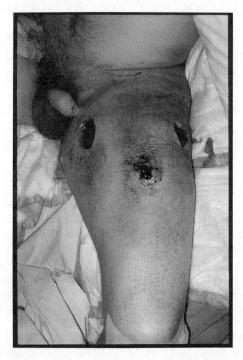

Fig. 11.8 Fasciotomies performed for decompression of compartment syndrome.

Fat embolism syndrome (FES)

Patients with FES have emboli of fat macroglobules in the pulmonary and systemic circulations. Organs with high blood flow, such as the heart, lungs, brain, and kidney, show evidence of capillary obstruction by fat or microaggregates of platelets, red cells and fibrin. The syndrome usually presents as respiratory insufficiency, cerebral dysfunction, and petechial skin haemorrhages.

FES is associated with bone fractures, particularly of the long bones and pelvis. These fractures result in fat and marrow entering the venous circulation. Massive trauma may also disrupt adipose tissue causing large fat globules to enter the bloodstream. The onset of signs and symptoms of the syndrome is generally at 24–48 hours post-injury.

Mechanical obstruction of the pulmonary capillaries rapidly causes dyspnoea and tachypnoea, hypoxaemia and, occasionally, production of blood-stained frothy sputum. A petechial rash develops classically over the upper thorax, neck, and soft palate and is seen in up to 50% of patients. Petechiae can sometimes be seen in the retina. A fever of up to 39 °C often develops with an associated tachycardia, Occlusion of cerebral vessels causes confusion, drowsiness, decerebrate signs, convulsions, and coma. If these signs become apparent other causes must be excluded by appropriate investigations (e.g. delayed post-traumatic intracranial injury by CT scanning). Obstruction of renal vessels causes oliguria or anuria and the diagnostic presence of fat globules in pulmonary artery blood or the urine. Coagulopathies are sometimes seen with increased fibrin degradation products, thrombocytopenia, and anaemia. There may be significant intrapulmonary haemorrhage. ECG changes may reveal right heart strain in fulminant FES. Biopsy of skin or kidneys may reveal microinfarcts associated with fat globules.

Treatment is largely supportive and the prognosis in fulminant FES is poor. Supplemental oxygen therapy is used to correct hypoxaemia but often mechanical ventilation ± PEEP is required. An adequate circulatory volume must be ensured, taking into account blood loss at fracture sites, and fluid loss from wounds. Careful monitoring of blood pressure, heart rate, CVP and, if possible, pulmonary artery pressures should be instituted. There is often a fall in cardiac output and an increase in pulmonary vascular resistance as the syndrome develops. Inotropic support may be required to maintain arterial pressure.

Renal support will be required if the patient becomes anuric or oliguric with rapidly deteriorating renal function. Close monitoring of serum electrolytes is essential.

The prevention of hypoxaemia reduces the severity of the syndrome. Early institution of oxygen therapy and maintaining good blood gas exchange are important preventative factors in the first 48 hours of patients at risk of FES. Anticoagulation with heparin is sometimes used.

Signs of fulminant fat embolism syndrome (FES)

- Hypoxaemia

- Respiratory rate ↑ Heart rate ↑ Temp ↑

- BP ↓ Cardiac output ↓ Urine output ↓

- Poor cerebral perfusion

- Petechiae

Air embolism

This results from air leaking from the lungs directly into the pulmonary vein and hence into the left heart. Massive air embolism may occur when patients with severe lung injury are mechanically ventilated and is due to a bronchopulmonary vein fistula or direct penetrating injury to the pulmonary veins. Major circulatory collapse follows; the patient is hypoxaemic and arterial blood samples may appear 'frothy'. Diagnosis is difficult in the presence of severe chest injuries or where there may be other causes of sudden cardiovascular collapse and hypoxaemia. Air embolism is uncommon and other causes, such as tension pneumothorax, should be excluded first. Treatment is by turning the patient on to his/her left side in a head-down, feet-up position so that air in the ventricle will not enter the systemic circulation. Air is then aspirated from the left ventricle followed by thoracotomy of the injured side.

Hypothermia

Hypothermia is defined as a sustained core temperature below 35 °C. It may be further classified as mild (32–35 °C), moderate (28–32 °C), or severe (< 28 °C).

In the patient with normal thermoregulation, accidental hypothermia may occur when the body is exposed to a cold environment or immersed in cold water. However, in the patient with abnormal thermogenesis a mild exposure to cold can cause hypothermia. This may occur for the following reasons:

- A reduced metabolic rate (e.g. myxoedema, hypopituitarism, or malnutrition, where heat production is insufficient to maintain the body's temperature).

- Spinal injury where muscle activity cannot be increased.

- Hypothalamic injuries (e.g. CVA), self-poisoning, alcohol abuse, and sedative drugs, which cause cutaneous vasodilatation and increased heat loss.

- The elderly, as a consequence of a reduced shivering response, immobility, poor living conditions, reduced subcutaneous fat, and a low metabolic rate.

Core temperature should be measured in hypothermic patients, ideally with an oesophageal temperature probe. Rectal temperature is less accurate because of heat-producing organisms in the bowel, the insulating effect of faeces, and cool blood returning from the legs may all affect the temperature. Typically, a rectal probe at 10 cm beyond the anal sphincter will record a temperature 0.25–0.5 °C below that of blood.

The clinical manifestations of hypothermia vary according to the core temperature, rate of cooling, and duration of hypothermia. Thermoregulatory mechanisms usually remain intact above 33 °C but below this there is progressive physiological deterioration. Loss of consciousness and pupillary dilatation occurs at 30 °C. The shivering mechanism is replaced by muscular rigidity at 33 °C and a rigor mortis-like appearance, with cessation of respiration at 24 °C.

The solubility of gases in plasma increases with hypothermia and the oxygen dissociation curve is shifted to the right (due to an increased affinity of haemoglobin for oxygen). It is debatable whether blood gas analysis should be corrected for temperature in the hypothermic patient.

Mortality varies from 6% to 85%, depending on the severity of hypothermia, duration, underlying disease conditions, and associated complications. (See Table 11.4 for physiological manifestations of hypothermia.)

Rewarming

The rate of rewarming depends on the degree of hypothermia. Rapid rewarming up to 15 °C per hour can be achieved by extracorporeal circuits but this is reserved for severe cases only who have life-threatening complications. Generally, rewarming is at a rate of 0.5–4 °C per hour. Rapid rewarming may precipitate 'rewarming shock' where sudden surface peripheral vasodilatation causes hypotension, an increase in metabolic acidosis, and a drop in temperature of up to 4 °C due to cool peripheral blood perfusing the central organs. Cool blood perfusing the myocardium may give rise to fatal arrhythmias, such as ventricular fibrillation, during rewarming. The elderly and those with underlying cardiac disease are particularly vulnerable so rewarming should be controlled and cautious.

Methods of rewarming
Passive. suitable for mild hypothermia. Rewarming takes place slowly (0.5–1.0 °C/h).

- warm environment (25–30 °C),

- reflective space blanket/warm air blanket,

- extra blankets,

- cover skin areas through which heat loss may occur (e.g. scalp).

Active: used in moderate hypothermia, those with impaired thermoregulation, and inability to shiver.

- heated humidified respiratory gases,

- warmed intravenous fluids,

- electrically heated mattresses or pads/warm air blanket,

- hot baths (40–45 °C) with limbs out of the water to avoid rewarming shock. These are only suitable for young adults and are usually not practicable. Monitoring is difficult in this situation.

Core warming: for severe hypothermia.

- peritoneal/haemodialysis,

- extracorporeal circuits,

- intragastric or bladder irrigation with warm fluids.

Burn injuries

Burn injuries may have psychological, systemic, and local effects on the patient. They can range from superficial, where the injury extends only partly into the skin and healing is spontaneous, to full thickness where the burn extends through the dermis, damaging the underlying fat and muscle tissue. Scarring will occur when a certain critical depth of damage to the dermis has occurred; this is permanent, often causing disability and disfiguration.

Assessment of the severity of the burn injury is traditionally by the percentage of the body surface area (BSA) involved. A major burn is considered to be > 10% BSA in a child and 15% BSA in an adult. Patients with > 20% BSA plus a severe smoke inhalation injury have a 50–80% mortality.

Table 11.4 Physiological manifestations of hypothermia

Problem	Cause	Treatment
Tachycardia Peripheral vasoconstriction ↑ cardiac output (in mild hypothermia)	Elevated levels of noradrenaline due to increased sympathetic activity	Monitor vital signs Passive rewarming
↓ cardiac output ↓ BP (moderate hypothermia)	Bradycardia	Active rewarming Intravenous fluids Monitor vital signs
Dysrhythmias • Bradycardia • Conduction disturbances • AF + SVT (<30 °C) • VF (<28 °C) VF may also be precipitated by stimulation (e.g. central venous catheter insertion, endotracheal intubation)	Decreased tissue perfusion, acidosis, underlying cardiac ischaemia, direct effect of cold on sinus node	Continuous ECG monitoring Avoid unnecessary stimulation Treat bradycardias with atropine/ isoprenaline/ pacing (as necessary) DC cardioversion is needed for VF, however, this may be resistant to electrical or pharmacological interventions until the core temperature >28 °C Note. In cardiac arrest situations, resuscitation must continue until the core temperature approaches normal. Hypothermia does have a cerebroprotective effect even though drugs and defibrillation may be ineffective
Hypoventilation Hypoxaemia	Decreased rate and depth of respiration Decreased gaseous diffusion capacity	Monitor blood gases Ensure patent airway Use supplemental oxygen and mechanical ventilation as necessary
Cerebral depression	Decreased cerebral blood flow (7% decrease per °C)	Neurological observations Maintain patent airway
Metabolic acidosis	Peripheral vasoconstriction and hypotension causing poor tissue perfusion. Lactate and other metabolites increase. Lactate clearance by liver is decreased. Decreased H^+ ion secretion by kidneys	Monitor blood pH Intravenous fluid therapy (±vasodilators) as patient warms up
Respiratory acidosis	Increased levels of CO_2 due to hypoventilation	Monitor blood gases. Mechanical ventilation may be necessary
Hyperglycaemia	Impaired peripheral circulation of glucose, decreased insulin release, glucose metabolized from liver glycogen Note. Pancreatitis may occur secondary to hypothermia	Monitor blood glucose Insulin infusion if necessary In prolonged hypothermia, glycogen stores may be depleted and hypoglycaemia may develop

Table 11.4 *contd*

Problem	Cause	Treatment
Polyuria Electrolyte imbalance	Impaired tubular function due to inhibition of enzyme systems and reduced responsiveness to ADH	Measure urine output and fluid input. Monitor urine specific gravity and electrolytes, vital signs, blood urea, and electrolytes Electrolyte replacement as necessary. Some patients develop renal failure: this is usually associated with hypotension Renal support (e.g. dialysis may be required)

Calculation of total percentage of burned skin: the 'Rule of 9'	
Head	9%
Arm	9% each
Front and back of trunk	18% each
Legs	18% each
Perineum	1%
Total	100%

The depth of the burn can be classified as follows:

Erythema
Redness of the skin, pain but no blistering

1st degree
The burn involves only the epithelial layer of the skin. The skin is red and blisters, blanches on pressure, and is painful. There is no residual scarring on healing.

2nd degree
The burn extends through the epithelial layer to the dermis. The skin appears red and blistered. Pain and residual scarring will depend on the depth of dermis damaged.

3rd degree
Involves full skin thickness. The skin is white. There is little or no pain as the sensory nerve endings are destroyed. Residual scarring usually occurs.

Areas of particular concern are burns to the face (especially around the nose and mouth which may indicate inhalational injury), circumferential burns of the limbs, and burns to the eyelids. The cause of the burn should be taken into account when assessment is made. These may be from a dry source (e.g. flames), wet source (e.g. scalds), electrical (e.g. household appliances, pylons), or chemical (acid, alkali, radiation).

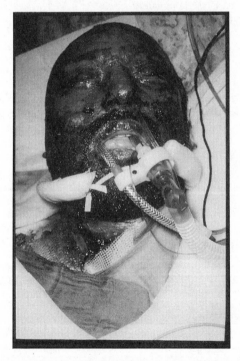

Fig. 11.9 Severe burn injury showing generalized swelling of face and upper airways.

Burn injuries cause an increase in metabolic rate which remains elevated for long periods of time. Nitrogen losses are greater than in any other form of trauma. Malnutrition may cause poor wound healing and an increase in mortality. Adequate and early institution of nutritional support is therefore vital. If enteral feeding is required, a fine bore polyurethane nasogastric tube should be passed as soon as possible after admission. Vitamin and mineral requirements, particularly zinc, iron, and vitamins B and C, increase in burn injuries and these may need to be supplemented. If the gut is inaccessible or non-functioning, total parenteral nutrition must be considered.

Initial management

If possible, the patient should be nursed in protective isolation and in an environment with humidity and temperature control. An air-fluidized bed may be required for severe burn injuries.

On arrival at the ICU, the patient must be assessed and vital signs recorded. A patent airway must be maintained and humidified oxygen therapy instituted. Patients with massive burns or inhalational injury may require urgent endotracheal intubation and mechanical ventilation. Intravenous access, preferably in a non-burned area, must be established. High fluid losses will occur from the burned area; central venous pressure and, occasionally, pulmonary artery wedge pressure monitoring may be required. An arterial line is useful for systemic pressure monitoring and blood sampling. A nasogastric tube and urinary catheter will also be required in severe cases. Insertion of tubes and cannulae should be carried out at an early stage as the patient will become grossly oedematous within 24 hours due to massive capillary leakage, thus making instrumentation extremely difficult. For this reason, scrupulous attention should also be paid to the airway and endotracheal intubation performed on early signs of respiratory distress. Massive swelling may occur around the face and/or neck resulting in respiratory difficulties; an inhalational injury need not necessarily be present.

Various formulae exist for fluid replacement but these should only be used as guidelines. Fluid losses are commonly underestimated and frequent assessment of vital signs, urine output, haematocrit, and base deficit are vital. Care must be taken not to overload the patient with fluid. In United Kingdom, the Muir Barclay (or Mount Vernon) formula is often used for guiding fluid resuscitation. The first 36 hours from the time of burn — not from the time of arrival in hospital — are divided into six periods of 4,4,4,6,6, and 12 hours. Over each period, 0.5 ml/g body weight/% burn of 5% human albumin solution is given with additional crystalloid as 5% dextrose at a rate of 1.5–2 ml/kg body weight/hour. Haemodynamic variables should be measured at the end of each period and the patient's intravascular fluid status reassessed and adjusted as necessary. A haematocrit of approximately 0.35 is considered satisfactory to ensure adequate oxygen carriage and a non-elevated blood viscosity. A high haematocrit may imply haemoconcentration and the need for more fluid. An increasing metabolic acidosis and a fall in urine output are signs of an inadequate intravascular volume. A low haematocrit is suggestive of fluid overload, however, blood loss should also be considered as a cause of a low haematocrit. This may either be from haemorrhage from non-burn injuries or from haemolysis of blood cells trapped in the burned areas. In general, blood transfusions are not needed in the first 24 hours unless escharotomies are performed.

Coagulation screens should be performed regularly as massive dilution may occur by the huge amount of fluid infused; clotting factors may also be consumed or production suppressed and replacement, usually as fresh frozen plasma, should be considered if significant derangement in coagulation occurs. Likewise, marked shifts may occur in electrolyte status; these should be measured regularly and corrected as necessary.

After 2–5 days the capillary leakage stops and the patient usually enters a diuretic phase. Excessive tissue fluid is reabsorbed back into the intravascular compartment and thence excreted via the kidney. This diuresis is spontaneous and may be massive; although fluid and sodium input should be reduced at this stage care must be taken not to allow intravascular depletion and electrolyte imbalance.

Subsequent management

Cardiovascular

The circulation of a burned patient is usually hyperdynamic with an elevated cardiac output. Shock can occur rapidly within the first 48 hours of the injury or later. Hypotension and a fall in cardiac output causes hypoperfusion of vital organs which may lead to single or multiple organ failure. Vascular permeability in the area of the burn increases and large amounts of fluid, similar in composition to plasma, leaks out and is lost through the burnt tissue. Oedema is related to vasoactive substances released as a consequence of the injury. This is not just limited to the affected areas; there is widespread generalized swelling indicative of the whole body inflammatory response to the burn. The circulating intravascular volume is thus depleted resulting in hypoperfusion. The released inflammatory mediators may also cause progression to multi-organ failure with cardiovascular collapse. The first step in management is to ensure adequate fluid resuscitation although vasoactive drugs, such as noradrenaline, may occasionally be required to maintain an adequate blood pressure.

Respiratory

Pulmonary injury may result from inhalation of irritant or noxious gases such as carbon monoxide and cyanide. Heat may cause damage to the upper and lower airways and lung tissue. Smoke inhalation causes thermal injury only to the larynx and pharynx, as hot gases have a low specific heat content. Steam has a much higher heat content and causes injury to the whole respiratory tract. ARDS and pneumonia may be secondary complications of the primary burn injury. There should be a low threshold for endotracheal intubation in patients with inhalational injuries as these patients can quickly progress to complete airway obstruction as oedema develops. Indications for intubation are:

- failure to maintain an adequate airway,

- respiratory failure,

- severe cyanide or carbon monoxide poisoning,

- convulsions,

- stridor,

- circumferential chest burns,

- severe facial burns or full thickness burns of nose or lips,

- endoscopic evidence of pharyngeal or laryngeal oedema/blistering/erythema/soot.

Arterial blood gas tensions must be monitored regularly and pulse oximetry used for continuous monitoring.

Soot in the airways should be promptly removed by aggressive per-endoscopic saline lavage to minimize local inflammation. Samples should be taken for bacteriological analysis and antibiotics (e.g. benzyl penicillin) commenced.

Carbon monoxide (CO) poisoning should be considered in any patient burned in an enclosed space such as a building or vehicle. Confusion, drowsiness, or coma may be present as may the characteristic cherry-red appearance. Carbon monoxide levels in the blood may be rapidly measured as carboxyhaemoglobin (COHb) using a haemoximeter. Both arterial blood gas tensions and pulse oximetry will be unreliable as neither will recognize the percentage of haemoglobin molecules being occupied by carbon monoxide rather than oxygen. Carbon monoxide has 200–250 times the affinity for haemoglobin as oxygen, therefore, oxygen transport to the tissues may be severely compromised. High-flow, high-concentration oxygen (100% by facemask or mask CPAP, if possible, or endotracheal tube) should be administered immediately and continued until COHb levels fall below 10%. The half-life of carboxyhaemoglobin is 4 hours when breathing air, and only 50 minutes on 100% oxygen.

Hydrogen cyanide poisoning prevents the uptake of oxygen at a cellular level. Treatment is to administer 100% oxygen as soon as possible. Antidotes, such as sodium thiosulphate or dicobalt edetate, have particular dangers in themselves and should be reserved for cases where cyanide poisoning is known to have occurred or is strongly suspected and the patient's condition is deteriorating. Clues to making the diagnosis include increasing drowsiness and a progressive metabolic acidosis despite adequate fluid resuscitation. Confirmation by measuring plasma cyanide levels will take in excess of 3 hours and there may be insufficient time to wait in life-threatening situations.

Renal

Renal failure usually results from hypoperfusion of the kidneys due to shock or, less commonly, the presence of haemoglobinuria (from intravascular haemolysis) or myoglobinuria (from tissue breakdown). Renal support in the form of dialysis or haemofiltration may be required. Close monitoring of urine output and blood electrolytes are essential.

Pain

Pain can be considerable in all but full thickness burns. Continuous intravenous opiate infusions are necessary and can be supplemented by benzodiazepines. There is often an increased need with dressing changes and physiotherapy.

Infection

Sepsis accounts for 50% of deaths from burn injuries. The immune system is generally depressed in severe injuries but prophylactic administration of antibiotics is not recommended unless there is evidence of an inhalation injury. In this case penicillin should be used as the main threat comes from pneumococcal infection.

Wounds should be swabbed and cultured regularly and antibiotics only begun when a specific pathogen has been isolated. Strict aseptic technique during wound redressing, protective isolation, good nutritional support, and avoidance of unnecessary instrumentation will help reduce the incidence of infection.

Acidosis

This may have respiratory and metabolic components. Metabolic acidosis develops from tissue hypoxia (usually secondary to hypoperfusion) and from the released products of damaged tissue. The possibility of cyanide poisoning should not be forgotten. Respiratory acidosis usually results from either a central cause, such as coma causing respiratory depression, or from direct injury.

Haematological

Anaemia may follow either haemolysis or blood loss. The plasma concentration of clotting factors may be diluted by the massive fluid replacement needed and disseminated intravascular coagulation can occur as part of the multi-organ failure syndrome. Treatment is by appropriate replacement of blood products.

Surgical

Urgent escharotomy (or limb amputation) may be required soon after admission. Escharotomy is the surgical release of a constricting area or circumferential burn by incising down to the fatty layer. Anaesthesia is not normally required as the skin area affected is usually dead. Debridement and grafting (using cadaveric tissue or the patient's own split skin from an unburnt site) will be indicated for full thickness burns. If this area is large, debridement may be advisable in the first few days with tangential excision of the necrotic area. Massive bleeding can occasionally occur both during and following this procedure.

Dressings

Dressing procedures will vary considerably from unit to unit. The following notes are thus intended as guidelines only.

Prior to any dressing procedure ensure that analgesia is adequate. Dressings should be changed every 24 hours except for recipient graft sites which remain intact for 5 days post-operatively. Clean burned areas with normal saline using a strict aseptic procedure. Flamazine cream can be applied directly to full thickness burns of the limbs, trunk, hands, feet, and ears. Hands and feet can then be lightly secured in plastic bags. This will allow

passive exercises and physiotherapy to be carried out. Flamazine can be applied to a Lyofoam sheet for burns to the back. Partial thickness burns of the limbs and trunk can be dressed with paraffin gauze. Following the application of Flamazine or paraffin gauze, the area is covered with Lyofoam, then gauze or absorbent dressing, and then a light bandage. Burns to the perineum may be dressed with Flamazine or paraffin gauze and nursed exposed with the legs abducted. Eyes should be cleansed hourly with sterile water, chloramphenicol eye ointment applied, and moistened gauze swabs or Geliperm applied. Limbs should be elevated to reduce oedema. Following escharotomy the wound should be dressed with tulle gras (or any non-adherent dressing), gauze, and crêpe bandages.

Physiotherapy

This is important in all burn patients in order to maintain joint mobility, muscle strength, and functional joint positions. Chest physiotherapy is indicated for inhalational injuries, trunk burns (especially circumferential), bed-bound patients, and before and after surgery. Correct positioning of the patient will reduce oedema and prevent contracture formation. Passive exercises should be carried out frequently to maintain a full range of movement at joints and to maintain muscle power. Prior to physiotherapy ensure that pain control is adequate. Reassure and explain the procedure to gain co-operation from the patient.

Psychological aspects

Psychological problems following the injury and helping the patient and family come to terms with disfigurement or disablement pose a major challenge. Considerable psychological support will be required over a prolonged period. Many ICUs have access to specially trained counsellors who should be involved at an early stage.

Near-drowning

Near-drowning is usually the result of submersion in fresh or salt water. However, aspiration of fluid is not always necessary to 'drown' — the so-called 'dry drowning' (see later).

Alcohol and epilepsy are sometimes major contributing factors. Deliberate hyperventilation prior to prolonged underwater swimming is also a common cause. Hyperventilation causes hypocarbia and the low levels of

P_{CO_2} suppresses respiratory effort, even in the presence of severe hypoxaemia, thus consciousness is lost whilst underwater.

'Dry drowning' occurs when little or no fluid is aspirated into the lungs while underwater. It is thought that a reflex laryngospasm is caused by the presence of water in the larynx and this prevents fluid entry into the lungs. This glottic spasm persists until death from asphyxiation occurs. The prognosis for near drowning victims who have not aspirated fluid is fairly good, provided they are promptly resuscitated, since they are not then subject to the secondary complications of fluid inhalation.

The diving reflex and hypothermia are potential protective mechanisms in submersion victims. The diving reflex is initiated by cold water on the face and consists of apnoea, bradycardia, and intense peripheral vasoconstriction. Blood flow is preferentially diverted to essential organs such as heart and brain. Hypothermia decreases cardiac output, cellular metabolism, and oxygen consumption. It is especially protective if it precedes anoxia. Survival without neurological damage has been reported after periods of submersion of longer than 20 minutes — the longest reported to date is 66 minutes. Neither a long submersion time nor the death-like appearance of the victim are reasons for not resuscitating. It is thus recommended to commence resuscitation in every victim who has been underwater for less than one hour, and to stop on the basis of objective diagnostic criteria only when the patient has reached hospital and has been warmed to normothermia. Cervical spine injuries are frequently associated with diving accidents and these must be considered during resuscitation.

Submersion is primarily a ventilatory disturbance with hypoxaemia the cause of cardiac arrest. The nature of the inhaled fluid will cause different physiological effects. In freshwater drowning, fluid in the lungs is quickly absorbed into the circulation causing dilutional effects that may lead to haemolysis. Pulmonary surfactant is denatured and widespread atelectasis can result. Electrolyte disturbances are usually mild and transient. Salt water contains higher levels of sodium and chloride and this causes mucosal injury and loss of surfactant. This fluid is hypertonic and thus water and plasma proteins move rapidly into the alveoli and interstitium, resulting in an osmotic pulmonary oedema.

In most drowning victims, the stomach also fills with water and there is a high risk of inhalation of gastric contents. This is particularly likely during resuscitation and cardiac compression. Inhalation of gastric contents will produce further inflammatory reactions in the alveolar-capillary membrane.

Management

There is little difference in management between saltwater and freshwater drowning. Therapy is directed at restoring the circulation and oxygenation, correcting electrolyte imbalance, and maintaining cerebral perfusion.

Problems

1. Hypoxaemia

Full cardiopulmonary resuscitation will usually be required initially and comatose patients will require endotracheal intubation. The presence of severe hypoxaemia and, possibly, pulmonary oedema mean that mechanical ventilation, high inspired oxygen concentrations, and PEEP are usually needed. CPAP via a facemask may be used if the patient is conscious and able to maintain a patent airway and an adequate arterial oxygen saturation. Hypoxaemia and intrapulmonary shunting can occur with the inhalation of as little as 2.5 ml fluid/kg body weight. Hypoxaemia is usually the major problem in submersion victims. Pulmonary oedema may occur soon after endotracheal intubation following relief of the larygoscopy and the very high intrathoracic pressures. Therapy with high levels of PEEP is usually effective. Secondary pulmonary oedema can occur after 24 hours and patients should therefore be closely observed for at least this period of time. Denaturation of surfactant can continue even after resuscitation and ARDS and pulmonary infection are common. The type of immersion liquid may influence the type of inhaled organism and, in many instances, mud, sand, and particulate matter are aspirated. Multiple abscess formation may ensue.

High inflation pressures may be required during ventilation due to bronchospasm caused by water aspiration and altered surfactant activity, atelectasis, and pulmonary oedema which cause a decrease in lung compliance.

2. Circulatory failure

Positive inotropic agents may be required if the patient is hypotensive. Fluid replacement should be guided by central venous or pulmonary artery wedge pressure measurements. In theory, salt water should cause hypovolaemia and fresh water should increase the circulatory volume. However, in practice, such small amounts of fluid are aspirated that significant changes in blood volume are not seen.

Dysrhythmias may result from acidosis, hypoxaemia, hypothermia, and electrolyte imbalance. These should revert to a normal rhythm once these abnormalities have been corrected.

3. Hypothermia

Hypothermia is common in submersion victims. Core temperature must be maintained and passive/active rewarming instituted (see hypothermia section, p.337).
Note. Dysrhythmias may occur during rewarming.

4. Electrolyte imbalance

Plasma levels of sodium and chloride may be elevated in salt-water drowning but serious disturbances are unusual. Electrolyte abnormalities may be associated with acute renal failure and magnesium levels may be elevated in salt-water drowning.

5. Renal failure

In freshwater drowning haemolysis may cause haemoglobinuria and consequent acute renal failure. Urine output must be closely monitored.

6. Neurological damage

Ischaemic cerebral damage can follow prolonged hypoxaemia and some patients will develop cerebral oedema. Attempts should be made to reduce raised intracranial pressure and maintain cerebral perfusion. Pyrexia must be reduced, oxygenation and circulation maintained, and blood glucose monitored (see Chapter 9). The patient must be observed for seizures and frequent neurological assessments made.

7. Gastric dilatation

Submersion victims often swallow large amounts of water. A nasogastric tube should be inserted to prevent inhalation.

8. Metabolic acidosis

This may develop following intense peripheral vasoconstriction and hypoxaemia. Lactate levels rise as oxygen delivery to the tissues falls. The acidosis should improve as the patient is rewarmed and hypoxaemia corrected.

The success rate of resuscitation in submersion victims is relatively high but a multitude of fatal complications may develop, in particular, ARDS and multi-organ failure, septicaemia, and pneumonia. Prognosis is poor if the patient is comatose following resuscitation.

Diving injuries

Too rapid an ascent from depth will result in nitrogen bubbles coming out of solution. This can result in neurological consequences including coma and seizures, and excruciating abdominal and joint pains ('the bends'). Treatment is by placing the patient in a hyperbaric chamber where a slow and gradual decompression from the raised pressure experienced at depth to the lower atmospheric pressure of sea level can be performed. This may take several days.

Trauma scoring

Trauma scoring is a means of classifying the severity of injury. Various scoring systems have been devised (32 between 1974 and 1987) and these usually combine both anatomical and physiological variables. Some are simple and specific for a particular type of injury such as the Glasgow Coma Scale (GCS) for head injuries. Others are complex and may even combine several individual scoring systems (see below).

Trauma scoring will allow an evaluation of trauma care provided and a means of comparing outcome, either over time or between different hospitals. It can aid the planning and provision of resources in special units and identify those patients who will benefit most from the specialized care that can be provided in these areas. Scoring is helpful in triage where patients are categorized into treatment hierarchies, enabling identification of the most severely injured patients who may require immediate transfer to specialized units or priority treatment. It may also distinguish those with a poor chance of survival and when resources are overwhelmed (e.g. following disasters, where treatment could be directed initially at those critically ill patients with a better prognosis).

TRISS

One method of trauma scoring called TRISS (Trauma Score–Injury Severity Score) has a world-wide reputation for consistency and reasonable predictions of outcome. It combines two scoring systems: the Revised Trauma Score (RTS), and the Injury Severity Score (ISS).

The threat to life can be measured by the extent of the

anatomical injury and the degree of physiological derangement. However, the age of the patient and the method of wounding also influence mortality. The TRISS method of scoring takes into account the patient's age and if the injury was blunt or penetrating. TRISS combines four elements:

1. Revised Trauma Score (RTS)

2. Injury Severity Score (ISS)

3. Patient's age.

4. Penetrating or blunt injury.

The score provides a measure of predicted outcome — the probability of survival (Ps).

The Revised Trauma Score (RTS) is composed of Glasgow Coma Scale (GCS) (see Chapter 9) and measurements of cardiopulmonary function. Each variable is given a number and multiplied by a weighting factor (See Table 11.6) derived from regression analysis of a large US database. This reflects the relative value of that variable in determining survival. The numbers are then totalled to provide the patient's RTS, which should be recorded on arrival in hospital. (See Table 11.5.)

Calculation of probability of survival (Ps)

$$Ps = \frac{1}{1 + e^{-b}}$$

where
Ps = probability of survival
e = 2.718282
b = Revised Trauma Score (RTS) + Injury Severity Score (ISS) + age coefficient (age coefficient = 0 if age ⩽ 54 years, or +1 if age ⩾ 54 years)

Table 11.6 Weighted coefficient values

Injury	Constant	RTS	ISS	Age
Blunt	−1.2470	0.9544	−0.0768	−1.9052
Penetrating	−0.6029	1.1430	−0.1516	−2.6676

Although this scoring method appears complicated, a TRISS chart has been devised to allow rapid determination of the probability of survival.

Despite being able to predict outcome reasonably well,

Table 11.5 The Revised Trauma Score (RTS)

Variable	Score					
	4	3	2	1	0	Weighting factor
Systolic BP (mmHg)	>89	76–89	50–75	1–49	Pulseless	× 0.7326
Respiratory rate (/min)	10–29	>29	6–9	1–5	0	× 0.2908
GCS	13–15	9–12	6–8	4–5	3	× 0.9368

Note. Add the combined scores for each variable to obtain the RTS.

The Injury Severity Score (ISS) provides a numerical measure of the injury severity in patients with multiple injuries. Every injury is given an AIS-85 code and classified into one of seven regions: head and neck; face; thorax; abdomen and pelvic contents; extremities; pelvic girdle; external and burns. The AIS-85 code is an abbreviated injury scale last revised in 1985 by the American Association for Automotive Medicine. It incorporates codes for assessment of blunt and penetrating injuries. Each injury is assigned a 6-digit code based on anatomical site, nature, and severity. The ISS is the sum of the squares of the highest AIS scores from three of the seven body regions. There is a significant correlation of ISS with mortality, morbidity and length of hospital stay.

the survivors' quality of life can vary considerably. At present, there are no methods that measure the quality of life after major trauma. However, trauma scoring will allow audit and, one hopes, improvement in the quality of care and outcome for trauma patients.

References and bibliography

AAAM (American Association for Automotive Medicine). (1985). *The abbreviated injury scale*, (revised). AAAM, Arlington Heights, IL.

ACS (American College of Surgeons) (1984). *Committee on Trauma. Advanced trauma life support course*, (student manual). ACS, Chicago.

Bickerstaff, E.R. (ed.) (1977). *Neurology for nurses*, (2nd edn). Hodder & Stoughton., London.

Bierens, J.J., van Zanten, J.J., and van Berkel, M. (1991). Resuscitation of submersion victims; wet CPR. In *Update in intensive care and emergency medicine*, Vol. 14, (ed. J.L. Vincent), pp. 11–17. Springer, Berlin.

Borel, C., Hanley, D., Diringer, M., and Rogers, M. (1990) Intensive management of severe head injury. *Chest*, **98**, 180–6.

Boyd, C.R., Tolsen, M.A., and Copes, W.S. (1987) Evaluating trauma care; the TRISS method. *Journal of Trauma*, **27**, 370–8.

Brunner, L. and Suddarth, D. (ed.) (1975). *Textbook of medical–surgical nursing*, (3rd edn). Lippincott, Philadelphia.

Bullock, R. and Teasdale, G. (1990). Head injuries: I. *British Medical Journal*, **300**, 1515–18.

Bullock, R. and Teasdale, G. (1990). Head injuries: II. *British Medical Journal*, **300**, 1576–79.

Champion, H.R., Sacco, W.T., Carnazzo, A.T., *et al.* (1981). Trauma score. *Critical Care Medicine*, **91**, 672–6.

Cope, A. and, Stebbings, W. (1990). Abdominal trauma. *British Medical Journal*, **301**, 172–6.

Copes, W.S. (1988). *Major Trauma Outcome Study (MTOS)*. Report of the American College of Surgeons. Chicago.

Deane, A. (1990). Trauma of the lower urinary tract. *British Medical Journal*, **301**, 545–7.

Gibson, R.M. and Stephenson, G.C. (1989). Aggressive management of severe closed head trauma; time for reappraisal. *Lancet*, **ii**, 369–70.

Green, J.H. (1978). *An introduction to human physiology*, (4th edn). Oxford University Press, New York.

Hutchinson, I., Lawlor, M., and Skinner, D. (1990). Major maxillofacial injuries. *British Medical Journal*, **301**, 595–9.

Johnston, R.A. (1989). Management of old people with neck trauma. *British Medical Journal*, **299**, 633–4.

Mendelow, A.D. (1990). Management of head injury. *Hospital Update*, **10**, 195–206.

Oh, T.E. (ed.) (1990). *Intensive care manual* (3rd edn). Butterworth, Sydney.

Smith, E.J., Ward, J., and Smith, D. (1991). Trauma scoring methods. *British Journal of Hospital Medicine*, **44**, 114–18.

Swaine, A., Dave, J., and Baker, H. (1990) Trauma of the spine and spinal cord: I. *British Medical Journal*, **301**, 595–9.

Terry, T. (1990). Trauma of the upper urinary tract. *British Medical Journal*, **301**, 485–7.

Trevor-Roper, P.D. (1978). *Lecture notes on ophthalmology*, (5th ed). Blackwell, Oxford.

Van Niekerk, J. and Goris, R.J.A. (1990). Management of the trauma patient. *Clinical Intensive Care*, **1**, 32–5.

Westaby, S. and Brayley, N. (1990). Thoracic trauma: I. *British Medical Journal*, **300**, 1639–43.

Westaby, S. and Brayley, N. (1990). Thoracic trauma: II. *British Medical Journal*, **300**, 1710–12.

Willett, K.M., Darrell, H. and Kelly, P. (1990). Management of limb injuries. *British Medical Journal*, **301**, 229–33.

Yates, D.W. (1990). Scoring systems for trauma. *British Medical Journal*, **301**, 1090–4.

12. Haematological problems

Physiology of the blood cells

The basic cellular components of the blood are:

1. Erythrocytes (red cells)

2. Leucocytes (white cells)

3. Thrombocytes (platelets)

See Table 12.1 for a summary of types of blood cells.

Table 12.1 Types of blood cells

Cell type	Normal adult value	Function
Erythrocyte	5×10^{12}	Oxygen transport
Leucocyte	$4–11 \times 10^9/l$	Resistance to infection and antibody production
• neutrophil	40–75%	
• eosinophil	1–6%	
• basophil	<1%	
• monocyte	2–10%	
• lymphocyte	1.5–4%	
Thrombocyte	$150–300 \times 10^9/l$	Blood clotting

Erythrocytes (red cells)

These cells have no nucleus and consist mostly of cytoplasm and haemoglobin. Haemoglobin constitutes about 34 per cent of the erythrocyte cell mass but may fall to 20 per cent when its formation in the bone marrow is deficient. Each cell is biconcave in shape with a cell membrane considerably larger than is required; this surplus allows the cell to change shape as it passes through narrow capillaries.

All blood cells are derived from a single cell type in the bone marrow known as a pluripotent stem cell. The pluripotent stem cell gives rise to a myeloid stem cell and a lymphoid stem cell from which erythrocytes, leucocytes and thrombocytes develop (Fig. 12.1).

Red cell formation is stimulated by the hormone erythropoietin which is produced in the kidneys. The release of erythropoietin is thought to be influenced by the presence of renal hypoxia but the maximum rate of red cell production is only seen five days after its release

and is therefore a long-term rather than an immediate response. Lack of erythropoietin, as seen in patients with renal failure, can cause severe anaemia.

Several vitamins and elements are vital for the maturation of red cells. Vitamin B_{12} is essential for nuclear maturation and cell division while folic acid is required for the formation of DNA. Vitamin B_6, thiamine, riboflavin, manganese and, cobalt are also important. Iron is vital for the formation of haemoglobin and is obtained either by absorption from the gastrointestinal tract or from the breakdown of old red blood cells by the reticuloendothelial system.

The prime function of erythrocytes is that of oxygen transport. Haemoglobin has a great affinity for oxygen with one gram of haemoglobin capable of combining with 1.34 millilitres of oxygen. Oxygen combines with haemoglobin in the lungs to form oxyhaemoglobin and readily dissociates from it in the tissues where the cellular oxygen concentrations are lower than that of the blood (for full details of oxygen transport see Chapter 3).

Red blood cells also have high levels of the organic phosphate 2,3-diphosphoglyceric acid (2,3-DPG) which plays an important part in oxygen transfer. In the middle range of oxygen tensions this compound combines with reduced haemoglobin and decreases the affinity of haemoglobin for oxygen. The more 2,3-DPG present, the more oxygen will be released at a given oxygen tension; the oxyhaemoglobin dissociation curve is thus shifted to the right. Anoxia increases the amount of 2,3-DPG in the red cell thus increasing the amount of oxygen given off when blood reaches the tissues (see Chapter 3).

Terms associated with erythrocytes
Anaemia: this is defined as a haemoglobin level of less than 11.5 g/dl in the adult female or less than 13.5 g/dl in the adult male.

Erythrocyte sedimentation rate (ESR): this is the rate at which red cells will settle under gravity in a sample of blood. The blood sample is placed in a standard 100 mm long test tube and after 1 hour the rate of sedimentation should be no more than 10 mm. Diseases involving inflammation, tissue destruction, or blood hyperviscosity will increase the sedimentation rate and it serves as a useful guide to disease progression.

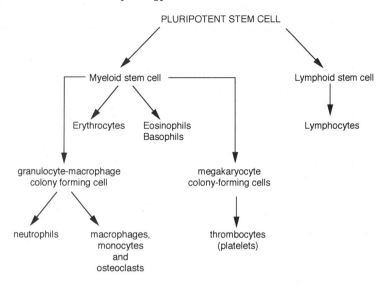

Fig. 12.1 Differentiation from the pluripotent stem cell.

Erythrocyte

Table 12.2   Erythrocyte disorders

Disorder	Result
Production	Increased (polycythaemia) • Primary • Secondary (e.g. altitude) Decreased due to: • Iron deficiency • Folate deficiency • Vitamin B_{12} deficiency • Erythropoietin (non-production) • Bone marrow failure
Membrane	Hereditary spherocytosis
Enzyme	Glucose-6-phosphate dehydrogenase deficiency
Haemoglobin	Sickle-cell anaemia Thalassaemia

Table 12.2 summarizes medical conditions associated with red blood cell disorders. Only those disorders relevant to treatment in the ICU are described in detail in the text (i.e. polycythaemia and sickle-cell anaemia.)

Polycythaemia
This is an increase in the red cell count $> 6 \times 10^{12}$l or Hb > 18 g/dl. 'Relative' polycythaemia is where the red cell mass is normal but the plasma volume is reduced (e.g. as in dehydration or diuretic therapy). 'True' polycythaemia is where the red cell mass is increased.

Secondary polycythaemia The red cell count is increased in response to chronic hypoxaemia and results from increased erythropoietin production. Conditions such as chronic obstructive airways disease or adaptation to high altitudes cause secondary polycythaemia.

Polycythaemia rubra vera. In this condition, the bone marrow becomes more proliferative and all cellular factors — red cells, white cells, and platelets — are increased. There is an increase in red cell mass and thus blood volume. The resulting increase in viscosity of the blood reduces flow leading to symptoms of headache, visual disturbances, and fatigue. The patient is at risk from angina, claudication, and cerebrovascular accidents. Immediate treatment is aimed at reducing the blood viscosity and this can be achieved by venesection to keep the haemoglobin below 17–18 g/dl. More definitive treatments include radioactive phosphorus or chemotherapy to depress bone marrow production. Occasionally, such a condition may transform into acute myeloid leukaemia.

Sickle-cell anaemia

Normal adult haemoglobin (HbA) contains two α- and two β-chains. There are two genes for the synthesis of each chain. Sickle-cell haemoglobin (HbS) has two α chains and two abnormal β-chains. The defect in the β-chain involves a single amino acid substitution and is inherited as an autosomal dominant gene. This defect leads to a chronic haemolytic anaemia.

Patients with sickle-cell trait have mainly HbA and less

than 50 per cent HbS. Sickle cell disease is found predominantly in Africa, the Middle East, India, and the Caribbean. The prevalence of the gene in these areas is probably because HbS protects against the serious effects of falciparum malaria.

Sickle-cell anaemia occurs in homozygotes (HbS/HbS) and the consequence of this abnormal haemoglobin is that when exposed to a low oxygen tension, the red cells become deformed, rigid and long in shape (sickle-shaped). These cells then become lodged and aggregate in small blood vessels in any part of the body, causing ischaemia or infarction. Patients with sickle-cell anaemia suffer chronic ill health, thrombotic crises, leg ulcers and infections. Many do not survive beyond 40 years of age. Those with sickle-cell trait are usually symptom-free unless the oxygen tension is very low since the HbA prevents the cells from sickling.

Acute haemolytic crises (sickle-cell crisis) occur from 6 months of age. There is haemolysis of the sickled cells and, by small vessel occlusion, infarction of tissues. These can cause bone, pulmonary or splenic infarcts, cerebrovascular accidents, priapism, haematuria, swelling (particularly of the toes and fingers), fever, and abdominal pain. The chronic anaemia is associated with tachycardia and cardiomegaly; heart failure and arrhythmias may develop in older patients.

Patients may be admitted to the ICU for management during these crises. Dehyration and hypoxia promotes sickling but the crises are unpredictable. Management is aimed at:

1. *Rehydration* — by IV fluids, at least 3 litres/day. Increasing the plasma volume dilutes the blood and decreases the agglutination of sickled-cells in small vessels. However, care must be taken not to overload these patients who usually have a cardiomyopathy and can thus be pushed into acute heart failure. CVP monitoring is usually necessary.

2. *Correction/prevention of hypoxaemia* — blood gases or pulse oximetry must be monitored closely, aiming to keep the oxygen saturation >95 per cent. Vigorous treatment of hypoxaemia is essential; this may initially be by oxygen mask or CPAP but mechanical ventilation may be required.

3. *Analgesia* — thrombotic episodes may cause severe pain in any part of the body. Continuous IV infusions of opiate analgesia such as pethidine or diamorphine should be given in a high enough dosage to control pain. Non-steroidal anti-inflammatory drugs such as diclofenac can be added. It should be remembered that high doses of pethidine can cause fits and in these circumstances subcutaneous diamorphine may be preferable.

4. *Infection* — often the patient will present with a fever and a raised white cell count during a crisis. Attempts must be made to rule out an underlying infection which, if found, requires appropriate treatment.

Splenic infarction is associated with recurrent sickle crises and patients are prone to capsulate organisms such as pneumococcus. Long-term prophylactic penicillin may be advocated.

5. *Blood transfusion* — if a crisis is severe, exchange blood transfusions may be carried out in order to dilute the number of sickle cells. This is usually reserved for patients who have a rapid drop in haemoglobin, those who develop chest or cerebral crises, a severe painful crisis not responding to other therapy, or pre-operatively if elective surgery is required.

Leucocytes (white cells)

The function of the leucocyte is to resist infection by phagocytosis or by forming antibodies against foreign material or agents. Phagocytosis is the process by which white cells engulf a foreign agent and then destroy it by the release of digesting enzymes within the cell.

Most of the white cells are formed in the bone marrow. There are five types:

1. Neutrophils

2. Eosinophils

3. Basophils

4. Monocytes

5. Lymphocytes

Note: neutrophils, eosinophils, and basophils are collectively known as granulocytes.

1. Neutrophils

When an area of tissue becomes inflamed it releases inflammatory mediators such as cytokines, for example interleukin-1 (IL-1), tumour necrosis factor (TNF), and histamine. These increase the number of neutrophils in the blood by up to fourfold. Neutrophils move into an inflamed area where they engulf and destroy foreign matter by phagocytosis.

'Neutrophilia' is a term used to describe an increase in the number of circulating neutrophils in the blood. Leucocytosis is also often used in this context although it strictly means an increase in the number of circulating white cells of all varieties, not just neutrophils. Neutrophilia will occur following infection, trauma, burn injury or tissue necrosis.

2. Eosinophils

These are weak phagocytes but collect at sites of antigen–antibody reactions in the tissues where they can phagocytose the antigen–antibody complex. They increase in number in allergic conditions (e.g. asthma and drug allergies), and parasitic infections, collecting around areas where histamine is released.

3. Basophils

These resemble the mast cells which are found just outside the capillaries and are responsible for liberating heparin into the blood. It is possible that basophils may, in fact, be cells that are transported to the tissues where they then become mast cells. However, basophils provide a similar function as mast cells in that they release heparin into the blood, which prevents coagulation, and also produce small quantities of bradykinin and serotonin.

4. Monocytes

These are very active phagocytes and large numbers will infiltrate areas of inflammation. The rate of monocyte production in the bone marrow increases with chronic infections (e.g. tuberculosis, endocarditis).

5. Lymphocytes

These are produced mainly in the lymph organs and nodes. B lymphocytes play an important part in the formation of antibodies and T lymphocytes are necessary for cellular immunity (e.g. in the non-rejection of transplant organs).

The inflammatory reaction is very complex. Tissue injury causes a local sympathetic reflex. This results in an increased blood flow, a consequent increase in blood cells, and redness in the area of injury. Macrophage monocytes release cytokines such as IL-1, TNF, serotonin, and histamine. Histamine causes local swelling. IL-1 and TNF stimulate an increase in basophils, eosinophils, and lymphocytes and cause an increase in production of granulocyte–macrophage colony-stimulating factor (GM-CSF), which, with histamine, results in increased neutrophil and eosinophil chemotaxia. The Gram negative bacteria cell wall also contains endotoxin. This stimulates inflammatory mediators (e.g. macrophages to release cytokines) and activates complement (catalysts which in turn stimulate other inflammatory mechanisms such as helping white cells to bind to bacteria).

Terms associated with leucocytes

Leucopenia — where the white cell count is less than 4×10^9/l. This may be due to a generalized bone marrow disorder (e.g. megaloblastic anaemia, aplasia, acute leukaemia, or metastatic tumour), viral or bacterial infections, or drug toxicity.

Leucocytosis — where the white cell count $> 11 \times 10^9$/l

Neutropenia — where the neutrophil count $< 1.0 \times 10^9$/l (severe neutropenia is $< 0.5 \times 10^9$/l)

Eosinophilia — where the eosinophil count $> 0.4 \times 10^9$/l

Lymphocytosis — where the lymphocyte count $> 3.5 \times 10^9$/l

Monocytosis — where the monocyte count $> 0.8 \times 10^9$/l

Agranulocytosis — a condition where the bone marrow stops producing white cells leaving the body open to overwhelming infection. It is often caused by irradiation or drug toxicity (e.g. carbimazole).

Leucocyte disorders

The leukaemias

The leukaemias are neoplastic disorders of the blood forming tissues (bone marrow, spleen, and lymphatic system). Commonly, there is unregulated and prolific accumulation of white cells in the bone marrow, liver, spleen, and lymph nodes with invasion of the gastrointestinal tract, meninges, skin, and kidneys. They are classified according to the cell line involved and are either acute or chronic. Leukaemia may be caused by irradiation but the cause is often unknown.

The symptoms of acute leukaemias reflect the infiltration of organs by white cells and/or bone marrow failure. Infiltration can cause local pain in the liver, spleen and lymph nodes as well as bone pain due to expansion of the marrow.

Bone marrow failure results in:

● anaemia causing lethargy and pallor;

● granulocytopenia causing increased risk of infection;

● thrombocytopenia causing increased risk of bleeding.

Summary of the types of leukaemia

Acute lymphatic leukaemia (ALL)

This type is more common in children. It is a severe disease where lymph nodes, bone and nervous tissue can become infiltrated. Therapy aims to induce a remission by cytotoxic agents and irradiation of the central nervous system. Fifty per cent of children between the ages of 2 and 11 years survive five years.

Chronic lymphatic leukaemia (CLL)

This occurs mainly in adults over 50 years of age and it is often discovered at a routine medical examination or blood test, as the patients are usually symptom-free. Occasionally, pleural or peritoneal effusions develop. If asymptomatic, no treatment is required but combined chemo- and radiotherapy can reduce the size of glands. Fifty per cent of patients survive five years.

Acute myeloid leukaemia (AML)

This affects people of any age, but is more common in adults. Until almost a decade ago the outcome was extremely poor. However, with intensive chemotherapy regimens and bone marrow transplantation, 30–50 per cent of patients may now have long-term survival.

Chronic myeloid leukaemia (CML)

This often occurs in the 30 to 50-year age group. Insidious onset with fever and weight loss. Splenomegaly, hepatomegaly, and thrombocytopenia may develop later in the disease. The white blood cell count is often very high. Treatment is with chemotherapy. Overall survival is about three years. However, with the use of allogenic bone marrow transplantation, particularly in younger patients, 50 per cent may have greater than five years survival. (See later for the care and management of malignant haematological disease (p. 364).

Thrombocytes (platelets)

Thrombocytes are actually fragments of a large type of white cell called a megakaryocyte. Megakaryocytes are formed in the bone marrow and the tip of the cells are thought to extend into the blood sinusoid. These tips are then nipped off and circulate in the blood as non-nucleated platelets. Platelets are essential for blood clotting, the mechanism of which is complex and is discussed later.

Thrombocyte disorders

Thrombocytopenia

A platelet count of $150 \times 10^9/l$ is the lower limit of the normal range but bleeding due to thrombocytopenia is unlikely to occur unless the count is below $50 \times 10^9/l$. However, bleeding can occur at higher levels if generalized infection is present. Thrombocytopenia can result from an increased destruction of platelets (e.g. idiopathic thrombocytopenic purpura and consumptive coagulopathies such as disseminated intravascular coagulation; DIC), or decreased production of platelets by the bone marrow (e.g. marrow aplasia, leukaemia, or tumour infiltration).

Idiopathic thrombocytopenic purpura

Idiopathic thrombocytopenic purpura (ITP) is a rare, autoimmune disorder where autoantibodies are directed against the platelets so that their lifespan is considerably shortened. It can affect any age group but is more common in young adults, particularly following respiratory or gastrointestinal viral infections. Symptoms usually begin suddenly with petechiae and mucosal bleeding. The platelet count is low, bleeding time prolonged, but coagulation times are normal. The acute form is usually post-infectious and recovery can take from weeks to months. The chronic form has a variable course and often does not recover.

There is no definitive treatment. Steroids are often tried with variable effect. In the acute form, steroids tend not to increase the platelet count but may have a role in reducing the incidence of bleeding. High dose gamma-globulin has also been advocated, particularly in patients with bleeding complications.

In the chronic form, a rise in platelets is usually seen within a week or so of commencing steroid therapy. Platelet transfusions may be required to control severe bleeding. In some patients unresponsive to medical management splenectomy may be required.

Thrombotic thrombocytopenic purpura

Thrombotic thrombocytopenic purpura (TTP) is a very rare condition and the aetiology is unknown. The mechanism may involve the vascular endothelium which becomes unable to produce a prostaglandin platelet inhibitor which normally prevents platelet aggregation. Haemolysis, widespread intravascular thrombosis, and thrombocytopenia occur, affecting, in particular, the gut and cerebral circulation but also the liver, kidney, and lung.

TTP usually affects young adults. The presenting features include abdominal pain, purpura, and fever. There may be hypertension and fluctuating (or permanent) neurological signs. Haematuria may develop and progress to renal failure. Mortality is high. The mainstay of treatment is plasma exchange (using fresh frozen plasma) in conjunction with steroids. However, once relapses occur treatment can be very difficult. If cerebral TTP occurs with renal failure, prostacyclin may be given but this therapy is controversial.

Drug-induced thrombocytopenia

Some drugs may cause thrombocytopenia, in particular, quinine, heparin, antituberculous drugs, thiazide diuretics, penicillins, sulphonamides, and anticonvulsants.

Heparin can sometimes cause the so-called heparin-induced thrombocytopenia syndrome (HITS). This is where an immune reaction occurs to the heparin, usually after 7–10 days of use. Thrombocytopenia will develop and platelet aggregation can cause venous and arterial thrombosis. Treatment is supportive, with platelet transfusions as necessary, and avoidance of all types of heparin administration, including the flushing of arterial lines. Low molecular weight heparin can occasionally be successfully substituted for heparin if anticoagulation is required.

Uraemia

Uraemia can cause defects in platelet function and bleeding can be a serious consequence of renal failure. These patients may have a prolonged bleeding time and develop gastrointestinal bleeding, nosebleeds, purpura, pericarditis, and cerebral haemorrhage. The prolonged bleeding time may be reduced by blood transfusion, DDAVP (1-deamino-8-D-arginine vasopressin) or dialysis. Low-dose heparin or prostacyclin should be used to maintain the patency of the circuit if haemodialysis is required.

The clotting mechanism and fibrinolysis

Rupture of a blood vessel leads to exposure of collagen fibres in the vessel wall. Platelets adhere to the collagen and roughened areas of the tear, forming a platelet plug. The platelets can then produce up to 40 substances, including catecholamines and coagulation factors; these initiate the cascade of reactions that will eventually form a fibrin clot. The damaged vessel vasoconstricts in response to the trauma and the release of noradrenaline, adrenaline, and serotonin by the platelets. Blood flow to the area is therefore reduced and a more durable effort to seal the tear begins. There are two pathways which may be activated, the intrinsic and extrinsic. These merge to form a common pathway (see Fig. 12.2).

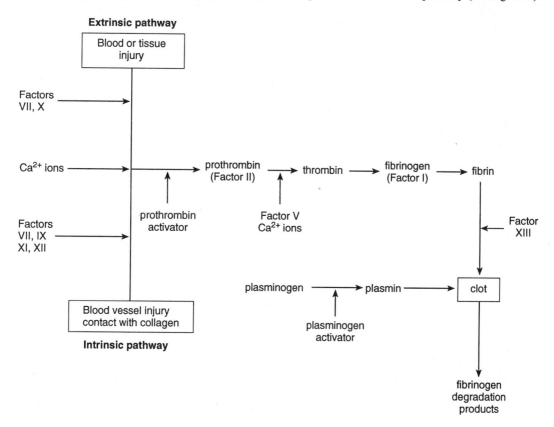

Fig. 12.2 The clotting mechanism and fibrinolytic pathway.

Intrinsic pathway

When the endothelium of the blood vessel is damaged a cascade of reactions involving factors V, VIII, IX, X, XI, and XII, in the presence of calcium ions, produces prothrombin activator. Prothrombin activator (also known as prothrombinase complex) is formed by factor Xa, V and platelet factor III (PF3). PF3 is a reaction surface or template for the clotting factors.

Extrinsic pathway

This is initiated by the release of tissue thromboplastin into the blood from damaged tissue outside the circulation. A series of reactions, involving factors VII and X, in the presence of calcium ions, produces prothrombin activator.

Common pathway

This pathway then begins, with prothrombin activator catalysing the conversion of prothrombin to thrombin. Thrombin acts as an enzyme to convert fibrinogen into fibrin threads, which forms the clot itself. (See Table 12.3 for blood-clotting factors.)

Table 12.3 Blood-clotting factors

Factor	Name
I	Fibrinogen
II	Prothrombin
III	Tissue thromboplastin
IV	Calcium ions
V	Labile factor
VII	Stable factor
VIII	Antihaemophilic factor
IX	Christmas factor
X	Stuart–Prower factor
XI	Plasma thromboplastin antecedent
XII	Hageman factor
XIII	Fibrin stabilizing factor

There must, however, be a balancing mechanism to control clotting within the body so that the clot can be dissolved when the injury is healed, and extensive clot formation prevented. The fibrinolytic system is responsible for the degradation of the clot and runs alongside the coagulation pathways. Its activation occurs immediately whenever the clotting cascade is triggered. Plasminogen may be activated intrinsically by the contact system via factor XII, or extrinsically by tissue plasminogen activator found in many cells including endothelial cells. The activation of plasminogen produces the enzyme plasmin which dissolves both fibrin and fibrinogen, thus lysing the clot.

The normal mechanisms of coagulation and fibrinolysis will complement each other until an underlying condition disturbs the body's homeostasis.

Clotting factor defects

Haemophilia

This is a sex-linked genetic disorder affecting men but carried by women. Haemophilia A is caused by deficiency of factor VIII and haemophilia B (Christmas disease) by a deficiency of factor IX. Clinically, they are indistinguishable. Haemophilia can cause severe bleeding from minor trauma and disabling muscle and joint haemorrhages.

Treatment is by administering purified factor VIII or IX concentrate as soon as possible after the bleeding has started, or prophylactically before dental extractions or surgery. The aim is to raise the factor to above 30 per cent of normal. Repeated infusions may be necessary every 8–12 hours.

Fresh frozen plasma (FFP) contains both factors but vast quantities are usually required. This is usually given only if the single factor concentrates are unavailable. Patients with haemophilia should never be given aspirin as this impairs platelet function and may cause gastric erosions. Intramuscular injections must be avoided and dental hygiene is important since dental extraction can be so hazardous.

Von Willebrand's disease.

This is an autosomal dominant disease affecting both males and females (these have different types of Von Willebrand's disease). It is due to a mild deficiency of factor VIII (15–50 per cent of normal). There is a prolonged bleeding time and poor platelet adhesion resulting in variable degrees of bleeding. Commonly, patients have nose bleeds, post-operative bleeding, and bleeding from cuts, but do not suffer from the massive soft tissue or joint haemorrhages seen in haemophilia. Treatment is by the transfusion of cryoprecipitate (which contains factor VIII) or by a purified concentrate of factor VIII. Mild Von Willebrand's disease may be treated soley by DDAVP infusion and this can also be used for prophylaxis prior to surgery.

Liver disease

The liver produces nearly all the factors involved in the formation and control of coagulation (except factor VIII). Bleeding associated with liver disease can be devastating and difficult to manage. Liver disease may result in the reduced synthesis of all of the coagulation factors. Fat-soluble vitamin K, which is necessary for the precursors of factors II, VII, IX, and X, may not be absorbed if there is concomitant cholestasis. Disseminated intravascular coagulation (DIC) can be initiated or exacerbated by the release of tissue thromboplastin from damaged liver cells. The prothrombin time (PT) and partial thromboplastin time (PTT) are both prolonged in liver failure and the platelet count low if there is splenomegaly. Fibrin degradation products (FDPs) may be elevated as a result of excessive fibrinolysis or because the liver fails to clear them from the blood.

Bleeding due to vitamin K deficiency may be reversed by the administration of vitamin K. Treatment of bleeding episodes associated with abnormal laboratory tests is by transfusions of FFP and platelets to maintain the platelet count $> 50 \times 10^9/l$ and to normalize the prothrombin time. Low fibrinogen levels usually indicate severe liver disease or the presence of DIC. Cryoprecipitate can be used to increase fibrinogen.

Anticoagulant therapy

Anticoagulants are used to prevent thrombus formation or the extension of an existing thrombus. Such therapy is commonly used in the ICU, but always carries the potential complication of haemorrhage. Patients having anticoagulant therapy must be observed closely for signs of bleeding. This may be overt, with active bleeding from cannulae sites, drains and wounds, or may be more occult (e.g. from the gastrointestinal tract: haematemesis, melaena).

Urine should be tested daily for blood and nasogastric aspirate also regularly observed or tested for blood. The skin should be observed for bruising, petechial or purpuric haemorrhages. Purpura is the extravasation of blood into the skin causing purple areas which may be variable in size. Pinhead sized spots are termed petechiae and larger areas ecchymoses (bruises). Purpura result from the increased fragility of the capillary due to a deficiency in the number or function of platelets or damage to the capillary wall due to antibodies (allergic purpura) or metabolic/bacterial toxins (bacterial endocarditis and uraemia).

In order to prevent haemorrhage the effect of the anticoagulant must be monitored carefully and regular laboratory coagulation screens will be required.

Anticoagulation is kept within a specific therapeutic range of values depending on the drug used. It is possible to measure activated clotting times (ACTs) at the bedside and this is a simple and quick procedure. ACTs are commonly recorded in the ICU in patients undergoing renal replacement therapy as such patients are frequently anticoagulated with heparin. The dose of heparin can then be titrated according to the ACT level. The value of the ACT aimed for will, however, vary according to the patient's clinical state and the purpose of the anticoagulation. Patients with extracorporeal circuits for renal replacement therapy usually require an ACT in the region of 170–200 seconds whilst those on cardiopulmonary bypass will need 400–600 seconds. The ACT cannot be used for determining the anticoagulant action of prostacyclin. (See Table 12.4 for coagulation tests.)

Anticoagulants commonly used in the ICU

Heparin

This is commonly used, for example, in patients with pulmonary embolus, deep vein thrombosis and those undergoing heart surgery or renal replacement therapy. Heparin is administered intravenously, acts rapidly but has a short half-life of about 90 minutes. Heparin may prolong the clotting time if heparin-induced antibodies block platelet aggregation. Heparin overdose may be corrected by stopping the heparin and, if necessary, by the intravenous administration of protamine sulphate. When used alone, protamine sulphate has an anticoagulant effect but when given in the presence of heparin, a stable salt is formed and the anticoagulant activity of both is lost: 1 mg of protamine sulphate will neutralize 100 iu of heparin, and is usually given in small doses with laboratory monitoring to assess the effect.

Warfarin

This is given orally and takes 36–48 hours' loading to achieve full anticoagulation. It is commonly used, for example, in patients with poorly controlled atrial fibrillation or prosthetic heart valves to prevent thrombus formation. Warfarin antagonizes the effects of vitamin K which is a co-factor for an enzyme essential for the synthesis of prothrombin and factors VII, IX, and X. It thus depresses the formation of the coagulation factors.

Warfarin readily combines with plasma proteins in the blood and can be displaced by some drugs (such as aspirin, chloral hydrate, and naladixic acid), so that levels of free warfarin in the blood rises. Other drugs, such as quinine, quinidine, and large doses of salicylates,

Table 12.4   Coagulation tests

Test	Abreviation	Normal value	Use
Prothrombin time	PT	13 s or < 2 s above control	Assesses the extrinsic pathway. Used as a guide to warfarin dosage. Prolonged levels indicate deficiency of factors V, VII and/or X,I,II.
Activated, partial thromboplastin time	APTT	40 s	Evaluates the intrinsic and common pathways. Prolonged level indicates deficiency of factors VII, IX, XI, or XII in the intrinsic pathway or factors II, V, or X in the common pathway.
Kaolin partial thromboplastin time	KPTT	< 7 s above control	Assesses the intrinsic and common pathway as for APTT. The only difference between APTT and KPTT is the type of activator used.
Thrombin time	TT	15s	Assesses the conversion of fibrinogen to fibrin. Prolonged levels due to inhibition of fibrin formation and is an indication of the presence of FDPs.
Fibrinogen degradation products	FDPs	< 10 mg/ml	FDPs result from the breakdown of fibrin.
Bleeding time		< 7 min	Measures the effectiveness of platelet clots and its interaction with the vessel wall.
Fibrinogen level		> 150 mg/dl	Reduced levels found in deficiency of fibrinogen or with inappropriate activation of fibrinolysis.

further depress prothrombin formation in the liver. Patients receiving such drugs in combination with warfarin, are subject to increased sensitivity and must be monitored carefully.

The dosage of warfarin is controlled by regular estimations of the international normalized ratio (INR) which is derived from the prothrombin time. The INR is a ratio that relates the sensitivity of the thromboplastin reagent used in the PT test to that of a World Health Organization standard. The INR should be kept between 2.0 and 4.5, depending on the reason for anticoagulation.

Warfarin overdose can be treated by the administration of phytomenadione (vitamin K). This antagonizes the effect of warfarin in the liver cells and is necessary for the production of clotting factors. This drug, however, may take up to 24 hours to act and a dose greater than 10 mg will prevent oral anticoagulants from acting for up to several weeks. If the patient is bleeding, fresh frozen plasma (FFP) can be transfused to provide an immediate supply of the deficient clotting factors.

Streptokinase and tissue plasminogen activator

Both are fibrinolytic drugs that are used to break down a thrombus that has already formed (e.g. in acute myo-

cardial infarction or pulmonary embolism). Tissue plasminogen activator (tPA) specifically activates fibrin-bound plasminogen while streptokinase can also activate circulating plasminogen.

Plasminogen is usually inactive until triggered. It is the precursor of plasmin, a proteolytic enzyme that dissolves fibrin. Allergic reactions to streptokinase can occur but are rare with tPA. Bleeding can be a major problem in fibrinolytic therapy and fibrinolysis can be corrected by the intravenous administration of tranexamic acid (plus FFP, cryoprecipitate, and blood transfusion, as necessary).

Epoprostenol sodium (prostacyclin)

Epoprostenol is a naturally occurring prostaglandin. It is a potent inhibitor of platelet aggregation and the degree of inhibition is dose-related. The effect on the platelets usually disappears within 30 minutes of discontinuing the infusion.

It is used as an alternative to heparin in renal support therapy (CVVHD, haemodialysis, etc.) where a high risk of bleeding from heparin exists. It must be given as a continuous infusion either intravenously or into the extracorporeal circuit.

Epoprostenol is also a potent vasodilator; hypotension and tachycardia may occur. If hypotension occurs the dose should be reduced or the infusion discontinued and supportive measures, such as plasma volume expansion, instituted.

Clotting disorders

Disseminated intravascular coagulation

Disseminated intravascular coagulation (DIC) is an inappropriate, accelerated, and systemic activation of the coagulation cascade in which both thrombus formation and fibrinolysis occur simultaneously. DIC never occurs as a primary disorder but always arises as a secondary complication of an underlying condition. Often, the primary condition that has induced the DIC will dominate the clinical picture, and the development of the syndrome provides a diagnostic and management challenge. The mortality of patients with DIC can be extremely high. (See Table 12.5.)

Table 12.5 Disorders which may trigger disseminated intravascular coagulation (DIC)

Infection
- viral diseases (varicella, rubella)
- bacterial infections
- parasitic infections (malaria)

Obstetric
- septic abortion
- eclampsia
- amniotic fluid embolism
- placental abruption

Malignant disease
- carcinoma
- leukaemia

Others
- Trauma (crush injuries, burns)
- shock states
- pulmonary embolism
- organ transplant rejection
- heat stroke
- ARDS
- liver disease
- ABO incompatible blood transfusions
- penetrating head injuries

The normal mechanism of coagulation and fibrinolysis complement each other until an underlying condition disturbs this fine balance. The causative factors of DIC can be grouped into three categories, described below.

1. The introduction of tissue coagulation factors
Tissue can be damaged by trauma, surgery, burns, or disseminated malignant disease. The damaged tissue allows the entry of tissue thromboplastin into the blood, triggering diffuse clotting, and overwhelming the inhibitory mechanisms. Penetrating head injury with extensive brain trauma may be followed by DIC, presumably by the absorption of thromboplastic materials. This may cause further brain damage due to haematoma formation.

2. Damage to the vascular epithelium
The normal intact endothelium has an anticoagulant effect due to the secretion of prostaglandins which prevent platelet aggregation. Vascular damage exposes collagen fibres, attracts platelets, and triggers the intrinsic pathway of coagulation. Endothelial damage can result from cardiothoracic surgery, dissecting aortic aneurysms, and viral infections. Bacterial endotoxins from Gram-negative bacteria can also damage the endothelium. Although the exact mechanism is not well understood, there is thought to be massive sloughing of the endothelial cells, exposing collagen and attracting platelets. ARDS may trigger DIC by injury to the pulmonary capillary membrane.

3. Stagnant blood flow
Prolonged hypotension, hypoxia, and acidosis lead to blood stasis which promotes intracapillary thrombosis and cell ischaemia. Blood stasis in the capillaries contributes to the aggregation of platelets, metabolites, and blockage by fibrin. The deposition of fibrin throughout the microcirculation predisposes the patient to a generalized coagulation defect.

In practice, the trigger mechanisms are often multiple and can be complicated by hypoxia, acidosis, and hyperpyrexia.

When the clotting cascade has been activated there is a rapid accumulation of thrombin. This in turn leads to the production of large amounts of fibrin. Fibrin is deposited throughout the small vessels of the body, leading to thrombi formation and, consequently, organ hypoperfusion, ischaemia, infarction, and necrosis. As the clotting process progresses, clotting factors and platelets are depleted, leading to generalized bleeding.

The natural defence against this widespread clotting is the fibrinolytic system. Activated factor XII, thrombin, and endothelial cells all stimulate the fibrinolytic system to release plasminogen activators. These stimulate plasmin to degrade fibrin into fibrin degradation products (FDPs). FDPs are potent anticoagulants and further potentiate the haemorrhagic cycle. The reticuloendothelial system, which normally removes FDPs, is overwhelmed and the patient has a self-perpetuating combination of thrombotic and bleeding activity.

There is no single laboratory test that will confirm the diagnosis of DIC. In order to make a diagnosis, the interpretation of a variety of laboratory tests must be correlated with the clinical presentation of the patient and an awareness of the conditions that predispose to DIC.

> **Laboratory values in DIC**
> (For normal values see Table 12.4)
> Prolonged prothrombin time > 15 s
> Prolonged partial thromboplastin time > 60–90 s
> Prolonged thrombin time > 15–20 s
> Low fibrinogen levels < 75–100 mg/dl
> Low platelet count < 20–75 × 10^9/l
> High FDPs > 100 mg/ml
> Raised levels of D-dimers

Treatment of DIC

The treatment of an individual presenting with DIC secondary to another disorder presents a considerable challenge. There is no single universally accepted treatment regimen and medical management is controversial (see Fig. 12.3). However, the agreed aims of therapy are the:

- elimination of the underlying cause;
- restoration of haemostasis;
- prevention of microemboli;
- the maintenance of blood volume and prevention of vascular stasis, hypoxia, and acidosis.

The method by which haemostasis is restored is controversial. Transfusions of blood, FFP, platelets and cryoprecipitate were once thought to be contraindicated because they would increase the clotting tendency of the blood. However, it is now an accepted form of therapy in order to restore the blood volume and consumed coagulation factors while the underlying condition is brought under control. FFP is particularly useful as it provides all the clotting factors required. A platelet count below $50 × 10^9$/l in a patient who is actively bleeding would be an indication for replacement therapy.

Heparin therapy may be indicated in situations of clear

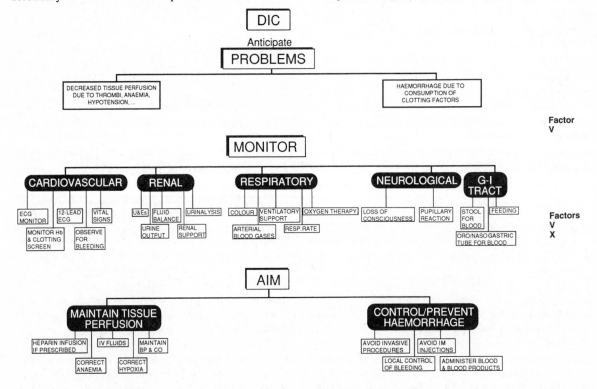

Fig. 12.3 The management of disseminated intravascular coagulation.

fibrin deposition in the form of dermal necrosis (e.g. venous thromboembolism), or when there is a retained dead fetus with decreased fibrinogen levels prior to induction of labour. However, in 95 per cent of cases of DIC, there is no indication for heparin.

Nursing management

The aims of management are to:

- identify the patient at risk of developing DIC (see trigger factors, p. 357);

- early detection and management of bleeding;

- prevent further bleeding;

- prevent the complications associated with decreased tissue perfusion or haemorrhage;

- treat the underlying cause of DIC (if possible).

Other DIC disorders

Cardiovascular disorders

Potential problems:

- Hypovolaemia due to haemorrhage.

- Skin necrosis due to decreased capillary refill or infarction.

Action: Haemorrhage may be acute or chronic, insidious or massive. Some degree of hypotension is likely in DIC if there is a fluid volume deficit. Vital signs must be monitored closely in order to detect hypovolaemia and must be vigorously treated in order to prevent vascular stasis and maintain organ perfusion.

Cannulae sites, puncture sites, wounds, drains, and mucosal membranes must be observed for bleeding and the skin for petechiae and bruising. Observe for necrotic areas (particularly on the toes and fingers).

Invasive procedures should be kept to a minimum in the patient with DIC. An arterial line *in situ* will avoid repeated puncturing of vessels for blood sampling and can be used to monitor blood pressure. If a blood pressure cuff is used it should be removed between recordings and alternate arms used if possible. Intramuscular injections should be avoided, but if essential, a small-gauge needle should be used. Mouth care must be gentle to avoid trauma to the gums. Use an electric razor in order to avoid nicks and cuts. Local pressure or haemostatic dressings may be necessary if there is bleeding from cannulae sites.

Respiratory disorders
Potential problems:

- Respiratory failure due to pulmonary haemorrhage.

- Haemothorax.

- Pulmonary embolus.

- Adult respiratory distress syndrome.

Action: Pulmonary bleeding will cause haemoptysis (in the self-ventilating patient) or blood-stained secretions on endotracheal suction. Respiratory function must be monitored closely (see Chapter 13). Oxygen therapy should be administered according to the arterial oxygen saturation but intubation and ventilation should not be delayed if the patient is hypoxaemic (despite the potential risk of bleeding associated with the procedure).

Renal disorders
Potential problem:

- Renal failure due to microemboli or hypovolaemia.

Action: the kidneys are a common site for microemboli and acute renal failure due to acute tubular necrosis often occurs. Urine output must be monitored and attempts made to maintain an output > 0.5 ml/kg/h in the adult. Oliguria can result from hypoperfusion of the kidney therefore hypovolaemia must be treated aggressively and efforts made to maintain an adequate blood pressure (with inotropic support if the cause of hypotension is not volume depletion). If renal failure becomes established renal support will be required (see Chapter 8) Urine should be tested regularly for protein and blood and renal function monitored by measurements of blood urea, creatinine, and electrolytes.

Neurological disorders
Potential problem:

- Cerebral ischaemia due to intercranial haemorrhage or thrombosis.

Action: the patient must be observed for changes in conscious level, restlessness, agitation, visual disturbances, headaches, and sensory or motor function. Monitor pupillary reaction (see Chapter 9).

Gastrointestinal disorders
Potential problem:

- Bleeding from the gastrointestinal tract.

Action: observe nasogastric aspirate, emesis, and stool for blood. Stools should be tested for occult blood. A mesenteric embolus may cause small bowel infarction and severe abdominal pain. Bleeding into the retroperitoneal space can result in varying degrees of pain, tingling or numbness due to secondary nerve compression.

Blood transfusion and blood component products

Transfusions of blood and blood products are common in the ICU, both for the management of acute haemorrhage, where circulating volume and oxygen transport needs to be restored, and in the treatment of a range of haematological disorders where specific components of the blood are needed.

Donated blood is collected and stored in closed plastic packs which can then be kept for up to 35 days at 4 °C. Whole blood can be separated into its component parts after donation and stored separately. This is an economical way of using a valuable resource as several different patients can benefit from a single unit of blood. Specific blood components, once separated, have different uses and storage needs and these are detailed later.

Blood screening

All donated blood is screened for infectious risk and cross-matched with the recipient's blood for immunological compatibility. The purpose of cross-matching blood before transfusion is to ensure that there is no antibody present in the recipient's plasma that will react with any antigen on the donor's cells. The most frequent cause of giving incompatible blood is incorrect labelling of samples, confusion between patients of the same name or failing to check from the label on the blood pack that the blood being transfused is the blood that has been cross-matched with the patient. Scrupulous and rigid checking procedures must be carried out at the bedside before any unit of blood or blood product is transfused. The patient identification details on the blood pack must be checked against those on the patient's wristband before the infusion is connected, no matter how urgent their need for the blood, as the consequences of giving mismatched blood can be dire (see transfusion hazards, p. 363)

Blood and blood products
Fresh whole blood

This is blood that is used within 24 hours of donation. It contains red cells, viable platelets, small amounts of all coagulation factors and plasma proteins. The use of fresh whole blood is usually restricted to neonates where it is used for top-up or exchange transfusions. Fresh blood carries a higher risk of transmitting cytomegalovirus (CMV) than stored blood.

Stored whole blood

Donated blood is stored at 4 °C in a special blood refrigerator from where it should not be removed for more than 30 minutes prior to the transfusion. Depending on the anticoagulant used in the blood pack, the red cells may remain viable for up to five weeks. The main use of stored whole blood is for the restoration of red cells and circulating blood volume in acute haemorrhage. It contains no therapeutic amounts of clotting factors, apart from fibrinogen, and no viable platelets or granulocytes. The consequences of giving large volumes of whole stored blood are discussed later.

Packed red cells (red cell concentrate)

Much of the plasma has been removed from whole blood leaving a concentrated solution of red cells. It is not given where volume replacement is needed but is used for chronic, persistent blood loss or bone marrow failure (e.g. aplastic anaemia, leukaemia). In the anaemic patient 1 unit of packed cells should raise the haemoglobin by approximately 1 g/dl in adults.

Leucocyte-depleted blood

This contains concentrated red cells with no neutrophil-specific antigens. Alternatively, red cell concentrate can be used with a specific leucocyte-depleting filter attached to the giving set. It is used to prevent non-haemolytic transfusion reactions demonstrated to be due to leucocyte antibodies in the recipient. It must be stored at 4 °C until its use and should be used within 12 hours of preparation. Check the pack carefully for expiry time and date.

Frozen red cells

These contain red cells, uncontaminated by other cells or plasma, in a suspending medium (usually saline). It is used in patients who have a rare blood group as a supply of blood; they donate blood and then the red cells are frozen for future use. Once frozen, these can be stored for an indefinite time but when thawed should be used within 12 hours.

Red cell concentrates can also be specifically CMV-negative or irradiated. CMV-negative products are from donors who have been screened for cytomegalovirus and are found to be sero-negative. They are used in patients who are recipients of bone marrow transplants or who may require one. Irradiation is actually used to destroy lymphocytes which can cause third-party graft verses host disease in the immunosuppressed patient. The CMV load can be reduced in leucocyte-depleted blood by using a filter.

Platelets

These are obtained by passing blood through a cell separator and may be from a single donor or random donors. A pack of random donor platelets contains platelet concentrate in 30–50 ml of donor plasma and is usually issued in pools of 6 packs. A single donor pack may contain up to 300 ml of platelets in plasma. Platelet transfusions are used in patients with thrombocytopenia due to bone marrow failure or who have congenital platelet defects. They also provide platelet replacement in patients who have undergone large, rapid blood transfusions or cardiopulmonary bypass surgery (see Chapter 7). Generally, infusions are given daily to maintain the platelet count $> 15 \times 10^9$/l by giving 1 unit of platelet concentrate per 10 kg body weight.

Platelet packs contain contaminating leucocytes, which may cause non-haemolytic febrile transfusion reactions, and contaminating red cells. ABO + RhD group-compatible platelets should be given where possible.

Once prepared, platelet function is best preserved at room temperature and must usually be used within 72 hours (check the expiry time carefully on the pack). Each pack of platelets should be transfused via a 170 mm in-line filter and specific platelet giving sets are available which have small filter surfaces and drip chambers to reduce the loss of platelets from volume left in the infusion line. Platelets can be infused as rapidly as the patient tolerates but should be completed within 30 minutes.

Fresh frozen plasma (FFP)

FFP is prepared in blood banks as a by-product of red cell concentrate preparation. The plasma is separated in a low temperature centrifuge at $4\,°C$ and is then deep frozen within 30 minutes to $-50\,°C$. It is stored at $-20\,°C$ and when needed can be prepared in about 15 minutes by immersion in a water bath at $37\,°C$.

After thawing, the potency of the replacement factors deteriorate and therefore should be given as soon as possible and at least within two hours.

FFP contains normal amounts of all clotting factors, plasma proteins, and some contaminating red cell fragments. The ABO + RhD group of the FFP must be compatible with that of the recipient. It is used as a source of clotting factors for the treatment of DIC and following rapid, large volume blood transfusions (1 unit of FFP is usually given per 5–6 units of stored blood, although replacement should be guided by clotting studies). FFP is also given to treat clotting factor deficiencies either when the deficient factor is not known or the specific factor is unavailable.

FFP is also useful in the treatment of liver disease where there is defective synthesis of coagulation factors. It is also beneficial in the treatment of thrombotic thrombocytopenic purpura (TTP), although the effective factor in the plasma has not been identified.

A pack of FFP is usually about 150–250 ml in volume. It should be given through an infusion set with a 170 mm filter. There is no added benefit in using microaggregate filters. It can be transfused as fast as the patient can tolerate.

Cryoprecipitate

This contains factor VIII and fibrinogen. It is used to provide these replacement factors in haemophilia and Von Willebrand's disease, or in patients with bleeding associated with hypofibrinogenaemia (< 0.8 g/dl), or uraemia. It is usually prepared in pools of 6 units, each unit containing approximately 20 ml of donor plasma with factor VIII, fibrinogen, and red cell fragments. ABO + RhD groups should be compatible between donor and recipient. Since six or more donors are usually involved in a single transfusion the likelihood of transmission of viral or bacterial infection is increased and anaphylactic reactions can occur to the plasma antigens.

Cryoprecipitate must be filtered because it contains cellular material from leucocytes, red cells, platelets, and fibrin. Transfuse through a 170 mm filter as rapidly as the patient's condition allows.

Notes on administering blood transfusions

1. If you have any queries when checking the identification details between the blood pack and the patient **always** seek the advice of the haematology department **before** you connect the transfusion.

2. Avoid skin contact with any blood or blood product.

3. Blood and component products should be administered through a 170 mm filter in order to remove particulate material. A fine 40 mm filter should be

used in patients who are neutropenic as these will also remove leucocytes and leucocyte debris.

4. Do not use if the pack is perforated.

5. Do not mix any drugs or calcium-containing infusion fluids with whole blood or red cell concentrate transfusions.

6. If a unit of blood is out of the storage refrigerator or cooled transport box for more than 30 minutes it should be returned to the laboratory.

7. Do not store blood in the ward or kitchen refrigerator, even temporarily. It must be stored at 4 °C ($\pm$ 2 °C) in a specified blood fridge.

8. When the transfusion is in progress be alert for transfusion reactions (see later).

Adverse reactions to blood transfusions

Blood transfusions are so common that it is easy to overlook the associated hazards. Unfavourable reactions usually occur within 20 minutes of starting the transfusion and it is during this time that particular attention must be paid. However, careful, continuous monitoring is vital throughout the transfusion, particularly in the ICU where circulatory overload can easily occur in patients with renal or cardiac impairment. Immediate transfusion reactions are usually due to pyrogens, allergens, bacteria, or incompatible blood, but delayed reactions can occur over a period of weeks or months.

Pyrexia

Monitoring of temperature is vital whilst a transfusion is in progress. Pyrexia may be due to pyrogens, leucocytes, or platelet antibodies. Pyrogens are polysaccharides produced by bacteria and can be present in distilled water, citrate, dextrose, and saline. Strict infection control procedures means that contamination has now been reduced, but febrile reactions may be caused by the presence of anti-HLA (human lymphocyte antibodies), granulocyte-specific and platelet-specific antibodies in the recipient as a result of sensitization during pregnancy or from previous transfusions. Since pyrexia due to pyrogens is now rare, if it occurs it should be presumed to be due to incompatibility of the red cells, white cells, or platelets that have been transfused or to plasma proteins. Plasma proteins are the main cause of transfusion reactions. The fever should respond to antipyretics, such as aspirin or paracetamol, and if mild the

transfusion may continue. However, if accompanied by rigors and the temperature exceeds 38 °C, the transfusion should be stopped.

Haemolytic reactions

These occur when the red cells are destroyed in the circulation (haemolysed) following the transfusion. As the red cells break down, haemoglobin is released, and complement activation causes smooth muscle contraction, platelet aggregation and release of vasoactive substances. The reaction may be delayed or immediate and the consequences can be fatal. Most delayed haemolytic reactions are immune and severity will depend on the red cell antibody involved. Most immediate reactions have an avoidable and identifiable cause and these can be the most dangerous. Immediate haemolysis can be caused by incompatible ABO blood groups, usually as a result of identification error (there is a 10 per cent mortality associated with this). Other immediate causes are incorrectly stored or out-of-date blood, over-heated, frozen, or infected blood, mechanical destruction of the red cells by administering the infusion under pressure, and the mixing of the blood with hypotonic infusion fluids.

The signs and symptoms of haemolysis can be immediate and severe. The patient may complain of pain at the infusion site, facial flushing, dyspnoea, headache, chest, abdominal, and loin pain. Nausea, vomiting, pyrexia, and rigors usually develop. Tachycardia and hypotension are common and may lead to complete circulatory collapse. Oliguria and consequent renal failure may follow. Other features of the reaction include the development of disseminated intravascular coagulation (DIC).

When a haemolytic reaction is suspected the blood transfusion must be stopped immediately. The blood bag must be retained and returned to the laboratory, together with samples of blood from the patient for checking the cross-match, full blood count, coagulation screen, and bacterial culture. Full resuscitative measures may be required in order to restore cardiovascular stability and maintain urine output. Urine should be tested for haemoglobin and, if DIC develops, replacement of clotting factors will be required.

Delayed haemolytic reactions are less severe and may occur over a period of days following the transfusion; symptoms include anaemia and jaundice.

Close monitoring of vital signs is essential for the early detection of immediate haemolytic reaction in any patients undergoing a blood transfusion. The sooner it can be identified, the transfusion stopped and supportive treatment begins, the better the prognosis. Careful and rigorous attention to the correct procedures of storing and checking may prevent many such reactions.

Circulatory overload

This is not usually a problem in patients with normal cardiac and renal function. However, those with impaired function, the elderly, or the pregnant patient may not tolerate the fluid load associated with blood transfusions, and this may lead to the development of pulmonary oedema and heart failure. Careful monitoring of vital signs is again essential if this is to be recognized early. Dyspnoea and tachypnoea, elevated blood pressure, CVP, and heart rate may indicate fluid overload. In patients at risk, this complication may be avoided by the administration of a diuretic at the time the transfusion begins, and by the use of red cell concentrate instead of whole blood, when volume replacement is not required.

Hazards of blood transfusion

Bacterial contamination

Contamination of the blood by bacteria is rare but may be lethal. Contaminants from the donor's skin may enter the blood while it is being donated. Usually, the bacteria responsible are staphylococci which do not grow at 4 °C and are killed during storage. However, any Gram-negative bacteria entering the blood will grow slowly at 4 °C (their number doubling in 8 hours), and over several weeks of storage may be sufficient to cause a lethal septicaemia. It is essential that blood is stored at 4 °C in order to minimize this risk as bacterial growth accelerates considerably at room temperature. The onset of pyrexia and circulatory collapse can be rapid if transfused blood is infected.

Transmission of disease

Donor selection criteria and the testing of donor blood for infectious agents has decreased the transmission of disease but can never completely eradicate it. Many of the organisms responsible for transmitting infection have a long incubation period and are stable in blood and blood products.

In 1983, the first deaths associated with transfusion-related HIV were reported. From 1986, those in high-risk groups were excluded from giving blood and all donor blood was tested for the presence of anti-HIV antibodies. However, the average delay in appearance of the anti-

body after the time of infection is 2–3 months, with 95% of infected people having sero-converted by 6 months. Thus donors giving blood within about 6 months of infection may not be detected. Factor VIII and IX concentrates used today in the United Kingdom carry a negligible risk of HIV transmission because of the use of anti-HIV screened plasma for their preparation. Furthermore, HIV appears to be inactivated by the heat treatment that such concentrates are now subjected to. Certain populations have a high incidence of viral carriers of hepatitis and post-transfusion hepatitis remains one of the most common hazards of blood transfusion. Screening tests have been devised for hepatitis B surface antigen and the incidence of such carriers in the United Kingdom is fairly low. Transmission of hepatitis C is the cause of the majority of cases of post-transfusion hepatitis and there is now a serological test to diagnose this.

Cytomegalovirus (CMV) is a herpes virus present in white cells and found free in the plasma. The virus can persist latently after infection and it is possible that up to 3.5% of units of blood have the potential for transmission of the virus. The main danger of transmission of CMV is to infants and immunocompromised patients, and the only way to avoid transfusion transmission is by using anti-CMV-negative blood.

Malaria can be transmitted via transfused blood or products that contain red cells as the parasites can remain viable for a week at 4 °C. Careful vetting of potential donors and screening for malarial antibodies is necessary now that travel to tropical countries is more widespread.

All donated blood in the United Kingdom is tested for syphilis and transmission by blood transfusion is now very rare.

Hazards associated with massive blood transfusion

Stored blood is deficient in platelets and coagulation factors. It is cold (4 °C), acid (pH 6.6–6.8), and contains citrate anticoagulant. Transfusions of large volumes of blood can therefore lead to metabolic and cardiac disturbances.

Hypothermia

A thermostatically controlled blood warmer should always be used when giving more than several units of blood to a normothermic patient as blood transfused at 4 °C can rapidly cool the patient. This will, of course, depend on the patient's temperature prior to starting the transfusion. If the patient is pyrexial, and the blood is not transfused rapidly, it may not be necessary to warm the blood until the patient is normothermic. Hypothermia increases the risk of cardiac arrhythmias, reduces metabolism, and shifts the oxygen dissociation curve to the left. Citrate toxicity (see below) is also more likely to occur when the patient is hypothermic.

Acid–base and electrolyte disturbances

Stored blood is acidic mainly due to the citric acid used as an anticoagulant and the lactic acid generated during storage. In the well-perfused patient, lactic and citric acid are rapidly metabolized, however, with hypoperfusion metabolism will be depressed and lactic acid production may continue increasing the metabolic acidosis. Frequent acid–base measurements are necessary to monitor this.

The sodium content of whole blood and FFP is higher than the normal blood level due to the sodium citrate anticoagulant (FFP contains approximately 35 mmol per unit and whole blood 49–53 mmol per unit, depending on the number of the days it has been stored). This should be remembered when giving such products to patients with renal failure.

Citrate toxicity

Citrate toxicity results from a reduction in ionized calcium in the patient's plasma caused by the binding of calcium by citrate which renders it inactive. A fall in ionized calcium may cause tetany, muscle tremors, and cardiac dysfunction. Prolongation of the Q–T interval is seen on the ECG.

The routine use of intravenous calcium supplements during large volume blood transfusion is controversial. Some authorities recommend that 2.2 mmol of calcium gluconate should be given for every 4 units of blood transfused. Others recommend that plasma ionized calcium levels should be monitored in the laboratory and supplements given as appropriate.

Haemostatic failure

Transfusion of the total body blood volume can lead to dilutional thrombocytopenia and haemostatic failure. Since stored blood contains no viable platelets and few of the clotting factors VIII and V, in these patients the platelet count will be reduced and the PT and KPTT increased. Laboratory monitoring is necessary to guide therapy however, if unavailable, it is recommended that 2 units of FFP should be given per 10 units of blood

transfused and platelet administration should be given according to the platelet count.

The ICU patient with haematological malignancy

Advances in supportive and antimicrobial therapy have meant that for many patients with malignant disease the long-term prognosis has improved. Although for some diseases mortality remains high, despite aggressive treatment, selected patients with life-threatening but potentially reversible complications can benefit from intensive care. Many of the reasons for their transfer to the ICU result from complications of the malignancy itself or from its treatment. These include:

1. Infection

2. Haemorrhage

3. Cardiac disturbances

4. Graft versus host reactions

5. Tumour lysis syndrome

6. Hypercalcaemia

7. Fluid overload / renal failure

8. Following extensive surgical procedures

9. Respiratory failure.

1. Infection

The most important cause of an increased susceptibility to infection is neutropenia. If the granulocyte count falls below $0.5 \times 10^9/l$ there is a very high risk of overwhelming infection. Most patients transferred to the ICU will have bone marrow suppression. Some hospital policies will require reverse barrier nursing though its benefit is contentious. Nevertheless, scrupulous attention to hand-washing is vital to minimize exogenous infection. Patients with neutropenia are susceptible to infection by bacteria (including atypicals such as mycobacteria), viruses, protozoa, and fungi. Most often the infection originates endogenously from the patient's own gut, airways, or skin. Broad-spectrum antibiotics suppress the normal bacterial flora; in the gut this can promote the overgrowth of pathogenic Gram-negative organisms. Chemotherapy can also cause areas of ulceration in the gastrointestinal tract and tracheobronchial mucosa. These areas can act as a focus for local colonization by organisms and may lead to invasion into deep tissues and septicaemia. There is a high incidence of fungal infection causing septicaemia and pneumonia (commonly *Candida* and *Aspergillus*). Herpes simplex and cytomegalovirus (CMV) are common viral infections and pneumocystis the most common protozoan infection.

Invasive procedures should be kept to a minimum and performed when the patient requires them rather than by virtue of being in ICU. Large-bore, soft Teflon catheters (such as Hickman lines) are often used for intravenous drug administration and are tunnelled subcutaneously to minimize infection from skin flora. Scrupulous attention must be paid to cannula insertion sites to keep them free of infection, and lines must be dated and changed according to hospital policy. Consider non-invasive methods of monitoring (e.g. pulse oximetry, see Chapter 4).

Decontamination of the gastrointestinal tract by the use of oral, non-absorbable antibiotics to reduce the endogenous flora has been advocated. However, this may promote the emergence of resistant organisms. Selective decontamination, where the antibiotics reduce only the aerobic organisms but leave anerobes to confer colonization resistance, has proved more sucessful but is costly, labour-intensive, and does not suppress all aerobic activity. Prophylactic antifungal drugs (such as 5-flucytosine) and antiviral drugs (such as acyclovir) have also been used with success in recipients of bone marrow transplants. In general, whatever antimicrobial therapy has been started on the ward is usually continued in the ICU.

Fungal infections (e.g. *Candida*) are common in warm, moist areas such as the groin, vagina, axilla, and in the mouth. Skin must be kept clean and dry and local antifungal therapy applied as appropriate.

Mouth care is very important and a variety of antifungal preparations are available (such as lozenges, suspensions, and mouthwashes) and should be used at least five times a day.

2. Hamorrhage

Thrombocytopenia is the most common cause of haemorrhage and can result from bone marrow suppression by cytotoxic drugs, bone marrow infiltration by tumour, or sequestration of platelets in the spleen (in patients with chronic lymphatic leukaemia). DIC is common and may be a complication of septicaemia or the malignancy itself. Patients with leukaemia often have reduced levels of factors V, VII, and X and, in patients with liver metastases, production of clotting factors by the liver may be impaired.

Most patients with bone marrow failure will require multiple transfusions, particularly of red cells, platelets, and clotting factors. If DIC is present, FFP and cryoprecipitate may also be required.

3. Cardiac disturbances

Cytotoxic drugs can cause serious cardiac disturbances. Adriamycin in large doses is particularly cardiotoxic causing congestive cardiac failure, direct endothelial damage with myocardial necrosis, and a cardiomyopathy. Some drugs cause a variety of acute dysrhythmias, particularly if the patient has existing cardiac disease. Cardiac tamponade can result from metastatic tumour, particularly those originating in the bronchus or breast. If the tumour extends around the heart a constrictive pericarditis can develop (this can also be caused by radiotherapy).

4. Graft versus host disease

This is an autoimmune reaction that can occur in allogenic bone marrow transplants. Immunocompetent donor T lymphocytes recognize the host histocompatability antigens as 'foreign' and produce a cell-mediated reaction against sensitive tissue, particularly the skin, gastro-intestinal tract, liver, and bone marrow. It causes fever, diarrhoea, severe skin rashes, and hepatitis. Mortality is high and management is with steroids and appropriate supportive care. Mortality rates are approximately 25 per cent.

5. Tumour lysis syndrome

The rapid lysis of malignant cells by cytotoxic drugs can cause hyperkalaemia, hyperuricaemia, hyperphosphataemia, and acute renal failure. This usually occurs in patients who present with a high white cell count ($> 100 \times 10^9$/l). The patient must be kept well hydrated and is usually given allopurinol prophylactically prior to commencing cytotoxic therapy. Allopurinol prevents tissue urate deposition and renal calculi which can occur secondary to elevated serum uric acid levels during cytotoxic therapy.

6. Hypercalcaemia

This is common in patients with malignant disease, particularly those with multiple myeloma. This can be due to invasion of the bone by tumour cells, or stimulation of osteoclastic activity by mediators, such as osteoclastic-activating factor, which causes bone reabsorption. Immediate treatment is aimed at reducing the calcium level by rehydration (3–6 1/24h), frusemide (which prevents calcium reabsorption in the loop of Henlé), calcitonin (which inhibits osteoclastic bone reabsorption), and sodium etidronate. Steroids are useful in reducing calcium reabsorption but this may take up to a week to show effect. Oral sodium phosphate is also effective but should be administered after hydration. For the long-term treatment of hypercalcaemia the cause must be removed by specific therapy (surgery, radiotherapy or chemotherapy).

Hypercalcaemia is discussed more fully in Chapter 13.

7. Fluid overload/renal failure (refer to Chapter 8).

8. Following extensive surgical procedures

Intensive care can benefit many patients undergoing lengthy, radical surgery to remove tumours. Such surgery (e.g. pelvic exoneration) can involve considerable blood loss and patients are often hypovolaemic on transfer from theatre. Continuous haemodynamic monitoring can permit optimal fluid replacement and pre-serve renal function. Analgesia can also be administered by intravenous infusion and titrated to achieve adequate pain control. Patients at high risk of respiratory failure are often electively ventilated post-operatively, especially if surgery is prolonged or the patient has pre-existing pulmonary disease.

Respiratory failure

There are a variety of factors that may precipitate respiratory failure in the patient with malignant disease and these are shown in Table 12.6.

Patients with malignant disease may also develop respiratory failure secondary to pleural effusions, fluid overload, cardiac failure, pneumothorax, or may require endotracheal intubation following diagnostic surgical procedures such as mediastiotomy.

Mortality rates are high in critically ill cancer patients and those requiring prolonged ventilation and/or renal support have a particularly poor prognosis. Before such patients are admitted to the ICU the nature and progress of the underlying malignancy must be taken into account

Table 12.6 Causes of respiratory failure

Infection:	**Bacteria** *Klebiella* *Escherichia coli* *Proteus* *Staphylococcus* *Pseudomonas* Pneumococcal **Fungal** *Aspergillus* *Candida* **Protozoan** *Pneumocystis carinii* **Viral** Cytomegalovirus
Drug-induced lung disease:	A variety of cytotoxic drugs (e.g. bleomycin) can cause interstitial inflammation
Radiation pneumonitis:	Occurs approximately 8 weeks following radiotherapy
Pulmomary haemorrhage:	Usually occurs only in patients with thrombocytopenia.
Malignant lung disease:	Metastatic spread of lymphoma or carcinoma
Tracheobronchial compression:	Due to airway compression by tumour or haematoma formation
Adult respiratory distress syndrome (ARDS):	Secondary to sepsis, DIC, pulmonary aspiration, radiation pneumonitis or haemorrhage

and the impact of ICU admission on the patient's quality of life must be considered. Invasive monitoring will limit mobility and intubation will prevent effective verbal communication. The requirements of life-sustaining therapy may simply prolong the patient's suffering. The admission of any of these patient's will almost certainly produce difficult ethical decisions which must be addressed on an individual basis for each patient.

Bibliography

Baughan, A.S., Hughes, A.S.B., Patterson, K.G., and Stirling, L. (1985). *Manual of haematology*. Churchill Livingstone, Edinburgh.

Epstein, C. and Bakanauskas, A. (1991). Clinical management of DIC, early nursing interventions. *Critical Care Nurse*, **11**, 42–51.

Gray, P.A. and Park, M.A. (1989). *Anaesthesia and intensive care*. Castle House, Tunbridge Wells, UK.

Green, J.H. (1978). *Introduction to human physiology*, (4th edn). Oxford University Press.

Guyton, A.C. (1984). *Physiology of the human body*, (6th edn). Holt Saunders, Japan/Philadelphia.

Hughe-Jones, N.C. and Wichramasinghe, S.N. (1991). *Lecture notes on haematology*, (5th edn). Blackwell, Oxford.

Isbister, J. (1986). *Clinical haematology*, pp. 23–4. Williams & Wilkins, Baltimore.

Jones, J. (1987). Abuse of FFP. *British Medical Journal*, **295**, 287.

Lewis, A. (1979). *Modern drug encyclopedia and therapeutic index*, (15th edn), pp. 973–4; 432–4.

Ludlam, C. (1990). *Clinical haematology*. Churchill Livingstone, Edinburgh.

Oh, T.E. (ed.) (1990). *Intensive care manual*, (3rd edn), Butterworth, Sydney.

Tinker, J. and Zapol, W. (1993). *Care of the critically ill patient*, (2nd edn). Springer, Berlin.

Young, L.M. (1990). DIC, The insidious killer. *Critical Care Nurse*, **10**, 26–53.

Virgilio, R.W. (1977). To filter or not to filter. *Intensive Care Medicine*, **31**, 144.

13. Endocrine, obstetric, and drug overdose emergencies

Endocrine disorders

Endocrine syndromes usually produce classical signs and symptoms but these may be difficult to identify in the severely ill patient. Appropriate investigations are essential in order to diagnose and treat these disorders promptly. Knowledge of the normal physiology of the endocrine glands is also vital in order to understand the systemic effects caused by their failure, the interactions between the glands and other body systems, and the effects of severe illness upon them.

Space does not permit a detailed account of the physiology of all the hormones produced by the endocrine glands or of every condition that may result from their dysfunction. Some conditions are rare or do not warrant admission to the ICU, therefore those discussed in detail are the endocrine emergencies and problems that are more commonly seen in the ICU.

The adrenal glands

The adrenal glands can be divided into two independent areas: the medulla and the cortex. Each produces different hormones with different functions.

The adrenal medulla (the inner core of the gland)

The cells of the medulla are derived from the sympathetic nervous system and secret the hormones adrenaline and noradrenaline in response to sympathetic stimuli. Noradrenaline is the transmitter substance of the sympathetic nervous system and preganglionic sympathetic fibres actually innervate the medulla. Events that activate the sympathetic nervous system (e.g. fear, hypoxia, hypotension, anger, cold, pain, etc.) cause the release of noradrenaline and adrenaline (collectively known as catecholamines). The joint action of the two hormones is to prepare the body for action ('fight or flight'). The immediate energy needs of the body must be met and blood flow and volume increased to essential organs.

Adrenaline

This constricts blood vessels in the skin and mucosa but dilates those in the skeletal muscle and the eye. It relaxes the bronchioles, thereby increasing lung capacity, and increases heart rate and cardiac output. Adrenaline also dilates the blood vessels of the brain, muscles, and myocardium, ensuring that blood flow is maintained to these crucial areas. Liver glycogen is mobilized and converted to glucose, providing an immediate source of energy, and the sphincters of the gut and bladder contract thus digestion is inhibited.

Noradrenaline

This raises the blood pressure by constricting arterioles and veins (except those in crucial areas where adrenaline counteracts this effect).

The adrenal cortex

The cortex secretes three categories of hormones: mineralocorticoids, glucocorticoids, and sex hormones. All are steroids and are similar in chemical composition to cholesterol.

Mineralocorticoids

These regulate sodium and potassium concentrations in the extracellular fluid. The most important is aldosterone which accounts for 95 per cent of mineralocorticoid secretion.

The effect of aldosterone is to increase the sodium and chloride ion concentration, and decrease the potassium ion concentration, of the extracellular fluid. Aldosterone causes the re-absorption of sodium in the distal loops and collecting ducts of the kidney (see Chapter 8). Since the sodium and potassium transport mechanisms in the epithelial cells are linked in a partial exchange process, potassium is also excreted at the same time. This sodium-potassium pump is stimulated by aldosterone. However, as the sodium–potassium ion exchange is unequal, this usually leads to more sodium being re-absorbed than potassium excreted.

A secondary effect of aldosterone is to decrease the amount of chloride ions lost in the urine. As there is an increase in sodium and chloride ion re-absorption in the tubules, water is also re-absorbed by an osmotic effect.

Aldosterone secretion can be stimulated by:

- elevated levels of potassium ions in the plasma;

- a persistently low plasma sodium level;

- a prolonged decrease in extracellular fluid volume;

- angiotensin: the plasma level of angiotensin rises when renin production by the kidney is increased as a result of a low plasma sodium level or reduced renal blood flow.

Glucocorticoids

These regulate the metabolism of fat, protein, and carbohydrate and can enhance resistance to physical stress.

The most important glucocorticoid is cortisol. Cortisol production is stimulated by adrenocorticotrophic hormone (ACTH) from the anterior pituitary via a negative feedback mechanism. It shows a diurnal variation in secretion — highest in the morning, lowest at about midnight. The primary stimulus for secretion is physical stress (injury) which activates the hypothalamus via nerve impulses from the site of injury. Cortisol causes increased availability of fats, glucose, and amino acids to repair the damage.

Effects of cortisol

- Increases fat metabolism

Cortisol mobilizes fat from adipose tissue cells and this provides an important source of energy in starvation. Excessive fat breakdown, however, can cause ketosis.

- Increases the use of protein

Cortisol suppresses the rate of protein production in non-liver cells, thus amino acids in the blood increase and these are available in times of injury. Chronically, this causes weakening of capillaries and skin atrophy.

The rate of protein formation in the liver cells is also increased (e.g. plasma proteins).

- Increases blood glucose

Cortisol increases the blood glucose level by two mechanisms:

1. It decreases the utilization of glucose by tissue cells thus raising glucose levels in the extracellular fluid.

2. It causes liver cells to convert fat and protein into glucose (by gluconeogenesis). Gluconeogenesis is increased because cortisol causes amino acids to be mobilized from tissue protein and fat (in the form of glycerol) from adipose tissue. This provides the liver with material that can be converted into glucose.

Excess cortisol can therefore cause diabetes mellitus.

- Decreases the absorption of vitamin D from the intestine

This may cause osteoporosis and impedes the development of cartilage.

- Decreases the number of lymphocytes and eosinophils in the blood. It suppresses the allergic responses and reactions to injury, inflammation, and infection.

- Can cause sodium retention and potassium depletion if synthetic cortisol is given in large doses or over long periods.

Sex hormones

Androgens, oestrogens, and progesterone are secreted by the adrenal cortex but are less important than those produced by the gonads. Occasionally, oestrogen-secreting tumours of the adrenal cortex develop.

Disorders of the adrenal medulla

Phaeochromocytoma

A phaeochromocytoma is a tumour of the adrenal medulla where high levels of adrenaline and noradrenaline are secreted. In 90 per cent of the patients the tumour originates in the medulla but in 10 per cent it may occur anywhere along the sympathetic chain (aorta, bladder, pelvis, abdomen, thorax).

It can metastasize and behave like a malignant tumour. The secretion of catecholamines is usually intermittent and during acute attacks the patient develops pulsating headaches, tachycardia, hyperglycaemia, blurred vision, bowel disturbances, and very severe hypertension (systolic blood pressure up to 300 mmHg).

Between attacks the blood pressure may be only slightly raised.

Diagnosis of a phaeochromocytoma

- Blood catecholamine levels;

- 24-hour urinary measurements of vanillylmandelic acid (VMA); a metabolic product of catecholamines.

- Computerized tomography.

The treatment of a phaeochromocytoma is surgical removal but the blood pressure must be controlled well in advance of surgery using alpha- and beta- adrenergic blocking agents. Alpha blockade must begin before beta blockade or a severe hypertensive crisis can be precipitated. Phentolamine or phenoxybenzamine are commonly used for short-term, pre-operative alpha blockade and propanolol for beta blockade. Alternatively, labetolol can be used as it has both alpha- and beta adrenergic blockade effects. During a severe hypertensive crisis an intravenous infusion of sodium nitroprusside can be used to control blood pressure.

Adrenoceptor blockade is usually withdrawn 12–36 hours pre-operatively. Post-operative care is as for any major abdominal surgery but continuous monitoring of blood pressure and heart rate is essential. Removal of the catecholamine source during surgery can cause hypovolaemic collapse unless the patient has been well prepared with alpha and beta blockade. If this occurs large volumes of fluid may need to be infused rapidly under CVP or pulmonary artery pressure monitoring in order to restore blood pressure.

Disorders of the adrenal cortex

Addison's disease

This disease results from a chronic deficiency of cortical hormones. This can be due to absence, atrophy or disease of the adrenal cortex or can occur secondary to hypopituitarism.

The symptoms of Addison's disease reflect the lack of cortisol, aldosterone and androgens.

Table 13.1 summarizes the tests used in the diagnosis of Addison's disease.

Effects of the lack of aldosterone

- Polyuria, dehydration, thirst.
- Hyponatraemia, hyperkalaemia.
- Hypotension (often postural).
- Cardiac arrhythmias.

Effects of the lack of androgens

- Loss of body hair.
- Loss of libido

Effects of the lack of cortisol

- Muscle weakness and fatigue, weight loss.
- Hypoglycaemia.
- Gastrointestinal disturbances (nausea, vomiting, diarrhoea, abdominal pain).
- Emotional disturbances (irritability, depression).
- Low resistance to infection, inability to cope with any type of stress.

Treatment of Addison's disease

The treatment of Addison's disease is by lifelong cortical hormone replacement therapy. Maintenance therapy consists of hydrocortisone, usually 20 mg in the morning and 10 mg in the evening. The difference in the 12-hourly dose reflects the normal diurnal variation in secretion of cortisol. Fludrocortisone may be added if a mineralocorticoid effect is required. This is a synthetic form of aldosterone and is given as a single dose in the morning (usually 0.05–0.3 mg). Dosages are prescribed according to plasma urea and electrolytes, and lying and standing blood pressure.

Table 13.1 Biochemical tests used for the diagnosis of Addison's disease

Test	Levels
Serum electrolytes and urea	Low sodium Raised potassium and urea
Serum ACTH levels 24-hour urinary 17-oxogenic steroids Serum cortisol (take at 0800 hours)	High in adrenal disease. Low in pituitary disease. Both may be in normal range — additional dynamic stress tests are performed if the disease is suspected.
Synacthen (tetracosactrin)	*Short test*: synacthen 250 µg is given IM and serum cortisol levels measured initially and then after 30 min. In normal patients, the initial level should be > 140 nmol/l and the level after 30 min. should be > 500 nmol/l. The difference between the two levels should not be less than 200 nmol/l. Longer tests can be performed where measurements are taken over 5 hours or 3 days.

In a healthy subject, cortisol levels are increased in times of stress. However, a patient with Addison's disease is unable to increase secretion of cortisol and the maintenance therapy maintains adequate levels only under normal conditions. In times of 'stress' (e.g. surgery, trauma, infection) the oral dosage of hydrocortisone must therefore be increased.

Addisonian crisis

If an acute demand for cortisol cannot be met, an Addisonian crisis may develop. This is one of the most life-threatening of all the endocrine emergencies. The signs and symptoms of an Addisonian crisis result mainly from the deficiency of aldosterone. There may be severe hypotension and tachycardia due to dehydration and arrhythmias, such as atrial fibrillation, are common. Serum sodium levels will be low and potassium and urea high. Hypoglycaemia is common in advanced cases. The patient will be in shock and will progress to complete circulatory collapse unless immediate treatment is instituted.

Immediate management of an Addisonian crisis.
Urgent rehydration with colloid followed by 0.9 per cent sodium chloride (3–4 litres will often be required over the first few hours). A central venous or pulmonary artery catheter is necessary to monitor the response and to ascertain fluid requirements.

Hypoglycaemia must be corrected by infusions of hypertonic glucose via a central venous catheter.

Cortisol must be administered without delay. The blood cortisol levels will not be known at the time but a blood sample should be taken, before treatment is instituted, for baseline cortisol levels. Hydrocortisone hemisuccinate 200 mg (or dexamethasone) is given intravenously for the immediate crisis followed after stabilization by an oral maintenance regimen of twice-daily hydrocortisone.

The precipitating cause of the crisis must be identified and treated.

Nursing management

- *Problem*: Cardiovascular instability (hypotension, tachycardia, arrhythmias) due to dehydration.

- *Management*: Continuous ECG monitoring. 12-lead ECG. Correct hypokalaemia. Administer IV fluids according to CVP or PAWP. If hypotension or low cardiac output persists after adequate rehydration, inotropic agents may be required (remember that the precipitating cause of the crisis may be sepsis).

- *Problem*: Oliguria due to hypotension and dehydration.

- *Management*: The patient should be catheterized and urine output measured hourly. Long periods of hypotension may precipitate renal failure. Oliguria should improve as the patient is rehydrated and becomes normotensive. Monitor blood urea and electrolytes.

- *Problem*: Respiratory failure.

- *Management*: Oxygen requirements and ventilatory support will be dictated by the patient's condition and blood gas analysis. Respiratory failure would not directly be caused by Addisonian crisis but may result from the underlying cause of the crisis (chest infection, pulmonary embolus).

There is an increased sensitivity to opiates and sedatives in patients with Addison's disease and these should be used with caution in the spontaneously breathing patient.

- *Problem*: Hypoglycaemia.

- *Management*: Regular monitoring of blood glucose. Continuous infusions of 10 or 20 per cent glucose may be required. Administer IV boluses of hypertonic glucose (20 or 50 per cent) as required. Aim for blood glucose level of 6–10 mmol/l.

- *Problem*: Pyrexia (if infection is the cause of the crisis).

- *Management*: Monitor core temperature. Identify source of infection by appropriate cultures. Give antibiotics as indicated. Cool patient (fanning, tepid sponging, antipyretics) and aim for temperature < 37.5 °C.

Addisonian crisis is rare but must always be suspected in a shocked patient who is resistant to conventional treatment and where the cause cannot be identified.

The thyroid glands

The thyroid gland consists of two lobes, one each side of the larynx and trachea, joined at the midline by an isthmus. It produces three hormones: thyroxine, triiodothyronine, and calcitonin.

The thyroid hormones

The thyroid gland removes iodine from the blood, concentrates it 40-fold and then stores it within the gland. Thyroxine (T_4) and triiodothyronine (T_3) are synthesized from iodine and the amino acid tyrosine.

T_3 and T_4 then combine to form thyroglobulin. Thyroglobulin is stored within the gland and released into the blood under the influence of thyroid-stimulating hormone (TSH) from the anterior pituitary. When released, T_3 and T_4 dissociate from the thyroglobulin and most combine with plasma protein, although a small amount circulates free in the plasma (normal level of plasma T_4 is 60–140 nmol/l).

Both T_3 and T_4 are responsible for the regulation of the metabolic rate in all the tissues of the body. They direct growth, tissue differentiation, and mental and physical development. T_3 and T_4 are virtually identical in action but T_3 acts much faster, has a shorter duration and is present in smaller amounts.

A third hormone, calcitonin, is also secreted by the gland, Calcitonin is not secreted by the same follicular cells that secrete T_3 and T_4 but by cells that lie between them. Calcitonin is responsible for lowering the serum calcium level. This is achieved by reducing the rate of calcium release from bone, removing calcium from the extracellular fluid by increasing deposition of calcium in the bones, and by reducing the rate of formation of new osteoclasts. Calcitonin can correct high serum calcium levels fairly quickly and its secretion is enhanced when blood calcium levels are elevated. Calcitonin is used by the body for the short term control of hypercalcaemia, while parathormone is used for more long term regulation (see parathyroid glands, p. 378).

Regulation of T_3 and T_4

The hypothalamus and anterior pituitary control the release of T_3 and T_4 by a negative feedback mechanism (see Fig. 13.1).

The anterior pituitary is stimulated to synthesize and secrete thyroid-stimulating hormone (TSH) by thyroid-releasing hormone (TRH) from the hypothalamus. TSH stimulates the thyroid gland to synthesize and secrete the thyroid hormones T_3 and T_4. The secretion of T_3 and T_4, in turn, inhibits the release of further TSH.

In hypothyroidism (where there is insufficient T_3 and T_4) the cause can be at the level of the hypothalamus, the anterior pituitary or the thyroid gland itself.

Classification of hypothyroidism

- Primary — due to disease of the thyroid gland.

- Secondary — where the anterior pituitary secretes insufficient TSH.

- Tertiary — where the hypothalamus does not secrete enough TRH.

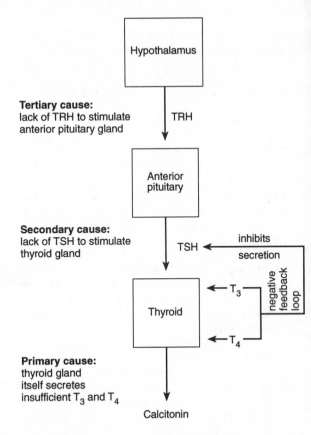

Tertiary cause: lack of TRH to stimulate anterior pituitary gland

Secondary cause: lack of TSH to stimulate thyroid gland

Primary cause: thyroid gland itself secretes insufficient T_3 and T_4

Fig. 13.1 Diagram showing negative feedback control of thyroid hormones.

Investigations of thyroid function determine at which level the cause of hypothyroidism is to be found.

Investigations of thyroid function

T_3 resin uptake

This test measures the unoccupied binding sites on thyroid-binding globulin (TBG) The number of binding sites increases in hypothyroidism (where there is little thyroid hormone) and in pregnancy (where there is excess TBG) but decreases in hyperthyroidism.

^{131}Iodine uptake

The patient is given radioactive iodine by mouth and this is taken up by the thyroid cells. The radioactivity of the gland is then measured after a set time. Uptake increases in hyperthyroidism and iodine deficiency and when taking certain drugs (e.g. phenothiazines).

Serum TSH

The serum TSH is increased in primary hypothyroidism (the pituitary gland is trying to stimulate the underactive thyroid) but decreased in secondary and tertiary hypothyroidism. For hyperthyroidism the serum TSH is decreased if there is primary thyroid overproduction, and increased if a pituitary tumour is responsible.

TRH test

TRH is given intravenously and the response of TSH release is measured. In pituitary hyperthyroidism there is a high basal level of TSH and a very marked increase in response to TRH. If hypothyroidism is caused by pituitary or hypothalamic disease there may be a reduction in response.

Disorders of the thyroid gland

Hypothyroidism (myxoedema)

This results from decreased thyroid hormone secretion.

Causes of hypothyroidism (myxoedema)

- Previous surgery to the thyroid gland (partial or complete thyroidectomy)

- Secondary to $[I^{131}]$ therapy for hyperthyroidism

- Spontaneous — the gland atrophies

- Hashimoto's thyroiditis — destruction of thyroid hormone-producing tissues

- Congenital absence of the thyroid gland

- Disease (or surgery) of the anterior pituitary or hypothalamus

---

Symptoms of hypothyroidism (myxoedema)
These reflect the lack of thyroid hormone and a hypometabolic state (see Table 13.2).

Once identified, hypothyroidism is treated by oral thyroxine (T_4) supplements but the cause of the disease must be ascertained by appropriate investigations. If the hypothyroid state continues myxoedema coma can result. Although rare, this would necessitate admission to the ICU.

Myxoedema coma

This arises when the patient with longstanding hypothyroidism encounters an additional stress that requires energy needs that cannot be met. Coma results from a combination of metabolic derangement, hypothermia, hypercapnia, and hypoxia.

Factors precipitating myxoedema coma

- Hypothermia

- Infection

- Trauma

- Cerebrovascular accident

- Myocardial infarction

- Drugs with an antithyroid action (e.g. lithium and amiodarone)

Table 13.2 Signs and symptoms of hypothyroidism (myxoedema)

Cardiovascular	Bradycardia
	Decreased cardiac output
	Decreased cardiac contractility
Central nervous system	Slow mental function
	Dementia
	Slowed speech
	Hoarse voice
	Fatigue
	Excessive sleep
Gastrointestinal tract	Anorexia
	Constipation
	Weight increase
Other	Dry, scaly skin
	Oedema of hands and feet
	Face puffiness and peri-orbital oedema
	Coarse, easily broken hair
	Poor wound healing
	Night blindness
	Coarse, fragile hair

Treatment of myxoedema coma

The aims of treatment are:

- Support of vital functions.

- Identifications of precipitating factors.

- Return to the euthyroid state.

Support of vital functions

- *Problem.* Hypoventilation (due to decreased conscious level) causing hypercapnia and a potential chest infection.

- *Management*. Ensure airway is protected. Endotracheal intubation may be required in deep coma. Administer humidified oxygen to maintain adequate oxygenation. If there is marked hypercapnia or hypoxaemia mechanical ventilation may be required. A respiratory acidosis is usually present and this should correct as efficient ventilation is restored. Aggressive physiotherapy to prevent/treat chest infection; culture sputum as appropriate (see Chapter 3).

- *Problem*. Hypotension and bradycardia.

- *Management*. Continuous ECG monitoring. No specific treatment is usually required for bradycardia as the heart rate should increase as treatment is instituted. Perform 12-lead ECG to exclude myocardial infarction.

  Monitor blood pressure. Patients in myxoedema coma are often resistant to inotropes and hypotension is initially treated with IV fluid infused under CVP or PAWP control. These patients are usually elderly and may have compromized cardiac function therefore fluids must be infused with caution. Sodium chloride 0.9% is used if the patient is hyponatraemic. Urinary retention can occur — catheterize bladder and monitor urine output. Oliguria should correct as the patient is rehydrated and normotensive.

  Pericardial effusion is a recognized problem and may progress to cardiac tamponade (see chapter 7).

- *Problem*. Hypoglycaemia.

- *Management*. Monitor blood sugar. Correct hypoglycaemia with glucose infusions or boluses of 50% glucose as required.

- *Problem*. Hypothermia.

- *Management*. Monitor core temperature. Re-warm patient ($0.5–1\,°C/h$ unless very hypothermic) using a re-warming blanket and, if necessary, warming IV infusion fluids. Nurse in a warm environment and warm humidified oxygen if administered. Observe ECG for potential arrhythmias while re-warming (see Chapter 11).

  A lactic acidosis is often present due to hypoperfusion of tissues. This should resolve as the patient is rehydrated, re-warmed, and adequately oxygenated.

- *Problem*. Convulsions due to hyponatraemia.
  Depressed level of consciousness due to cerebral hypoxia.

- *Management*. Assess level of consciousness.
  Observe and report fits. Maintain patient safety at all times (cot sides on bed, ensure patent airway during fits).

Monitor serum sodium levels. Aim to correct hyponatraemia slowly by IV infusion of 0.9% sodium chloride. If serum sodium is less than 110 mmol/l some authorities recommend more aggressive sodium replacement using small, frequent volumes of hypertonic saline.

The level of consciousness is always depressed and some patients may be deeply comatose. Regular neurological assessments should be performed (see Chapter 9). Note that a cerebrovascular accident may be the precipitating factor of the coma.

- *Problem*. Paralytic ileus due to decreased gut motility.

- *Management*. A nasogastric tube should be inserted, regularly aspirated, and left to drain freely.

Identification of precipitating factors

All potential sites of infection should be cultured (sputum, urine, blood, wounds, etc.). A 12-lead ECG should be recorded to exclude myocardial infarction and a full neurological examination performed to exclude a cerebrovascular accident although this is difficult in the comatose patient.

Other precipitating factors, such as hypothermia and trauma, will be obvious. The patient's own drug therapy should be considered as a potential precipitating factor.

Return to the euthyroid state

Thyroxine supplements will be required but sudden introduction of high plasma levels of thyroxine are dangerous. The consequent abrupt increase in metabolism can cause angina, myocardial infarction, and arrythmias. Many patients with long-term hypothyroidism have ischaemic heart disease to some degree. While oxygen demand to the heart is low in the hypothyroid state a reduction in blood supply has little effect. However, when thyroid hormone is administered oxygen demand is increased and requirements may not be met by delivery due to the atherosclerosis. Angina, infarction, or arrhythmias may result.

There are two differing schools of thought for administering thyroxine replacement. Some authorities propose that a large loading dose should be given followed by a small maintenance dose. Others suggest that this loading dose could be dangerous and recommend that small quantities of thyroxine are given initially and then gradually escalated.

If T_4 is administered it then has to be converted to T_3 by the body. This conversion is not efficient in the seriously ill and its half-life in the circulation can be more than 7 days. T_3 can be administered directly. Its onset of action is slow and takes several days to weeks to take effect. It can be given intravenously by slowly increasing dose.

Steroids. Patients in myxoedema coma usually have an impaired glucocorticoid response to stress since the adrenals share the general hypometabolism of the body.

The myxoedema coma may be secondary to hypopituitarism in which case there may also be an associated adrenal insufficiency. Corticosteroids (usually IV hydrocortisone) are therefore given until adrenal sufficiency can be demonstrated.

Hyperthyroidism (thyrotoxicosis)

Hyperthyroidism results from an excess of thyroid hormones (T_3 and T_4). It may be caused by primary disease of the thyroid gland or can be secondary to a pituitary tumour (where excess TSH is produced).

Causes of hyperthyroidism

- Autoimmune: antibodies called thyroid-stimulating immunoglobulins are found in 50–80 per cent of thyrotoxic patients. These cause structural and functional changes to the gland, the development of a goitre, and infiltration by lymphoid tissue. One of these antibodies is called long-acting thyroid stimulator (LATS) and causes prolonged stimulation of the thyroid cells.

- Thyroid adenoma: a tumour of the thyroid gland that secretes thyroxine independently of control by the anterior pituitary.

- Overtreated myxoedema.

- Self-administered thyroxine.

Effects of hyperthyroidism
These reflect the increase in metabolism caused by the thyroid hormones.

Cardiovascular:
- Increase in total blood volume.

- Increase in heart rate. Thyroid hormones are positive inotropes. They also increase sinoatrial firing and reduce the electrical threshold of atrial excitation. Atrial fibrillation or other tachyarrhythmias can develop and may further impair cardiac performance.

- Cardiac output is increased due to increased heart rate, preload and myocardial contractility. This hyper-

dynamic circulation imposes an increase in cardiac work which can lead to myocardial hypertrophy as the heart functions near to its limit. Heart failure can result from a combination of reduced myocardial contractile reserve, an increase in total blood volume, and tachyarrhythmias.

- Systemic vascular resistance (SVR) is decreased. Blood flow is not uniformly distributed in the body; it is greatly increased in the skin, skeletal muscle, and coronary arteries, although not to the cerebral, hepatic, or renal vessels. The effect of this is to change the loading conditions on the heart. The increase in total blood volume increases preload whereas the decrease in SVR reduces afterload.

Angina may be aggravated in patients with hyperthyroidism due to the increase in myocardial oxygen demand. The risk of thrombosis is also increased in patients with atrial fibrillation and prophylactic anticoagulation should be given.

Management of heart failure in patients with hyperthyroidism is by reduction of volume overload (by venodilators and diuretics), control of heart rate (digoxin for atrial fibrillation — often higher than normal doses are required), and treatment of the cause of the hyperthyroidism.

Gastrointestinal tract:
- Nausea, vomiting, diarrhoea (due to increase in gut motility).

- Increased glucose uptake into the cells.

- Weight loss.

Central nervous system:
- Nervousness, agitation, confusion.

- Hyperactivity.

- Tremors.

Other effects of hyperthyroidism
- Frequent micturition.

- Exophthalmus and corneal ulceration.

- Photosensitivity.

- Increased body temperature, warm, moist skin.

- Heat intolerance.

- Hyperpigmentation.

- Increased hair loss

- Goitre — may result in swallowing or breathing difficulties.

Exophthalmus. This results from an excess growth of tissue and the formation of oedema behind the eye sockets causing the eye balls to protrude. It is caused by the same autoimmune mechanism that causes the hyperthroidism. The tissue growth cannot be eliminated once formed and even with adequate treatment of the hyperthyroidism the exophthalmus will remain throughout life. The eyelid retracts and the patient is unable to lubricate the cornea by blinking. The cornea is then prone to drying and ulceration. Specialist advice must be sought at an early stage if the eyes appear inflamed as this is a serious complication and can cause blindness.

Goitre. This is an enlargement of the thyroid gland which becomes visible and palpable. This can be associated with hypothyroidism, hyperthyroidism, or the euthyroid state.

A non-toxic goitre occurs when the gland hypertrophies in response to an increase in secretion of TSH secondary to diminished output of thyroid hormones. In hypothyroidism the thyroid gland enlarges in an attempt to produce adequate quantities of thyroid hormone and in the euthyroid state a simple non-toxic goitre results from a dietary lack of iodine (also known as endemic goitre).

Some goitres become nodular and can cause hyperthyroidism (toxic goitre) or become malignant.

The enlarged gland can also compress the larynx and trachea causing hoarsness of the voice and an inspiratory stridor.

Treatment of hyperthyroidism

Treatment is by:

- Antithyroid drugs. Carbimazole is the drug of choice and acts by interfering with the synthesis of thyroid hormones. Iodine solution is also given as short-term treatment in thyrotoxic crisis or prior to surgery.

- Radioactive iodine [^{131}I]. Thyroid cells take up the radioactive iodine and are then destroyed by it. This reduces the vascularity of the gland and hence its size. It is a long-term treatment and results may not be apparent for several months.

- Propanolol to reduce sympathetic activity.

- Surgery to remove part of the gland.

Patients with hyperthyroidism will not usually require admission to the ICU unless symptoms are severe. Rapid atrial fibrillation may require synchronized cardioversion if this is unresponsive to digoxin. Severe heart failure will also require intensive monitoring. However, a thyroid crisis can develop in the untreated patient and, although rare, such patients will require management in the ICU.

Thyroid crisis ('thyroid storm')

This is an exaggerated form of hyperthyroidism. It occurs acutely, in any age group, and is an extreme, life-threatening condition.

Advances in diagnostic methods have made this condition very uncommon and it is usually only seen in patients who have undiagnosed or inadequately treated hyperthyroidism. Even in these patients predisposing factors are usually required to trigger the acute crisis.

Predisposing factors that may trigger a thyroid crisis

- Infection.

- Surgery, trauma.

- Myocardial infarction, cerebrovascular accident.

- Eclampsia, labour.

- Uncontrolled diabetes mellitus.

- Radioactive iodine if given to patients who are not euthyroid.

- Palpation of the thyroid gland or inadequate beta and adrenergic blockade pre-operatively may be a cause (this is disputed by some authorities).

Whatever the predisposing factor the features and management of the crisis are the same and treatment must be rapid and aggressive.

Features of thyroid crisis

- *Hyperpyrexia*: this may be extreme (> 40 °C) and could be wrongly attributed to sepsis.

- *Cardiac failure*: this is often refractory to conventional treatment and may be fatal. Cardiomegaly and ECG changes of left ventricular hypertrophy may be apparent.

- *Tachycardia*: can be sinus but frequently atrial fibrillation is seen in the middle-aged or elderly. Heart rate often exceeds 160 beats/min and there may also be ventricular arrhythmias.

- *Neurological features*: extreme agitation, tremors, and confusion which may lead to convulsions and coma.

- *Abdominal features*: epigastric pain, vomiting and diarrhoea, and later, liver dysfunction and jaundice.

- *Skin*: usually hot and moist with increased sweating.

- *Other symptoms* include those listed in Table 13.2.

Management of thyroid crisis

This is essentially aimed at reducing the effects of the thyroid hormones and supportive treatment until these effects can be bought under control. Before treatment begins blood samples are taken for measurement of TSH, T_3, and T_4. Treatment, however, is not delayed to await the results as this test is merely to confirm the presence of thyroid overactivity.

Drug therapy

Drugs are used to inhibit the catecholamine-like effects of the thyroid hormones and to inhibit their synthesis.

The large quantities of T_3 produced in a thyroid crisis have a similar effect to catecholamines and propanolol intravenously is the most commonly used beta-adrenergic receptor antagonist. Chlorpromazine is often used in combination with propanolol for its sedative effect.

Drugs, such as carbimazole (or propylthiouracil), are also used to inhibit the synthesis of T_3 and T_4, and work by blocking the reaction of tyrosine and iodine.

Iodine (in the form of Lugol's solution or potassium iodide) is given to inhibit the synthesis and release of thyroxine. This reduces the vascularity and size of the thyroid. It is usually given in milk as it is unpalatable. Lugol's iodine must be drunk through a straw (or placed down a nasogastric tube) to prevent staining of the teeth. Potassium iodide can be given intravenously but requires dilution in 500 ml of 0.9% sodium chloride and if heart failure is present this must be administered with care.

Hydrocortisone should also be administered intravenously.

Support of vital functions

- *Problem*. Tachycardia.

- *Management*. Continuous ECG monitoring. 12-lead ECG. Observe for arrhythmias. Atrial fibrillation can be resistant even to large doses of digoxin and amiodarone may be useful. Serum potassium must be monitored and hypokalaemia corrected, particularly before antiarrhythmic drugs are given. Administer propanolol — oral or intravenously according to severity of illness.

- *Problem*. Heart failure.

- *Management*. Monitor CVP. Pulmonary artery catheterization may be required as a guide to management as heart failure can be resistant to conventional treatment.

There may be considerable fluid loss from sweating and hyperpyexia and fluid administration will be determined by CVP and PAWP. Intravenous nitrate infusions can produce an improved cardiac performance by decreasing peripheral resistance (SVR) and preload. Hypotension is not usually a problem if the cardiac filling pressures are maintained but continuous blood pressure monitoring should be carried out, particularly if intravenous propanolol is being given.

- *Problem*. Hyperpyrexia.

- *Management*. Monitor core temperature. Actively reduce pyrexia by fanning, tepid sponging, and antipyretics. Salicylates should be avoided as they displace thyroid hormones from their binding proteins.

- *Problem*. Hypoglycaemia.

- *Management*. Monitor blood sugar levels. Give glucose infusions or boluses of 50% glucose as required. Early enteral nutrition should be encouraged but intestinal absorption is often impaired during a crisis.

- *Problem*: Agitation

- *Management*. These patients can be very irritable and apprehensive. Chlorpromazine intramuscularly should be given as required for sedation. If untreated, convulsions may occur and progress to coma. Observe for fitting, maintain patient safety (cot sides, airway control). Protect patient from additional stresses and nurse in a quiet environment.

- *Problem*. Dyspnoea (secondary to heart failure).

- *Management*. Monitor respiratory rate and blood gases. Treat heart failure. Administer humidified oxygen therapy as required. CPAP or mechanical ventilation may be required to maintain adequate oxygenation.

- *Problem*: Corneal ulceration due to exophthalmia or lid retraction.

- *Management*: Exophthalamos is due to swelling of the retro-orbital tissues and the sclera is visible above the lower lid. Lid retraction causes the sclera to be visible below the upper lid.

Protect the exposed cornea by frequent application of hypromellose eye drops.

Local or systemic steroids may be required for exophthalamos with tarsorraphy in severe cases. Lid retraction usually responds to treatment of the thyrotoxicosis.

Patients presenting in a thyroid crisis are extremely ill and mortality for this condition remains 15–20 per cent.

The parathyroid glands

Four parathyroid glands are situated adjacent to the posterior and lateral aspects of the thyroid gland. They produce parathyroid hormone (PTH, parahormone) which plays an essential part in the regulation of the plasma calcium level. Parathyroid hormone has several mechanisms by which it raises serum calcium and is itself regulated by a negative feedback mechanism so that calcium levels remain constant. The parathyroid glands can enlarge up to 10-fold if there is a long-term decrease in the plasma calcium level.

The parathyroid hormone (PTH)

Actions of parathyroid hormone (PTH)
PTH increases the plasma calcium level by:

- Decreasing the amount of calcium excreted by the renal tubules.

- Increasing ostoeclastic activity in the bone which causes release of calcium and phosphate.

- Decreasing osteoblastic activity in the bone thus reducing bone matrix formation.

- Increasing calcium absorption from the gastrointestinal tract.

Calcitonin released from the thyroid gland and PTH have opposing effects; together, they maintain in adults a plasma calcium level of 2.3–2.8 mmol/l and an ionized calcium level (non-protein-bound) of 1.18–1.3 mmol/l.

Functions of calcium
- Calcium decreases the permeability and increases the strength of capillary membranes. If the plasma calcium levels are low the membranes become very friable and there is increased permeability to fluid.

- At half the normal plasma calcium level the membranes of nerve fibres are more permeable to sodium ions and become partially depolarized. These fibres then transmit repetitive and uncontrolled impulses to the muscles resulting in spasm (tetany).

- Increased levels of calcium depress neuronal activity and the membranes will not depolarize easily.

- Calcium imbalances can have profound effects upon heart muscle. Low plasma levels cause the duration of systole to decrease and the heart dilates excessively during diastole. High calcium levels promote an overconstriction of the cardiac muscle causing it to contract too forcibly during systole and not relaxing satisfactorily during diastole. The reason for this is that when impulses pass through cardiac muscle small amounts of calcium ions are released into the sarcoplasm of the muscle fibres. These ions initiate the contractile process. If only small amounts are available in the extracellular fluid the intensity of the contraction is reduced, if excess is present there is overexcitation of the heart.

- Calcium is a vital component of the blood clotting process (see Chapter 12) and can occasionally be low enough to cause severe clotting abnormalities.

- There is no direct correlation between the severity of symptoms and the plasma calcium level. Generally, symptoms appear at a level above 3.0 mmol/l and can be fatal above 4–5 mmol/l.

- Vitamin D is essential for the absorption of calcium through the gut wall (hence in childhood rickets, where there is a lack of vitamin D, the bone is soft and deforms).

Hypercalcaemia

See Table 13.3 for symptoms of hypercalcaemia.

Management of hypercalcaemia
Symptomatic hypercalcaemia requires immediate treatment and, if severe, admission to the ICU will be necessary for monitoring purposes.
    The aims of treatment are to:

- Lower plasma calcium levels.

- Monitor and support vital functions.

- Identify the cause and treat where possible e.g. malignancy, hyperparathyroidism, sarcoidosis.

Plasma calcium levels
Table 13.4 indicates methods of reducing plasma calcium levels.

Table 13.3 Symptoms of hypercalcaemia

- Ureteric stones may form and can lead to obstructive uropathy
- Conjunctivitis due to calcium deposits on the cornea
- Damage to the renal tubular mechanism causes polyuria but later renal failure may develop as glomeruli are damaged
- Weakness and general malaise due to neuropathy
- Hypertension
- Headaches, confusion, myalgia
- Bone pain, joint effusions
- Abdominal pain, pancreatitis
- ECG changes: short Q–T interval, prolonged P–R interval, A–V block, VF
- Anorexia, vomiting, thirst, constipation, peptic ulceration
- Psychiatric disorders
- Osteoporosis

- Monitoring and support of vital functions
  Problem. Dehydration due to polyuria.

- *Management.* Monitor CVP or PAWP measurements. Rehydrate using colloid or 0.9% sodium chloride. Monitor urine output.

- *Problem.* Potential arrhythmias due to hypercalcaemia.

- *Management.* Continuous ECG monitoring. 12-lead ECG. Observe for and treat arrhythmias. Note that hypercalcaemia enhances the action of digoxin and can cause digoxin toxicity (particularly if there is concurrent renal impairment).

- *Problem.* Potential renal failure due to renal tubular damage or (long-term) stone formation/nephrocalcinosis.

Table 13.4 Methods of reducing plasma calcium levels

Treatment	Reason
Rehydration	Patients with hypercalcaemia are often dehydrated due to polyuria. This limits excretion of calcium by the kidneys and contributes to the maintenance of hypercalcaemia.
Oral phosphate and glucocorticoid therapy (hydrocortisone or dexamethasone)	Both drugs reduce the intestinal absorption of calcium and phosphate reduces osteoclastic activity.
Phosphate (IV)	This precipitates calcium phosphate in the tissues but can cause nephrocalcinosis and impairment of renal function.
Mithromycin (IV)	This inhibits mobilization of calcium from the skeleton and is probably the most rapidly effective drug. However, it cannot be given continuously for more than a few days due to its bone marrow toxicity and it can cause liver and renal failure.
Calcitonin (IV or SC)	Inhibits ostoeclastic activity. Not effective in all patients and may take several days to achieve effect.
Ethylenediaminetetraacetate acid (EDTA) (IV)	This is a calcium resin exchanger eliminated in the urine. Effective but nephrotoxic.
Peritoneal or haemodialysis	This effectively reduces the calcium level and avoids the dangerous side-effects of drug therapy *Note.* use calcium-free dialysate.

● *Management*. Monitor urine output, plasma urea and electrolytes, arterial pH and bicarbonate. Renal support therapy if required.

● *Problem*. Hypertension due to hypercalcaemia.

● *Management*. Correct hypercalcaemia. Monitor blood pressure. Antihypertensive therapy (e.g. calcium antagonists) if necessary.

Hypocalcaemia

See Table 13.5 for symptoms of hypocalcaemia.

Table 13.5   Symptoms of hypocalcaemia

● Tetany, muscle twitching, tremors, facial spasms
● Paraesthesiae (tingling) of extremities and mouth
● ECG changes: prolonged Q–T interval
● Stridor, bronchospasm
● Convulsions
● Haemorrhage
● (Long-term) cataracts, changes to teeth, nails, hair

Management of hypocalcaemia

Tetany is the major symptom of hypocalcaemia. The patient usually complains of numbness, stiffness, tremor, or tingling in the hands and feet. This progresses to generalized muscle hypertonia causing spasmodic and uncoordinated muscle contractions, particularly of the elbows, wrist, and carpophalangeal joints (carpopedal spasm). If untreated, this progresses to photophobia, bronchospasm, laryngeal spasm, cardiac arrhythmias, dysphagia and, ultimately convulsions. There may also be psychiatric disturbances such as anxiety, irritability, and neuroses.

Hypocalcaemia is generally better tolerated than hypercalcaemia, however, the onset of tetany or myocardial dysfunction requires rapid treatment.

This is relatively easy to correct by the administration of calcium salts. If hypocalcaemia is symptomatic this is given by intravenous infusion of 10–20 ml of 10% calcium chloride, if asymptomatic, calcium supplements can be given orally (calcium gluconate tablets, Sandocal).

Nursing assessment

● *Problem*. Neuromuscular instability/anxiety

● *Management*. Reassure patient and use calm manner. Nurse in an environment with minimum noise and avoid bright lights. Protect patient from injury (padded cot sides, remove articles that may cause harm).
Anticonvulsive therapy may be required.

● *Problem*. Potential cardiac arrhythmias.

● *Management*. Continuous ECG monitoring. Note that calcium potentiates the effect of digoxin and both increase systolic contractions. Observe for arrhythmias and monitor blood pressure.

● *Problem*. Dyspnoea due to bronchial or laryngeal spasm

● *Management*. Observe respiratory rate and effort. Monitor oxygen saturation using pulse oximetry, administer oxygen therapy and bronchodilators as required. Intubation and respiratory support may be necessary.

Disorders of the parathyroid glands

Hyperparathyroidism

Excess parathyroid hormone (PTH) is produced by the gland causing hypercalcaemia and hypophosphataemia (PTH causes increased excretion of phosphate ions by the kidney).

Causes of hyperparathyroidism

● Primary hyperparathyroidism
  – parathyroid adenoma or hyperplasia
  – carcinoma of the parathyroid (rare)
  – ectopic PTH (may be produced by a tumour elsewhere, e.g. lungs, kidney)

● Secondary hyperparathyroidism
  – can occur in response to hypocalcaemia resulting from another disease (usually chronic renal failure)

● Tertiary hyperparathyroidism
  – longstanding secondary hyperparathyroidism can lead to autonomous function in one or more parathyroid adenomas.

Investigations for the diagnosis of primary hyperparathyroidism
Biological tests are given in Table 13.7.

Hypoparathyroidism

This is caused by insufficient secretion of parathyroid hormone.

Table 13.6 Biochemical tests for the diagnosis of primary hyperparathyroidism

Test	Level
Plasma ionized calcium	Raised
Plasma calcium*	Raised
Plasma phosphate	Low
Serum PTH	Raised
Serum alkaline phosphatase	Raised

* Corrected for serum albumin concentration.
Note. for every 6 g/l albumin below 42 g/l add 0.1 mmol/l to the calcium level.

Causes of hypoparathyroidism

- Primary idiopathic and autoimmune disease.
- Secondary to thyroid surgery.

Investigations for the diagnosis of hypoparathyroidism tests are given in Table 13.7.

Table 13.7 Biochemical tests for the diagnosis of hypoparathyroidism

Test	Level
Plasma ionized calcium	Low
Plasma calcium*	Low
Plasma phosphate	High
Serum alkaline phosphatase	Normal

* Corrected for serum protein or albumin concentration.

The pancreas

The pancreas secretes two hormones, insulin and glucagon, from the islets of Langerhans. The islets consist of two types of cell, alpha and beta, and there are many thousands of these throughout the pancreas. Insulin is secreted by the beta cells and glucagon by the alpha cells. Both hormones have a profound effect upon metabolism.

Insulin

Functions of insulin

- Promotes the transport of glucose into most cells of the body (particularly liver, fat and muscle cells) by activating the carrier mechanism by which glucose is transported into the cells. Insulin therefore lowers the blood sugar. Lack of insulin causes hyperglycaemia.

- Promotes glycogen storage in the liver and muscle. Insulin activates liver enzymes (glucokinase and glycogen synthetase) to enable storage of glucose either by combining glucose with phosphate ions, or combining many glucose molecules to form glycogen. When insulin is absent, phosphorylase is activated within the liver; this depolymerizes glycogen, releasing glucose back into the circulation. Glycogen therefore provides a store of glucose for use when immediate energy requirements cannot be met by the body (e.g. during periods of starvation, increased exercise).

- Converts glucose into fat. Excess glucose in the circulation is firstly stored as glycogen but when these stores are filled it is then converted into fat. Most of the glucose is converted into fat by the liver and then released as lipoprotein for storage in fat tissues. However, some is synthesized directly by the fat cells.

- Inhibits fat metabolism (except for the storage and synthesis of fat from glucose). Cells preferentially use glucose for energy rather than fat because of the nature of their enzyme systems. In times of insufficient circulating glucose, stored glycogen in the liver and muscle cells is broken down to release glucose. Insulin inhibits hormone-sensitive lipase which is responsible for splitting fatty acids from stored fat before release into the blood. Therefore, once stored, fat is usually unavailable as a primary source of energy whilst there are sufficient levels of insulin and energy requirements can be met from stored glycogen. However, when insulin is lacking, fat metabolism is greatly increased and large amounts of fatty acids are released into the blood. These fatty acids are used as an immediate energy source by the cells as they are unable to utilize glucose due to the lack of insulin.

  Blood lipid levels greatly increase when insulin is lacking as the free fatty acids are transported to the liver and converted into cholesterol, triglycerides, and phospholipids (lipoproteins).

  This rapid and massive metabolism of fatty acids by the liver causes large amounts of acetoacetic acid and other ketones to be released into the blood. This causes a severe acidosis and, if untreated, coma and death ensues.

- Promotes protein deposition in cells. Insulin increases the formation of RNA in cells, the formation of protein by ribosomes and increases the rate that amino acids are transported into cells for the synthesis of protein.

When insulin is lacking, protein as well as fat is used as a source of energy. Lack of insulin therefore affects growth as tissue formation (which utilizes protein) is inhibited.

Insulin secretion

Insulin is secreted from the pancreas as a direct effect of raised levels of glucose on the beta cells. As insulin facilitates transport of glucose into the cells the glucose level falls and secretion is inhibited (negative feedback mechanism).

Glucagon

Many of the actions of glucagon are opposite to that of insulin and its effect is to raise the blood glucose level. This is achieved by causing the breakdown of stored glycogen (glycogenolysis) and by converting proteins into glucose (gluconeogenesis).

Glucagon secretion is stimulated when the beta cells detect subnormal blood glucose levels. Once released, glucagon causes blood glucose levels to rise within minutes as glucose is released from stored glycogen. As the blood glucose rises to normal, glucagon secretion is inhibited.

By the opposing actions of insulin and glucagon blood glucose levels can be kept within a fairly constant range.

Functions of insulin

- Promotes transport of glucose into cells, hence lowers blood glucose level

- Promotes glycogen storage in liver and muscle cells.

- Converts glucose into fat.

- Inhibits fat metabolism.

- Promotes tissue growth by protein deposition.

Functions of glycogen

- Raises blood glucose level

- Glycogenolysis

- Gluconeogenesis

Disorders of the pancreas

Diabetes mellitus

This is hyperglycaemia due to the deficiency, destruction (due to antibodies), or impaired effectiveness of insulin.

There are two types.

Type I: insulin-dependent diabetes (IDDM)
This accounts for approximately 20 per cent of diabetics and usually has its onset in childhood or adolescence (also called juvenile diabetes). It results from destruction of the beta cells in the pancreas and there may be both a genetic disposition and a viral trigger (e.g. cocksackie B, mumps).

IDDM often presents acutely as hyperglycaemic keto-acidosis. Lifelong insulin therapy will be required.

Type 2: non-insulin-dependent diabetes (NIDDM)
This usually affects those over 40 years of age (also called maturity onset diabetes) and tends to occur in the over-weight. Patients are often asymptomatic and may first present with related complications (see later).

This type of diabetes is usually controlled by a combination of diet, weight loss (if appropriate), and oral hypoglycaemic drugs.

Secondary diabetes

This occurs secondary to drug therapy or metabolic/endocrine disease.

Causes of secondary diabetes

- Drugs: glucocorticoids, adrenaline, thiazide diuretics, thyroid hormones, oral contraceptives

- Metabolic/endocrine: Cushing's syndrome, Conn's syndrome (primary hyperaldosteronism), phaeochromocytoma

- Other: acute or chronic pancreatitis, pancreatic cancer, pregnancy, 'stress' — major trauma, burns, infection, head injury (due to high endogenous catecholamine response)

Diabetic emergencies

There are three main diabetic emergencies:

1. Diabetic ketoacidosis (DKA) — characterized by hyperglycaemia, ketosis and acidosis, often with coma.

2. Hyperosmolar, hyperglycaemic non-ketotic coma (HHNKC) — characterized by hyperglycaemia but minimal ketosis.

3. Hypoglycaemic coma.

1. Diabetic ketoacidosis (DKA)

Approximately one-third of patients presenting with the symptoms of DKA are newly diagnosed diabetics. The causes of DKA in diabetics include infection, myocardial infarction, thromboembolic episodes or non-compliance with treatment. Coma is not always a feature of the illness but the conscious level will vary according to the severity of ketoacidosis. Hyperglycaemia and ketosis are, however, always features of DKA. This condition is life-threatening, even if the patient is not comatose.

Principal features of DKA

● Hyperglycaemia
Insulin facilitates the transfer of glucose into the cells, therefore lack of insulin means that the tissue cells are unable to utilize the glucose derived from carbohydrate metabolism.
Other 'stress' hormones, such as adrenaline, noradrenaline, glucagon, cortisol, and growth hormone are also released and their catabolic action further exacerbates the hyperglycaemia.

● Dehydration
When the concentration of glucose in the blood is above the renal threshold (approximately 8.5–10.5 mmol/l) the kidney does not reabsorb the excess glucose and this is excreted in the urine. An osmotic diuresis results and large volumes of water and electrolytes are lost. The patient experiences extreme thirst and becomes polydipsic but, nevertheless, still rapidly dehydrates. Dehydration initially depletes the intracellular compartment as this is the largest of the body's fluid spaces. At first there is little effect on intravascular volume but as the fluid loss becomes more severe, the intravascular volume falls and the patient progresses to hypovolaemic shock (hypotension, tachycardia).

Fluid is not only lost through an osmotic diuresis but also via hyperventilation, nausea, vomiting, fever, and decreased fluid intake due to coma.

● Electrolyte loss
This is associated with polyuria. In particular, sodium, potassium, phosphate, and magnesium ions are lost via the urine. Hypokalaemia can be a fatal complication of DKA and this results mainly from haemodilution following fluid resuscitation, the correction of hyperglycaemia by insulin infusion and inadequate potassium replacement. Low serum concentrations of potassium, phosphate and magnesium can cause cardiac arrhythmias or asystole, particularly if there is pre-existing cardiac disease. Hypophosphataemia can cause serious complications such as decreased level of consciousness, generalized muscle weakness, respiratory failure and impaired myocardial contractility.

● Ketoacidosis
Lipolysis (fat breakdown) causes weight loss and, although extremely hungry, the patient cannot utilize glucose derived from dietary carbohydrate. Some of the free fatty acids released by lipolysis are converted into ketones by the liver and can cause a profound metabolic acidosis. The patient compensates for this acidosis by hyperventilation (Kussmaul respiration — see Chapter 3). A sustained pH below 6.8 will be incompatible with life.

Management of DKA

In the management of DKA there is no place for rigid regimens of fluid and insulin. Every patient will differ in their degree of hypovolaemia, blood glucose levels, and level of consciousness. They may also have an underlying condition, such as sepsis, which has triggered the illness or suffer chronic disease, such as renal failure or cardiac impairment. Resuscitation must be guided by measured cardiovascular parameters and response to treatment. The patient requires intensive monitoring, (routinely a central venous line and, if indicated by the precipitating condition or past medical history, a pulmonary artery catheter) and frequent reassessment. Mortality remains approximately 10 per cent but can be as high as 43 per cent in patients over the age of 50.

Nursing management

● *Problem.* Inadequate airway protection due to decreased level of consciousness.

● *Management.* Ensure patent airway — endotracheal intubation may be necessary. Mechanical ventilation is rarely required. A nasogastric tube should be inserted as gastric atony, which is associated with DKA, increases the risk of aspiration.

Observe respiratory rate and pattern. Monitor blood gases and give oxygen therapy as indicated. Note that elderly patients may have underlying respiratory disease or may have been immobile at home prior to admission thus increasing the risk of atelectasis or infection (this may also be a precipitating factor).

● *Problem.* Hypovolaemia due to dehydration.

● *Management.* This must be rapidly corrected, particularly in patients with pre-existing renal dysfunction where adequate organ perfusion must be maintained.

Care should be taken not to overload the patient, especially if there is a pre-existing cardiac history.

Average fluid requirements will be 5–10 litres in the first 24 hours but replacement must be governed by CVP or PAWP measurements. The choice of fluid used for replacement is controversial but should logically depend on the degree of hypovolaemia. Fluid is not lost equally from the three body spaces: (1) intracellular (ICS), (2) interstitial (ISS) and, (3) intravascular (IVS). Fluid is initially lost from the largest space (ICS) and least of all from the IVS. Therefore, it is logical to rehydrate using a fluid similar in sodium concentration to the fluid lost (i.e. hypotonic saline, 0.45%). If dehydration is more severe and has caused hypovolaemia and shock (hypotension, tachycardia, low CVP or PAWP) then fluid has also been lost from the intravascular space. The circulating fluid must be rapidly replaced; use of a colloid solution aids fluid retention in the IVS (only one-quarter to one-third of crystalloid will remain in the IVS, the remainder enters the ISS). Resuscitating the severely hypovolaemic patient with crystalloid fluids only may cause a massive expansion of the ISS and ICS, compared to the IVS, and can result in peripheral, pulmonary, or cerebral oedema.

All cardiovascular parameters — HR, BP, CVP, PAWP, CO — must be continuously monitored during rehydration. The rate of infusion of colloid can be gauged by measuring the variables before and after 200 ml aliquots are given and assessing the response.

Total body water losses are difficult to assess and will differ with each patient. If intravascular replacement needs are high then water loss will generally be high. A range of 50–200 ml/h of 5% glucose is given for 48 hours or until the patient can take oral fluids. (*Note*: there is minimal extra glucose in 5% glucose and this will have a negligible effect on the blood glucose level.)

See Table 13.8 for a summary of fluid replacement in DKA.

Table 13.8 A summary of fluid replacement in DKA:

- If hypovolaemic, rapidly restore lost intravascular volume using colloids.
- When dehydration is less severe (normal BP, HR, CVP) replace intracellular losses with hypotonic or normal saline (e.g. 100–200 ml/h).
- Replace total body water losses concurrently with 5% glucose.
- Adjust rates and volumes of infusion according to cardiovascular parameters and response.

- *Problem.* Hyperglycaemia.

- *Management.* Hourly blood glucose measurements initially. A continuous infusion of insulin should be titrated according to glucose levels, aiming for a smooth, slow return to normal over the next 24–48 hours. A reduction in blood glucose of 2–4 mmol/h is satisfactory. Rapid correction of hyperglycaemia should be avoided and an initial intravenous bolus of insulin is unnecessary. Insulin not only reduces the blood glucose level but also moves water and other ions into the cells. A rapid movement of water can increase CSF pressure and cause cerebral oedema. The movement of water out of the IVS into the ICS also exacerbates hypovolaemia.

  Rigid regimens of insulin should be avoided as patients vary in their response. A low rate infusion of 2–5 units/h is commenced initially and can be increased as necessary. Initial insensitivity in some patients may be related to dehydration.

  Some authorities recommend that insulin for infusions is mixed with a carrier solution, such as albumin, to prevent the absorption of insulin on to the plastic syringe. This is unnecessary as it is not the amount of insulin given that matters but the patient's response to it.

  Urine should be tested regularly for ketones and glucose.

- *Problem.* Electrolyte depletion due to polyuria

- *Management.* Continuous ECG monitoring, observe for arrhythmias. Monitor potassium levels one to two hourly. Give IV supplements accordingly (usually 5–30 mmol/h are required).

  Serum phosphate and magnesium levels should be measured on admission and thereafter daily until normal. Supplements of both can be given IV until levels are normal.

- *Problem.* Metabolic acidosis due to ketosis

- *Management.* Measure arterial pH, bicarbonate and base excess/deficit hourly initially. IV sodium bicarbonate is not currently recommended for routine use due to the dangers of paradoxical intracellular acidosis, sodium overload, and rebound alkalosis. However, if the blood pH < 6.9 then aliquots of bicarbonate (e.g. 50 ml of 8.4% solution) can be considered. The acidosis will correct naturally when insulin therapy and fluid replacement are established.

- *Problem.* Potential thrombosis due to dehydration and possible pre-existing vascular disease.

- *Management.* Observe for thrombotic episodes (DVT, pulmonary embolus). Give prophylactic subcutaneous heparin.

In the patient with DKA every attempt should be made to identify the cause of this illness. Potential sites of infection (urine, sputum, wounds, etc.) should be cultured. A 12-lead ECG should be taken to exclude a myocardial infarction.

2. Hyperosmolar, hyperglycaemic non-ketotic coma (HHNKC)

HHNKC commonly occurs in undiagnosed patients with NIDDM and typically the patient is older. Often there is a predisposing factor that triggers the condition.

Factors predisposing to HHNKC

- Elderly

- Myocardial infarction

- Trauma (including burns)

- Infection

- Pancreatitis, hepatitis

- Renal failure

- Hypothermia

- Carbohydrate overload (enteral feeding, dextrose solutions)

- Drugs: phenytoin, thiazides, adrenaline (all inhibit insulin release)

- Other:
  - glucagon (elevates blood glucose)
  - propanolol, frusemide, cimetidine (all antagonize insulin)
  - mannitol (produces an osmotic diuresis)
  - glucocorticoids, growth hormone (stimulate gluconeogenesis)

HHKNC differs from DKA in that the level of free fatty acids and counter-regulatory hormones are lower although the pathophysiology of this is still uncertain. Lipolysis may be inhibited by the hyperosmolar state itself, by the higher levels of circulating insulin, or the hepatic synthesis of ketones may be restricted. Although circulating levels of insulin are higher than in DKA, they are not high enough to prevent hyperglycaemia.

Ketosis may be absent or mild.

Mortality is higher at 40–70 per cent and is often due to pulmonary embolus. However, it is much less common than DKA.

Management of HHNKC

The management is similar to that for DKA. However, the principal differences are as follows.

- Level of consciousness
  The patient may stay in coma longer — up to six days, therefore active management is longer. The incidence of coma is higher than in DKA. Airway maintenance and prevention of pneumonia is paramount. Early endotracheal intubation is recommended for airway protection, tracheal toilet, and intensive physiotherapy. There may be a higher incidence of chest infection in these patients since they are usually elderly, have been immobile or semi-comatose prior to admission, and the coma may last longer.

  Whereas patients with DKA often do not require supplemental oxygen, these patients usually do and may benefit from mask CPAP if intubation is not required. Hyperventilation is not a feature of HHNKC since the acidosis, if present, is mild.

- Insulin therapy
  Although hyperglycaemic, patients with HHNKC are more sensitive to insulin than patients with DKA. Insulin infusions should therefore be commenced at a lower dose (e.g. 2 units/h) and the dose altered according to response, aiming to reduce the blood glucose level over 36–48 hours.

- Fluid replacement
  Dehydration is often more severe than in DKA and the patient is more likely to be hypovolaemic and shocked. However, the same principles of fluid replacement apply. Colloid is given to resuscitate the patient in shock. The rate of overall rehydration should be slower than for DKA because of the danger of rapid intracerebral fluid shifts precipitating cerebral oedema. The plasma sodium level is often elevated and, despite appropriate treatment, may even continue to rise for a few days, sometimes exceeding 170 mmol/l. The total body sodium is, however, grossly depleted so the patient usually requires either 0.45 or 0.9% saline for electrolyte replacement. Potassium supplementation is also necessary to correct the large potassium deficit. Particular care must be paid to

titrate fluid replacement against cardiovascular para-meters since these patients are often elderly and may have existing cardiac or renal dysfunction.

- Anticoagulation

Pulmonary embolus is considered to be the major cause of mortality in these patients. It arises due to prolonged immobility and to the hyperviscosity of the circulating blood. Most authorities recommend anti-coagulation with heparin, although whether this should be full intravenous heparinization or merely subcutaneous is still contentious.

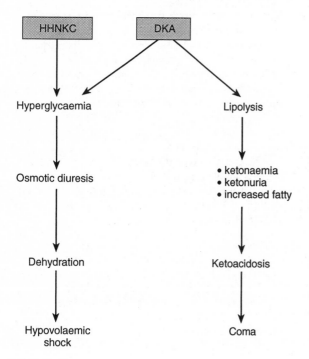

Fig. 13.2 Diagram showing the effects of HHNKC and DKA.

3. Hypoglycaemic coma

Patients who develop hypoglycaemia are usually known diabetics controlled by insulin or oral sulphonylurea hypoglycaemics (e.g. glibenclamide).

Occasionally, Addison's disease, liver failure or an insulinoma may also precipitate hypoglycaemia.

Hypoglycaemic symptoms (Table 13.9) result from a low blood glucose level. This may be caused by an insulin overdose (deliberate or accidental), when the diabetic patient takes excessive exercise, has an inadequate food intake or ingests excess alcohol.

The onset of coma is usually rapid but most patients are aware of the onset of symptoms and can prevent an impending hypoglycaemic attack by taking sugar.

Table 13.9 The symptoms of hyperglycaemia and hypoglycaemia

Hyperglycaemia	Hypoglycaemia
Restlessness	Headache
Thirst	Hunger
Vomiting	Faintness
Abdominal pain	Cool, moist skin
Hot, dry, flushed skin	Sweating
Drowsiness	Slurred speech
Tachycardia	Tachycardia/bradycardia
Deep sighing (Kussmaul) respirations	Irrational behaviour, agitation
Hypotension	Coma
Coma	

Patients admitted to the accident and emergency department in coma can easily be diagnosed by bedside blood glucose analysis. Treatment must be rapid as hypoglycaemia can cause irreversible brain damage. Symptoms can be reversed in minutes by the adminis-tration of aliquots of 20–50ml IV of 50% glucose.

Such patients rarely require ICU care once the coma is reversed except those patients who have taken an insulin overdose (particularly if a long-acting insulin) where close monitoring of blood glucose levels will be required.

The pituitary gland

The hypothalamus and pituitary gland are anatomically and functionally closely linked.

The hypothalamus lies below the third ventricle of the brain and extends down as the pituitary stalk to join the posterior pituitary gland. The anterior pituitary gland lies adjacent to the posterior pituitary but secretions and functions are independent. The pituitary stalk contains nerves and capillaries through which hormones produced in the hypothalamus pass into the posterior pituitary gland.

The anterior pituitary gland

Hormones produced by the anterior pituitary are as follows:

- Growth hormone (GH) — affects fat, protein, and carbohydrate metabolism.

- Thyroid-stimulating hormone (TSH) — stimulates the thyroid gland to secrete thyroid hormones.

- Adrenocorticotrophic hormone (ACTH) — controls the secretion of adrenocortical hormones.

- Prolactin — produced during pregnancy and stimulates breast growth and secretory functions.

- Gonadotrophic hormones — involved in sexual functions.

In women — follicle-stimulating hormone (stimulates development of follicles in the ovary) and luteinizing hormone (causes oestrogen and progesterone secretion by ovary and allows rupture of follicle).
In men — interstitial cell-stimulating hormone stimulates the testes to produce androgens.

The posterior pituitary gland

Two hormones are released from the posterior lobe. These are produced in the hypothalamus and stored in the posterior pituitary gland.

- Oxytocin — stimulates contraction of the uterus and the muscles of the milk ducts in the breast.

- Antidiuretic hormone (ADH) — stimulates the reabsorption of water from the distal tubules of the kidney.

Fig. 13.3 shows the hormones secreted by the pituitary gland.

Disorders of the posterior pituitary

Diabetes insipidus

Diabetes insipidus results from a lack of ADH causing polyuria, excessive thirst, and polydipsia.

Nephrogenic diabetes insipidus is a primary renal tubular defect of water reabsorption in which there is a poor response to ADH (a hereditary disorder). Water balance in the body is regulated by a complex negative feedback system involving thirst, ADH secretion, and responses by the kidney which maintains the plasma osmolality at 275–295 mOsmol/kg. There are many factors which influence ADH secretion (see later). One of the most important is a change in plasma osmolality; above 280 mOsmol/kg there is a steady increase in ADH response.

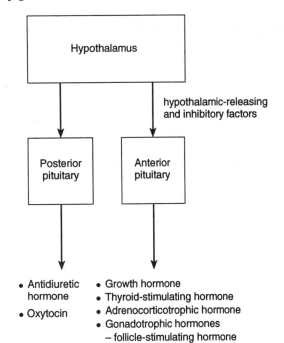

- Antidiuretic hormone
- Oxytocin

- Growth hormone
- Thyroid-stimulating hormone
- Adrenocorticotrophic hormone
- Gonadotrophic hormones
  – follicle-stimulating hormone

  – luteinizing hormone

  – interstitial cell-stimulating hormone

- Prolactin

Fig. 13.3 Diagram showing the anterior and posterior pituitary hormones.

Causes of diabetes insipidus

- Neurosurgery

- Head injury

- Infarction of a pituitary tumour (pituitary apoplexy).

- Also, rarely, following meningococcal meningitis, penetrating thoracic trauma, coronary artery bypass surgery, amiodarone therapy.

Note. All the above can cause complete or partial destruction of the hypothalamus or posterior pituitary

Actions of ADH

- Induces reabsorption of water in renal tubules.

- Vasoconstriction, particularly of skin, mesenteric and coronary vessels.

- Stimulates prostacyclin production and increases fibrinolytic activity.

- Increases factor VIII coagulant activity.

Factors influencing ADH secretion
Table 13.10 shows factors that influence ADH secretion.

Effects of diabetes insipidus
Failure of adequate secretion of ADH in response to plasma hyperosmolality results in the passage of huge volumes of dilute urine (4–20 litres/day). If the thirst mechanism or water intake is impaired the plasma will become hyperosmotic and hypernatraemic. Total body sodium is, however, decreased due to renal losses and inadequate intake. Gross dehydration will cause hypovolaemic shock and death. Hypernatraemia will cause delirium, lethargy, convulsions, and coma.

Other causes of polyuria should be excluded by appropriate investigations; in particular hyperglycaemia, recovery from fluid overload, polyuric renal disease, and psychogenic polydipsia.

Investigations
See Table 13.11 for the diagnosis of diabetes insipidus.

Management of diabetes insipidus
Mild polyuria (< 250 ml/h) may be observed and fluid output replaced with a crystalloid infusion. Plasma and

Table 13.10 Factors that influence ADH secretion

Increased by:	Inhibited by:	Potentiated by:	Antagonized by:
Drugs • cholinergic • β-adrenergics • nicotine • barbiturates • chlorpropamide • angiotensin II	Causes of diabetes insipidus (see p. 387)	Drugs: • thiazide diuretics • chlorpropamide • carbamazepine • clofibrate • prostaglandin synthetase inhibitors (e.g. indomethacin)	Drugs: • amphoteracin B • lithium carbonate
Hyperosmolality	Opioid antagonists		Hypokalaemia
Hypotension			Hypercalcaemia
Trauma, surgery, stress, pain			Excess vasopressinase
Hyperthermia			Prostaglandin (PGE$_2$)
Positive pressure ventilation			
Exercise			

Table 13.11 Investigations for the diagnosis of diabetes insipidus

Test	Normal value	Diabetes insipidus
Plasma osmolality*	275–295 mOsmol/kg	< 280 mOsmol/kg
Urine osmolality	300–1300 mOsmol/kg	< 150 mOsmol/kg

* Plasma osmolality can be also be calculated from serum sodium, potassium glucose, and urea (all values in mmol/l):

Osmolality in mOsmol/kg = 1.86 (Na^+ + K^+) + glucose + urea.

urine osmolality must be measured frequently. If the urine output is persistent or more severe, specific drug therapy will be required. In this case, DDAVP (desa-mino-D-8-arginine-vasopressin), a specific synthetic anti-diuretic hormone, given intravenously or by nasal snuff is the drug of choice. The dose and frequency depends on the clinical effect and can be variable. When the urine volume has been lowered to about 2 ml/min an infusion of 0.9% sodium chloride should be used to maintain the plasma osmolality at 280–300 mOsmol/kg. Measurements of plasma and urine osmolality should be made every 8 hours.

Cardiovascular parameters (CVP, BP, HR) and urine output must be monitored closely. Urine specific gravity should be measured regularly.

(See Chapters 9 and 11 for diabetes insipidus in head injury.)

Obstetric emergencies

The pregnant patient near term is unique because the feto-placental unit has radical effects on maternal physiological function. When treating the critically ill pre-term woman, the welfare of the fetus must always be considered. Pregnancy-associated emergencies that require admission to the ICU are uncommon but an understanding of the pathological mechanisms underlying the disorders is essential.

The major physiological changes that occur during pregnancy

Respiratory changes

- A decrease in functional residual capacity (FRC) in the second half of pregnancy. This is due to elevation of the diaphragm by the developing fetus. In late pregnancy, airway closure occurs above or closer to the FRC than in the non-pregnant state and may adversely affect gas exchange.

- Minute ventilation can be increased up to 50 per cent by term due to hyperventilation and an increase in tidal volume caused by the central respiratory stimulant effects of progesterone.

- Oxygen consumption increases by up to 15 per cent by term due to demands from the developing fetus, uterus, placenta and breasts. This is met by an increase in minute ventilation, an increase in cardiac output and a shift of the maternal oxyhaemoglobin dissociation curve to the right.

Cardiovascular changes

- Maternal blood volume increases from the first trimester and reaches its maximum by weeks 24–34. This increase is necessary to compensate for blood lost at delivery and for the placenta. About one-third of the extra blood fills the sinuses of the placenta and the remainder stays in the circulation. The volume of increase varies with the number of fetuses and can be up to 50% greater than in the non-pregnant state.

  The increase in plasma volume exceeds that of red cell volume creating a physiological anaemia.

- Cardiac output rises gradually from the first trimester due to the increase in blood volume and an increase in heart rate (up by 20 per cent) and stroke volume. By 30 weeks it can be 30–50 per cent above non-pregnant values.

  During labour, cardiac output is further increased by autotransfusion induced by each uterine contraction.

- Systemic vascular resistance decreases. This is induced by oestrogen and progesterone which cause smooth muscle relaxation and ensure oxygen and nutrition needs are met for the developing fetus.

- Immediately after delivery, cardiac output rises due to autotransfusion by uterine contractions and the relief of venocaval obstruction.

- Within three weeks of delivery the expanded blood volume has been reabsorbed and cardiac output is restored to normal values.

Utero-placental perfusion

- The utero-placental circulation is a pressure-dependent system without its own regulatory mechanism. Any factor that decreases venous return or cardiac output in the mother will impair uterine flow (e.g. mechanical ventilation or aortocaval compression).

- Hypotension can develop due to compression of the iliac vessels, inferior vena cava and aorta due to the enlarging uterus. This is evident during the second half of pregnancy and is maximal when the patient is supine. Hypotension can critically impair utero-placental blood flow and in any instance of hypotension the patient should be placed in the left lateral position to relieve compression. If this is not possible the right hip should be elevated to displace the uterus leftward to minimize venacaval and aortic compression. This should also be the position in which cardiopulmonary resuscitation is carried out.

- Hypoxaemia, acidosis, and vasopressors all cause utero-placental constriction and impair perfusion.

- Utero-placental perfusion can be increased by correct positioning, volume infusion, and leg raising.

Obstetric disorders

Amniotic fluid embolism

This is an uncommon disorder but one of the most dangerous — more than 80 per cent of episodes are fatal. It results from entrance of amniotic fluid and particulate matter into the maternal circulation and causes maternal pulmonary embolism and a syndrome of haematological and cardiovascular manifestations.

Predisposing factors for amniotic fluid embolism

- Multiparity

- Intra-uterine death

- Hypertonic labour

- Caesarean section

- Amniocentesis

- Cervical tears

- Use of oxytocics

- Premature placental separation

- Meconium in the amniotic fluid

The most likely route of the amniotic fluid into the maternal circulation is by laceration or rupture of the uterus, cervix, endocervical veins, or abnormal uteroplacental sites. Amniotic fluid is rich in lipid particulate material and may contain meconium and fetal debris — these can cause vascular obstruction.

The patient presents with the sudden onset of respiratory distress and circulatory collapse.

The initial response of the pulmonary vasculature to amniotic fluid and debris is intense vasoconstriction producing pulmonary hypertension, right heart failure and severe hypoxia. Patients who survive this phase (many die within the first hour) then develop left ventricular failure, pulmonary oedema and haemorrhage. Haemorrhage (particularly uterine) results from disseminated intravascular coagulation in approximately 40 per cent of patients.

Management of amniotic fluid embolism

There is no specific treatment; management is largely supportive.

- Respiratory

  Oxygenation must be maintained. In less severe cases, oxygen via a facemask may suffice but, more often, endotracheal intubation and mechanical ventilation will be necessary.

- Cardiovascular

  Full haemodynamic monitoring may be required, including pulmonary artery pressures and cardiac output.

  Treatment of heart failure and hypotension (by inotropic support, nitrates, diuretics) must be guided by haemodynamic measurements.

- Haemorrhage

  Fluid replacement should be guided by haemodynamic measurements. Treat coagulopathy using blood component therapy (fresh frozen plasma, platelets, cryoprecipitate). Blood transfusion to correct anaemia.

Pre-eclampsia and eclampsia

Pre-eclampsia is defined as acute hypertension, oedema, and proteinuria (> 300 mg/day).

It occurs in the latter half of pregnancy, is more common in the first pregnancy and up to 10 per cent of all pregnancies are affected. This disorder remains a significant cause of fetal and maternal morbidity and mortality and outcome is worse if pre-eclampsia develops in the second trimester.

Eclampsia is the convulsive phase of pre-eclampsia and may occur after delivery.

The precise aetiology is still unclear but it is postulated that there is some imbalance between the placenta and blood flow causing placental ischaemia and the release of vasopressors (in response to a decrease in perfusion pressure). A further hypothesis is that the disorder is primarily a trophoblast-dependent process mediated by platelet/endothelial cell dysfunction and damage. An imbalance has been found in women with pre-eclampsia in the production of thromboxane and prostacyclin by the placental vascular bed. There is a decrease in production of prostacyclin and an increase in thromboxane. This leads to clotting activation, platelet aggregation, local vasoconstriction, and the release of vasopressor substances (causing intense vascular smooth muscle sensitivity) in the placental and maternal circulations. Fibrin deposition in the placenta and maternal organs can cause impaired utero-placental blood flow and organ dysfunction in the mother.

Manifestations of pre-eclampsia

- Hypertension

- Proteinuria

- Oliguria

- Oedema

- Visual disturbances

- Heart failure

- Pulmonary oedema

- Disseminated intravascular coagulation (DIC)

- Hyperexcitability of the central nervous system

- Related liver disease

Pre-eclampsia can be classed as mild or severe according to the degree of hypertension and proteinuria but eclampsia can occur suddenly even when the blood pressure is mildly raised.

Management of severe pre-eclampsia
Delivery of the baby is the only definitive treatment of severe pre-eclampsia. If the fetus is too immature for delivery management is aimed at:

- Control of hypertension.

- Maintenance of placental perfusion.

- Prevention of eclamptic convulsions.

Induction should only be postponed for as long as the maternal condition allows. Severe uncontrollable hypertension, impending liver failure, severe coagulopathy, seizures, and pulmonary oedema are indications for early delivery.

Nursing management

- *Problem*: Hypertension.

- *Management*. Monitor blood pressure. Continuous ECG monitoring. Administer anti-hypertensive drug therapy. There is no clear consensus on the drug of choice but intravenous hydralazine (a peripheral vasodilator) or labetalol (an alpha and beta adrenergic blocker) are commonly used.

  Sudden falls in mean blood pressure or hypotension must be avoided as this will be detrimental to uteroplacental perfusion. Diastolic blood pressure should not be reduced below 90 mmHg.

Intravenous nitrates should be avoided as the reduction in blood pressure can be abrupt and is at the expense of a reduced cardiac output (an exception to this is when there are high ventricular filling pressures and a low cardiac output). Sodium nitroprusside should also be avoided due to the risk of fetal toxicity from cyanide poisoning, although it is useful for acute hypertensive crises complicated by pulmonary oedema and left ventricular failure.

The patient should remain on bedrest, preferably nursed in the left lateral position.

- *Problem*. Oliguria due to decreased renal blood flow.

- *Management*. Monitor urine output.
  Oliguria is usually due to inadequate cardiac output and this may be as a result of decreased circulatory volume or severe systemic vasoconstriction. Optimal circulatory volume must be maintained by fluid infusion and afterload reduction.

  This must be guided by CVP or pulmonary artery catheter monitoring. Diuretics should only be used with proven intravascular fluid overload.

  Acute tubular necrosis is rare but in such cases renal support may be required.
  Monitor blood urea, electrolytes, and creatinine.
  Test urine daily for proteinuria.

- *Problem*. Potential haemorrhage due to DIC.

- *Management*. Observe for evidence of bleeding. Correct the coagulopathy using fresh frozen plasma and cryoprecipitate. Significant thrombocytopenia will require platelet transfusion.

  There is a significant risk of *abruptio placentae* in these patients.
  Cerebral haemorrhage can occur if blood pressure and coagulopathy are not controlled.

- *Problem*. Dyspnoea due to pulmonary oedema.

- *Management*. Monitor respiratory rate. Continuous pulse oximetry or arterial blood gases to monitor oxygen saturation. Treatment of pulmonary oedema should be guided by pulmonary artery catheter monitoring. Large volumes of crystalloid should be avoided and afterload reduced by vasodilators. Diuretics may be necessary. If hypoxaemic, supplemental oxygen by mask, CPAP, or mechanical ventilation may be required.

- *Problem*. Potential eclamptic convulsions.

- *Management*. Observe for convulsions. These are attributed to microemboli in the cerebral circulation or to local vasospasm and can occur irrespective of elevated blood pressure. Prophylactic intravenous phenytoin is advocated for patients with moderate to severe pre-eclampsia.

However, if convulsions occur the priorities of care are maintenance of the airway, oxygenation and control of the fits (usually by IV magnesium, diazepam, or phenytoin). Endotracheal intubation and ventilatory support may be required. If the patient remains in coma, cerebral oedema or haemorrhage must be suspected. The neurological management of these patients includes maintenance of cerebral perfusion pressure and control of intercranial pressure. Hypertension must be brought under control and prompt caesarean section considered.

Magnesium acts as a central nervous system depressor and can be used (IV or IM) to prevent or control convulsions. It is now the first-line drug for eclamptic fits. Therapeutic maternal blood levels are 2–3.5 mmol/l but respiratory paralysis can occur when levels are greater than 5 mmol/l. Careful observation of respiratory pattern and depth will be required to avoid respiratory arrest. Magnesium also increases patient sensitivity to all neuromuscular blocking agents and passes across the placenta (can cause a flaccid new-born).

Liver disease associated with pregnancy

Two syndromes will be mentioned briefly. They are viewed as part of pre-eclampsia, because they have the same underlying causative mechanism but primarily affect the liver. They are uncommon and are termed the syndromes of HELLP and AFLP.

HELLP Syndrome: Haemolysis, Elevated Liver function tests, Low Platelet count
This syndrome is associated with haemolytic anaemia, elevated liver enzymes, and low platelet count but not necessarily hypertension or proteinuria. It usually occurs in the third trimester or post-partum and 40 per cent of patients are multigravid. Symptoms include epigastric or right upper quadrant pain and nausea. The liver disturbance is of major concern since encephalopathy, liver haemorrhage, necrosis, or rupture can occur.

Prognosis is unpredictable and immediate delivery is usually indicated. There may be particular problems with haemorrhage and transfusions of red cells, fresh frozen plasma, cryoprecipitate, and platelets may be necessary.

AFLP syndrome: Acute Fatty Liver of Pregnancy
This is characterized by cholestasis and histologically by microvesicular fat. Symptoms include nausea, right upper quadrant pain, jaundice, encephalopathy, and fulminant hepatic failure. Coagulation disorders such as DIC occur and there may be persistent hypoglycaemia.

Early delivery may improve maternal survival and liver function.

Peri-partum cardiomyopathy

This disorder presents in the last month of pregnancy or the first six months after delivery. It is a dilated cardiomyopathy that is more common in older, multiparous, black women. The aetiology is uncertain but several mechanisms have been proposed including hormonal changes of pregnancy, nutritional deficiencies, and autoimmune or viral processes.

The patient usually presents with classical signs of left or biventricular failure.

There is a severe reduction in left ventricular performance and gross dilatation of the left ventricle.

A major complication is pulmonary or cerebral emboli. Mortality is 25–50 per cent and death can be caused by ventricular arrhythmias, diminished cardiac output, or the consequences of emboli.

There is a tendency for this condition to recur with subsequent pregnancies, particularly in patients whose heart size does not return to normal within six months.

Management is by systemic anticoagulation and the conventional treatment for congestive cardiac failure.

Effects of drugs on the fetus

- *Inotropes*: adrenaline in high doses increases uterine contractility, but at low doses decreases it. Most inotropes reduce uterine blood flow.

- *Vasopressors*: these raise maternal blood flow but have less effect on uterine flow.

- *Anticoagulants*: heparin does not cross the placenta but warfarin does and can cause fetal abnormalities.

- *Antiarrhythmics*: propanolol can cause premature labour, neonatal bradycardia, hypoglycaemia, and respiratory depression. Therapeutic levels of digoxin and lignocaine have no adverse effects on the fetus.

Drug overdose and toxic substance ingestion

Poisoning may be accidental or iatrogenic. Self-administered drug poisoning accounts for over 10 per cent of acute medical admissions to hospital. Death from acute poisoning is relatively uncommon except in children under 4 years where accidental poisoning remains an important cause of death.

In deliberate drug overdose, often more than one drug will be ingested and alcohol is a common co-agent. Complications can be unexpected and require prompt action and specific treatments. Supportive therapy in the ICU can be life-saving.

Conditions that require ICU admission

Admission to ICU will be required if the patient is or may become:

- Cardiovascularly unstable (hypotensive, cardiac arrhythmias).

- Unconscious.

- Requires endotracheal intubation or mechanical ventilation.

- Requires specialist therapy (haemodialysis/filtration, temporary pacing, peritoneal dialysis).

- Suffers convulsions.

Assessment

Self-poisoning is the cause of undiagnosed coma in 15 per cent of patients aged between 15 and 55 years and although other causes of coma must be excluded this should always be suspected.

A careful history must be obtained from the patient (if conscious), ambulance personnel and relatives or friends. Empty bottles, drugs or a suicide note may have been found with the patient and the patient's general practitioner can provide details of recently prescribed medication or any history of depressive illness.

A physical examination can provide important evidence:

- Venepuncture marks may indicate the patient is a drug-abuser.

- Cherry pink skin and mucosa may be due to carbon monoxide poisoning.

- Bullous skin lesions can occur in overdose of barbiturates.

- Pin-point pupils can result from opioid overdose.

- Dilated pupils occur in tricyclic or amphetamine overdose.

Urine, blood, and gastric contents should be sent for analysis but urgent drug screening is usually limited to paracetamol and salicylate screening. A more comprehensive drug screen can be carried out by a poisons laboratory. When the cause of a coma is unknown a blood sugar should always be performed urgently. Other investigations (such as LP or CT scan) must not be delayed while the results are awaited.

General principles

The signs and symptoms of drug overdose depend on:

- The patient's size, age, health.

- The drug.

- The route.

- How long ago the drug was taken or over what period of time.

- The quantity taken.

- Whether other drugs were taken at the same time (e.g. alcohol).

For some drugs that require specific treatment (e.g. antidotes) recovery is dependent on the time interval between ingestion and the time that treatment begins. Definitive treatment must therefore begin as soon as resuscitation is completed.

Resuscitation

- The airway must be kept patent. If the patient is comatose with no cough or gag reflex then endotracheal intubation will be required.

- Establish intravenous access.

- Give oxygen by mask or if spontaneous respiration is inadequate, ventilatory support will be required.

- Take baseline measurements of heart rate, rhythm, and blood pressure. Assess peripheral perfusion, skin colour, body temperature.

- Correct hypovolaemia.

- Carry out a bedside blood glucose test.

- Assess conscious level.

- Take blood samples for glucose, urea, creatinine and electrolytes, liver function tests, full blood count, coagulation screen, arterial blood gases, and drug assays.

- Chest X-ray (if indicated).

Treatment

After basic resuscitation, treatment is aimed at:

- Decreasing further drug absorption.

- Increasing drug excretion.

- Administration of specific antidotes.

- Supportive therapy.

Treatment strategies are given in Table 13.12.

Further management

The action and side effects of the drug taken (if known) should be documented in order to anticipate and observe for problems that may occur. Specific supportive treatments will vary according to the drug taken (see later).

The basic principles are:

- Respiratory
  - Maintain airway (depends on level of consciousness): oropharyngeal (Guedel) airway, endotracheal intubation, patient positioning.
  - Monitor blood gases, acid–base status, and oxygen saturation. Give oxygen therapy or ventilatory support as indicated.
  - Hypoxaemia may indicate additional pulmonary pathology such as aspiration, infection, oedema, atelectasis.

- Cardiovascular
  - Monitor cardiovascular status: continuous ECG recording, observe for arrhythmias, perform 12-lead ECG, monitor BP.

Circulatory failure can result from a variety of causes (hypovolaemia, myocardial insufficiency, vasodilatation, or reduced cardiac output due to cardiac arrhythmias). The mechanism of shock must be ascertained by appropriate monitoring of cardiovascular parameters and acid-base staus in order to institute effective treatment.

- Neurological
  - Assess neurological status. Perform full neurological assessment, document regular neurological observations until fully conscious. Observe for and report convulsions.
  - Convulsions may occur as an effect of the poison taken or following a hypoxic episode.

Table 13.12: Treatment strategies for drug overdose

Aim of treatment	Method	Comments
Decreasing further drug absorption	• Inducing emesis — using ipecacuanha syrup.	Use in fully conscious patients only. Never use if poisoning is by paraffin or corrosives.
	• Gastric lavage — using large volumes of 0.9% sodium chloride instilled via a large-bore orogastric tube.	Should be performed within 6 hours of ingestion. Airway must be protected — may necessitate endotracheal intubation.
	• Activated charcoal — charcoal is instilled after gastric lavage and adsorbs the poison.	Can be given in repeated doses for certain drugs. Must be given as soon as possible to be effective.
Increasing excretion of the drug	• Forced diuresis: IV fluids and diuretics are used to promote a diuresis and prevent time for drug reabsorption in the kidney.	Can be very hazardous in patients with renal or cardiac dysfunction. Requires vigilant haemodynamic, respiratory, fluid and electrolyte monitoring. Drug must be renally excreted for this to be effective.
	• Alkalinization of the urine (enhances excretion of salicylate and phenobarbitone)	Sodium bicarbonate 8.4% is give as IV boluses to maintain the urinary pH 7–8. Monitor blood pH carefully.
Specific antidotes	Available for certain drugs.	
Alteration of drug metabolism	Metabolic pathways can be saturated, preventing formation of toxic metabolites.	Metabolic pathways of methylene and ethylene can be saturated using IV ethylene. N-acetylcysteine is used for paracetamol poisoning.

• Renal

– If unable to take oral fluids an IV infusion will be required. Monitor urine output, blood urea, electrolytes, and creatinine. Perform urinalysis.

– Consider nutritional status (need for enteral/parenteral nutrition).

– Rhabdomyolysis can be a complication of some poisonings, particularly when the patient is comatose but also when drugs are taken that cause 'hyper-exercise' (strychnine, cocaine, amphetamines including Ecstasy). Diagnosis is usually confirmed by a grossly elevated CPK and myoglobinuria. Circulatory and renal failure can develop (for further details see Chapter 8).

• Monitor blood glucose

• Body temperature

Monitor body temperature. Hypothermia is a common manifestation of many poisonings (often accompanied by hypotension and oliguria). Such patients must be re-warmed with close monitoring of CVP. In some cases (e.g. in poisoning with hypnotic agents) the patients are rarely dehydrated. If plasma expanders are vigorously infused they may cause circulatory overload and pulmonary oedema. Caution is required, especially when the core temperature is $< 32\,°C$. (See Chapter 11 for further details of hypothermia).

Specific management of common drug overdoses

Table 13.13 details the management of drug overdose.

During the recovery period patients who have made a deliberate suicide attempt may become withdrawn and uncommunicative or aggressive and uncooperative. Skill and understanding is needed by the nurse during this difficult period. A psychiatric referral should be arranged as soon as possible so that the acute problem can be alleviated and further suicide attempts prevented. Assistance from other support agencies may be required (social workers, ministers of religion).

Table 13.13 Specific management strategies for drug overdose and poisons

Poison	Features	Management
Antidepressants: • Tricyclics	Dilated pupils, dry mouth, urinary retention, ileus, agitation, convulsions, hyperpyrexia. Cardiotoxic effects may appear after up to 3 days: A–V conduction disturbances, ST, VF, VT.	Supportive Maintain pH > 7.5 with bicarbonate if cardiotoxic
• Monamine Oxidase inhibitors (MAOIs)	Hypertensive crisis when taken with tyramine containing foods and sympathomimetic agents.	Phentolamine, sodium nitroprusside or diazoxide to control hypertension.
Anticholinergics and antihistamines	As for tricyclics. Cardiotoxic effects after 48 hours.	*Antidote*: physostigmine (target competitor).
Barbiturates	CNS depression — coma. Skin blisters and red wheals on pressure points of limbs. Hypothermia CVS depression — hypotension, peripheral vasodilation. Dilated pupils.	Supportive. Correct hypovolaemia Alkalinization of urine hastens elimination of phenobarbitone.
Benzodiazipines	Drowsiness, potentiated by alcohol.	*Antidote*: flumazenil (receptor antagonist) *Note*: this is short-acting and may also precipitate convulsions.
Beta blockers	Cardiotoxic effects within 48h: sinus bradycardia, AV conduction disturbances. Circulatory failure, respiratory depression.	Supportive Temporary venticular pacing may be required Inotropes and/or glucagon may be needed.
Carbon monoxide	Displaces oxygen from Hb, causing carboxyhaemoglobin and hypoxaemia and blocks cellualr mitochondrial respiration. Hypertonicity, pulmonary oedema, coma, agitation. May have cherry pink skin and mucosae.	100% oxygen. Mechanical ventilation often necessary Hyperbaric oxygen (if readily available) should be considered at levels of $> 25\%$ COHb or if the patient is symptomatic.

Table 13.13 *contd*

Poison	Features	Management
Cyanide	Prevents mitochondrial cellular respiration — circulatory failure due to cellular hypoxia even though P_aO_2 normal. Convulsions and respiratory failure. Death often rapid.	100% oxygen *Antidotes*: dicobalt edetate or sodium nitrite when diagnosis certain. If uncertain, sodium thiosulphate.
Chloroquine	Cardiotoxic effects 2–6 h: AV conduction disturbances, VF. Negative inotropic effect, vasodilation, hypotension. Sudden cardiac arrest.	Supportive — adrenaline for hypotension.
Digoxin	May take 24–76 h for toxic effects. SB, VT, VF, and A–V conduction problems. Vomiting.	*Antidotes*: antidigoxin Fab (receptor antagonist). Phenytoin can also be given. Pacing if necessary.
Ethylene glycol (antifreeze)	Severe metabolic acidosis due to oxalic acid. Acute renal failure. Inebriation	*Antidote*: ethanol (metabolic competitor).
Heavy metals:		
● Iron	Corrosive to gastrointestinal tract. Nausea, haematemasis, abdominal pain, malaena. Gastric perforation may occur.	*Antidote*: desferrioxamine mesylate
● Lead	Liver and renal failure. Diarrhoea, vomiting, abdominal pain, convulsions, coma.	*Antidote*: EDTA (calcium disodium edetate)
● Mercury	Burns to skin if local contamination. CNS damage — tremor, ataxia, dysarthria.	*Antidote*: acetyl penicillamine
● Arsenic	Causes increased permeability of blood vessels and vasodilation. Abdominal pain, nausea, vomiting, profuse diarrhoea, profound electrolyte disturbances (hypokalaemia, hyponatraemia). Circulatory collapse, cellular enzyme disturbances.	*Antidote*: *N*-acetyl penicillamine
Methanol	Methanol is metabolized to formaldehyde and then formic acid which causes blindness and metabolic acidosis.	*Antidote*: ethanol (metabolic competitor).
Opiates	CNS depression. Pin-point pupils. Respiratory depression — hypoxia.	*Antidote*: naloxone (receptor antagonist). Supportive treatment including IPPV.
Organophosphates	CNS depression — hypoxia. Muscular paralysis/fasciculations. Bradycardia, asystole. Hypothermia, abdominal pain, diarrhoea. Bronchospasm, salivation.	*Antidote*: atropine to control parasympathetic activity. Supportive — mechanical ventilation.

Table 13.13 *contd*

Poison	Features	Management
Paracetamol	Liver necrosis with ingestion of > 10 g. Nausea, vomiting for first 24 h, liver failure 3–6 days after ingestion.	Gastric lavage and activated charcoal. *Antidote*: N-acetylcysteine. Protective effect is time-dependent — if given up to 36 h after overdose. Toxicity can be assessed by referring to a graph of plasma paracetamol levels against time after ingestion.
Paraquat	Causes local irritation to mucosal membranes — vomiting, abdominal pain, diarrhoea, difficulty swallowing, and oesophageal ulceration. Multi-organ failure. Pulmonary fibrosis develops within 10–14 days. Death usually ensues within 24–48 h. 10 ml can be fatal.	*No antidote.* Supportive treatment. After gastric lavage instillation of Fullers Earth or betonite with magnesium sulphate can lessen absorption. Haemodialysis or haemoperfusion should be instituted if within about 6 h of ingestion.
Phenothiazines	As for tricyclics	Supportive. May require diazepam for fits.
Salicylates	Flushing, sweating, tinnitus, deafness, hyperventilation. Cellular hypoxia. Acid–base disturbances. Hypokalaemia, pulmonary oedema.	Alkalinization of urine increases elimination. Haemodialysis in severe poisoning.

References and bibliography

Behi, R. (1989). Treatment and care of thyroid problems. *Nursing*, **3**, 4–6.

Brunner, L.S. and Suddarth, D.S. (1979). *Textbook of medical-surgical nursing* (3rd edn). Lippincott, Philadelphia.

Byth, P.L. (1990). Obstetrical emergencies. In *Intensive care manual*, (ed. T.E. Oh), (3rd edn). Butterworth, London.

DHSS (1983). *Pesticide poisoning*. HMSO, London.

Dugernier, T. and Reynaert, M. (1991). Cardiocirculatory emergencies related to pregnancy. *Clinical Intensive Care*, **2**, 163–71.

Evangelisti, J. and Thorpe, C.J. (1983). Thyroid storm — a nursing crisis. *Heart and Lung*, **12**, 184–93.

Green, J.H. (1978). *An introduction to human physiology*, (4th edn), pp. 159–69. Oxford University Press.

Guyton, A.C. (1984). *Physiology of the human body*, (6th edn). Holt-Saunders, Philidelphia.

Hardcastle, W. (1989). Management of Addison's disease. *Nursing*, **3**, 7–9.

Hillman, K. (1991). Management of acute diabetic emergencies. *Clinical Intensive Care*, **2**, 154–61.

Mathewson, M.K. (1987). Thyroid disorder. *Critical Care Nurse*, **7**, 74–85.

Rubenstein, D., and Wayne, D. (1985). *Lecture notes on clinical medicine*, (4th edn). Blackwell, Oxford.

Smallridge, R.C. (1992). Metabolic and anatomic thyroid emergencies: a review. *Critical Care Medicine*, **20**, 276–91.

Shulham, C. (1985). Diabetic ketoacidosis — an endocrine emergency. *Nursing* **2**, 246–9.

Stover Leske, J. (1985). Hyperglycaemic hyperosmolar nonketotic coma: a nursing care plan. *Critical Care Nurse*, **5**, 49–56.

Tinker, J. and Zapol, W.M. (1992). *Care of the critically ill patient*, (2nd edn), 546–49, 761–92. Springer, Berlin.

Vedig, A. (1990). Adrenocortical insufficiency. In *Intensive care manual*, (ed. T.E. Oh). (3rd edn). Butterworth, London.

Weekes, J. (1990). Drug overdose. In *Intensive care manual*, (3rd edn), (ed. T.E. Oh). Butterworth, London.

14. The systemic inflammatory response and multiple organ dysfunction

Introduction

One of the greatest challenges currently facing those who work in the ICU is the care of the patient suffering from multiple organ dysfunction and the systemic inflammatory response syndromes. The patients are usually acutely ill with many wide-ranging problems requiring an array of the most complex forms of organ support and intervention. At present, there is no definitive form of treatment and a variety of therapies may be tried.

A major factor in the problem is that any organ or system in the body may be affected (although some are more vulnerable such as the lungs, kidneys, and clotting system) and each individual will have differing degrees of organ dysfunction producing different requirements. The development of specific definitions of the condition is important in clarifying and comparing information from different patients and different manifestations of the problem (Table 14.1).

Definitions

Systemic inflammatory response syndrome (SIRS) and multiple organ dysfunction syndrome (MODS) have been known previously under a variety of different names. SIRS has been referred to as sepsis, septicaemia, septic syndrome, and septic shock (terms that suggest an underlying infective component), until it was confirmed that infection was only one of the many triggers involved in the response. The use of these terms was considered misleading and an alternative definition suggesting an inflammatory component was put forward (ACCP/SCCM 1992). In the circumstance where SIRS is the result of a probable infectious process, the term 'sepsis' is still used.

MODS was previously known as multiple organ failure, progressive/sequential organ failure, or multi-system organ failure. This was felt to denote a situation that was either present or absent rather than a progressive devel-opment along a continuum of physiological derangement and the term 'multiple organ dysfunction syndrome' was introduced (ACCP/SCCM 1992).

Systemic inflammatory response syndrome (SIRS)
The systemic inflammatory response to a variety of severe clinical insults, manifested by two or more of the following conditions:

- Temperature $> 38\,°C$

- Heart rate > 90 beats/min

- Respiratory rate > 20 breaths/min or hyperventilation with a P_aCO_2 < 4.3 kPa (32 mmHg)

- WBC $> 12\,000$ or < 4000 cells/mm^3, or 10 per cent immature neutrophils

---

Multiple organ dysfunction syndrome (MODS)
Presence of altered organ function in an acutely ill patient such that homeostasis cannot be maintained without intervention. This can either occur directly as the result of a well-defined insult or as a secondary result of the host response induced in SIRS.

Sepsis syndrome (after Bone *et al.* 1989)
Hypo- or hyperthermia ($< 35.6\,°C/96\,°F$ or $> 38.3\,°C/101\,°F$)
Heart rate > 90 beats/min
Respiratory rate > 20 breaths/min
Evidence of inadequate organ perfusion/function:

- alteration in mental status

- arterial hypoxaemia (P_aO_2 < 9.6 kPa/72 mmHg)

- an elevated plasma lactate level

- urine output below 0.5 ml/kg/h for at least 1 hour

Sepsis syndrome does not require the presence of a positive blood culture nor hypotension.

Toxins and degradative substances associated with bacteria

Exotoxins

These are proteins released into the environment following their synthesis in the cytoplasm of the cell. They often react with a single target tissue to cause specific damage (e.g. nerves, cardiac muscle). They are produced by Gram-negative and positive bacteria.

Endotoxins

These are structural components of bacterial cells; an integral part of the cell wall and are released as the cell lyses. They are large lipopolysaccharides, usually associated with the lipopolysaccharide layer of Gram-negative bacteria. Toxicity is associated with the lipid A portion of the molecule.

Enzymes

Gram-negative bacteria contain a periplasmic space in the cell wall which produces hydrolytic enzymes including lipases, phosphatases, and proteases.

Gram-positive bacteria produce hydrolytic exoenzymes as they do not have a periplasmic space.

Examples of specific degradative substances:

Streptokinase (streptococci): dissolves fibrin clots thus preventing isolation of infection.

Hyaluronidase (pneumococci, streptococci, staphylococci): digests hyaluronic acid in the basement membrane permitting tissue penetration.

14.1 Table of definitions

Term	Definition
Bacteraemia	The presence of viable bacteria in the blood.
Septicaemia	An imprecise term used in a number of different ways to describe: (1) the presence of microorganisms or their toxins in the blood, (2) sepsis syndrome (see box). Its use is no longer recommended.
Septic shock	Sepsis-induced hypotension (systolic BP < 90 mmHg or reduced by > 40 mmHg from baseline without other cause), which is unresponsive to fluid resuscitation with manifestations of hypoperfusion, such as oliguria, altered mental state, etc.

> **Triggers of SIRS**
>
> - Trauma
> - Pancreatitis
> - Major burns
> - Major surgical procedures
> - Infection
> - Haemorrhage/major blood-transfusion
> - Ischaemic tissue
> - Periods of inadequate perfusion

Leucocidin (staphylococci, streptococci): disintegrates phagocytes.

Haemolysin (clostridia, staphylococci): dissolves red blood cells, inducing anaemia, and limiting oxygen delivery.

Pathophysiology of SIRS and MODS

Development of the systemic inflammatory response syndrome occurs as a result of an insult which triggers the exaggerated, generalized inflammatory response and leads to the clinical and pathological sequelae of organ dysfunction and failure.

The response was first described in association with infective triggers but it has since been shown to be present without infection and as a result of a variety of different insults.

Sepsis (the infective trigger) remains the most common single cause of development of MODS but 40–50 per cent of patients do not have positive blood cultures or an identifiable septic focus (Huddleston 1992).

The effect of these factors is to initiate a common pathway of response. This is the inflammatory/immune response resulting in the release of inflammatory mediators. Following the insult, specific primary events will effect release of these mediators into the circulation. These primary events are as follows:

Inflammatory/immune response

A series of complex interactive mechanisms are activated via humoral (non-cellular) and cellular mediators. In normal circumstances these are subject to extensive inhibitory regulators such as feedback loops and redundant pathways. In the overwhelming inflammatory response, these inhibitory systems fail to control activation and a cycle of continuous re-activation may occur.

Activation of the inflammatory response often leads to concomitant activation of coagulation or alterations in haemostatic balance. Several circulating components play a role in both processes: kallikrein/kinin cascade, complement, Hageman factor, and platelets.

Endothelial damage

The endothelium is highly susceptible to damage, particularly by white blood cell/endothelial cell interactions. Other inflammatory mediators, such as tumour necrosis factor (TNF) — released from monocyte/macrophages, will also damage the endothelium.

The endothelium has a major function in anticoagulation. When damaged, it loses many properties integral to anticoagulation and can become the source of procoagulant substances such as tissue thromboplastin.

The three major effects of endothelial damage are:

(1) release of further mediators and potent vasoactive substances, e.g. prostaglandin, thromboxane, nitric oxide;

(2) potentiation of coagulation;

(3) increased capillary permeability.

If damage is widespread then coagulation abnormalities are likely and altered capillary permeability will produce diffuse interstitial oedema and alterations in intravascular fluid volume as fluid passes into the interstitial space.

Neuroendocrine activation

Release of ACTH, glucocorticoids, adrenaline and noradrenaline, growth hormone, endorphin, and prolactin results in increased cardiac output and blood flow to vital organs, decreased blood flow to secondary organs, increased capillary permeability, and increased blood glucose (for full details see Chapters 2 and 13).

Components of the inflammatory response (Fig. 14.1)

Humoral (plasma enzyme cascades)
   (i) *Complement* — classically, this is activated by antigen/antibody complexes or alternately by specific microorganisms. It is a complex cascade

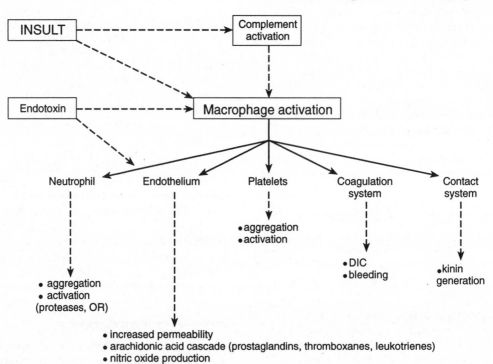

Fig. 14.1 Diagram showing inflammatory pathways (DIC, disseminated intravascular coagulation; NO, nitric oxide; OR, oxygen radicals).

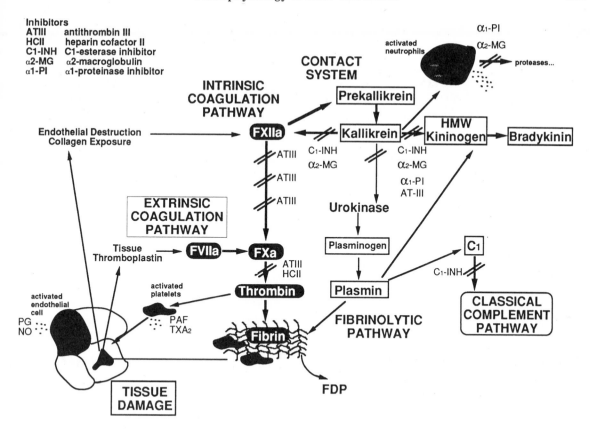

Fig. 14.2 The coagulation, contact, and fibrinolysis pathways.

through a series of approximately 20 circulating proteins. The major physiological function in normal circumstances is to initiate and enhance the inflammatory response.

Activities of the complement cascade

- Induction of inflammation

- Opsonization (coating with opsonin to enhance binding to phagocytic cells) of foreign particles

- Cellular activation of phagocytic cells (neutrophils, macrophages/monocytes)

- Direct target cell lysis (rupture of the cell membrane)

The effect is protective if complement activation is regulated and localized to the site of injury. If large amounts of complement activation occur and appear systemically then actions become detrimental. This effect is manifested by overwhelming vasodilatation, increased capillary permeability, and phagocytic activation with concomitant release of toxic by-products.

(ii) *Coagulation* and (iii) *fibrinolysis* — the mechanisms of coagulation and fibrinolysis work interdependently, producing a fine balance of haemostasis which once disrupted, can be difficult to control. Activation of coagulation occurs in response to injury, localized inflammation, and damage to the endothelium. The localized response provides an excellent protective mechanism which, in unregulated circumstances leading to systemic involvement, will rapidly produce coagulopathy and disseminated intravascular coagulation (DIC). The effects are seen as an increased incidence of vascular obstruction, tissue ischaemia and organ damage and, in DIC, the combined problems of intravascular coagulation and haemorrhage.

(iv) *Kallikrein/kinin* — the contact system is activated at the same time as the coagulation cascade through factor XII (Hageman factor). Although the role of this system is not clearly defined, it includes enhancement of the inflammatory response and the fibrinolytic cascade and a possible role in renal blood flow and blood pressure regulation. Bradykinin is the major metabolite produced by the cascade. It has a potent vasodilator effect and has also been shown to increase capillary permeability in some tissues. The kinins also indirectly activate complement, further propagating the inflammatory response.

Cellular (white blood cells, platelets, endothelium, mast cells, and fibroblasts)

1. *White blood cells* — these include neutrophils, monocytes (macrophages), and lymphocytes. The primary function of the neutrophil is surveillance and phagocytosis of foreign pathogens. They are drawn to the site of injury by chemotactic attraction to chemical products of cell destruction or foreign organisms. The neutrophil phagocytoses the pathogen by releasing proteases (cytotoxic enzymes such as elastase and catalase), and converting to oxidative metabolism. This produces highly reactive oxygen-related molecules collectively referred to as oxygen-derived free radicals. These radicals attack the pathogen in combination with the proteases secreted from the neutrophil causing cell death and phagocytosis.

There is usually some release of these highly toxic substances into the extracellular environment and this can result in local tissue damage and organ dysfunction.

Effects of mediators synthesized and released by activated neutrophils include vascular endothelial damage and parenchymal damage.

Proteases, such as elastase, can damage the extracellular matrix. The normal function of proteases is to digest bacteria and other foreign protein matter but they will also act as enzymatic catalysts for four enzyme cascades: complement, coagulation, kallikrein/kinin, fibrinolysis. Their action is potentiated by the presence of oxygen radicals which damage enzymes normally responsible for breaking down and eliminating proteases.

The primary functions of macrophages (mature tissue-based monocytes) and monocytes (immature mobile cells circulating in the blood) are: (a) to engulf and phagocytose foreign pathogens or antigens and process them for presentation to lymphocytes, thus stimulating specific lymphocytic proliferation, and (b) to produce inflammatory mediators known as monokines (cytokines).

Mediators released by activated neutrophils
- Oxygen-derived free radicals
- Proteases (collagenase, elastase)
- interleukins
- platelet-activating factor
- prostaglandins
- leukotrienes
- tissue factor (thromboplastin)
- nitric oxide (NO)

Mediators released by macrophages
- Tumour necrosis factor
- Interleukins
- Interferons
- Platelet-activating factor
- Leukotrienes
- Proteases
- Oxygen-derived free radicals
- Nitric oxide

Lymphocytes form sensitized cells and antibodies which are highly specific to a particular foreign pathogen. In cell-mediated immunity the T lymphocytes proliferate in response to presentation of the antigen surface of a macrophage to T cell lymphoid tissue. This is stimulated to produce numerous antigen-specific cells by macrophage release of interleukin-1 (IL-1). In humoral immunity the B lymphocytes recognize the antigen and differentiate into antibody-producing cells. The antibodies bind with the antigen producing the antigen/antibody immune complex which is removed by phagocytic cells in the reticuloendothelial system. Lymphocytes also produce mediators which are known as lymphokines.

2. *Platelets* — these react to disruption of the endothelium and exposure of the underlying collagen basement

---

Mediators released by lymphocytes
- Antibodies
- Tumour necrosis factor
- Colony-stimulating factors
- Gamma-interferon
- Interleukins

membrane. The shape of the platelet alters from the normal disc to a swollen sphere and they develop numerous projections known as pseudopods. These two manoeuvres expand the surface area available for adhesion and increase the likelihood of aggregation. During the shape change adenosine diphosphate (ADP) is released which initiates platelet aggregation. Thromboxane A_2 (TXA_2) is also extruded and causes vasoconstriction and further stimulation of platelet aggregation. This effectively activates platelet surface stickiness but the Von Willebrand factor must be present for adhesion to the exposed collagen and fibrinogen must be present for formation of the platelet plug. In addition, release of platelet surface procoagulant from the platelet initiates formation of a fibrin plug. The liberated ADP and TXA_2 activate more platelets until the aggregate is large enough to plug the vessel effectively.

Uncontrolled and excessive platelet activation triggered by a major insult will result in disruption of the normal coagulation mechanisms and development of DIC.

3. *Mast cells* — these are found in almost all tissues. The mast cell mediates the inflammatory response to injury by releasing mediators (see below) following stimulation either from direct injury, or the presence of endotoxin, complement, or bradykinin. The effects include vasodilation (histamine and prostaglandins), increased capillary permeability (histamine and leukotrienes), chemokinesis — increased white blood cell movement (histamine), and bronchoconstriction (histamine and leukotrienes).

Effects of mediators produced by the inflammatory response

There are numerous mediators produced by the inflammatory response and it is beyond the scope of this chapter to describe the function and actions of all of them. However, there are a number of important mediators which will be described. Mediators are produced primarily by immune cells although some are also generated in the endothelium.

Arachidonic acid metabolites
Arachidonic acid (AA) is a normal constituent of cell membranes that is released as a result of the contact of the enzyme phospholipase A_2 with injured cell walls. Arachidonic acid metabolism produces mediators known as eicosanoids which are essential for activation of macrophages. The two pathways of AA metabolism are the cyclooxygenase and lipooxygenase pathways. Their action is summarized in Fig. 14.3.

Mediators produced by the inflammatory response

- Arachidonic acid metabolites (prostaglandins, leukotrienes, thromboxanes)
- Nitric oxide
- Oxygen-derived radicals
- Clotting factors
- Plasminogen
- Colony-stimulating factors
- Plasminogen activators
- Complement
- Platelet-activating factor
- Hageman factor
- Proteases
- Heparin
- Tissue factor
- Histamine
- Tumour necrosis factor
- Interferon
- Interleukins

Tumour necrosis factor
Tumour necrosis factor (TNF) is a polypeptide cytokine produced primarily by activated macrophages. TNF release is stimulated by endotoxin, microorganisms, ischaemic tissue, and tissue debris. It may well have a central role in the pathogenesis of multiple organ dysfunction and its actions include:

(i) neutrophil activation to produce oxygen-derived free radicals and proteases,

(ii) platelet – neutrophil – endothelial interactions,

(iii) endothelium activation leading to increased vascular permeability and release of endothelial-derived inflammatory mediators.

TNF also has valuable functions in the normal inflammatory/immune response.

Interleukins (including IL-1,-6,-8,-10)
Interleukins are released in a number of inflammatory conditions, such as rheumatoid arthritis, haemodialysis, and transplant rejection, as well as sepsis and trauma.

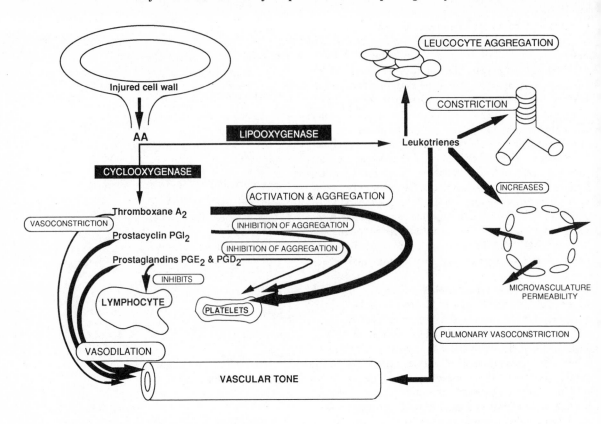

Fig. 14.3 Diagram showing arachidonic acid metabolism.

Like TNF, interleukin-1 (IL-1) is responsible for many beneficial effects in the normal inflammatory/immune response. It is released by macrophages, and other cells and is associated with inducing procoagulant activity in the endothelium, decreased vascular responsiveness to catecholamines, increased muscle proteolysis, and negative nitrogen balance. IL-1 also produces leucocytosis, fever, enhanced T cell, B cell, natural killer cells, macrophages, and polymorphonuclear (PMN) activity and proliferation, enhanced antibody production and stimulation of production of acute phase proteins.

Interleukin-6 (IL-6) is probably a second stage messenger released by macrophages, endothelial and other cells in response to TNF or IL-1. Its most important actions are the stimulation of acute phase protein production and antibody production, and the maintenance of the metabolic response to surgical stress.

Platelet activating factor
Platelet-activating factor (PAF) is a lipid mediator produced from the cell membrane of many different

inflammatory response cells and damaged endothelium following phospholipase A_2 activation.

Once in the circulation, PAF initiates platelet activation and the morphological changes associated with the ability to aggregate. Other actions include

● promotion of neutrophil adhesion,

Physiological functions of TNF

● Enhancement of phagocytic activity of neutrophils and macrophages

● Initiation of hepatocyte resistance to invasion (particularly parasitic)

● Enhancement of lymphocyte activity

● Stimulation of interleukin-1, platelet-activating factor, and gamma-interferon release

● Induction of fever

● Stimulation of collagenase production leading to tissue remodelling

- stimulation of respiratory burst,

- degranulation (release of oxygen-derived radicals and digestive enzymes)

- induction of release of leucotrienes and free radicals from neutrophils. Once PAF enters the systemic circulation, excessive platelet activation leads to clot formation and platelet plugs, as well as vasoconstriction. This results in abnormalities of the microcirculation as well as exacerbation of any pre-existing coagulopathies.

Nitric oxide

Nitric oxide, formerly known as endothelium derived relaxant factor, is a potent vasodilating mediator which is released from many different cell types as well as endothelium. It has other properties including cytotoxicity and neural transmission. Sepsis is associated with very high levels of NO caused by increased expression of the inducible form of NO synthase. NO is currently thought to be the major mediator involved in producing sepsis-related hypertension.

The numerous mediators provoke pathophysiological changes in three major areas of body function:

1. *Maldistribution of circulating volume.* The factors involved in maldistribution of circulating volume are numerous. Many of the mediators cause vasodilatation while others vasoconstrict. Some affect capillary vascular permeability. This causes intravascular fluid to move both into peripheral venous vessels where it pools, or to pass through the capillary membrane into the interstitial space (known as the third fluid space). Another factor in maldistribution is the obstruction to blood flow within the microvasculature caused by clumping of white cells in response to the initial injury and development of microthrombi stimulated by kallikrein, PAF, and thromboxanes. Normal peripheral vascular autoregulatory mechanisms are also dysfunctional during the hyperdynamic phase of SIRS resulting in vasodilatation and localized vasoconstriction with inappropriate closure of pre-capillary sphincters. It appears that normal tissues have the ability to regulate the density of perfused capillaries inversely with the tissue PO_2 (Schumacker and Cain 1987). This may also contribute to defective intra-organ blood flow distribution.

2. *Imbalance of oxygen supply and demand.* In healthy tissue, decreases in oxygen delivery do not initially lower oxygen consumption because tissue oxygen extraction is increased proportionately (see Chapter 5).

Table 14.2 Pathophysiological derangements associated with mediators and the neuroendocrine response

1. Maldistribution of circulating blood volume
   - Systemic vasodilatation
   - Increased microvascular permeability
   - Vascular obstruction related to cellular aggregation, microthrombi, and tissue oedema
   - Selective vasoconstriction
   - Endothelial damage
   - Coagulation/microvascular thrombi
   - Loss of autoregulation

2. Imbalance of oxygen supply and demand
   - Maldistribution of circulating volume
   - Microvascular abnormalities
   - Increased oxygen demand due to pain, fever, tachycardia, restlessness, etc.
   - Oxygen extraction defects
   - V/Q mismatch
   - Intrapulmonary shunt
   - Excessive cellular activity
   - Myocardial depression

3. Alterations in metabolism
   - Hypermetabolism
   - Hyperglycaemia
   - Protein catabolism and gluconeogenesis
   - Resistance to insulin
   - Excessive cellular activity
   - Fatty acid mobilization and increased oxidation
   - Hepatic dysfunction and lactate production

When available oxygen to the tissues falls below a critical level, tissue extraction can no longer increase to compensate and oxygen consumption will fall when there is a further fall in oxygen delivery. This is known as supply-dependent oxygen consumption.

It is postulated that in SIRS an impairment of tissue oxygen extraction capacity occurs which may lead to oxygen supply dependency at normal or increased levels of overall oxygen delivery (Schumacker and Cain 1987).

Pathological supply dependency in SIRS may be due to:

(i) Maldistribution of blood flow (see above).

(ii) Cellular defects. An impairment of oxidative metabolism has been demonstrated in sepsis in some studies but others have shown normal mitochondrial oxidative capacity (Dantzker 1989).

(iii) Impaired oxygen diffusion. This is hypothesized to be due to:

- an increase in interstitial fluid widening the distance between capillaries and cells,

- shorter capillary transit time (due to low SVR and high cardiac output) preventing unloading of oxygen from haemoglobin (Dantzker 1989),

- 'shunting' of blood away from the nutrient capillaries.

3. *Catabolic alterations in metabolism.* Principal alterations seen in SIRS are hypermetabolism, hyperglycaemia, protein catabolism, resistance to utilization of exogenous substrates, and inadequate reserves of substrates. The majority of these alterations are associated with the hypothalamic and sympathetic nervous system response to a major stress (for details see Chapters 2 and 13).

Central nervous system involvement in MODS

Central nervous system (CNS) failure in multiple organ dysfunction is defined as a decreased level of consciousness ranging from confusion to coma that cannot be explained by physical, drug, or metabolic abnormalities.

Sepsis, circulatory, and microcirculatory perfusion deficits and reperfusion injury are all significant factors in the process of development of CNS failure. The exact mechanism in sepsis is still unclear; suggested factors include:

1. Disordered amino acid transport and metabolism. Increased plasma levels of aromatic and sulphur-containing amino acids (specifically phenylalanine and glutamine) are found in the brain and cerebrospinal (CSF) of patients with sepsis. Accumulation of these substances could play a role in vasodilatation and altered cerebral function.

2. Altered neurotransmitter concentration. Increased levels of serotonin (5-HT) and 5-hydroxyindoleacetic acid (5-HIAA) have been found in animal studies. Their effects are compatible with the encephalopathic changes associated with MODS.

3. Brain microabscesses. These are produced by blood-borne contaminants which may block cerebral arterioles causing ischaemia. They may also initiate hyperaemia, oedema, and petechial haemorrhages.

Circulatory and microcirculatory perfusion deficits

Cerebral cellular metabolism relies on adequate supplies of oxygen and glucose. If the supply of both oxygen and glucose is inadequate due to perfusion deficits, anaerobic metabolism takes place producing lactic acid accumulation and eventual intracellular acidosis. When intracellular pH falls below 5.5, or ATP is exhausted, irreversible cell damage occurs.

However, if in incomplete ischaemia the supply of glucose continues but that of oxygen is inadequate, anaerobic metabolism (glycolysis) will continue with a rapid build-up of lactic acid and early cellular acidosis.

Cellular acidosis decreases the uptake of calcium ions (Ca^{2+}) by the mitochondria thus increasing intracellular levels of Ca^{2+}. This activates enzymes, such as phospholipases and proteases, which are capable of destroying cell membranes and intracellular organelles. Cellular acidosis will also inhibit mitochondrial respiration, further blocking ATP synthesis.

ATP depletion occurs and calcium shifts, prostaglandin synthesis, release of oxygen-derived radicals, and membrane damage result.

The excitatory neurotransmitters glutamine and aspartate may also have a role in the ischaemic process.

Cerebral reperfusion injury

Reperfusion injury refers to damage occurring after circulation has been restored due to generation of toxic oxygen-derived radicals as a by-product of oxygen-supported conversion of hypoxanthine to xanthine and uric acid. Cell damage also results from the accumulation of free fatty acids and prostaglandins (see Fig. 14.4).

Two processes have been associated with reperfusion injury: (1) post-ischaemic hypoperfusion, and (2) the no-reflow phenomenon.

Post-ischaemic hypoperfusion

This occurs after periods of complete global ischaemia and is seen as a 15–20 minute period of hyperaemia followed by vasospasm-induced hypoperfusion. The hyperaemia occurs as a result of loss of autoregulation and from the difference in blood viscosity of stagnant blood and circulating blood reperfusing the microcirculation.

Vasospasm lasts 6–34 hours and is thought to be a response to calcium activation and increased production of thromboxane A_2.

The no-reflow phenomenon

This is less common and occurs for 1–3 days after ischaemia. There is a continued decrease in cerebral blood flow despite normal mean arterial and cerebral perfusion pressures.

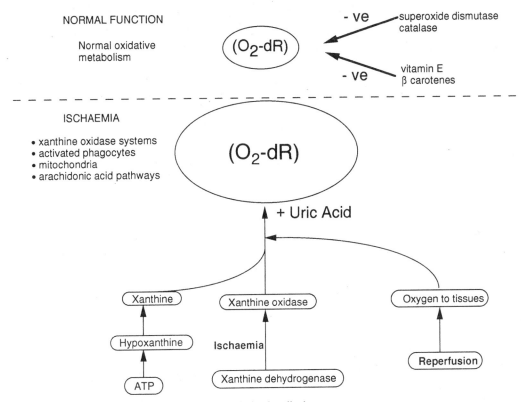

Oxygen-derived free radical production (O_2-dFR)

NORMAL FUNCTION

Normal oxidative metabolism

(O_2-dR)

- ve ← superoxide dismutase catalase

- ve ← vitamin E, β carotenes

ISCHAEMIA

- xanthine oxidase systems
- activated phagocytes
- mitochondria
- arachidonic acid pathways

(O_2-dR)

+ Uric Acid

Xanthine   Xanthine oxidase   Oxygen to tissues

Hypoxanthine   Ischaemia   Reperfusion

ATP   Xanthine dehydrogenase

Fig. 14.4 Diagram showing the generation of oxygen-derived radicals.

Processes contributing to the no-reflow phenomenon

- Oedema
- Vasospasm
- Increased blood viscosity with red blood cell sludging
- Hypermetabolism
- Membrane damage
- Intracellular or mitochondrial calcium shifts
- Release of oxygen-derived free radicals

Dysfunctions associated with CNS involvement

CNS involvement in MODS is not always associated with a period of hypoxia and metabolic causes are still unknown. It is generally an indicator of poor prognosis (Sprung *et al.* 1990).

Three distinct types of dysfunction are seen:

(1) septic encephalopathy,

(2) critical illness polyneuropathy,

(3) neuroendocrine exhaustion or failure.

(1) In septic encephalopathy neurological alterations are diffuse ranging from altered concentration and intermittent confusion to coma. EEG changes are also variable but the degree of abnormality correlates with the degree of encephalopathy. A mortality rate of 49 per cent has been associated with severe encephalopathy in sepsis (Sprung *et al.* 1990) and this may simply be a reflection of the severity of the MODS seen in these patients.

(2) Critical illness neuropathy increases patient mortality and can double or triple recovery time. It is associated with primary axonal degeneration of motor and sensory fibres and denervation atrophy of limb and skeletal muscles (Witt *et al.* 1991). This usually presents clinically as profound limb and chest wall weakness, although sensory deficits can occur alone or in combination.

(3) Neuroendocrine exhaustion or failure is associated with the following problems:

- glucose intolerance;

- failure to mount a febrile response;

- neurogenic pulmonary oedema;

- low T_3 (triiodothyronine) syndrome;

- hypoadrenal response, producing a relative adreno-cortical insufficiency which is associated with poor outcome (Rothwell *et al.* 1991).

Presence of these problems suggests that the body is no longer able to mount an effective response to the neuroendocrine triggers associated with SIRS.

Patient assessment for CNS involvement

Assessment should include the following:

Conscious level (although this can be impossible to assess due to the levels of sedation required to maintain ventilation). A high index of suspicion should be maintained if the patient appears unresponsive when sedation is reduced. Sedation should be reduced when the patient appears totally unresponsive, even during unpleasant procedures such as suction or turning (for further details see Chapter 9).

Mental agitation and confusion. This is often apparent when the patient is first admitted and other causes must be excluded (e.g. hypoxaemia). It can herald a further septic episode in a patient who has previously been recovering with no evidence of mental confusion.

Profound weakness and muscle wasting may only become apparent as the patient is recovering from MODS. It can be distinguished from simple weakness related to normal catabolic muscle wasting by electrophysiological studies which will show evidence of primary axonal degeneration of both sensory and motor fibres.

EEGs may exhibit evidence of changes consistent with *metabolic or anoxic encephalopathy* and a few will show evidence of profound abnormalities.

Respiratory system involvement in MODS

Respiratory system involvement in MODS is termed 'acute respiratory distress syndrome' (ARDS). (A full description of ARDS is given in Chapter 3).

ARDS is defined by the following clinical findings:

(1) diffuse acute pulmonary infiltrates seen on CXR associated with decreased pulmonary compliance,

(2) increased alveolar–arterial oxygen difference (despite supplemental oxygen),

(3) pulmonary artery wedge pressure of < 18 mmHg (i.e. non-cardiogenic origin),

(4) a precipitating factor.

There is usually evidence of respiratory failure (dyspnoea, tachypnoea, tachycardia, agitation).

Definition of respiratory failure

Blood gases

- PO_2 < 8.0 kPa patient breathing air and at rest

- $+/-$ PCO_2 > 6.5 kPa in the absence of primary metabolic alkolosis

- $+/-$ pH < 7.25 in the absence of primary metabolic acidosis

Patient

- Respiratory rate > 40 or < 6–8 breaths min

- Deteriorating vital capacity (< 15 ml/kg)

The underlying pathophysiology consists of disruption of the alveolar epithelium and endothelial damage, releasing mediators that cause increased capillary permeability, neutrophil and platelet aggregation, and pulmonary vasoconstriction. This results in alterations to microcirculatory flow and V/Q mismatch. Capillary membrane disruption also allows movement of fluid and protein into the interstitium. Atelectasis occurs as a result of interstitial oedema compressing alveoli. This compounds the decreased lung compliance caused by decreased surfactant production. Finally, direct parenchymal damage occurs as a result of mediator and macrophage action and necrosis from hypoxia. This damage ultimately causes fibrosis in alveolar tissue, further decreasing lung compliance. The net result is progressive alveolar collapse, intrapulmonary shunting, and hypoxaemia.

Patient assessment for ARDS

General appearance

Patient colour, respiratory function and pattern, level of fatigue, mental state, signs of sweating and distress. (see Chapter 3 for details).

Lung fields

Ausculatation in ARDS may sound clear or will detect isolated or generalized crackles or wheezes (see Chapter 3 for details).

Chest X-ray — antero-posterior, either erect (if possible) or supine. The typical early ARDS picture is non-specific with clear lung fields or scant infiltrates. There may also be unilateral lobar consolidation or diffuse lung involvement. In late ARDS the picture is one of diffuse alveolar infiltrates, sometimes termed 'white-out'.

Pulse oximetry

Patients are usually hypoxaemic from the early stages of ARDS and S_aO_2 will be <90% on air. Additional inspired oxygen will improve S_aO_2 initially, but requirements will continue to rise until CPAP or mechanical ventilation are necessary.

Pulmonary secretions

Volume, colour, and texture should be assessed. There are usually minimal, loose white secretions present in the early stages of ARDS. As the disease progresses secretions become thicker and more profuse. A specimen should be sent for culture.

Arterial blood gases

In the early stages of ARDS, the patient's P_aO_2 will be low and the P_aCO_2 will be either normal or low if the patient is hyperventilating in response to hypoxaemia. The pH will be normal or slightly alkalotic if the P_aCO_2 is low.

In the later stages, as the patient tires and respiratory failure ensues, the P_aCO_2 will rise with a decrease in pH due to a mixed respiratory and metabolic acidosis. The P_aO_2 will remain low in spite of increased inspired oxygen concentrations of up to 1.0.

Ventilator observations

Compliance will be decreased usually to a static compliance of less than 20–30 ml/cmH$_2$O.

The decreased compliance will produce high airway pressures causing barotrauma and increasing alveolar damage if not pressure limited to less than 35–40 cmH$_2$O. The overall goal of intervention is to re-open and stabilize closed, but potentially functional, alveolar units while minimizing barotrauma and variations in expansion of different areas of the lung caused by the disease process (see Chapter 3 for details).

Inspired oxygen requirements are often increased to a F_iO_2 of 0.6 or greater in order to achieve oxygen saturations of >90 per cent, though there are concerns about oxygen toxicity at this level.

Heart rate

The patient will be tachycardic due to hypoxaemia as well as a number of other factors (mediator and catecholamine release, pyrexia, low systemic blood pressure).

Pulmonary hypertension

Pulmonary artery pressures show increased pulmonary systolic and diastolic pressures with normal pulmonary artery wedge pressures. Pulmonary artery wedge pressures may rise if there is associated cardiac dysfunction.

Cardiovascular involvement in MODS

A major part of the cardiovascular response to MODS is related to: (1) the loss of peripheral vasoautoregulatory mechanisms, and (2) the need to maintain tissue oxygenation in spite of increasing hypoxaemia. A confounding factor in the ability of the myocardium to respond is the depressant effect often associated with SIRS.

The loss of peripheral autoregulation and excess NO production leads to inappropriate vasodilatation, maldistribution of flow, and decreased oxygen extraction. The response to this tissue hypoxia is to increase cardiac function by increasing heart rate, and contractility in an attempt to meet tissue demands. Preload and afterload are reduced by the fall in arterial and venous tone. The decreased preload leads to a decreased contractility (Starling effect) which is compensated by the reduction in resistance to flow. If adequate intravascular volume is maintained then cardiac output rises to meet tissue oxygen demands and the hyperdynamic response is evident.

The hyperdynamic response

- Increased cardiac output
- Increased heart rate
- Decreased systemic vascular resistance

Myocardial dysfunction

This is evident early in the course of sepsis and several factors and mediators have been implicated in its development:

1. Loss of autoregulation of coronary blood flow — resulting in excessive vasodilatation, high coronary blood flow, and reduced oxygen extraction.

2. Maldistribution of coronary blood flow — micro-circulatory disturbances and scattered necrosis have been reported.

3. Alterations in myocardial substrate extraction — reliance on lactate and endogenous cardiac reserves as a major fuel source rather than the normal free fatty acids.

4. Myocardial oedema and altered calcium metabolism.

5. Altered response to sympathetic nervous system stimuli — decreased sensitivity to circulating catecholamines due to down-regulation of β-adrenergic receptors.

6. Myocardial depressant factor — there is strong evidence supporting the presence of myocardial depressant factors but they have not as yet been isolated. The factors appear to reduce ventricular contractility by up to one third.

7. Endotoxin — may play a role in depressing myocardial function but the mechanism has not as yet been fully established.

8. TNF — may indirectly affect myocardial function.

9. Interleukin-2 has been shown to induce heart failure and haemodynamic changes when used as immunotherapy in cancer patients.

Many other mediators are thought to be implicated in myocardial dysfunction but their roles have yet to be clarified.

The net result of this is that while cardiac output may remain normal or even increased there is a decrease in ventricular ejection fraction with accompanying ventricular dilatation (Parker and Fink 1992). In addition, there is an abnormal response to fluid volume loading showing a smaller increase in left ventricular end diastolic volume and stroke work index for an increase in pulmonary artery wedge pressure (Ognibene et al. 1988). This is reversible as the patient recovers.

Patient assessment of cardiovascular dysfunction
Heart rate and rhythm

Tachycardia is a feature of the patient with SIRS. Atrial and occasionally ventricular arrhythmias can occur which may diminish cardiac output and exacerbate hypotension.

Mean arterial pressure (MAP)

Mean arterial pressure is not a good indicator of flow. A mean arterial pressure of at least 60 mmHg is usually necessary to maintain the perfusion pressure of vital organs.

Urine output

Urine output in a catheterized patient allows continuous assessment of renal perfusion as a marker of general organ perfusion. The aim is to maintain >0.5 ml/kg/h urine output. However, the quality of the urine produced may be poor and daily measurement of plasma urea and creatinine levels are required for assessment of renal function.

Cardiac output (CO) and pulmonary artery wedge pressure (PAWP)

Ideally, a pulmonary artery catheter should be placed to obtain PAWP, CO, and stroke volume (SV). Fluid resuscitation should then be carried out as a series of fluid challenges against serial measures of PAWP, CO, and SV.

In general, PAWP is maintained at between 12 and 15 mmHg, but greater pressures may be required to maintain stroke volume if ventricular compliance falls. Cardiac output can either be normal or more usually raised if the patient has been adequately fluid resuscitated. In most ICUs the thermodilution technique is the established method of determining cardiac output. It will also allow calculation of oxygen delivery and consumption. However, it is also possible to use the Doppler ultrasound or transthoracic bioimpedance techniques, both of which offer a less invasive method of determining cardiac output (although not oxygen delivery and consumption).

Gut tonometry

This is a method of monitoring regional (gut) perfusion (see Chapter 4). A thin silicone balloon wrapped around the end of a fine-bore tube is placed in the stomach. The balloon is filled with 0.9% saline which is allowed to equilibrate for at least 15 minutes. During this time carbon dioxide (CO_2) released from the gut mucosa crosses the semi-permeable membrane of the balloon into the saline. A value of the pH of the gut mucosa (pH_i) can then be determined from calculations using measurement of the amount of CO_2 in the saline and arterial bicarbonate (from an arterial blood sample). Use of pH_i to guide fluid resuscitation in order to improve perfusion has been shown to improve survival in patients with a normal pH$_i$ on admission to the ICU (Gutierrez *et al.* 1992). As the splanchnic bed is one of the first areas of hypoperfusion in low perfusion states it could provide an early indicator of poor regional levels of oxygenation.

Arterial base deficit

A rapidly developing arterial base deficit, measured doing routine blood gas analysis is highly suggestive of tissue hypoxia, ischaemia or infarction. Correction of the metabolic acidosis is achieved by treating the underlying cause rather than by giving bicarbonate.

Lactate

Blood lactate levels may be a good indication of global ischaemia. Levels >2 mmol/l reflect increased lactate production and is often associated with tissue hypoxia. Blood lactate is an end-product of anaerobic respiration which occurs when pyruvate entry into the TCA (Krebs) cycle is blocked by lack of oxygen. It is now recognized that hyperlactataemia may also be due to a variety of other causes including accelerated glycosis, ATP hydrolysis and inactivation of pyruvate dehydrogenase (which blocks pyruvate entry into the mitochondrial Krebs cycle). However, a normal blood lactate level does not necessarily indicate that all organs are adequately well perfused.

Temperature

The septic patient may exhibit either pyrexia or occasionally, a hypothermic response. Pyrexia may be accompanied by tachycardia and hypotension associated with vasodilatation and efforts may be necessary to cool the patient in order to reduce metabolic demands.

Gastrointestinal involvement in MODS

Splanchnic hypoperfusion occurs as a part of the compensatory mechanisms associated with a decrease in cardiac output. Perfusion is reduced as a result of the vasoconstrictive response and blood flow diversion which produce supply-dependent oxygen consumption and an oxygen deficit causing intracellular acidosis.

Effects on gastrointestinal organs are severe, particularly at mucosal level where rapidly proliferating cells have a high oxygen and substrate requirement.

Stomach — disruption of the mucosal barrier occurs with development of mucosal and submucosal ischaemia. This leads to an increased risk of ulceration. Gastric motility is also reduced.

Small intestine — disruption of the mucosal barrier occurs and there is a loss of gut mucosal integrity which may lead to translocation of luminal organisms (see Chapter 10 for further information).

Pancreas — pancreatitis (an inflammatory response resulting from premature activation of pancreatic enzymes) can occur (see Chapter 10 for further information). Pancreatitis is itself a trigger for a further systemic inflammatory response.

Gallbladder — acalculous cholecystitis (inflammation unrelated to gallstones) can develop.

Colon — disruption of the mucosal barrier and an increased translocation of luminal organisms may result. Colitis may also develop.

Patient assessment for gastrointestinal involvement

Abdomen

Palpation, ausculation, and observation should be carried out for evidence of distension, discomfort and pain, and presence of bowel sounds (see Chapter 10 for further information).

Faeces

Note the presence of diarrhoea — colour, consistency, frequency. Note the presence of blood.

Gastric intolerance

The following can occur: nausea, vomiting and large aspirates (>200 ml) from the nasogastric tube.

Pancreatic enzymes

Test for serum amylase (see Chapter 10 for further information).

Gut tonometry

This can be used as a monitor of gut hypoperfusion and a possible indicator of tissue oxygenation (see Chapter 4 for). However, this is still only a research tool.

Liver involvement in MODS

Liver dysfunction is not usually seen until several days after the development of hypermetabolic and hyperdynamic changes. The serum bilirubin is >20–30 μmol/l and is associated with other markers of hepatic dysfunction such as increased hepatic enzymes (see box) or hepatic encephalopathy.

Clinical markers of hepatic dysfunction

- Raised serum bilirubin (> 20–30 µmol/l), jaundice
- Raised AST and LDH (at least twice normal levels)
- Abnormal prothrombin time or INR
- Hepatic encephalopathy

At present, there is no clearly identified mechanism of liver dysfunction in MODS, although a number of theories have been put forward. It seems likely that a contributing cause is hypoperfusion resulting in liver cell ischaemia. However, even in hyperdynamic states there are signs of liver dysfunction and it is thought that the effects of various mediators released by neutrophils and damaged tissue may cause shunting, altered vascular permeability, and further platelet activation within the liver itself, thus producing localized areas of ischaemia.

An alternative theory suggests Kupffer cells are the source of hepatic dysfunction. They are stimulated by endotoxin or other inflammatory mediators circulating from either the trigger or secondary dysfunction sites, to release toxic mediators. These mediators act on the closely situated hepatocytes altering their function but not causing cell death. The presence of any pre-existing liver disease is likely to precipitate liver dysfunction.

Effects of liver dysfunction

Demands placed on the liver's metabolic functions (see Chapter 10) during the hypermetabolic phase are enormous. In conjunction with this, the combined effect of circulating mediators and hypoperfusion on hepatic cell function is highly damaging. The result is deranged carbohydrate, protein, and lipid metabolism as well as dysfunctional immune response, protein synthesis and impaired detoxification processes.

Protein metabolism

The liver increases the rate of gluconeogenesis, (with concomitant rises in protein catabolism and urea production) and urinary nitrogen excretion increases.

Ultimately, the ability of the liver to clear amino acids is decreased and high levels of phenylalanine and tyrosine result.

Lipid metabolism

Lipolysis and lipogenesis may occur, resulting in high levels of serum lipids compounded by decreased peripheral lipid clearance. Hepatocyte utilization of ketones produced from lipid conversion is reduced.

Hepatic protein synthesis

Synthesis of acute-phase reactant proteins is increased at the expense of synthesis of albumin and transferrin. Fibronectin, which has an important role in enhancing phagocytosis, is partially synthesized by the liver and levels become depleted due to hepatic dysfunction.

Detoxification of drugs, toxins, and hormones

High levels of hormones normally detoxified by the liver such as antidiuretic hormone (ADH) and aldosterone can occur as a result of liver dysfunction.

Detoxification of drugs metabolized by the liver is also affected and may produce higher serum levels, prolonged duration of action and increased toxicity as a result.

Clotting factors

Hepatic failure may accentuate bleeding and DIC by limiting the removal of activated clotting factors and reducing clotting factor synthesis.

Patient assessment for liver involvement

Conscious level and neurological status

This should take other factors such as sedation and neuro-trauma into consideration.

Conjunctival and skin colour

These should be observed for a yellow tinge indicating jaundice (see Chapter 10 for details).

Skin, mucous membranes, and invasive line sites

Evidence of coagulation abnormalities which give rise to bleeding from gums, purpura, bleeding from line sites, etc.

Urinalysis

Daily urinalysis should be done for bilirubin levels

Liver function tests

These should be carried out at least every 2–3 days in the acute phase.

Clotting tests

These should be carried out on a daily basis.

Renal involvement in MODS

Either pre-renal failure leading to acute tubular necrosis (ATN) or direct renal damage by toxins can develop in MODS. Pre-renal failure occurs as a result of decreased renal perfusion. This can be reversed if perfusion is restored but if not, then ATN will result. ATN develops as a result of ischaemia, toxins such as endotoxin and mediators or as a drug-related response. Full details of the pathogenesis of acute renal failure and ATN are given in Chapter 8.

There are three likely causes of the renal failure seen in MODS:

1. Acute pre-renal problems seen during the early stages of hypoperfusion

2. ATN related to profound ischaemia during later stages. This is associated with decreased cardiac output and renal blood flow.

3. ATN resulting from toxic microbial products of sepsis, endogenous inflammatory mediators, and drug therapy for MODS.

The clinical course of ATN has four phases:

1. Onset — a potentially reversible stage, which may correspond with pre-renal failure. It may last hours to days depending on the cause. The disease course following post-ischaemic causes is shorter than for toxic causes.

2. Oliguric–anuric phase — lasts 1–6 weeks. The glomerular filtration rate is significantly reduced with fluid overload, high blood urea and plasma creatinine levels, electrolyte abnormalities, and resulting metabolic acidosis. Evidence of uraemic symptoms are also present.

3. Diuretic phase — an increased urine output is accompanied by a gradual increase in renal function. Urine output may be more than 2–3 litres per day with little or no evidence of concentration or excretion. Gradually, the urinary urea increases and sodium falls. Acidosis and electrolyte imbalance begin to improve.

4. Recovery phase — glomerular filtration returns to 70–80 per cent of normal within 1–2 years. Mild to moderate residual renal damage may remain.

Patient assessment for renal involvement

The patient should be assessed for:

● Oedema (peripheral and pulmonary), nausea, vomiting, pruritis, and other symptoms of uraemia (see Chapter 8),

● urine output (the aim is > 0.5 ml/kg/h),

● urinalysis for specific gravity, protein, glucose, and blood; ±urinary sodium and urea; ±urine: plasma osmolality,

● blood urea,

● plasma creatinine,

● blood potassium,

● blood pH,

● intravascular fluid volume status (see also cardiac assessment, p. 410).

Haematological involvement in MODS

The manifestations of coagulopathy most commonly seen in MODS are:

1. Bleeding from line sites and wounds due to depletion of clotting factors.

2. Disseminated intravascular coagulation (DIC).

DIC is a pathological overstimulation of normal coagulation which paradoxically causes both microvascular thrombi (which deplete normal stores of clotting factors and activate the fibrinolytic system) and bleeding due to the resultant lack of clotting factors and overactive fibrinolysis. (Full details are given in Chapter 12.)

Although DIC occurs as a result of almost any severe disease process, there are a number of particular factors which pre-dispose to its development. These are:

(1) arterial hypotension,

(2) inadequate tissue perfusion,

(3) stasis of capillary blood flow (Hudak *et al.* 1990).

DIC represents a dysfunction of the haematological system and can often occur as a response to SIRS. (A list of trigger factors for DIC can be found in Chapter 12.)

Table 14.3 Summary of manifestations of organ failure associated with SIRS and MODS

Central nervous system
- Encephalopathy
- Peripheral neuropathy

Respiratory system
- Acute respiratory distress syndrome (ARDS)

Renal system
- Acute renal failure

Gastrointestinal
- Pancreatitis
- Gastric and intestinal stasis
- Acalculous cholecystitis
- Stress ulceration and gastrointestinal bleeding

Hepatobiliary
- Elevation in liver function enzymes to > twice normal levels
- Serum bilirubin > 20–30 µmol/l

Cardiovascular
- Central myocardial depression
- Decreased response to catecholamines
- Loss of microvascular regulatory tone and peripheral vasodilatation

Coagulation
- Disseminated intravascular coagulation (DIC)
- Thrombocytopenia
- Clinical evidence of bleeding

Patient assessment for haematological involvement

The following should be assessed/observed:

- skin for evidence of petechiae, purpura, bruising and haematomas,

- gums and mucous membranes for bleeding,

- sclera and conjunctiva for haemorrhage,

- intravenous cannulae sites, arterial cannulae sites, chest drain sites, wounds, tracheostomy sites for bleeding,

- sputum during suction for bleeding,

- urinalysis for evidence of haematuria,

- stools for evidence of melaena and nasogastric aspirate for evidence of gastric bleeding,

- measurement of haemoglobin, platelet count, thrombin time, prothrombin time, D-dimer levels (the fibrin-

specific degradation fragment D is measured using monoclonal antibodies), fibrinogen level, partial thromboplastin time (PTT).

Priorities and principles of management

Priorities

As with any critical illness the initial resuscitation response is to assess and support the Airway, Breathing, and Circulation.

Airway. A patent airway is likely to be threatened in the patient who is comatose and aspiration is a high risk in the obtunded patient. Intubation should be considered early rather than following a catastrophic event.

Breathing. Oxygen therapy and, if necessary, ventilatory support should be instituted to maintain oxygen saturations of 90–95 per cent. If ventilation is required the aim is to limit the risk of barotrauma using alternative modes and, in some circumstances, allowing carbon dioxide levels to rise.

Circulation. The main aim is rapid restoration of organ perfusion and perfusion pressure. Initially, fluid volume status should be optimized using colloid challenges (aliquots of 200 ml) followed by measurement of CVP or PAWP, and stroke volume. If this is unsuccessful in restoring perfusion pressure, vasoactive drugs are used.

Early interventions

Once the patient is stabilized any injuries should be actively treated with particular reference to the removal of any necrotic tissue, debriding burn eschar, and stabilizing fractures. If these are not dealt with they will form a focus for further stimulation of the inflammatory/immune response.

Further soft tissue damage and inflammation should be minimized.

Blood, urine, and other cultures, as indicated, should be sent to attempt identification of any source of sepsis.

Appropriate antibiotics should be prescribed and administered either as a broad spectrum cover prior to microbiological results or according to culture sensitivities if these are available.

Further interventions

These are aimed at supporting failing organs or preventing further dysfunction.

Metabolic

Any metabolic derangement should be corrected as quickly as possible. Body temperature should be maintained within the normothermic range of 36.0–37.5 °C.

Infection

Any focus of infection, such as abscesses, should be located and drained. Prevention of secondary infection is essential and strict asepsis, care of intravenous cannulae, and all aspects of infection control should be observed.

Renal

Continuous haemofiltration and diafiltration can be used to support renal dysfunction and, if metabolic acidosis is severe to normalize pH.

Nephrotoxic and hepatotoxic drugs should be avoided where possible or levels monitored (for example, gentamicin).

Gastrointestinal tract

Prophylaxis against GI bleeding including H_2 antagonists, sucralfate, and enteral feeding may be considered. Restoration of adequate organ perfusion is paramount.

Provision of appropriate nutrition based on individual requirements and monitoring and maintenance of electrolyte and trace element levels should be carried out.

Haematological

Haemoglobin levels of $\geqslant 10$g/dl should be maintained and any clotting abnormalities should be corrected using clotting factors, etc.

Musculoskeletal

Pressure areas should be protected from damage by position change where possible or the use of special support beds where necessary.

Further insults capable of triggering the immune/inflammatory response should be avoided; particularly hypoxaemia and hypotension.

Circulation

A major objective in management of the patient with SIRS is the maintenance of tissue perfusion. As discussed previously in the chapter, the inflammatory response is associated with three distinct pathophysiological problems.

1. Maldistribution of circulating volume.

2. Imbalance of oxygen supply and demand.

3. Alterations in metabolism.

All of these affect the ability of the cardiovascular system to respond to tissue oxygen requirements. In addition, the myocardial depressant factor associated with SIRS reduces the myocardial response still further.

Monitoring circulatory disturbance (see also Chapter 4)

It is necessary at the outset to use comprehensive haemodynamic monitoring to establish the extent of cardiovascular derangement. Ideally, the patient should have a pulmonary artery thermodilution catheter placed to allow monitoring of cardiac output, PAWP, and systemic vascular resistance. If a fibre-optic thermodilution catheter with continuous S_vO_2 monitoring is available this can be useful to provide an assessment of therapeutic interventions when cardiac output is decreased.

Evidence of global tissue hypoxia can be monitored by measuring blood lactate or base deficit. The aim is to reduce blood lactate to < 2.0 mmol/l (Armstrong et al. 1991). The degree of ischaemia in the gut can be measured by the gastric intramucosal pH which may be a marker of hypoperfusion and hypoxia (Gutierrez et al. 1992).

Supporting the circulation

Optimizing intravascular fluid volume
Serial measurements of cardiac output, stroke volume and PAWP can be used to assess the response to fluid resuscitation (see Chapter 5 for details). The aim is to continue volume loading until the cardiac output and stroke volume show no further improvement. Occasionally, in cases of severe ARDS, the intravascular volume may be kept purposefully lower to reduce the extracapillary fluid shift.

The mean arterial pressure should be maintained at > 60–70 mmHg. This is the lowest level compatible with continued renal and cerebral perfusion. Other markers of renal perfusion are continued urine output of > 0.5 ml/kg/h and measures of blood urea and creatinine. Other markers of cerebral perfusion are more difficult to obtain but conscious level and alertness are useful indicators if the patient is not fully sedated and/or paralysed.

If fluid administration does not improve the stroke volume further but the MAP remains below 60 mmHg then vasopressors or inotropes must be considered. Vasopressors (e.g. noradrenaline) are used in high output states with low SVR and inotropes (e.g. dobutamine) in low output states. Adrenaline is both an inotrope and a vasopressor and can be used for either effect. The choice of drug will depend on the individual ICU and the patient; commonly, dobutamine or noradrenaline are used initially, with adrenaline added in at a later stage if MAP remains low.

The use of 'supranormal' levels of cardiac output and oxygen delivery

Shoemaker *et al.* (1988) showed that high-risk surgical patients who were maintained at high levels of cardiac output and oxygen delivery using fluid and inotropes pre- and peri-operatively had a greatly improved outcome compared to those who were not. It was theorized that higher (so-called 'supranormal') levels of cardiac output and oxygen delivery were required in order to cope with the stress of surgery and that these patients might otherwise have been unable to respond to this. The design of the study has been criticized and the conclusions are not accepted by all authorities. However, this concept was then adopted for patients in septic shock (Edwards *et al.* 1989) with the goals of:

(1) an increased oxygen delivery of > 600 ml/min/m^2,

(2) a cardiac index of > 4.5l/min/m^2

(3) an oxygen consumption > 170 ml/min/m^2.

Patient mortality was 48 per cent, which was less than other published outcomes where patients required inotropic support for hypotension. However, this was an uncontrolled study (using historical controls). More recent controlled studies have failed to establish any connection between improvement in outcome and use of 'supranormal goals' in critically ill as opposed to high-risk patients.

Currently, the management aim is to maintain patients with a cardiac output and oxygen delivery necessary to support organ perfusion.

The theory of oxygen supply dependency in sepsis

In 1987, Schumacker and Cain developed the concept of a critical oxygen delivery. This concept postulated that, in conditions causing a pathological supply dependency (such as sepsis), tissue oxygen extraction capacity is impaired leading to an oxygen supply dependency despite normal or raised overall oxygen delivery. The critical level at which tissues become oxygen supply-dependent is therefore higher than normal in these patients (Fig. 14.5).

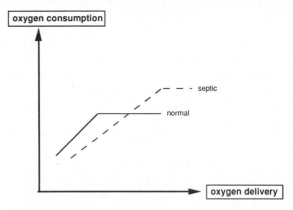

Fig. 14.5 Oxygen supply-dependency relationship in septic and normal patients.

Causes for this were hypothesized as either:

(i) loss of autoregulatory capacity by disrupted blood flow distribution secondary to peripheral micro-embolization or alterations in vasomotor tone, or

(ii) other factors interfering with efficient tissue distribution of oxygen delivery with respect to oxygen consumption.

These hypotheses fitted well with the concept of 'supranormal' levels of oxygen delivery being associated with an increased survival. In a retrospective review of 78 patients with septic shock, Tuchschmidt *et al.* (1989) found significant differences in cardiac index and oxygen delivery in survivors as opposed to non-survivors. However, these may reflect inherent properties of the individual rather than the ability of the patient to respond to attempts to increase oxygen delivery. Overall, the concept of 'supranormalization' and oxygen supply dependency is still the subject of considerable debate and controversy.

Supporting respiration

Physical measures supporting gas exchange and alternative modes of ventilation are employed to achieve the aims of:

(1) maintaining saturations > 90 per cent,

(2) minimizing the incidence of barotrauma by keeping airway pressures below 35–40 cmH$_2$O.

The overall goal of intervention is to re-open and stabilize closed, but potentially functional, alveolar units while minimizing barotrauma and variations in expansion of different areas of the lung caused by the disease process.

Secondary goals are to: (1) reduce F_iO_2 to the minimum acceptable level, (2) allow adequate carbon dioxide excretion, (3) avoid haemodynamic compromise, (4) maintain adequate oxygen transport.

The conventional approach to ventilatory support in the patient with ARDS is volume-cycled ventilation with tidal volumes of 10–15 ml/kg and flow rates that maintain an inspiratory–expiratory ratio of 1:2 to 1:4. Increments of PEEP are added to both improve recruitment of non-aerated alveoli and to prevent airway closure and alveolar collapse.

The disadvantages to this approach are: (1) too short an inspiratory time will increase peak airway pressures, (2) peak airway pressure is increased by increments of PEEP with increased risk of barotrauma, (3) dead space may be increased by increments of PEEP at constant tidal volume; mean airway pressure increases and carbon dioxide excretion is reduced. If oxygenation continues to be a problem and airway pressures rise above the generally accepted upper limit of 40 cmH$_2$O then other modes of ventilation must be employed.

One alternative mode of ventilation is pressure-controlled inverse ratio ventilation (PC-IRV). Controlled studies have yet to show its superiority (Matthay 1989). However, most uncontrolled studies have reported improved oxygenation (Sassoon 1991) (for details see Chapter 3).

Specific therapies

There are currently a wide range of possible therapies being studied for their effect on sepsis, SIRS, and the development of MODS.

Anti-endotoxin products

Anti-endotoxin (HA-1A) monoclonal antibody

Endotoxin has been identified as a potent activator of various inflammatory responses following Gram-negative sepsis. Consequently, a monoclonal antibody specific to endotoxin (HA-1A) was developed and a major double-blind, randomized, controlled trial for the treatment of patients with clinical evidence of Gram-negative sepsis was carried out (Ziegler et al.

1991). The results were somewhat equivocal apart from those patients with ultimately proven Gram-negative bacteraemia. In this subset, a reduction in mortality from 52% to 37% between placebo and antibody was found. However, a further trial of the antibody was halted after interim analysis showed an increase in mortality among patients treated with HA-1A who did not have Gram-negative bacteraemia. This increase was statistically significant compared to the placebo control group (Chang et al. 1993). The problem of identifying patients who would benefit from the use of HA-1A is compounded by the need for early administration and the difficulty in correctly diagnosing endotoxaemia and Gram-negative bacteraemia at the bedside. The cost of the drug and its possible detrimental effects are too high to consider treating all those with suspected or potential Gram-negative bacteraemia prophylactically. Thus, HA-1A has been withdrawn from general use, although it is still available on individual request.

Bactericidal permeability-increasing protein (BPI) and endotoxin receptor antagonists

Polymorphonuclear leucocytes (PMN) are able to secrete a number of antimicrobial proteins in response to endotoxin. BPI is released from the PMN and binds to the outer membrane of Gram-negative bacteria. As a result, changes occur in the organism's outer membrane permeability with arrested growth of the organism. Cytoplasmic membrane changes are then induced and the organism dies. Infusion of BPI may act as a protective mechanism in high-risk patients. Endotoxin receptor antagonists have an anti-endotoxin capability and are being developed.

Anti-TNF (tumour necrosis factor) antibody

This antibody is being studied in two large, multi-centre, placebo-controlled trials in patients with SIRS or septic shock. Work in animals showed improved early survival and reduced hypoxaemia but there is concern about the possibility of blocking the protective effect of TNF. Early reports indicate no major benefit (Fisher et al. 1993).

Interleukin-1 receptor antagonist

This naturally occurring inhibitor of (interleukin-1) IL-1 which has been successfully cloned, blocks the cell-surface receptor to which IL-1 binds. It has also been evaluated in critically ill patients. A pilot study showed encouraging results but a follow-up larger study showed no significant benefit (Lynn 1993). This agent has now been withdrawn from further experimentation.

Pentoxifylline

This is a phosphodiesterase inhibitor (i.e. it inhibits phosphodiesterase which breaks down cyclic AMP) which is used to decrease blood viscosity in chronic vascular disease. It is also reported to decrease the sequestration of neutrophils, inhibit TNF activity, and decrease severe morbidity in animals given intravenous endotoxin (Huddleston 1992). The precise mode of action in multiple organ failure is uncertain (Bennett 1991). Currently, there is little published evidence to support any improvement in outcome following its use in critically ill patients.

Nitric oxide (inhaled)

Work is currently being carried out into the effect of inhaled low concentration (< 40 ppm) nitric oxide on the pulmonary circulation. Nitric oxide is an endogenous mediator synthesized from L-arginine by the vascular endothelium. It stimulates guanylate cyclase which dilates blood vessels and inhibits platelet aggregation and adhesion. The problems of high pulmonary artery pressures and intrapulmonary shunting associated with ARDS can be reduced by direct inhalation of nitric oxide (Rossaint et al. 1993). Nitric oxide gas dilates the pulmonary circulation by relaxing muscular arteries and veins but as it is immediately bound to haemoglobin it does not affect the systemic circulation. There is also an improvement in the degree of ventilation–perfusion mismatch as a result of redistribution of pulmonary blood flow away from nonventilated regions. Currently, the only studies have been carried out on small groups of patients (Rossaint et al. 1993) and randomized controlled trials are required to evaluate the potential of this drug. Concern has been voiced regarding possible toxicity as nitric oxide is a recognized air pollutant and will combine with oxygen to form nitrogen dioxide which can be further oxidized to nitric and nitrous acids.

Nitric oxide antagonists

The role of nitric oxide as a mediator of the systemic vasodilatation and hypotension seen in sepsis has prompted studies into the blockade of nitric oxide production. At low doses the inhibitor has been shown to reverse endotoxin-induced hypotension in rats (Naval et al. 1991) and an early anecdotal report in patients

showed rapid reversal of hypotension (Petros et al. 1991). However, some concern has been expressed that there may be the loss of various protective functions of nitric oxide (such as regulation of visceral flow, platelet aggregation, cytotoxicity and antimicrobial activity) that would be lost and may prove ultimately harmful (Sinclair and Singer 1993).

Steroids

The use of steroids in patients in septic shock has largely been discontinued as a result of two large randomized controlled multi-centre trials (Bone et al. 1987b, The Veterans Administration Systemic Sepsis Cooperative Study Group 1987). The results showed no improvement in overall outcome, moreover there was increased mortality due to secondary infection in the group treated with steroids. However, there is some evidence of improvement following early administration and in certain subgroups such as those in the fibroproliferative phase of ARDS (Meduri et al. 1991) and those with meningococcal meningitis (Tauber and Sande 1989). There may also be a place for steroid administration in patients who remain dependent on vasoactive drugs (Voerman et al. 1990), possibly as a result of adrenal insufficiency (Rothwell et al. 1991). The role of steroids in septic shock requires further clarification and considerable work before their full therapeutic capability is established.

Plasmapheresis

It is possible that the exchange of plasma, resulting in the removal of circulating mediators and replacement of depleted levels of protease inhibitors, may have a beneficial effect on patients with septic shock and multiple organ failure. Studies to date are small or anecdotal but there is some evidence to suggest a reduction in mortality in patients treated with sequential plasmafilter dialysis with slow continuous haemofiltration (Barzilay et al. 1989).

Arachidonic acid cascade modulators: ibuprofen, prostacyclin, and prostaglandin

Ibuprofen preferentially blocks thromboxane synthesis by inhibiting the cyclooxygenase pathway. Studies in animals have shown attenuation of most adverse consequences of endotoxin when ibuprofen is given before or during endotoxin challenge (Bone 1992). However, when given post-challenge results are not as consistent.

In patients with sepsis syndrome and septic shock, a

randomized, controlled trial (Bernard *et al.* 1991) found improved blood pressure and heart rate, temperature, minute ventilation, and peak airway pressures as well as an increased frequency of shock reversal (88 vs. 43 per cent). A large multi-centre trial is in progress in the United States. However, there are concerns regarding the use of ibuprofen in the light of its potential nephrotoxicity and increased incidence of gastric ulceration.

Prostacyclin (PGI_2) and prostaglandin (PGE_1) are thought to exert primarily beneficial effects in sepsis by reversing the actions of thromboxanes and leukotrienes. In a study of 100 patients given PGE_1 versus placebo, no difference in survival rate was found although oxygen transport variables were improved (Bone *et al.* 1989*b*). Studies of controlled trials of PGI_2 in humans have yet to be performed.

Protease inhibitors

The release of supraoxide radicals and proteases, such as elastase and catalase, occurs as a result of complement and neutrophil activation. These substances act as catalysts for the major enzyme cascades.

Circulating protease inhibitors protect the body from excess protease action.

Naturally occurring protease inhibitors include:

- Antithrombin III (ATIII), a potent inhibitor of the coagulation cascade and contact system.

- C_1-esterase inhibitor (C_1-INH) which also inhibits contact activation as well as complement activation.

- α_1-proteinase inhibitor will combine with elastase released by neutrophils to block its action.

ATIII and C_1-INH have been produced synthetically. Administration of ATIII and C1-INH have shown attenuation of the effects of endotoxin in animals. Trials of ATIII supplementation are currently underway. Aprotinin is a non-specific inhibitor of proteases including trypsin, chymotrypsin, plasmin, and also has an inhibitory effect on kallikrein. It may be useful as an alternative means of limiting the effects of some plasma proteases, although no trials are currently forthcoming.

Bradykinin antagonists are also being developed and are undergoing clinical trials.

Antioxidants

Oxygen derived free radical scavengers, xanthine oxidase inhibitors, and iron-chelating agents have all been studied for possible beneficial effects in SIRS. Oxygen derived free radicals incite lipid peroxidation of cell membranes which means that the radical reacts with the polyunsaturated fatty acid in the cell membrane. This alters membrane fluidity, secretory function, and ionic gradients causing increased permeability and oedema. A more potent radical (the hydroxyl ion) is generated by combination of free iron with other free radicals such as hydrogen peroxide.

Allopurinol inhibits xanthine oxidase production but also appears to scavenge radicals as well.

Superoxide dismutase, catalase and peroxidase have been administered to remove radicals; iron-chelating agents (desferrioxamine) which bind with free iron, thus reducing its ability to produce the hydroxyl ion, have also been investigated. Although some improvement in animal studies has been shown (Malcolm and Zaloga 1990) further study is still required.

N-acetylcysteine also has anti-oxidant properties and is currently being studied in a multi-centre trial.

Platelet-activating factor (PAF) antagonists

PAF is produced by a wide range of inflammatory cells including monocytes, macrophages, mast cells, and platelets as well as by vascular endothelial, glomerular, and gastrointestinal epithelial cells. Secretion of PAF occurs in response to a wide range of stimuli including many of the mediators in the SIRS response. Its actions include aggregation of platelets, neutrophil activation, stimulation of macrophages to release TNF, interleukin-1, and eicosanoids, and increased vascular permeability. Use of PAF antagonists have been studied in a number of large multi-centre trials with no obvious benefit.

It seems likely from the complexity of the pathways involved in the systemic inflammatory response that a single therapeutic answer is unlikely. What is certain is that considerable further work is required to understand the mechanisms involved and to catalogue the effect of each therapy. Until this is carried out and effective interventions are identified the mainstay of patient care will remain the support of failing organs and the prevention of further damage and infection.

References and bibliography

ACCP/SCCM consensus panel (1990): Ethical and moral guidelines for the initiation, continuation and withdrawal of intensive care. *Chest*, **97**, 949–958.
ACCP/SCCM (American college of Chest Physicians/Society of

Critical Care Medicine) (1992). Consensus Conference: definitions for sesis and organ failure and guidelines for the use of innovative therapies in sepsis. *Critical Care Medicine*, **20**, 864–74.

Armstrong, R.F., Bullen, C., Cohen, S., Singer, M., and Webb, A.R. (1991). *Critical care algorithms* pp. 80–2. Oxford University Press.

Barzilay, E., Kessler, D., Berlot, G., Gullo, A., Geber, D., and Zeev, I. (1989). Use of extracorporeal supportive techniques as additional treatment for septic-induced multiple organ failure patients. *Critical Care Medicine*, **17**, 634–7.

Bennett, E.D. (1991). New agents — pentoxifylline and dopexamine. *Clinical Intensive Care* (suppl.), **2**, 72–82.

Bernard, G.R., Reines, H.D., Halushka, P.V., Higgins, S.B., Metz, C.A., Swindell, B.B., *et al.* (1991). Prostacyclin and thromboxane A$_2$: Formation is increased in human sepsis syndrome. *American Review of Respiratory Disease*, **144**, 1095–101.

Bone, R.C. (1992). Phospholipids and their inhibitors: A critical evaluation of their role in the treatment of sepsis. *Critical Care Medicine*, **20**, 884–90.

Bone, F.C., Fisher, C.J., Clemmer, T.P., Slotman, G.J., Metz, C.A., and Balk, R.A. (1989*a*). Sepsis syndrome: A valid clinical entity. *Critical Care Medicine*, **17**, 389–93.

Bone, R.C., Slotman, G., Maunder, R. and the Prostaglandin E$_1$ Study Group (1989*b*). Randomized double-blind, multicenter study of prostaglandin E$_1$ in patients with the adult respiratory distress syndrome. *Chest*, **96**, 114–19.

Chang, R.W.S., Beale, R., Smithies, M., Bihari, D. (1993). A preliminary cost-performance evaluation of HA-IA (centoxin) with an addendum on its demise. *Clinical Intensive Care*, **4**, 208–16.

Clarke, G.M. (1990). Severe sepsis. In *Intensive care manual*, (ed. T.E. Oh), pp. 401–8. Butterworth, Sydney.

Dantzker, D. (1989). Oxygen delivery and utilisation in sepsis. *Critical Care Clinics*, **5**, 81–98.

Edwards, J.D. (1993). Management of septic shock. *British Medical Journal*, **306**, 1661–64.

Edwards, J.D., Brown, C.S., Nightingale, P., Slater, R.M., and Faragher, E.B. (1989). Use of survivors' cardiorespiratory values as therapeutic goals in septic shock. *Critical Care Medicine*, **17**, 1098–103.

Fisher, C.J., Opal, S.M., Dhainaut, J.F., *et al.* (1993). Influence of an anti-tumour necrosis factor monoclonal antibody on cytokine levels in patients with sepsis. *Critical Care Medicine*, **21**, 318–27.

Gutierrez, G., Bismar, H., Dantzker, D., and Silva, N. (1992). Comparison of gastric intramucosal pH with measures of oxygen transport and consumption in critically ill patients. *Critical Care Medicine*, **20**, 451–7.

Hazinski, M.F., Iberti, T.J., NacIntyre, N.R., *et al.* (1993). Epidemiology, pathophysiology and clinical presentation of Gram-negative sepsis. *American Journal of Critical Care*, **2**, 224–37.

Hudak, C.M., Gallo, B.M., and Benz, J.J. (1990). *Critical care nursing: A holistic approach*, p. 818. Lippincott, Philadelphia.

Huddleston, V.B. (1992). *Multisystem organ failure: Pathophysiology and clinical implications*, p. 308. Mosby–Year Book, St Louis.

Lynn, W.A. (1993). Prospects for the immunotherapy of septic shock. *Current Opinion on Investigational Drugs*, **2**, 973–81.

Malcolm, D.S. and Zaloga G.P. (1990). Adjunctive pharmacotherapy in sepsis. *Infections in Medicine*, **10**, 41–48.

Marcy, T.W. and Marini, J.J. (1991). Inverse ratio ventilation in ARDS: Rationale and implementation. *Chest*, **100**, 494–504.

Matthay, M.A. (1989). New modes of mechanical ventilation for ARDS: How should they be evaluated. *Chest*, **95**, 1175–6.

Meduri, G.U., Belenchia, J.M., Estes, R.J., Wenderink, R.G., Torky, M., and Leeper, K.V. (1991). Fibroproliferative phase of ARDS: Clinical findings and effects of corticosteroids. *Chest*, **100**, 943–52.

Nava, E., Palmer, R.M.J., and Moncada, S. (1991). Inhibition of nitric oxide synthesis in septic shock: how much is beneficial? *Lancet*, **338**, 1555–7.

Ognibene, F., Parker, M., Natanson, C., Shelhamer, J.H., and Parrillo, J.E. (1988). Depressed left ventricular performance: Response to volume infusion in patients with sepsis and septic shock. *Shock*, **93**, 903–11.

Parker, M.M. and Fink, M.P. (1992). Septic shock. *Journal of Intesive Care Medicine*, **7**, 90–100.

Petros, A., Bennett, D., and Vallance, P. (1991). Effect of nitric oxide synthase inhibitors on hypotension in patients with septic shock. *Lancet*, **338**, 1557–8.

Rossaint, F., Falke, K.J., López, F., Slama, K., Pison, U., and Zapol, W.M. (1993). Inhaled nitric oxide for the adult respiratory distress syndrome. *New England Journal of Medicine*, **328**, 399–405.

Rothwell, P.M., Udwadia, Z.F., and Lawler, P.G. (1991). Cortisol response to corticotropin and survival in septic shock. *Lancet*, **337**, 582–3.

Sassoon, C.S.H. (1991). Positive pressure ventilation: Alternate modes. *Chest*, **100**, 1421–9.

Schumacker, P.T. and Cain, S.M. (1987). The concept of a critical oxygen delivery. *Intensive Care Medicine*, **13**, 223–9.

Shoemaker, W.C., Appel, P.L., Kram, H.B., Waxman, K., and Lee, T. (1986). Prospective trial of supranormal values of survivors as therapeutic goals in high-risk surgical patients. *Chest*, **94**, 1176–86.

Sinclair, S. and Singer, M. (1993). Reviews in medicine: Intensive care. *Postgraduate Medical Journal*, **69**, 340–58.

Sprung, C.L., Peduzzi, P.N., Shatney, C.H., Schein, R.M., Wilson, M.F., Sheagren, J.N., *et al.* (1990). Impact of encephalopathy on mortality in the sepsis syndrome. *Critical Care Medicine*, **18**, 801–6.

Tuchschmidt, J., Fried, J., Swinney, R., and Sharma, O.P. (1989). Early hemodynamic correlates of survival in patients with septic shock. *Critical Care Medicine*, **17**, 719–23.

Vaca, K.J., Reedy, J.E., Lohmann, D.P., Moroney, D.A., and

Swartz, M.T. (1993). Nursing Care of the patient with an intravascular oxygenator. *American Journal of Critical Care*, **2**, 478–88.

Veterans' Administration Systemic Sepsis Co-operative Study Group (1987). Effect of high-dose glucocorticoid therapy on mortality in patients with clinical signs of systemic sepsis. *New England Journal of Medicine*, **317**, 659–65.

Villar, J. and Slutsky, A.S. (1991). Alternative modalities for ventilatory support. In *Update in intensive care and emergency medicine*, Vol. 14, (ed. J.L. Vincent), pp. 345–6. Springer, Berlin.

Voerman, H.J., Strack van Schijndel, R.J.M., and Thijs, L.G. (1990). Endocrine disturbances in the critically ill: The role of growth hormone and cortisol. In *Update in intensive care and emergency medicine*, Vol. 10, (ed. J.L. Vincent), pp. 809–22. Springer, Berlin.

Wilt, N.J., Zochodne, D.W., Bolton, C.F., Grand' Maison, F, Wells, G., Young, B., and Sibbald, W.J. (1991). Peripheral nerve function in sepsis and multiple organ failure. *Chest*, **99**, 176–84.

Ziegler, E.J. Fisher, C.J. Sprung, C.L., *et al.* (1991). Treatment of Gram-negative bacteremia and septic shock with HA-1A human monoclonal antibody against endotoxin. *New England Journal of Medicine*, **324**, 429–436.

15. Evaluating care in the ICU

Introduction

Intensive care is expensive and labour-intensive, it carries a high cost for the patient in physical and mental distress and may offer only limited benefit. In spite of this, little work has been carried out on evaluating the cost–benefit implications of intensive care. In a report on intensive care in the United Kingdom, the King's Fund Panel (1989) found a serious lack of evidence. It recommended:

1. that those responsible for intensive care should collect and evaluate data on the clinical outcome and costs, in general and of the care of individual patients,

2. research should focus on the data required to allow proper audit and the evaluation of specific practices in intensive care.

Currently, no guidelines exist as to who should be admitted to the ICU, what treatment is considered appropriate in what circumstances, and to what lengths that treatment should extend. These are some of the most difficult ethical dilemmas faced by intensive care staff. The problem is intensified as technology progresses offering more intervention at greater cost while resources remain static or dwindle.

One of the most important responsibilities of those working in this area is evaluation of the effect and efficacy of the care they offer. This applies to all types of care offered by the multidisciplinary team.

This chapter will address the following issues:

- Audit and quality assurance.

- Cost versus outcome.

- Recovery and follow-up.

- Ethics

Audit and quality assurance

Audit has been defined as the systematic and public examination of factors which affect the delivery of good care. Quality assurance has been defined as a planned system of activities which, if carried out correctly, should provide a product or service satisfying agreed standards within agreed resources and timescales (Five Regions Consortium 1991).

Management of quality can be controlled on three levels (Macfarlane 1989):

(1) 'pre-action control' (setting the standards or goals of care);

(2) 'concurrent control' (monitoring the care given);

(3) 'feedback control' (evaluating the level of practice).

Maxwell's (1984) dimensions of quality allow one method of reviewing quality cited in Redfern and Norman (1990) issues in health care. There are six dimensions: (1) access, (2) equity, (3) relevance to need, (4) social acceptability, (5) efficiency, (6) effectiveness.

This approach allows far more input from the consumer and is specific to formulating the service to their needs. It does, however, produce problems in application to the intensive care area because many of the criteria involved may have different standards in differing circumstances. For example, desired outcomes of the consumer may alter from recovery when the patient is first admitted, to a peaceful and dignified death when recovery is no longer possible.

Measurement of quality is a complex and difficult task. This is particularly so in nursing where many of the skills are problematic to quantify, and quality almost always carries value judgements based on socialisation (Norman and Redfern 1992). (See Fig.15.1 which is a diagram of the quality assurance cycle.)

Measurement of quality in nursing is associated with two approaches:

(1) the objective quantitative measurement of care criteria;

(2) the qualitative analysis of caring.

The first approach is by far the easiest to measure, but the second may be a truer reflection of real quality in terms of nursing care. If these factors can be measured then comparison can be made between levels of quality and cost between different units, wards, and hospitals.

Redfern and Norman (1990) suggest that quality incorporates not just consumer satisfaction, but also all the considerations of equity, accessibility, acceptability, efficiency, effectiveness, appropriateness of the care

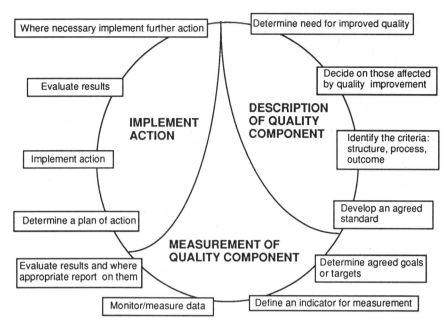

Fig. 15.1 The quality assurance cycle.

offered. They believe that 'these considerations highlight the point that high-quality health care or, more specifically, high quality nursing care is influenced predominantly by social values'.

Measurements of quality assessment

Currently, a number of generic quality assessment instruments are available. They are based on expert opinion of components of nursing related to quality and attempt to transfer levels of key criteria into scores. Examples include Monitor (Goldstone *et al.* 1983), Qualpacs (Wandelt and Ager 1974), and the Nursing Audit (Phaneuf 1976). However, none are specifically designed for intensive care and only one has been adapted for use in intensive care. They have not been validated in this or many other areas. There is a need for valid tools to assess the quality of care so that changes in methods of delivery of care and in organization of care can be evaluated.

Monitor

This is a nursing audit requiring simple yes or no answers to a series of questions on the presence or absence of quality-related items of care. It uses over 200 criteria that apply to a variety of specialist settings. The criteria are divided into four areas corresponding to four levels of

patient dependency. Within each area are four further sections on: (1) planning nursing care, (2) meeting physical needs, (3) meeting non-physical needs, and (4) evaluating nursing care. A trained nurse observer gathers information about the ward structure, facilities, and policies, classifies the patients into dependency levels, observes their care, and records activities. Staff are given questionnaires to rate their satisfaction and the observer examines patient records and interviews patients. This extremely comprehensive survey of ward practice is then assessed overall and fed back to the staff.

Monitor is available specifically for the intensive care area and is thought to provide a clear indication of deficiencies in care although it is debatable as to whether it can distinguish the patient care in one ICU as better than that in another.

Qualpacs

The quality patient care scale uses observation by trained observers of the care of a small group (up to five patients) over a period of two hours. Further information about these patients' care is also obtained from care plans and nursing records as well as nursing handovers. Details of the patient dependency and ward staffing levels are also collected to put care into context. The two observers use a form covering 68 items under six categories (physical care, psychosocial care, communication, professional implications, etc.). A scale from 1 to 5 is used to indicate worst (1) to best (5) care.

Advantages of its use include:

● it is reasonably simple to use;

● it requires only 3–4 hours of time for two observers;

● it focuses on the delivery of care.

Disadavantages of its use include:

● the ability only to see a small group of patients for a short space of time;

● the use of subjective clinical judgement to rate nursing care;

● one poor quality carer can reduce the overall quality of the score considerably.

Nursing Audit

Nursing audit is a method of evaluating nursing care through records and as such is a retrospective approach. The records reviewed include nursing care plans, observation and prescription charts, medical notes, and any other record used by nursing staff.

A trained reviewer checks for a series of 50 items under seven headings. These include carrying out doctor's orders, observing patients' signs and symptoms, supervising patients and carers, and promoting physical and emotional health. A judgement is made about the quality of care as recorded using five standards: excellent, good, incomplete, poor, unsafe.

Advantages include:

● records can be assessed on a regular basis;

● records provide a fair comparison;

● records reflect the unit as a whole if they are examined in sufficient numbers.

Disadvantages include:

● only the quality of recording may be being assessed;

● it is difficult to know how well records reflect care;

● it is a retrospective tool.

Quantitative audit

Areas that can be assessed quantitatively are useful objective measures for audit of practice.

Quantitative indicators of quality

● Rates of nosocomial infection:
  – cannulae
  – urinary tract infection
  – wound infection
  – chest infection

● Incidence of pressure sores evaluated against severity of illness and chronic health problems

● Patient's or relatives' complaints and/or satisfaction

● Achievement of pain relief using visual analogue scoring

● Amount of time spent on non-nursing duties

● Number of drug errors

● Incidence of sharps injuries, back injuries etc

● Critical incident analysis

Standard of care

This is a professionally agreed level of performance appropriate to the population addressed which is achievable and desirable. Donabedian (1966), in a seminal paper on evaluating quality in medical care, divided it into three categories: structure, process, and outcome. Structure includes the fabric and facilities of the environment, the staffing and organization, and the resources. Process includes the delivery of care, the values and philosophy of the caregivers and the way care is organized. Outcome includes survival, the quality of life of survivors, and relative satisfaction with care. This has come to be regarded as an appropriate framework for developing standards in all areas of care.

Outcome is probably the easiest and most frequently audited area but depends heavily on factors involved in both structure and process.

Process can be examined using established standards against which comparisons of practice can be made. This is the area the generic nursing quality assessment tools are designed to cover based on expert professional opinion.

Intensive care has some specific disadvantages which make audit more complex. These are, the lack of a satisfactory definition of what constitutes intensive care, the heterogeneity of the patients involved, and the difficulty of establishing a link between particular therapies and survival.

There are however, considerable data available in intensive care on all aspects of the patient's illness and response to interventions. In fact, recording of observations about the patient can occupy up to 20 per cent of the nurses' time (Price and Mason 1986). This wealth of information would provide considerable insight into many aspects of the patient's care if it could be collated and analysed in a structured format. The use of clinical information systems for the future may well allow such complex data analysis to be performed regularly providing a clearer view of the effects of therapeutic interventions.

Sources of data for quality criteria

- Patient observation
- Patient interview
- Environmental observation
- Nurse interview
- Patient record review
- Ancillary staff interview
- Family and relatives interview

Illness severity scoring systems

The scoring system has been one of the most useful developments in terms of assessing the patient's relative severity of disease. The scoring system allows an objective assessment of severity which can then be used to compare a wide range of disorders or disease states. Most systems are designed to define the extent of deviation from normal of acute and chronic disease variables. These include physiological, functional, and psychosocial variables.

Outcome prediction

Some scoring systems are used to predict outcome. This outcome applies only to a patient population and cannot be applied to the individual. The aim is to reduce prognostic uncertainty by giving the probability of an outcome. It cannot therefore be used as the basis for denying or withdrawing treatment from a patient. This is valuable for comparison of the predicted outcome with the actual outcome and can be used to assess the efficacy of therapeutic intervention or other factors such as the environment, organization, staffing, etc.

A variety of scoring systems have evolved in intensive care to provide:

- an index of disease severity — either general (e.g. APACHE) or specific (e.g. Glasgow Coma Score, Trauma Score),

- an index of workload and consumption of resources (e.g. TISS),

- a means of comparison for: (i) audit of performance (either in the same unit over time or between Units), and (ii) research (e.g. evaluation of new products and treatment regimens),

- patient management objectives (e.g. sedation, pressure area care).

Severity scoring systems

These have been devised either for specific conditions, e.g. trauma (Trauma Score, Injury Severity Score), sepsis (Sepsis Score), pancreatitis (Ransom Score), and head injury (Glasgow Coma Score); or for the general ICU patient (e.g. APACHE, SAPS). Most systems rely to a great extent on physiological and clinical assessment though are often complemented by readily obtainable laboratory measurements such as haematocrit and white blood cell count,

The APACHE (acute physiology and chronic health evaluation) classification devised by Knaus *et al.* was first described in 1981. Now known as 'APACHE I', this was a score derived from the degree of abnormality of 34 physiological and biochemical variables, age, and chronic health status (e.g. severe heart failure, cirrhosis, immunosuppression). The amount of physiological scoring proved rather unwieldy so a simplified version — 'APACHE II' — was developed and published in 1985. APACHE II uses the most extreme levels recorded in the first 24 hours following admission of the 12 most commonly measured physiogical and biochemical variables in addition to age and chronic health grading (Table 15.1). The level of risk of subsequent death from a wide range of admission disorders was computed, although burns and cardiac surgery were specifically excluded from analysis. Validation of this risk stratification was performed in 6000 patients in 13 American intensive care units. This validation study has been recently repeated in 26 British ICUs to see whether the American model was applicable to British patients (Rowan 1993). Although a generally good agreement was noted some significant differences were found. For example, the British study performed better in acute surgical conditions but worse in acute medical admissions. Age also had a greater impact on outcome in Britain.

Table 15.1 APACHE II score
Acute physiology score

Variable	+4	+3	+2	+1	0	+1	+2	+3	+4
Temp (rectal) (°C)	≥41	39–40.9		38.2–38.9	36–38.4	34–35.9	32–33.9	30–31.9	≤29.9
Mean BP (mmHg)	≥160	130–159	110–129		70–109		50–69		≤49
Heart rate (bpm)	≥180	140–179	110–139		70–109		55–69	40–54	≤39
Resp rate (/min)	≥50	35–49		25–34	12–24	10–11	6–9		≤5
If $F_iO_2\geq0.5$: A-aDO$_2$ (mmHg)	≥500	350–499	200–349		<200				
If $F_iO_2<0.5$: PO$_2$ (mmHg)					>70	61–70		55–60	≤55
Arterial pH	≥7.7	7.6–7.69		7.5–7.59	7.33–7.49		7.25–7.32	7.15–7.24	<7.15
Serum Na (mmol/l)	≥180	160–179	155–159	150–154	130–149		120–129	111–119	≤110
Serum K (mmol/l)	≥7	6–6.9		5.5–5.9	3.5–5.4	3–3.4	2.5–2.9		<2.5
Serum creatinine (µmol/l) (double if acute renal failure)	≥300	171–299	121–170		50–120		<50		
Haematocrit (%)	≥60		50–59.9	46–49.9	30–45.9		20–29.9		<20
Leucocytes (/mm^3)	≥40		20–39.9	15–19.9	3–14.9		1–2.9		<1
Neurological = (15: Glasgow Coma Score)									

Age points:

Years	≤44	45–54	55–64	65–74	≤75
Points	0	2	3	5	6

Chronic health points—
2 pts for elective post-operative admission or 5 pts if emergency operation or non-operative admission, if patient has either cirrhosis, heart failure (NYHA Grade 4), respiratory failure, dialysis-dependent renal disease, or is immunocompromised.

The APACHE system has been refined still further with the introduction of 'APACHE III' in 1990. The APACHE III database contained an initial 17457 patients from 40 American hospitals. However, it is being continually expanded and now includes a dataset of non-US patients. APACHE III attempts to improve the statistical predictive power by: (1) adding five new physiological variables (albumin, bilirubin, glucose, urea, urine output), (2) changing the thresholds and weighting of existing variables, (3) comparing both admission and 24-hour scores, (4) incorporating the source of admission (e.g. casualty, ward, operating theatre), and (5) reassessing the effect of age, chronic health, and specific disease category. Comparative studies between APACHEs II and III have yet to be published to confirm the superiority of the modified system. Furthermore, the APACHE III risk stratification is now proprietary and has to be purchased; this may limit its general acceptance.

SAPS (simplified acute physiology score), devised by Le Gall and colleagues in 1984, is very similar to the APACHE II system though uses 14 readily measured clinical and biochemical variables. It too has been modified ('SAPS II') (Le Gall 1993).

Chang (1989) developed the Riyadh Score — a computer model based on trends of daily APACHE II scores and organ system failures — to refine further outcome prediction.

However, none of the above systems (APACHE, SAPS, Riyadh) are totally infallible; the individual very poor outcome patient may well defy the odds while the expected survivor may still die. For this and other more emotive reasons, outcome prediction systems have yet to be used to instigate early withdrawal or refusal of intensive care treatment. Proponents, however, claim that progressive rationalization of health care resources will eventually force the institution of this decision-making process and a refined scoring system will be vital.

The therapeutic intervention scoring system (TISS) provides an index of workload activity by attaching a score to procedures and techniques being performed on an individual patient (e.g. use and number of vasoactive drug infusions, renal replacement therapy, administration of enteral nutrition). This system has been used by some ICUs to develop a means of costing individual patients by attaching a monetary value to each TISS point scored. A discharge TISS score can also be used to estimate the amount of nursing interventions required for a patient in step-down facilities (e.g. a high dependency unit) or on the general ward. TISS does not accurately measure nursing workload activity as it fails to cater for tasks and duties such as coping with the irritable or confused patient or dealing with grieving relatives. A number of nursing workload scoring systems have been developed in order to assess nurse staffing requirements (e.g. GRASP). Although not developed specifically for intensive care, GRASP determines the type and amount of care required for a patient rather than measure severity of illness or bed occupancy.

Table 15.2 Simplified Acute Physiology Score (SAPS) II (point score in brackets)

Age	<40 (0); 40–59 (7); 60–69 (12); 70–74 (15); 75–79 (16); ⩾80 (18)
Heart rate (bpm)	<40 (11); 40–69 (2); 70–119 (0); 120–159 (4); ⩾160 (7)
Systolic BP (mmHg)	<70 (13); 70–99 (5); 100–199 (0); ⩾200 (2)
Body temp (°C)	<39 (0); ⩾39 (3)
P_aO_2/F_iO_2 (kPa) [only if ventilated or CPAP]	<13.3 (11); 13.3–26.5 (9); ⩾26.6 (6)
Urine output (l/day)	<0.5 (11); 0.5–0.999 (4); ⩾1 (0)
Serum urea (mmol/l)	<10 (0); 10–29.9 (6); ⩾30 (10)
White blood count (/mm³)	<1 (12); 1–19.9 (0); ⩾20 (3)
Serum potassium (mmol/l)	<3 (3); 3–4.9 (0); ⩾5 (3)
Serum sodium (mmol/l)	<125 (5); 125–144 (0); ⩾145 (1)
Serum bicarbonate (mEq/l)	<15 (6); 15–19 (3); ⩾20 (0)
Serum bilirubin (μmol/l)	<68.4 (0); 68.4–102.5 (4); ⩾102.6 (9)
Glasgow Coma Score	<6 (26); 6–8 (13); 9–10 (7); 11–13 (5); 14–15 (0)
Chronic disease	metastatic cancer (9); haematological malignancy (10), AIDS (17)
Type of admission	scheduled surgical (0); medical (6); unscheduled surgical (8)

The GRASP score indicates the sum of estimated time units needed to perform a variety of nursing duties, including the provision of emotional support to patient and/or family.

Unfortunately, other than the Glasgow Coma Score (see Chapter 9), there is no universally accepted system practised by every ICU. Competing systems have often been developed simultaneously. For example, APACHE and SAPS are both widely used for scoring disease severity — APACHE is the predominant system in America and Britain, while SAPS is more popular in mainland Europe. Each system has its devotees not prepared to shift allegiance and, due to considerable financial implications, a common system is unlikely to be agreed upon.

Specific scoring systems:

Trauma
Trauma scoring systems have been utilized for a variety of purposes:

- performing rapid field triage to direct the patient to appropriate levels of care;

- quality assurance;

- developing and improving trauma care systems by categorizing patients and identifying problems within the systems;

- making comparisons between groups from different hospitals, in the same hospital over time, and/or undergoing different treatment strategies.

The Injury Severity Score (ISS) is a severity scoring system for trauma patients based on the anatomical injuries sustained. The Revised Trauma Score (RTS) utilizes measures of physiological abnormality to predict survival (see Table 15.3). A combination of ISS and RTS — TRISS — was developed to overcome the shortcomings of anatomical or physiological scoring alone. The TRISS methodology uses ISS, RTS, patient age, and whether the injury was blunt or penetrating to provide a measure of the probability of survival. It is the current system of choice in Britain for auditing effectiveness of care in trauma patients admitted to hospital for more than three days, managed in an intensive care area, referred for specialist care; or who die in hospital.

Head injury
The Glasgow Coma Scale, first described by Teasdale and Jennett in 1974 utilizes eye opening, best motor response, and best verbal response to categorize the severity of head injury. It is probably the only system used universally in ICUs. Apart from its ability to prognosticate, it is also frequently used for therapeutic decision-making (e.g. elective ventilation in patients presenting with a GCS score of less than 8).

Table 15.3 Revised Trauma Score

	Coded value	× weighting	= Score
Respiratory rate (breaths/min)			
10–29	4	0.2908	
> 29	3		
6–9	2		
1–5	1		
0	0		
Systolic blood pressure (mmHg)			
> 89	4	0.7326	
76–89	3		
50–75	2		
1–49	1		
0	0		
Glasgow Coma Scale			
13–15	4	0.9368	
9–12	3		
6–8	2		
4–5	1		
3	0		

Total = Revised Trauma Score

Sepsis/multiple organ failure/ARDS
A variety of definitions exist for ARDS and for multiple organ failure. Knaus produced his definitions for MOF which are frequently cited though others are also quoted. Recent attempts to clarify the area have been made by Bone *et al.* (1992) who coined the terms systemic inflammatory response syndrome (SIRS) and multiple organ dysfunction syndrome (MODS) (see Chapter 14).

A more surgically oriented definition of sepsis — the Sepsis Score — was proposed by Elebute and Stoner in 1983 for grading the severity of sepsis from the local effects of infection, pyrexia, secondary effects of sepsis, and laboratory data.

Sedation

A variety of scoring systems have been developed for gauging and recording the level of sedation of a mechanically ventilated patient. The aim is to enable the staff to titrate the dose of sedative agents to avoid either over- or under-sedation. The Ramsay Sedation Score developed in 1974 consists of a six-point scoring system separated into three awake and three asleep levels where the patient responded to a tap or loud auditory stimulus with brisk, sluggish, or no response at all. The main problem lies in achieving reproducibility of the tap or loud auditory stimulus. Bion (1990) developed a more complex score by combining analogue scales representing sedation: from alert to unrousable; distress, from calm to agitated; and comprehension, from orientated to uncomprehending. A set of observations could be recorded and linked by three lines to form a triangle. Triangles can be produced from subsequent observations of the same patient to indicate whether or not the change in sedation was better or worse. Bion also included the APACHE II score as the need for sedation is naturally linked to the degree of disease. Combining these analogue scales with the APACHE II score makes the whole concept too complex to be used in daily ICU practice, however, it does provide a good illustration of changes in the quality of sedation in an individual patient.

The Cambridge Sedation Score allocates a number from 1 to 7 ranging from agitated to unresponsive. Level 3 describes a patient who is awakened when spoken to with a normal voice

Injury Severity Score

This system has the following scoring system:

1. Use the AIS90 (Abbreviated Injury Score 1990) dictionary to score every injury

2. Identify the highest abbreviated injury scale score for each of the following:

   - head and neck

   - abdomen and pelvic contents

   - bony pelvis and limbs

   - face

   - chest

   - body surface

3. Add together the squares of the three highest area scores.

Cost versus outcome

The escalation in costs for intensive care has engendered a need to examine financial outlay in the light of outcome and effectiveness. The ultimate benefit of prolonging meaningful quality life must be weighed against the huge cost of treatment. In particular, length of survival following discharge and the quality of life for survivors are key factors. Dragsted (1990) has stated that evaluation of intensive care medicine may be expected to have the following consequences:

1. An improvement of procedures which might lead to an improvement in the quality of ICU care.

2. Modifications in teaching.

3. Reduction of the economic costs for society.

4. An increased efficiency as an effect of a better control of the organization.

Parno et al. (1982) investigated hospital charges and long-term survival in ICU and general hospital patients in the United States. The average total hospital charge was nearly five times greater for ICU patients compared with general patients and the mortality rate in hospital was 17.3 per cent for ICU patients as opposed to 3.4 per cent for general patients. Following discharge, the two-year survival rate was 83 per cent of ICU patients and 89 per cent of non-ICU patients suggesting that, providing patients survive their hospital stay, the likelihood of a reasonable extension of life is good. However, there was some difference in age and sex distribution between the two groups which casts doubt on the validity of the observation.

In a smaller study in the United Kingdom, Shiell et al. (1990) compared survival and long-term outcome in two ICU care units. Mortality rates at discharge were 15 and 25 per cent in each unit, rising to 38 and 31 per cent 6 months after admission. Thus, mortality post-discharge from the ICU in the short term was 23 per cent for one unit and 6 per cent for another. Mortality was positively associated with severity of illness and age. Cost was heavily weighted towards a small group of 10 patients who had significantly longer lengths of stay and who were responsible for over 45 per cent of total expenditure.

In a study of 337 ICU patients following both emergency and elective admission, Sage et al. (1986) found that those patients who did not survive until follow-up incurred the greatest cost, in this instance, due to greater intensity of treatment.

Significant factors in outcome for emergency admissions were APACHE II scores and TISS scores indicating severity of illness and intensity of intervention. However, factors in outcome following discharge were age and chronic health suggesting that once intensive care is successful then subsequent events may be determined by pre-existing factors.

High usage of resources and therefore high costs were associated with hospital mortalities of 30–45 per cent and cumulative mortalities of 35–60 per cent. There is an important obvious difference in outcome between emergency and elective admission to the ICU. The French multicentre study (1989) showed that mortality in the emergency surgical admission group was 27 per cent compared with a mortality of 5 per cent in the elective group.

Factors influencing outcome from intensive care

- Age

- Previous health status

- Severity of acute illness

- Diagnosis

Cost therefore, is, usually related to severity of illness, length of stay, and intensity of treatment. It is unfortunate that this is frequently associated with the greatest mortality rate. Detstky *et al.* (1981) found that those patients attracting the highest cost were those with the least expected outcomes (i.e. survivors who had been expected to die and non-survivors who had been expected to live). They suggest that refining prognostic accuracy may reduce inappropriate treatment.

The cost per survivor may seem high but if viewed as the cost per extended life-year the investment may seem a reasonable one.

Quality of life

Shiell *et al.* (1990) investigated quality of life in survivors assessed using the Nottingham health profile which shows how the patients' current health is affecting their daily lives. One-third of the patients had problems with employment, carrying out housework, and sexual relations; almost one-half had difficulty pursuing personal interests, socializing or going on holiday. In all, 22 per cent of patients reported substantial levels of disability and 19 per cent reported substantial levels of distress.

Sage *et al.* (1986) found quality of life was good in the 140 patients who responded to follow-up questionnaires

16–20 months after discharge from the ICU. This was only 41 per cent of the initial sample, with an 11 per cent hospital mortality and a post-discharge mortality of 24.6 per cent, and it is possible that some bias was introduce (only those patients satisfied with their outcome responded). Goldstein *et al.* (1986) studied functional outcomes in 2213 patients admitted to an ICU. Unlike other studies they grouped the patient's according to their pre-admission functional status and found that mortality was clearly related to prior functional status. However, they found that activity level was reduced in 74 per cent of those initially admitted with an active level functional status, although 60 per cent of the previously employed returned to work. This is consistent with the results of Zaren and Hedstrand (1987) who found that 75 per cent of those in employment prior to ICU admission were back at work within one year and concluded overall that there was no great deterioration in quality of life among long-term survivors of intensive care.

Dragsted and Qvist (1989) followed-up 1308 patients for 12 months following ICU admission and found that 44 per cent of the survivors returned to their pre-hospital activity level within one year. Increasing age and chronic disease were found to influence functional outcome significantly.

Factors influencing functional outcome following ICU admission

- Age

- Chronic disease/previous health status

- Previous functional level

Although there is some variation in the groups of patients studied and the criteria used to define quality of life, there are some fairly consistent results among several studies. Most interestingly, it would appear that quality of life as denoted by activity and return to employment is high, including up to three-quarters of those working prior to ICU admission.

However, there are clear indications that those whose life quality is limited prior to admission either by chronic health problems or age are less likely to regain an acceptable level of function and more likely not to survive the admission.

Recovery and follow-up

Until recently, little work had been undertaken in following up and identifying problems in post-intensive patients. The need for justifying the benefits of ICU care has ensured that clinicians are starting to use the ultimate quality of life of the patient rather than simply their condition at transfer to the ward as the end-point of their interventions.

Some ICUs now run follow-up clinics for ex-patients who have spent a period of time in intensive care (Griffiths 1992). The purpose of these clinics is two-fold. One function is to allow assessment, diagnosis, treatment, counselling, and support of the individual patient and their families. The other purpose is to allow collection of data regarding specific problems, both short- and long-term, associated with the interventions used in the ICU and evaluation of the efficacy of treatment.

Long-term problems associated with prolonged ICU admission

The effect of intensive care on the patient is overwhelming and there are few patients who spend longer than 2–3 days in intensive care who do not continue to suffer mental and physical problems as a result.

Physical problems

Weight loss and muscle wasting. Skeletal muscle loss during illness is due to inactivity, catabolism, and frequently inadequate nutrition. In many patients, this loss will take months to recover and other pathology may limit the patient's ability to exercise and rebuild muscle bulk.

Reduced respiratory function. Diaphragmatic and intercostal muscle loss may contribute to this as well as residual pulmonary pathology from infection or other problems. Patients may remain short of breath on exertion due either to respiratory problems or cardiac insufficiency.

Complications of endotracheal intubation or tracheostomy. Patients may experience vocal disturbance due to vocal cord damage or stridor and wheezing due to tracheal stenosis.

Neurological problems. Sensory and motor neuropathies may occur and there may be disturbances of fine motor control. Some patients experience visual deficits and auditory problems such as tinnitus.

Psychological problems

These can be severe and are often associated with hallucinations and nightmares experienced during the period in intensive care. Many patients continue to suffer nightmares and sleep disturbance for many years after their illness. Friedman *et al.* (1992) surveyed 46 patients following ICU discharge and found that 24 per cent of patients contacted after a mean of eight months had sleeping problems and ICU-related dreams. The adjustment of role from total dependence to relative independence can be traumatic and coming to terms with the nearness of their own mortality may also cause problems. Some patients have complete memory loss of the time spent in intensive care and this may lead to false expectations of their ability to recover from their illness. Patients may also suffer loss of concentration, mental fatigue, and difficulty in following a line of reasoned thought. Short-term memory may also be affected. There may be abrupt mood swings and periods of severe depression.

Social factors

Relationships with family and friends may suffer as a result of the patient's experiences and the associated psychological problems. There may be personality changes and difficulty in relating to people.

General problems

Loss of appetite, alteration in taste sensation, altered body image, and sexual dysfunction can all cause problems in the long-term recovery period. Friedman *et al.* (1992) recorded only 54 per cent of patients had returned to their daily routine.

The extent of problems which may be experienced by these patients requires a broad range of professional expertise in providing advice and assistance. If a clinic is to function successfully it should involve a multi-disciplinary approach to problems and assessment.

Members of the multidisciplinary team involved in an ICU follow-up clinic

- ICU clinician
- ICU nurse
- Physiotherapist
- Psychologist
- Dietitian
- Social worker
- Occupational therapist

Follow-up service for bereaved relatives

A recent study (Jackson 1992) found that only 12 per cent of ICUs in the United Kingdom offered a formal follow-up service for bereaved relatives. They are often left to cope with sudden and traumatic death after a variable length of time spent in the ICU. Coming to terms with this sudden loss may prove difficult especially after the period of hope (sometimes false) offered by admission to the ICU. There may be difficulty separating from what was a safe, supported environment (the ICU) to face the problems of home and its accompanying memories.

Most ICUs offer a high degree of support, advice and information at the time of death but this is unlikely to be taken in or remembered.

Collins (1989) recommends that families receive a follow-up visit by a nurse or chaplain within two weeks of the death. This is not usually a practical alternative and it may be more appropriate to ask the relative to visit the ICU or an area close by. The nurse or appropriate person can then discuss problems, answer questions and supply information, as well as listening and expressing empathy for their grief. In units where primary nursing is carried out, it may be most appropriate that the primary nurse follows-up the family.

Ideally, a trained bereavement counsellor would be available to support the family but this resource is not always available.

Jackson (1992) suggests a phone follow-up service where the responsible nurse rings the bereaved family and offers condolence and further support where necessary.

Sources of further help

- Bereavement support groups

- Chaplains or ministers of other religions

- Bereavement counsellor (if available)

- Citizen's Advice Bureau (for assistance with practical difficulties)

Ethics

The exact definition of 'ethics' is the philosophical study of the moral value of human conduct and the rules and principles that govern it. However, it has come to be regarded as the morals or code of conduct of particular social groups such as the professions.

Morals are the principles of behaviour actually held or followed by individuals or groups in accordance with standards of right and wrong.

Ethics in intensive care are an important issue partly due to the increasing sophistication of medical science and technology balanced by a growing emphasis on the autonomy of the individual. The effect of financial constraints on resources have also lead to an upsurge in ethical dilemmas in this expensive area of care.

Among the many ethical dilemmas facing staff in intensive care a number are encountered with reasonable frequency. These are:

- determining the point of withdrawal of treatment;

- withholding resuscitation measures;

- deciding when the burdens of further therapeutic measures outweigh the benefits;

- when resources are limited, deciding which patient will receive intensive care;

- evaluating when intensive care is an appropriate measure.

Although the final decision in most cases will rest with the consultant involved, the situation will usually be discussed beforehand among the staff, with the patient's relatives and, where appropriate, with the patient. The establishment of a consensus view is an important part of acceptance of the final decision. If those heavily involved in the patient's care have no opportunity to explore and express their feelings there may be a loss of trust in the validity of the decision and resentment about its outcome.

Ethical decision-making is complex, stressful, and extremely difficult. The same decision must be re-appraised for each case and guidelines can only be broad and non-specific. Ethical decisions depend on moral judgements and these will be based on personal values and social pressures.

Use of a decision-making process may help in clarifying the pros and cons of the situation. The unit philosophy will also provide a record of the attitudes and values that the staff generally hold and can be useful in providing some clear ideals with which to examine the ethical dilemma.

Knowledge of the basic principles of ethics may help to provide a foundation on which to base decisions.

Ethical theories

There are two major theories for determining whether an action is right or wrong. The first refers to the consequences of the action (consequentialist) and the second to the moral rules or guidelines governing that action (deontological).

Consequentialist theory

Moral or ethical dilemmas are resolved by calculating the good over harm expected to be produced by each alternative. Utilitarianism is the best known consequentialist philosophy (John Stuart Mill 1867) and is based on the need for human beings to act in bringing about the best outcome for all concerned.

Deontological theory

Moral or ethical dilemmas are resolved by considering the action in its own right according to duties, rights, and justice. The act itself is judged right or wrong and the consequences of the action do not matter. The greatest proponent of this was the German philosopher, Immanuel Kant, who advocated using the individual's moral sense to judge each act.

Tschudin (1986) quotes the principles of ethics established by the philosopher Thiroux as a readily applicable formulation of ethical theory. The five principles are:

1. The value of life — humans should revere life and accept death.

2. Goodness or rightness — promote good over bad, cause no harm, prevent harm.

3. Justice or fairness — egalitarianism over scarce resources,

4. Truth-telling or honesty — there may be circumstances when this is not always best.

5. Individual freedom — freedom to choose and to choose what may not always be best.

These principles act as foundations for ethical decision-making and may help to clarify the decision although they cannot direct the choice itself. (See also Fig. 15.2.)

Withdrawing treatment.

One of the most difficult decisions in intensive care is deciding the point at which treatment is no longer likely to bring benefit to the patient either in terms of relief of symptoms or in terms of recovery. The emphasis of intervention must then be changed from cure to care and the goals redefined to allow death within a comfortable, humane, and peaceful environment.

In the irreversible illness, LIFE is neither the absolute good nor DEATH the absolute evil (Hugh Casson).

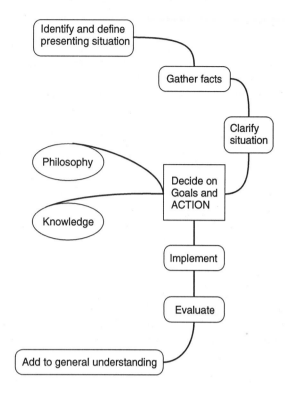

Fig. 15.2 The ethical decision-making process.

It is frequently difficult to accept that all the technological and pharmaceutical interventions and support that have been so important to the patient up till now are no longer going to benefit him or her. This may be more of a problem to the medical than nursing staff due to the values and ethos attached to each profession. In a convenience sample of readers the *Nursing Times* (1988) found that 91 per cent would agree with removing life support in the case of prolonged and irreversible coma.

The Society of Critical Care Medicine consensus report on the ethics of foregoing treatment (1990) recommends discussion in the following situations:

1. When the patient has a diagnosis with a grave prognosis.

2. When the burdens of therapy outweigh the benefits.

3. When the quality of the patient's life is expected to be unacceptable to the patient.

Frequently, it is the nursing staff who will first bring up the possibility of withdrawing treatment. They are usually closest to both the patient and family and have a very clear view of the burden of treatment. In these circumstances, the nurse will act as advocate on the patient's behalf and these skills can be vital in limiting the length of unnecessary and unproductive treatment.

Advocacy is seen by Brown (1985) as a means of transferring power back to the patient to enable him to control his own affairs. It is not about taking over for the patient but about assisting the patient so that his needs and rights are met.

Criteria to be considered when discussing withdrawal of treatment

- Prognosis

- Age

- Chronic health status

- Attainable quality of life

- Family

- Social support

- Cultural and religious background

Expanding intensive care nursing

If intensive care nursing is to continue to progress and improve there must be an expansion of knowledge and understanding of the effects of critical illness and the intensive care environment on the patient. Alternative methods of structuring care and of delivery must be explored and made known. This will only be achieved by a programme of structured research which is co-ordinated, repeated, and validated in a variety of settings and institutions. The multi-disciplinary approach which is so important in the delivery of care must also encompass the approach to research. Currently, few institutions offer the facility for nursing involvement in research and the studies undertaken are usually performed by individuals with a commitment to research or as part of a thesis leading to a higher education award. There is an urgent need for a structure that will allow collaborative research looking at all angles of care in numerous situations and applying a logical approach to testing different methods of treatment and care.

References and bibliography

ACCP/SCCM Consensus Panel. (1990). Ethical and moral guidelines for the initiation, continuation and withdrawal of intensive care. *Chest*, **97**, 949–50.

Baggs, J.G., Ryan, S.A., Phelps, C.E., Richeson, J.F., and Johnson, J.E. (1992). The association between interdisciplinary collaboration and patient outcomes in a medical intensive care unit. *Heart and Lung*, **21**, 18–24.

Baker, S.P., O'Neill, B., Haddon, W., and Long WB. (1974). The Injury Severity Score: a method of describing patients with multiple injuries and evaluating emergency care. *Journal of Trauma*, **14**, 187–96.

Bion, J. (1990). Audit in intensive care. In *Update in intensive care and emergency Medicine*, Vol. 10, (ed. J.L. Vincent), pp. 851–6. Springer, Berlin.

Bone, R.C., Balk, R.A., Cerra, F.B., *et al.* (1992). Definitions for sepsis and organ failure and guidelines for the use of innovative therapies in sepsis. The ACCP/SCCM Consensus Conference Committee. American College of Chest Physicians/Society of Critical Care Medicine. *Chest*, **101**, 1644–55.

Boyd, C.R. Tolson, M.A., and Copes, W.S. (1987). Evaluating trauma care: the TRISS method. *Journal of Trauma*, **27**, 370–8.

Brown, M. (1985). Matter of commitment. *Nursing Times*, **81**, 26–7.

Champion, H.R., Sacco, W.J., Copes, W.S., *et al.* (1989). A revision of the Trauma Score. *Journal of Trauma*, **29**, 623–9.

Chang, R.W.S. (1989). Individual outcome prediction models for intensive care units. *Lancet*, **ii**, 143–6.

Collins, S. (1989). Sudden death counselling protocol. *Dimensions of Critical Care Nursing*, **8**, 375–83.

Cullen, D.J., Civetta, J.M., Briggs, B.A., and Ferrara, L.C. (1974). Therapeutic intervention scoring system: a method for quantitative comparison of patient care. *Critical Care Medicine*, **2**, 57–60.

Detsky, A.S., Stricker, S.C., Mulley, A.G., and Thibault, G.E. (1981). Prognosis, survival and the expenditure of hospital resources for patients in an intensive care unit. *New England Journal of Medicine*, **305**, 667–72.

Donabedian, A. (1966). Evaluating the quality of medical care. Millbank Memorial Fund Quarterly, **44**, 166–206.

Dragsted, L. (1990). Long-term outcome from intensive care. In *Update in intensive care and emergency medicine*, Vol. 10, (ed. J.L. Vincent), pp. 865–9. Springer, Berlin.

Dragsted, L. and Qvisk, J. (1989). Outcome from intensive care III. A 5 year study of 1308 patients activity level. *European Journal of Anaesthesiology* **6**, 385–96.

Elebute, E.A. and Stoner, H.B., (1983). The grading of sepsis. *British Journal of Surgery*, **70**, 29–31.

Five Regions Consortium with Greenhalgh and Co. Ltd. (1991). Quality. In *Using information in managing the nursing resource*. H. Charlesworth, Huddersfield.

French Multicenter Group of ICU Research (1989). Factors related to outcome in intensive care: French multicenter study. *Critical Care Medicine*, **17**, 305–8.

Friedman, B.C, Boyce, W., and Bekes, C.E. (1992). Long-term follow-up of ICU patients. *American Journal of Critical Care*, **1**, 115–17.

Goldstein, R.L., Campion, E.W., Thibault, G.E., Mulley, A.G., and Skinner, E. (1986). Functional outcomes following medical intensive care. *Critical Care Medicine*, **14**, 783–8.

Goldstone, L.A., Ball, J.A and Collier, M. (1983). *Monitor: An index of the quality of nursing care for acute medical and surgical wards*. Newcastle upon Tyne Polytechnic, Newcastle upon Tyne.

Griffiths, R.D. (1992). Development of normal indices of recovery from critical illness. In *Intensive care Britain*, (ed. M. Rennie), pp 134–7. Greycoat, London.

Jackson, I. (1992). Bereavement follow-up service in intensive care. *Intensive and Critical Care Nursing*, **8**, 163–8.

Keene, A.R., and Cullen, D.J. (1983). Therapeutic intervention scoring system: update. *Critical Care Medium*, **11**, 1–3.

King's Fund Report (1989). *Intensive care in the United Kingdom*: Report from the King's Fund. King's Fund Centre. London.

Knaus, W.A., Draper, E.A., Wagner, D.P., and Zimmerman, J.E. (1986). An evaluation of outcome from intensive care in major medical centers. *Annals of Internal Medicine*, **10**, 410–18.

Knaus, W.A., Draper, E.A., Wagner, D.P., and Zimmerman, J.E. (1985). APACHE II: a severity of disease classification system. *Critical Care Medicine*, **13**, 818–29.

Knaus, W.A., Wagner, D.P., Draper, E.A., *et al.* (1991). The APACHE III prognostic system. Risk prediction of hospital mortality for critically ill hospitalized adults. *Chest*, **100**, 1619–36.

Knaus, W.A., Zimmerman, J.E., Wagner, D.P., Draper, E.A., and Lawrence, D. (1981). APACHE — acute physiology and chronic health evaluation: a physiologically based classification system. *Critical Care Medicine*, **9**, 591–7.

Le Gall, J., Brun-Buisson, C., Trunet, P., Latournerie, J., Chantereau, S., and Rapin, M. (1982). Influence of age, previous health status, and severity of acute illness on outcome from intensive care. *Critical Care Medicine*, **10**, 575–7.

Le Gall, J.R., Lemeshow, S., and Saulnier, F (1993). A new Simplified Acute Physiology Score (SAPS II) based on a European/North American multicenter study. *Journal of the American Medical Association* **270**, 2957–63.

Le Gall, J.R., Loirat, P., Alperovitch, A. *et al.* (1984). A simplified acute physiology score for ICU patients. *Critical Care Medicine* **12**, 975–7.

Macfarlane J. (1989), cited in Redfern, S. and Norman, I.J., (1990). Measuring the quality of nursing care: a consideration of different approaches. *Journal of Advanced Nursing*, **15**, 1260–71.

Maxwell, R. (1984) Quality assessment in health, *British Medical Journal* 1470–72.

Meyers, D. (1978). *GRASP, a patient information and workload management system*. MCSI, Morgantown, NC.

Norman, I., Redfern, S, Tomalin, D., and Oliver, S. (1992). Applying triangulation to the assessment of quality of nursing. *Nursing Times*, **88**, 43–46.

Mill, J.S. (1867). *Utilitarianism*. Longmans, London.

Nursing Times (1988). Euthanasia, what *you* think? *Nursing Times*, **84**, 38–39.

Parno, J.R., Teres, D., Lemeshow, S., and Brown, R.B. (1982). Hospital charges and long-term survival of ICU versus non-ICU patients. *Critical Care Medicine*, **10**, 569–74.

Phaneuf, M. (1976). *The nursing audit*. Appleton Century Crofts, New York.

Price, D.J. and Mason, J. (1986). Resolving the numerical chaos at the bedside. In *Current perspectives in health care* (ed. J. Bryan, T. Roberts, and P. Windsor), p. 147–57. British Journal of Health Care Computing, Weybridge, Surrey.

Redfern, S. and Norman, I. (1990). Measuring the quality of nursing care: a consideration of different approaches. *Journal of Advanced Nursing*, **15**, 1260–71.

Ridley, S., Jackson, R., Findlay, and J., and Wallace, P. (1990). Long-term survival after intensive care. *British Medical Journal*, **301**, 1127–30.

Rowan, K.M., Kerr, J.H., Major, E., McPherson, K., Short, A., and Vessey, M.P. (1993). Intensive Care Society's APACHE II study in Britain and Ireland–II: Outcome comparisons of intensive care units after adjustment for case mix by the American APACHE II method. *British Medical Journal* **307**, 977–81.

Sage, W.M., Rosenthal, M.H., and Silverman, J.F. (1986). Is intensive care worth it? An assessment of input and outcome for the critically ill. *Critical Care Medicine*, **14**, 777–82.

Shiell, A.M., Griffiths, R.D., Short, A.I.K., and Spiby, J. (1990). An evaluation of the costs and outcome of adult intensive care in two units in the UK. *Clinical Intensive Care*, **1**, 256–62.

Teasdale, G. and Jennett, B., (1974). Assessment of coma and impaired consciousness. *Lancet*, **ii**, 81–4.

Tschudin, V. (1986). *Ethics in nursing. The caring relationship*. Heinemann Nursing, Oxford.

Wandelt, M. and Ager. J. (1974). *Quality patient care scale*. Appleton Century Crofts, New York.

Zaren, B. and Hedstrand, U. (1987). Quality of life among long-term survivors of intensive care. *Critical Care Medicine*, **15**, 743–7.

Index

Page numbers in **bold** type refer to figures, and those in *italics* to tables.